Nutrition, health and disease

A lifespan approach

Simon Langley-Evans, BSc, PhD, DSc, PGCHE, RNutr, FAfN

School of Biosciences
University of Nottingham

SECOND EDITION

WILEY

This edition first published 2009 © 2015 by John Wiley & Sons, Ltd

Registered Office
John Wiley & Sons, Ltd, The Atrium, Southern Gate, Chichester, West Sussex, PO19 8SQ, UK

Editorial Offices
9600 Garsington Road, Oxford, OX4 2DQ, UK
1606 Golden Aspen Drive, Suites 103 and 104, Ames, Iowa 50010, USA

For details of our global editorial offices, for customer services and for information about how to apply for permission to reuse the copyright material in this book please see our website at www.wiley.com/wiley-blackwell

10 07473842

Library of Congress Cataloging-in-Publication Data

Langley-Evans, S. C., author.
  [Nutrition]
  Nutrition health and disease : a lifespan approach / Simon C. Langley-Evans. – Second edition.
    p. ; cm.
  Preceded by Nutrition : a lifespan approach / Simon Langley-Evans. 1st ed. 2009.
  Includes bibliographical references and index.
  ISBN 978-1-118-90709-2 (pbk. : alk. paper)
  I. Title.
    [DNLM: 1. Nutritional Physiological Phenomena. 2. Growth and Development– physiology. 3. Nutrition Assessment. QU 145]
    QP141
    612.3–dc23
                            2015006387

A catalogue record for this book is available from the British Library.

Wiley also publishes its books in a variety of electronic formats. Some content that appears in print may not be available in electronic books.

Cover image:

    istockphotos/vegetables/
    11-15-06 © jgroup
    http://www.istockphoto.com/photo/vegetables-2446716

    istockphotos/Cheerful senior couple choose vegetables in the supermarket/
    05-09-11 © RapidEye
    http://www.istockphoto.com/photo/cheerful-senior-couple-choose-vegetables-in-the-supermarket-16526341

    istockphotos/healthy pregnancy/
    08-10-11 © YanLev
    http://www.istockphoto.com/photo/healthy-pregnancy-17389949

    istockphotos/Mother breastfeeding her baby girl/
    06-22-12 © svetikd
    http://www.istockphoto.com/photo/mother-breastfeeding-her-baby-girl-20676102

    istockphotos/school lunch time/
    05-22-13 © SolStock
    http://www.istockphoto.com/photo/school-lunch-time-24615068

Set in 8.5/11pt Meridien by SPi Global, Pondicherry, India
Printed in Singapore by C.O.S. Printers Pte Ltd

1   2015

Contents

Preface

The modern science of nutrition has arisen from humble beginnings, moving from a poorly respected side-shoot of many older established disciplines, such as biochemistry and physiology, to become an active entity in its own right. Nutrition is now rightly seen as being at the forefront of modern understanding of health and disease. It receives constant attention in the media and is highly visible as a clinical, educational and societal issue. Many of the established academics in the field have come to nutrition tangentially through many disparate routes, usually becoming immersed in the subject through research interests based in other fields. My own background was in biochemistry and microbiology, and my early interest in nutrition came from tantalizing, but sadly vague, mentions in textbooks that suggested that key processes such as the development of cancers might be, 'regulated by nutrition'.

The lack of specific nutrition training of the current crop of academics in the field reflects the fact that 20–30 years ago there were no degree courses in the subject. Interest in nutrition has increased exponentially since the early 1990s, and it is pleasing to see that degrees in nutrition have blossomed across all regions. In the United Kingdom alone, a prospective undergraduate considering training in nutrition will enter a competitive market, with a choice of over 250 university courses with a nutrition component. Nutrition is now rightly recognized as a key element in the training of all health professionals.

But what is nutrition? Everyone in the field may hold a different view which is shaped by their own specialism and the networks that the work within. In my view it is a hybrid subject which crosses over disciplines as disparate as politics and economics (which are the global drivers determining the food security of populations), food science and agriculture, the social sciences, psychology and sociology (which govern eating behaviours and food choices of individuals), biochemistry, physiology, medicine and pharmacology. The second edition of this book aims to provide a basic text for undergraduate students in all disciplines that impinge upon the nutritional sciences, including those training as health professionals as well as those reading nutrition as their core subject. It covers nutrition from a range of perspectives including those of the physiologist, the molecular biologist and the public health nutritionist. I have mostly assumed that the reader will have an understanding of the basics of the subject, and have focused my attention upon how nutrition-related factors shape human health and disease across all stages of the life course. This second edition, however, has an appendix with basic material (the general properties, classification and chemical nature of the nutrients) to assist readers coming at the subject from other backgrounds.

One of the main challenges for the modern nutritionist is to translate complex scientific concepts into simple advice about food and health that can be understood by the lay public. The conditional nature of the subject, namely the way in which our understanding advances and throws up controversies and contradictions, is a constant theme running through this book. A major component of the writing of this new edition has involved looking for significant changes in the evidence base for each topic and updating accordingly. For each chapter I have attempted to provide a balanced view of the evidence base, but inevitably the chapters will reflect my own personal view of the subject matter. The reader is directed to the extensive bibliographies that accompany each chapter to obtain a more detail. This second edition also signposts to other texts which may provide an alternative perspective on the material in each chapter.

Simon Langley-Evans
University of Nottingham
September 2014

Acknowledgements

It is a huge pleasure to have the opportunity to revise and update this book from the first edition. I would like to thank Alison for her endless support through the trials and tribulations of editing and revision.

The anytime, anywhere textbook

Wiley E-Text

Your book is also available to purchase as a **Wiley E-Text: Powered by VitalSource** version – a digital, interactive version of this book which you own as soon as you download it.

Your **Wiley E-Text** allows you to:

Search: Save time by finding terms and topics instantly in your book, your notes, even your whole library (once you've downloaded more textbooks).

Note and Highlight: Colour code, highlight and make digital notes right in the text, so you can find them quickly and easily.

Organize: Keep books, notes and class materials organized in folders inside the application.

Share: Exchange notes and highlights with friends, classmates and study groups.

Upgrade: Your textbook can be transferred when you need to change or upgrade computers.

Link: Link directly from the page of your interactive textbook to all of the material contained on the companion website.

The **Wiley E-Text** version will also allow you to copy and paste any photograph or illustration into assignments, presentations and your own notes.

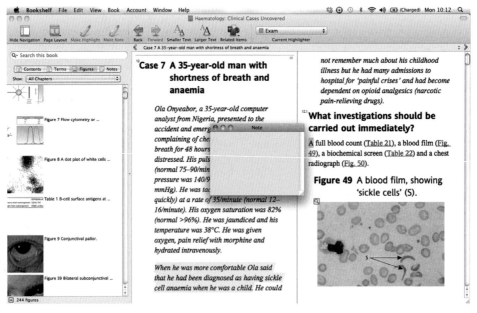

To access your Wiley E-Text

To access your Wiley E-Text

- Visit www.vitalsource.com/software/bookshelf/downloads to download the Bookshelf application to your computer, laptop, tablet or mobile device.
- Open the Bookshelf application on your computer and register for an account.
- Follow the registration process.

CourseSmart

CourseSmart gives you instant access (via computer or mobile device) to this Wiley-Blackwell e-book and its extra electronic functionality, at 40% off the recommended retail print price. See all the benefits at: **www.coursesmart.com/students**

Instructors … receive your own digital desk copies!

CourseSmart also offers instructors an immediate, efficient and environmentally friendly way to review this book for your course.

For more information visit **www.coursesmart.com/instructors**.

With CourseSmart, you can create lecture notes quickly with copy and paste, and share pages and notes with your students. Access your **CourseSmart** digital book from your computer or mobile device instantly for evaluation, class preparation, and as a teaching tool in the classroom.

Simply sign in at **http://instructors.coursesmart.com/bookshelf** to download your Bookshelf and get started. To request your desk copy, hit 'Request Online Copy' on your search results or book product page.

We hope you enjoy using your new book. Good luck with your studies!

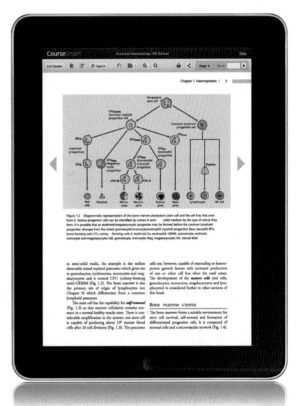

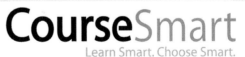

About the companion website

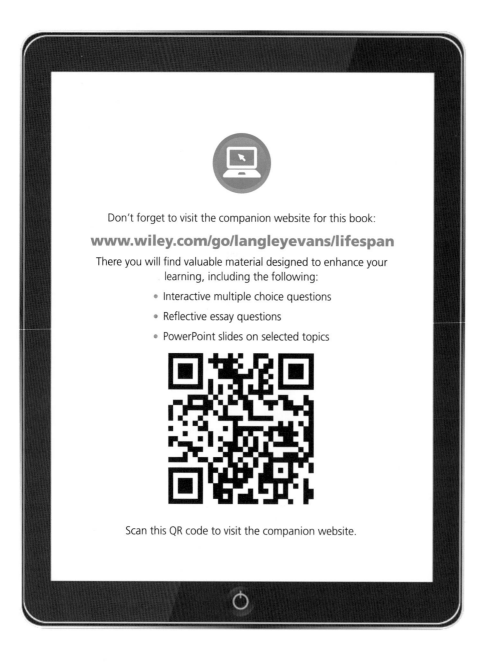

Don't forget to visit the companion website for this book:

www.wiley.com/go/langleyevans/lifespan

There you will find valuable material designed to enhance your learning, including the following:

- Interactive multiple choice questions
- Reflective essay questions
- PowerPoint slides on selected topics

Scan this QR code to visit the companion website.

Abbreviations

ADHD	Attention-deficit hyperactivity disorder	**LRNI**	Lower Reference Nutrient Intake
AN	Anorexia nervosa	**LTL**	Leukocyte telomere length
AZD	Alzheimer's disease	**MC4R**	Melanocortin receptor 4
BFHI	Baby Friendly Hospital Initiative	**MRC**	Medical Research Council
BMC	Bone mineral content	**MI**	Myocardial infarction
BMD	Bone mineral density	**MODY**	Maturity onset diabetes of the young
BMI	Body mass index	**MTHFR**	Methylenetetrahydrofolate reductase
BMR	Basal metabolic rate	**MUFA**	Monounsaturated fatty acid
BN	Bulimia nervosa	**NHANES**	National Health and Nutrition Examination Study
CHD	Coronary heart disease	**NICE**	National Institute for Health and Care Excellence
CI	Confidence interval	**NTD**	Neural tube defect
CMACE	Centre for Maternal and Child Enquiries	**NVP**	Nausea and vomiting of pregnancy
CR	Caloric restriction	**OR**	Odds ratio
CRC	Colorectal cancer	**PCOS**	Polycystic ovary syndrome
CVD	Cardiovascular disease	**PE**	Preeclampsia
DBP	Diastolic blood pressure	**PKU**	Phenylketonuria
DHA	Docosahexaenoic acid	**PPAR**	Peroxisome proliferator-activated receptor
DNA	Deoxyribose nucleic acid	**PPH**	Postpartum haemorrhage
DNMT	DNA methyltransferase	**PUFA**	Polyunsaturated fatty acid
DoH	Department of Health	**RAEs**	Retinol activity equivalents
DRVs	Dietary reference values	**RCT**	Randomized controlled trial
DXA	Dual X-ray absorptiometry	**RDA**	Recommended Daily Allowance
EAR	Estimated Average Requirement	**REE**	Resting energy expenditure
EFSA	European Food Safety Authority	**RNI**	Reference Nutrient Intake
EPIC	European Prospective Investigation into Cancer	**ROS**	Reactive oxygen species
FAO	Food and Agriculture Organisation	**RR**	Relative risk
FAS	Foetal alcohol syndrome	**SACN**	Scientific Advisory Committee on Nutrition
FSH	Follicle-stimulating hormone	**SBP**	Systolic blood pressure
GDA	Guideline daily amount	**SCFAs**	Short-chain fatty acids
GDM	Gestational diabetes mellitus	**SES**	Socioeconomic status
GI	Glycemic index	**SGA**	Small for gestational age
GnRH	Gonadotrophin-releasing hormone	**SIDS**	Sudden infant death syndrome
GPx	Glutathione peroxidase	**SMR**	Sexual maturity rating
GR	Glucocorticoid receptor	**SNP**	Single nucleotide polymorphism
hCG	Human chorionic gonadotrophin	**T2DM**	Type 2 diabetes mellitus
HDL	High-density lipoprotein	**TEE**	Total energy expenditure
HG	Hyperemesis gravidarum	**TNFα**	Tumour necrosis factor α
HIV	Human immunodeficiency virus	**UL**	Upper limit
HR	Hazard ratio	**UN**	United Nations
IL1	Interleukin 1	**UNICEF**	United Nations Children's Fund
IL6	Interleukin 6	**USDA**	United States Department of Agriculture
IL10	Interleukin 10	**VCAM**	Vascular cell adhesion molecule
IQ	Intelligence quotient	**VDR**	Vitamin D receptor
IU	International units	**VLCD**	Very low-calorie diet
LCPUFA	Long chain polyunsaturated fatty acid	**VLDL**	Very low-density lipoprotein
LDL	Low-density lipoprotein	**WCRF**	World Cancer Research Fund
LGA	Large for gestational age	**WHO**	World Health Organisation
LH	Luteinizing hormone		

Glossary of terms used in this book

Adipocyte: A fat containing cell found in adipose tissue.

Adipokines: Cytokines secreted by the adipose tissue.

Adiponectin: A hormone secreted by adipose tissue. It enhances insulin sensitivity and promotes glucose uptake.

Adipose tissue: The site of body fat deposition. Cells within adipose tissue store and release fat.

Adiposity rebound: Body mass index rises rapidly in the first 2 years of life and then declines until a point between the age of 4 and 6 years when it starts to increase again. This point where the trend reverses is termed the 'adiposity rebound'.

Adrenal glands: Endocrine organs located above the kidneys. The adrenals are the sites for production and release of adrenaline, noradrenaline and steroid hormones such as cortisol and aldosterone.

Adrenarche: The maturation of the adrenal cortex into three distinct zones, resulting in secretion of androgenic hormones during adolescence.

Aflatoxins: Mycotoxins formed by fungi such as Aspergillus. Aflatoxins are important contaminants on peanuts and groundnuts stored in humid climates.

Alkaloids: Toxic compounds found in plant foods (e.g. potatoes) or as contaminants on cereals, produced by mildew.

Allergic sensitization: The process through which exposure to foreign materials, either through ingestion, inhalation or skin contact, elicits immune responses that will manifest as allergic symptoms (rash or asthma). Initial contact with allergens may not produce a response but instead primes (sensitizes) to produce responses at further contacts.

Allergy: Adverse reaction to antigens (for example proteins in certain foodstuffs), that is mediated by the immune system (production of antibodies).

Allium: Plants of the onion family. Includes onions and garlic.

Alzheimer's disease: An irreversible and progressive neurodegenerative disorder leading to memory loss, altered behaviour and dementia. The disease is characterized by the formation of plaques of amyloid beta peptide in the brain.

Amenorrhea: The absence of a menstrual period in a woman of reproductive age.

Ames Test: A test used to determine the potential carcinogenicity of chemicals. The test uses cultures of Salmonella typhimurium that must undergo a mutation to be able to grow on a limiting medium. Presence of colonies in the medium indicates potential mutagenicity of test compounds.

Anaemia: Deficiency of red blood cells or haemoglobin.

Androgens: The male sex hormones. The main androgens are the steroid hormones, testosterone and dehydroepiandrosterone.

Anencephaly: A defect of the formation of the embryonic neural tube, which results in the non-formation of the cerebral arches.

Angina pectoris: Chest pain caused by the partial occlusion of the coronary arteries due to atherosclerosis.

Angiogenesis: The process through which new blood vessels branch off from existing vessels.

Anorexia nervosa: An eating disorder characterized by body image distortion and fear of weight gain. Anorexics, who are typically underweight, may voluntarily starve, indulge in excessive exercise, vomit or purge after eating and abuse laxatives or anti-obesity drugs.

Anovulation: The absence of ovulation in women of reproductive age.

Anterior pituitary: One of two lobes of the pituitary gland. This endocrine tissue responds directly to signals from the hypothalamus and plays a key role in regulation of the production of hormones from the adrenals and reproductive organs.

Anthropometry: The measurement of the human body in terms of the dimensions of muscle, and adipose (fat) tissue. Simple measures of height and weight, supplemented with measurements of skinfold thicknesses, mid-upper arm circumference, waist and hip circumferences can be used to estimate body composition and distribution of body fat.

Antioxidants: Molecules that are capable of quenching the reactivity of free radicals and other oxidizing agents (e.g. hydrogen peroxide). Antioxidants may be scavenging antioxidants, which are destroyed in reactions with reactive oxygen species, or enzymes that are capable of rapid metabolism of high quantities of reactive oxygen species.

Apoptosis: Programmed cell death which involves a coordinated series of biochemical events leading to the death of the cell and removal of resulting debris.

Arrhythmia: Condition in which the heart beat is irregular, or excessively slow or fast. Arrhythmias are the product of damage to the heart during myocardial infarction.

Arterial intima: The innermost layer of the arterial wall.

Ataxia telangiectasia: An immunodeficiency disorder.

Atherosclerosis: The process through which the artery accumulates a plaque containing cholesterol, collagen and calcium. Atherosclerotic plaques cause stiffening and narrowing of the arteries and act as a focus for clots. Atherosclerosis is the basis of all cardiovascular disease (coronary heart disease, stroke, peripheral artery disease).

Atopy: A predisposition to allergic responses.

Attention-deficit hyperactivity disorder: A neurological disturbance in children, which leads to inattention and impulsive behaviour.

Axillary hair: Hair in the underarm region.

Bacterioides: One of the six main genera of bacteria which contribute to the human intestinal microflora.

Bariatric surgery: Surgery to promote weight loss through restriction of the stomach capacity in order to limit food intake.

Basal metabolic rate (BMR), resting metabolic rate (RMR): The energy cost associated with maintaining the basic physiological processes of the body at rest (i.e. respiration, circulation, nerve and muscle tone). BMR is in proportion to body size, since it is determined by the amount of metabolically active tissue.

Betel chewing: The habit of chewing betel quid. The quid is a mixture of areca nut and leaves. This habit is most common in Pacific communities and in some parts of Asia (e.g. Taiwan).

Bifidobacteria: One of the six main genera of bacteria which contribute to the human intestinal microflora.

Bioimpedance: The measurement of body fat content through determination of the resistance of the body to the flow of an electrical current.

Biomarker: A measurement used to assess the state of a biological system. In nutrition biomarkers may include measurements of nutrient concentrations in suitable samples (e.g. blood and urine), or measurements of nutrient-dependent physiological functions.

Bisphonates: A class of drugs used in the treatment of osteoporosis. Bisphonates inhibit the action of osteoclasts.

Blood pressure: The pressure generated within the arteries due to the pumping of the heart. Between beats the vessels are at rest and the pressure is at the lowest point (diastolic pressure). Maximum pressure occurs with ejection of blood from the left ventricle (systolic pressure).

B-lymphocytes: Cells of the immune system which are responsible for the production of antibodies.

Body Mass Index (BMI): A measure of weight in relation to height (weight in kg/height in m²). BMI is widely used as a tool to determine whether an individual is of healthy weight (BMI between 20 and 25), underweight (BMI < 20), overweight (BMI 25–30) or obese (BMI < 30).

Bone mineral density: A measure of bone mass. Reduced BMD is generally indicative of conditions such as osteoporosis, in which fracture risk is increased.

Bulimia nervosa: An eating disorder linked to body image distortion and fear of weight gain. Affected individuals periodically binge-eat, and then compensate for excessive intake through excessive exercise, vomiting and purging.

Cachexia: Severe loss of weight and muscle mass, often accompanied by loss of appetite.

Caffeine: A methyl xanthine compound found in tea, coffee, chocolate and over-the-counter medications. Caffeine is a central nervous system stimulant.

Cancer: Disease involving the uncontrolled growth of cells to form a tumour. Cancer cells can invade tissues and organs at the point where they are first formed (primary tumours), or can spread to other organs through the process of metastasis, forming secondary tumours.

Carcinogen: Any agent that is capable of directly initiating the formation of a tumour, or which can promote the development or spread of existing tumours.

Carcinogenesis: The process through which exposure of cells to carcinogens initiates the formation of tumours, leading to cancer.

Cardiac output: The volume of blood pumped by the blood in a given unit of time. Cardiac output is generally measured in litres per minute. Cardiac output is one of the determinants of blood pressure.

Cardiovascular disease: The term used to collectively describe the diseases that involve the heart or blood vessels. Most clinically significant cardiovascular disease (coronary heart disease, stroke, peripheral artery disease) is related to atherosclerosis.

Carotenoids: Organic pigments found primarily in plants. This group of tetraterpenoids includes α- and ß-carotene, lutein, lycopene and zeaxanthin.

Carotid intima-media thickness: A clinical measurement of the extent of atherosclerosis in the carotid artery. Development of plaques results in increased thickness of the arterial wall.

Case-control studies: An epidemiological study design in which characteristics of a group of individuals suffering from a disease (cases) are compared to those of a group of healthy individuals (controls).

Catabolism: The metabolic breakdown of macromolecules to release energy.

Catch-up growth: Accelerated growth which follows a period of growth restriction.

Chondrocyte: Cells found in cartilaginous tissues that are responsible for secreting the characteristic proteins of cartilage.

Chorion: A membrane that surrounds the embryo and foetus during development. Processes formed in this membrane develop into the chorionic villi, which invade the uterine lining during placentation.

Claudication: Pain, usually in the lower legs, caused by poor circulation due to peripheral artery disease.

Clotting factors: Factors which promote the coagulation of blood. In humans the major clotting factors are fibrinogen, factor VII, factor VIII, pro-thrombin and von Willebrand factor.

Coeliac disease: An autoimmune disorder of the bowel in which an inflammatory response occurs in response to the ingestion of the gliadin portion of gluten.

Cohort studies: An epidemiological study in which a group of individuals is followed over a period of time in order to determine how characteristics observed early in the study might influence the later development of disease. Prospective cohort studies define the characteristics of the population as soon as individuals are recruited, and follow-ups are performed as the study progresses. Retrospective cohort studies assess population characteristics after the disease data is collected.

Colonic microflora: The bacterial species that colonise the human digestive tract. The human colon is home to over 500 species of bacteria, some of which are pathogenic, whilst others have benefits for human health.

Colostrum: The first milk produced by the mammary glands after giving birth. Colostrum is a protein-rich, thick fluid, that is an important source of immunoprotective factors.

Complement: An element of the immune system which involves a cascade of enzyme-mediated events that kill infected cells and pathogens.

Complementary feeding: Weaning. Complementary foods are foods added to the diet of breastfed infants during the transition from full breastfeeding to family foods.

Complex carbohydrates: Carbohydrates with a complex chemical structure. The complex carbohydrates include the soluble and insoluble starches and those components of the diet that are generally referred to as dietary fibre (cellulose, lignans, chitin).

Confidence interval: All measurements are subject to error and summary statistics such as odds ratios, relative risk or estimated means lie within a range of values for the estimate. They are in fact 'best estimates' of the true value. The level of confidence of the confidence interval indicates the probability that the confidence range includes the true value. This level of confidence is represented by a percentage. Ninety-five per cent confidence indicates that 95% of the observed confidence intervals will hold the true value of the measurement.

Confounding factor: A factor in an epidemiological study, that can lead to a false conclusion regarding an apparently causal association between a risk factor and disease endpoint, unless controlled for statistically.

Constipation: Impaired bowel function in which small hard stools are formed, which are difficult to egest.

Coronary heart disease: Disease of the coronary arteries caused by the formation of atherosclerotic plaques. Plaques and associated clots can prevent blood and oxygen from reaching the muscles of the heart. Cells of the heart subsequently die, leaving a damaged area called an infarct.

Corpus luteum: The remnant of the Graafian follicle after the release of an egg during mammalian ovulation. The corpus luteum becomes a temporary endocrine organ, producing progesterone to maintain the uterine wall should pregnancy occur.

Cortical bone: Bone with a dense structure. Also termed compact bone.

Cross-sectional study: An epidemiological approach in which the prevalence of disease (outcomes) or determinants of health (exposures) are measured in a population at the same point in time, or over a short period.

Cruciferous vegetables: Vegetables of the plant family Brassicaceae, which includes cabbage, Brussels sprouts, kale, cauliflower and broccoli.

Cryptorchidism: Condition in which the testicles fail to descend during normal male reproductive development.

Cytochrome P450 system: A large and diverse superfamily of enzymes, which are largely responsible for the metabolism of xenobiotics. Most reactions catalyzed by cytochrome P450s involve the addition of a hydroxyl group from water, which facilitates the subsequent conjugation and excretion of the agent.

Cytokines: Chemical messengers that can be produced by almost all cell types (unlike hormones that are produced by specific endocrine cells). Cytokines are especially important in mediating inflammatory and immune responses.

Dementia: Progressive loss of cognitive functions including memory, language and problem-solving skills. Dementia represents extreme loss of these functions that goes beyond normal age-related declines.

Developed countries: The economically successful countries, in which the national income translates into significant advantages for the health and education of the population. The developed nations include Japan, Canada, the United States, Australia, New Zealand and the nations of Western Europe, along with Singapore, Hong Kong, South Korea and Taiwan.

Developing countries: Countries with a low industrial base and lacking economic wealth to invest in the health, education and welfare of the population.

Diabetes mellitus: A metabolic disorder characterized by raised circulating glucose concentrations, attributable to defects of glucose homeostasis. Type 1 diabetes is due to insufficient insulin production, whilst Type 2 diabetes arises from impaired responses to insulin, which may be present in very high concentrations.

Diaphysis: The shaft portion of a long bone.

Dietary fibre: One of several terms used to describe the non-digestible matter present in food. Cellulose, chitin and insoluble starches all pass through the digestive tract largely unchanged. Fibre is also referred to as non-starch polysaccharides and complex carbohydrates.

Dieting: The process of restricting food intake with the intention of losing weight. Dieting may involve a reduction of all foods consumed, or the exclusion of particular food items, or groups of nutrients.

Dietitian: A health professional who uses dietary change as a tool for the management and treatment of disease states in her/his patients.

Diuretic: A pharmacological agent which stimulates the excretion of water.

Diverticular disease: A condition of the large intestine whereby small sacs or pouches called diverticula form in the wall of the large intestine. Diverticula may become infected, leading to a condition known as diverticulitis.

Dizygotic twins: Non-identical twins.

DNA methylation: Chemical modification of DNA that can be inherited without changing the DNA sequence. DNA methylation plays an important role in the silencing of gene expression and is an element of epigenetic regulation.

Doubly labelled water: A method for measuring energy expenditure, in which subjects are administered water labelled with deuterium and ^{18}O. Elimination of the isotopes allows determination of CO_2 production, which is a marker for total energy expenditure.

Dual X-ray absorptiometry: DXA. An X-ray technique in which patients are subjected to X-ray scans in two different planes. The absorption of the X-ray energy by soft tissues and by bone allows accurate determination of bone mineral content and density. DXA can also be used to estimate the fat mass of the body.

Dyslipidaemia: Disruption of the normal concentrations of lipids (mostly triglycerides and cholesterol) in circulation. The most commonly noted dyslipidaemias involve increases in circulating lipid concentrations (hyperlipidaemia).

Dysphagia: Difficulty in swallowing.

Eclampsia: A life-threatening complication of pregnancy, characterized by uncontrolled hypertension and multiple organ failure.

Ecological studies: A type of study design in nutritional epidemiology. Ecological studies utilize observations of the trends in disease prevalence either over time, or between different populations/geographical areas, and attempt to relate these trends to variation in nutritional markers or other risk factors. Ecological studies are the weakest and least discerning approaches to studying diet–disease relationships and should always be followed up with more robust methods.

Ectopic pregnancy: An abnormal pregnancy in which the embryo implants outside the uterus.

Eicosanoids: Components of the inflammatory and immune responses, which are synthesized from the long-chain fatty acids of the n-3 and n-6 series.

Embryogenesis: The process through which an embryo forms and develops through mitotic divisions.

Emetic: An agent which stimulates vomiting.

Endocrine disruptors: Chemical agents that have the capacity to interfere with normal hormone action, either by mimicking the action of particular hormones (e.g. oestrogen mimics) or antagonizing the action of hormones (e.g., anti-androgens).

Endometriosis: Condition in which the cells that normally line the uterus and slough off with each menstrual cycle, grow on the outside of the uterus. Endometriosis can be a cause of infertility and pelvic infections.

Endothelial dysfunction: Abnormal function of the cells that comprise the inner layer surrounding the lumen of arterial tissue. Altered function in terms of clotting, immune and inflammatory responses, production of nitric oxide and vasoconstriction or vasodilation to maintain normal blood pressure, is a key step in the development of atherosclerosis and cardiovascular disease.

Enteral feeding support: The provision of nutrients via a tube directly into the gastrointestinal tract. Enteral tube feeding can be directed to the stomach, or if necessary to lower levels of the digestive tract.

Epigenetic regulation: The expression of genes can be modified by the environment to produce different phenotypes. Epigenetic gene regulation is the process through which patterns of gene expression can be modified through methylation of DNA or by altering chromosome packing rather than by differences in DNA sequence.

Epiphysis: The end portion of a long bone, for example the head of the femur.

Erectile dysfunction: Impotence. The inability for a man to develop or maintain an erection.

Erytrhopoiesis: The process through which the red blood cells are formed from stem cells in the bone marrow.

Escherichia coli: One of the bacterial species which contribute to the human intestinal microflora.

Essential amino acids: The amino acids that are required within the diet as they cannot be synthesized within the human body. Some amino acids are conditionally essential as the ability to synthesize enough to meet demand cannot be sustained in circumstances such as pregnancy.

Essential fatty acids: The fatty acids that cannot be synthesized within the human body and which are therefore required within the diet. The essential fatty acids are linoleic acid (n-6) and linolenic acid (n-3).

Estimated Average Requirement (EAR): One of the dietary reference value terms used in the United Kingdom. The EAR for a nutrient is the level of intake that should meet the requirements of 50% of individuals within a population.

Expressing milk: The process of drawing milk from the breast through manual stimulation of the let-down reflex. Many women express milk using specially designed breast pumps in order to leave breast milk for other individuals to feed to their infants via a bottle and teat. Expressing milk may also be necessary to maintain lactation when mother or child are ill, or if the mother requires brief treatment with drugs that may be toxic to suckling infants.

Faddy eating: A common eating behaviour of young children, in which food is periodically refused or only a very narrow range of food items is habitually consumed.

Fatty acids: Organic acid molecules with long hydrocarbon tails. Fatty acids can be saturated or unsaturated (having double-bonded carbons within the hydrocarbon chain). The fatty acids are the basic building blocks of lipids within the body.

Fatty streak: The earliest stages of atherosclerosis are characterized by the appearance of deposits of macrophages bearing cholesterol and other fats in vesicles within the cytoplasm.

Foam cells: Foam cells are derived from macrophages within the intimal layer of arteries. Foam cells are the basic constituents of atherosclerotic plaques.

Follicle-stimulating hormone (FSH): A hormone of the anterior pituitary, which in both men and women regulates the production of sex steroids from the gonads. In women FSH stimulates maturation of follicles. In men FSH has a critical role in the production of spermatozoa.

Follicular phase: The early phase of the menstrual cycle in which the Graafian follicles mature in preparation for ovulation.

Food allergy: An adverse reaction to proteins in food. Allergies arise due to immune responses directed at allergenic proteins.

Food groups: Food groups are a means of classifying foods of similar types in order to simplify health promotion advice for the population. For example, within the UK Eatwell model, there are five food groups: fruits and vegetables; breads, cereals and potatoes; meat and alternatives; milk and dairy produce; foods containing fat and sugar.

Food intolerance: An adverse reaction to particular food items or components of food. Intolerance reactions are distinct from food allergies as there is no involvement of the immune system. Intolerances often arise due to a lack of digestive enzymes or secretions necessary to process particular items.

Food neophobia: A food behaviour often seen in children. Neophobia involves the rejection of foods that have not been previously encountered, often based purely on their appearance or aroma.

Food tables: Databases showing the macronutrient and micronutrient composition of foods.

Fortification: The process through which a nutrient is added to a staple foodstuff at the point of production in order to increase intakes of that nutrient within the whole population. In the United Kingdom, for example, margarines have been fortified with vitamin D to maintain intakes at similar levels to those associated with consumption of butter.

Fortifiers: Nutrient supplements that can be added to milk products used in infant nutrition. Fortifiers are mixed with human milk when feeding some premature infants to ensure that intakes of protein, micronutrients and energy are optimal.

Free radical: A free radical is any atom or molecule that has one or more unpaired electrons within its orbitals. The presence of unpaired electrons makes free radicals highly reactive, and they have the capacity to bond to, or remove constituents from other molecules in their vicinity. In biological systems this reactivity can be highly damaging to cells, and is the basis of many major disease processes.

Functional foods: Foods which have been developed to have ingredients that have health promoting properties.

Galactosaemia: An inherited disorder in which sufferers lack the enzyme galactose-1-phosphate uridyl transferase, which prevents the normal metabolism of galactose. Unmanaged, this will lead to renal failure, enlarged liver and brain damage.

Gallstones (choleliths): Solid, crystalline accretions of bile components that form within the gall bladder or bile duct.

Gastric parietal cells: Cells of the stomach epithelium which secrete intrinsic factor and hydrochloric acid.

Gastric reflux: Escape of acidic gastric secretions into the oesophagus. Also termed 'heartburn'.

Gastritis: Inflammation of the lining of the stomach.

Genomic imprinting: Process through which epigenetic marking of genes ensures that they are expressed in a specific manner. For example certain genes in mammalian systems are expressed in a parent of origin-specific manner. This process allows paternally derived alleles that could be harmful to maternal health to be suppressed.

Genomic instability: Events associated with ageing and cancer. Genomic instability results in abnormalities in the chromosomal arrangement of DNA, often due to defects of DNA repair or high background levels of damage.

Glitazones: A class of drugs developed to treat type 2 diabetes. The glitazones are agonists of peroxisome proliferator activated receptor (PPAR)γ and promote expression of insulin-sensitive genes.

Glomerular filtration rate: The rate at which blood is filtered through the kidney.

Gluconeogenesis: The metabolic pathway leading to the generation of glucose from non-sugar substrates, including pyruvate, lactate, glycerol, and the glucogenic amino acids (e.g. glycine, serine, aspartate, glutamate).

Glucose homeostasis: Homeostasis is the regulation of metabolic and physiological systems in order to maintain a normal steady state function in response to environmental fluctuations. Glucose homeostasis describes the processes which maintain circulating and tissue glucose concentrations within optimal ranges.

Glucosinolates: Secondary products of plants of the Brassicaceae family. Glucosinolates are derivatives of glucose, with side chains containing sulphur and nitrogen.

Glutathione: A tripeptide synthesized from glycine, cysteine and glutamine. Glutathione is one of the most abundant compounds within the mammalian body and plays a key role in antioxidant defences and the metabolism of xenobiotics. The antioxidant capacity of glutathione is due to its role as a substrate for glutathione peroxidase.

Glycaemic control: A term used to describe the ability of patients with diabetes to maintain blood glucose concentrations within optimal ranges, either through dietary change or use of pharmacological agents.

Glycaemic index (GI): A system used to rank foodstuffs in order of their ability to increase blood glucose concentrations following consumption. Foods with high GI contain simple sugars that are rapidly absorbed and lead to a rapid peaking of blood glucose. Foods with low GI contain complex carbohydrates which release glucose to the bloodstream more slowly.

Glycosylated haemoglobin A1c: HbA1c is a form of haemoglobin which is generated in the presence of excessive concentrations of blood glucose. Glucose binds to the haemoglobin and the glycosylated haemoglobin begins to accumulate on red blood cells. Measurement of HbA1c provides a good measure of the quality of habitual glycaemic control of diabetic individuals.

Gonadotrophin-releasing hormone (GnRH): Peptide hormone released in a pulsatile manner by the hypothalamus. GnRH is the principal regulator of the reproductive axes in both males and females.

Great Apes: Species belonging to the family Hominidae. This includes gorillas, orangutans, chimpanzees, bonobos and humans.

Growth hormone: A polypeptide hormone with largely anabolic functions. Growth hormone stimulates growth, increases muscle mass, promotes protein synthesis and hepatic glucose uptake and gluconeogenesis.

Haemochromatosis: An inherited disorder in which iron accumulates within organs, particularly the liver and pancreas.

Haemorrhoids: Blood-filled swellings around the anus, caused by dilation of varicose veins.

Hayflick limit: All differentiated cells have a limited capacity to divide. The number of divisions that can occur before cell death is termed the 'Hayflick limit'. In humans the Hayflick limit is 52 divisions.

Height velocity: The rate at which height is increasing during growth, usually measured as centimetre gained per year.

Helicobacter pylori: A bacterial species that can colonize the human stomach and small intestine. H. pylori infection is associated with gastritis and peptic ulcers and is a major risk factor for stomach cancer.

Hepatic steatosis: Fatty liver.

Heterocyclic amines: Carcinogenic compounds that are generated during the cooking of meat.

High-density lipoprotein (HDL) cholesterol: HDL is one of the lipoprotein transporters that are required to carry cholesterol around the body. HDL transports cholesterol from peripheral tissues back to the liver for reutilization or excretion, and as such higher concentrations of HDL cholesterol are associated with lower risk of atherosclerosis.

Hirsutism: Excessive growth of hair in women. Hirsutism generally occurs in response to increased production of androgens and is associated with growth of facial or chest hair, or increased growth of hair on the legs and arms.

Hyperemesis gravidarum: Intractable and excessive nausea and vomiting associated with pregnancy.

Hyperglycaemia: Circulating glucose concentrations that are above normal ranges. Blood glucose concentrations that are persistently over 126 mg/dl (7 mmol/l) are generally accepted as indicative of hyperglycaemia.

Hyperhomocysteinaemia: Elevated plasma homocysteine concentrations (in excess of 15 μmol/l). A risk factor for cardiovascular disease.

Hyperphagia: An abnormally increased appetite leading to habitually excessive consumption of food.

Hypertension: Raised blood pressure. In clinical settings hypertension is generally defined as a systolic pressure over 140 mmHg and diastolic pressure over 90 mmHg)

Hypertriglyceridaemia: Elevated plasma triglyceride concentrations (over 1.7 mmol/l).

Hypocalcaemia: Low circulating concentrations of calcium.

Hypospadias: A congenital defect of the penis in which the urethral opening is misplaced.

Hypothalamic–pituitary–adrenal axis: Hormonal cascade that regulates stress responses, the immune system, metabolism, appetite and sexual behaviour.

Hypothalamic–pituitary–gonadal axis: Hormonal cascade that regulates reproductive physiology. Elements of this axis also regulate skeletal development, body composition and immune functions.

Hypothalamus: A region of the brain seated above the pituitary gland. The hypothalamus is the central integrator of sensory input and responses to maintain homeostasis. The hypothalamus plays a critical role in the control of temperature, circadian cycles, thirst, appetite and reproductive functions.

Immunoglobulins: Immunoglobulins are also known as antibodies. These globular proteins occur in several different classes (isotypes, IgG, IgA, IgM, IgE), all of which mediate specific functions within the immune system.

Incontinence: Involuntary leakage of urine or faeces.

Infertility: The inability of a man or woman to conceive a child. Infertility is clinically defined on the basis of failure to conceive within 12 months of attempting to do so.

Inflammatory bowel disease: Chronic disease states involving inflammation of the small or large intestines. Crohn's disease generally impacts upon the ileum and parts of the large intestine, whilst ulcerative colitis affects the wall of the bowel within the colon and rectum.

Insulin resistance: The condition in which normal circulating concentrations of insulin are insufficient to allow normal responses to the hormone.

Intelligence quotient (IQ): IQ is a measure of performance in tests designed to assess intelligence. IQ tests are normalized against the typical performance of the population, with a score of 100 rated as average.

Intervention studies: Epidemiological studies in which the impact of limiting a potentially harmful exposure (e.g. reduction of red meat intake), or of increasing exposure to a potentially beneficial agent (e.g. increasing intake of dietary fibre) upon disease risk can be evaluated.

In vitro fertilization: The process through which eggs are fertilized to create embryos outside the body. In vitro fertilization is one of the techniques used in assisted reproduction.

Junk food: Foods which are high in sugar and fat, but which contain few micronutrients. Many nutritionists dislike the use of this term as it is a poor means of defining the composition of food and is only selectively applied to convenience foods.

Ketosis: The metabolic state in which the liver switches to the breakdown of fatty acids to ketones. This state is usually associated with the response to starvation, but can also be initiated by trauma and inflammation.

Kwashiorkor: A form of protein–energy malnutrition, characterized by oedematous swelling, fatty liver, bleaching of the hair and dermatitis. Classically defined as protein deficiency.

Lactation: The secretion of milk from the mammary glands.

Lactobacillus: One of the six main genera of bacteria which contribute to the human intestinal microflora.

Lactose intolerance: Condition in which a deficiency of lactase prevents the digestion of lactose. Consumption of dairy produce will lead to abdominal distension and diarrhoea.

Laxative: A pharmacological agent that loosens stools and induces defecation.

Let-down reflex: Hormonal response to stimulation of the nipples in breastfeeding women. Stimulation of mechanoreceptors leads to release of oxytocin (stimulates milk release) and prolactin (stimulates milk synthesis).

Leydig cells: Cells of the testis which synthesise testosterone.

Life expectancy: The average number of years a human is expected to live. This figure is conventionally calculated from the time of birth and is highly dependent on infant mortality rates in the region of birth.

Lignans: Polyphenolic compounds formed in plants. In the human diet lignans are generally consumed via seeds and certain vegetables (broccoli and other Brassicacae). Lignans are one of the major classes of phytoestrogens.

Lipid hydroperoxides: Stable forms of oxidized lipids that are formed via the peroxidation cascade following free radical activity.

Lipolysis: The breakdown of fat stores to release free fatty acids to the circulation.

Lipoproteins: Complexes of lipids and proteins which are primarily involved in the transport of cholesterol and other fats. Lipoproteins may also be structural proteins, adhesion molecules and transmembrane receptors.

Low-density lipoprotein (LDL): LDL is one of the lipoprotein transporters that are required to carry cholesterol around the body. LDL transports cholesterol from the liver to peripheral tissues. LDL cholesterol is vulnerable to oxidation within the arterial endothelium, and this process is one of the prerequisite events for the development of atherosclerotic plaques.

Lower Reference Nutrient Intake (LRNI): One of the dietary reference value terms used in the United Kingdom. The LRNI for a nutrient is the level of intake that should meet the requirements of just 2.5% of individuals within a population.

Luteal phase: The phase of the menstrual cycle which follows ovulation.

Luteinizing hormone (LH): A hormone of the anterior pituitary, which in both men and women regulates the production of sex steroids from the gonads. In women LH promotes ovulation. In men LH has a critical role in the production of testosterone.

Lymphocyte: A class of white blood cell, operative within the mammalian immune system. There are three major types of lymphocyte: T cells, B cells and natural killer cells.

Macrophages: Phagocytes of the immune system. Macrophages are derived from monocytes.

Macrosomia: A term used to describe a baby that is large-for-gestational age.

Malnutrition: State in which an individual is chronically deprived of the macro- and micronutrients required to maintain normal physiological functions at an optimal level.

Mammary alveoli: The glandular tissues of the breast, which are the sites of milk synthesis.

Marasmus: A form of protein–energy malnutrition, characterized by hunger, weight loss, muscle wasting and loss of adipose tissue reserves. Classically defined as energy deficiency.

Maturity onset diabetes of the young (MODY): Rare hereditary forms of type 2 diabetes, caused by mutations of transcription factors and enzymes involved in the normal response to insulin. There are at least six identified MODY defects.

Menarche: The onset of reproductive cycling in females. The first menstrual bleeding.

Menopause: The end of reproductive cycling in females triggered by the cessation of ovarian function.

Meta-analysis: A statistical approach which overcomes problems of small sample size in epidemiological studies by combining the results of several studies that all address a related research hypothesis.

Metabolic syndrome: Cluster of metabolic disorders (hyperinsulinaemia, hypertriglyceridaemia), cardiovascular disorders (hypertension) and obesity, driven by insulin resistance. Metabolic syndrome is a major risk factor for cardiovascular disease.

Metabolomics: The systematic study of metabolites to obtain a profile of the metabolic response to a particular challenge.

Metastasis: The spread of cancerous cells from the initial site of tumour formation to other parts of the body.

Metformin: A drug used in the control of type 2 diabetes. Metformin increases insulin sensitivity and delays the uptake of glucose from the digestive tract.

Methyl-tetrahydrofolate reductase (MTHFR): Enzyme responsible for generation of 5-methyltetrahydrofolate from 5,10-Methylenetetrahydrofolate. This is an essential step in the removal of potentially harmful homocysteine. Polymorphisms of the MTHFR play an important role in establishing an individual's risk of cardiovascular disease and certain cancers.

Microalbuminuria: The leakage of albumin into the urine. This is indicative of kidney damage, which increases the permeability of the glomeruli.

Micronutrient deficiency: The micronutrients are the vitamins, minerals and trace elements required by the body. Where the supply of these nutrients is insufficient to meet demands over a sustained period, deficiency may result. True deficiencies of micronutrients will be associated with clinically important disorders, each being characteristic of the nutrient concerned (e.g. ascorbate deficiency leads to scurvy, niacin deficiency leads to pellagra).

Miscarriage: The spontaneous loss of an embryo or foetus at a time before it is capable of survival.

Mitogen: An agent that stimulates cell division.

Monocytes: An immature form of phagocytic white blood cell. Monocytes have the capacity to differentiate into macrophages as they mature.

Monozygotic twins: Genetically identical twins derived from a single fertilized egg that subsequently splits into two.

Morbidity: The state of being diseased.

Morphogenesis: The process through which the cells of the embryo become organised into specialist structures and organs, and by which it develops a human shape and form.

Mullerian ducts: The early embryonic structures that eventually develop into the reproductive tract. In the absence of androgenic factors the ducts develop into the female reproductive organs.

Myocardial infarction: A heart attack. Occlusion of the coronary arteries due to formation of blood clots at atherosclerotic plaques starves the heart muscle of oxygen. This causes damage to the heart tissue (infarction) and can lead to death.

n-3 fatty acids: The family of fatty acids with the shared property of having a double-bonded carbon at the ω-3 position. α-linolenic acid is the essential precursor of the n-3 series.

n-6 fatty acids: The family of fatty acids with the shared property of having a double-bonded carbon at the ω-6 position. Linoleic acid is the essential precursor of the n-6 series.

Natural killer cell: A type of lymphocyte. Natural killer cells contain enzymes and cytokines which are capable of killing tumour cells and microbial agents.

Negative feedback: A term used in endocrinology to describe the process through which a hormone switches off the processes that lead to its own synthesis or release.

Neural tube defects: Birth defects in which the embryonic neural tube, which is destined to become the spinal cord and brain, fails to close over. This means that the effected individual will either have exposed nerves in the spinal cord (spina bifida) or will lack the bone covering for the cerebral tissues (anencephaly).

Non-starch polysaccharides: An alternative term used to describe dietary fibre.

Nutrient density: A term used to describe the ratio of the content of specific nutrients to energy within a foodstuff.

Nutrigenomics: The study of the molecular relationships between nutrition and the gene expression.

Nutritional analysis software: Software developed to provide simple access to food table based databases. An important tool in the analysis of food records and food frequency questionnaires.

Nutritional epidemiology: The study of how nutrients and nutrition-related factors influence patterns of disease within human populations.

Nutritional status: The state of a person's health in relation to the nutrients in their diet and subsequently within their body.

Obesity: A state of excessive body fat storage. Obesity can be diagnosed using a variety of anthropometric measures, such as body mass index, and is associated with increased risk of death due to cardiovascular disease and cancer.

Occult bleeding: Loss of blood in the faeces. Occult bleeding is a symptom of gastrointestinal diseases including colon cancer, inflammatory bowel disease, oesophagitis or gastritis.

Odds ratio: A measure of association between an exposure (e.g. diet) and an outcome (disease). The odds ratio represents the odds that an outcome will occur given a particular exposure, compared to the odds of the outcome occurring in the absence of that exposure.

Oedema: The swelling of organs or the extremities due to movement of water from intracellular to extracellular compartments. Oedema is often a response to inflammation, as seen in protein–energy malnutrition.

Oesophagitis: Inflammation of the oesophagus, generally resulting from gastric reflux or injury to the oesophagus during radiotherapy.

Oligorrhea: Defective menstrual cycling in which the normal 28 day cycle is extended for periods of up to 90 days.

Oncogenes: A gene, or mutated gene, that encodes a protein which promotes cancer. Proto-oncogenes are genes that have the potential to become oncogenes if mutated. Anti-oncogenes are genes that encode proteins that block development and progression of cancer.

Oral glucose tolerance test: A test used to diagnose diabetes mellitus. Patients are given an oral load of glucose and blood sampled at baseline and at intervals up to 3 h. Failure to restore baseline glucose concentrations within this time is indicative of diabetes and/or insulin resistance.

Organic farming: The production of foodstuffs (animal and plant) without the use of synthetic pesticides, fertilizers or feed additives.

Ossification: The process through which cartilaginous tissue becomes mineralised and transformed to bone tissue.

Osteoblast: A cell responsible for bone formation through the production of collagen and deposition of bone mineral.

Osteoclast: A cell responsible for the removal of bone tissue during skeletal repair or remodelling.

Osteopenia: Low bone density. In children this may be due to a failure to deposit minerals such as calcium. In adults osteopenia may be a precursor of osteoporosis, caused by loss of calcium and other minerals from bone.

Osteoporosis: Condition of bone in which loss of bone mineral leads to increased risk of fracture.

Overnutrition: Condition in which the supply of nutrients (usually nutrient intakes) exceeds the physiological requirement for those nutrients. Over-nutrition may be associated with adverse health consequences.

Ovulation: The process through which a mature Graafian follicle ruptures to release an ovum during the menstrual cycle.

Oxidative damage: The cellular and tissue damage that is caused by free radicals and other reactive oxygen species. All components of cells are vulnerable to such damage, which may include peroxidation of lipids, protein strand scission or DNA mutation.

Oxidative phosphorylation: The metabolic pathway found within mitochondria, through which energy substrates generate ATP through the donation of electrons to the electron transport chain.

Pagets disease of bone: A chronic disease of the skeleton in which the bones become enlarged and weaker, creating an increased risk of fracture.

Palatability: The acceptability of a food to the senses. Aroma, taste and texture all determine palatability.

Pancreatitis: Inflammation of the pancreas, often caused by other conditions of the gastrointestinal tract, such as gallstones.

Parenteral nutrition: A form of nutritional support in which simple nutrients are delivered to the body intravenously.

Periodontal disease: Inflammatory disease of the gum caused by infection with bacterial species. Severe periodontitis will result in loss of teeth and has been linked to systemic inflammation and infection.

Peripheral resistance: The resistance of the arterial system to the flow of blood. Resistance is one the determinants of blood pressure.

Pernicious anaemia: A consequence of vitamin B12 deficiency, arising due to the loss of gastric parietal cells and hence intrinsic factor.

Personalized nutrition: An approach to providing nutritional advice which is based on assessment of genetic background and how this will determine the response to nutrients, and of measures of biomarkers of risk of disease.

Phase I xenobiotic metabolism: Xenobiotics are exogenous chemicals such as drugs, toxins and pollutants, which may be harmful to the body. These agents are removed in two steps. In Phase I metabolism the cytochrome P450 add hydroxyl groups to xenobiotics, facilitating their removal in Phase II metabolism.

Phase II xenobiotic metabolism: Xenobiotics that have been modified in Phase I metabolism can be readily conjugated to sulphonates or glucuronic acid, to yield soluble products that are excreted via the urine.

Phenylketonuria: An inherited disorder in which individuals lack the enzyme phenylalanine hydroxylase. Accumulation of phenylalanine can lead to mental retardation, so the condition requires restriction of the intake of this amino acid.

Phospholipids: Lipids comprising a hydrophilic head group (e.g. phosphatidyl choline, phosphatidylserine) and hydrophobic fatty acid tails. Phospholipids are the principle components of biological membranes.

Phytoestrogens: Plant-derived molecules that can mimic the actions of oestrogens.

Pica: The consumption of non-nutritive substances such as clay or laundry starch.

Placental abruption: A complication of pregnancy in which the placenta breaks away from the uterine wall.

Placental previa: A dangerous complication of pregnancy in which the placenta lies close to or across the cervix and hence blocks access of the baby to the birth canal.

Plasticity: The ability of an organism adapt in response to changes in the environment.

Polycystic ovary syndrome: Disease of the ovaries characterized by the formation of cysts, leading to disruption of normal menstrual cycling and infertility.

Polymorphisms: Polymorphisms are multiple variables of a gene within a population. Individuals with variant alleles may be at greater, or lesser, risk of disease depending upon interactions with environmental or dietary factors.

Polyphenolics: Plant products comprising two or more phenol rings. The polyphenolics include the flavonoids, tannins and lignin. Many polyphenolics are antioxidants and may have other bioactivities within the human body.

Ponderal index (PI): An alternative to BMI which is sometimes applied to infants. PI is calculated as weight (kg)/length (m^3).

Positive feedback: A term used in endocrinology to describe the means through which a hormone stimulates the processes that drive its own production.

Posterior pituitary: One of two lobes of the pituitary gland. This endocrine tissue responds directly to nerve signals from the hypothalamus and has two main products: vasopressin and oxytocin.

Post-partum haemorrhage: Excessive maternal bleeding after the delivery of the baby and placenta.

Prebiotics: Substances added to food to induce the multiplication of beneficial bacterial species in the colon.

Pre-eclampsia: A hypertensive disorder of pregnancy, characterized by elevated blood pressure and proteinuria.

Premature infant: A baby born before full-term gestation. Full-term is 40 weeks and prematurity is generally defined as birth before 38 weeks.

Prevalence rates: A measure of the level of a disease within a population. The prevalence rate is usually expressed as the number of disease cases per 100 000 people in the population. Prevalence rates should not be confused with incidence rates, which are defined as the number of new cases arising within a population over a given period of time.

Probiotics: Bacterial cultures added to foodstuffs to increase the populations of those bacteria within the human digestive tract.

Programming: The process through which exposure of the developing foetus to an insult during a critical period of development, permanently alters the structure and function of tissues and organs.

Protein–energy malnutrition: Chronic undernutrition arising through insufficient intakes of protein and energy to meet metabolic and physiological demands. Protein–energy malnutrition is the most common form of clinically significant malnutrition and may arise due to inadequate food supply (as in developing countries) or high nutrient requirements associated with trauma.

Proteolysis: The degradation of proteins through the actions of proteases.

Pseudotumour cerebri: A medical condition characterized by persistent headache. It is often caused by increased blood and cerebrospinal fluid pressure within the brain.

Pubarche: The first appearance of pubic hair during sexual maturation.

Puberty: The process of physical change that marks the transition from childhood to sexual maturity.

Publication bias: A form of bias in research reports which arises from the tendency for researchers and journal editors to highlight study results that are positive rather than study results that are inconclusive.

Public health nutrition: The application of the science of nutrition for the benefit of the population. Public health nutritionists are involved in investigation of the links between human nutrition and disease states, and the development of suitable disease prevention and health promotion strategies.

Pulmonary thromboembolism: Blockage of the pulmonary artery due to a clot from another site becoming dislodged and transferring to the lungs.

Quartile: Populations may be divided into equally sized groups based on key characteristics such as their nutrient intake, body mass index, height or weight. Where the division is into four groups, each group is termed as a quartile.

Quiescence: A resting state, or state of dormancy.

Quintile: Populations may be divided into equally sized groups based upon key characteristics such as their nutrient intake, body mass index, height or weight. Where the division is into five groups, each group is termed as a quintile.

Reactive oxygen species: Collective term used to describe free radicals and other oxidizing species that are formed in biological systems through the use of oxygen in metabolic processes, such as respiration.

Reference nutrient intake (RNI): One of the dietary reference value terms used in the United Kingdom. The RNI for a nutrient is the level of intake that should meet the requirements of 97.5% of individuals within a population.

Relative risk: A measure of association between an exposure (e.g. diet) and an outcome (disease). Relative risk is calculated as the ratio of the probability of an event occurring (developing a disease) in an exposed group compared to the probability of the event occurring in a non-exposed group.

Retinol activity equivalents: As vitamin A exists in different forms (retinol, α-carotene, ß-carotene) and as each form difference in biological potency, retinol activity equivalents are used to define the standard units of vitamin A intake.

Reverse transcription: The process of generating a double-stranded copy DNA from single-stranded RNA using the enzyme reverse transcriptase.

Rooting reflex: The innate ability of the human infant to locate and grasp the breast in preparation for suckling.

Safe intake: One of the dietary reference value terms used in the United Kingdom. Safe Intake is applied to certain nutrients, for which there is insufficient evidence to define more detailed references. The safe intake would represent an intake expected to meet demands without posing a risk associated with excess.

Sarcopenia: Age-related degeneration of muscle mass and strength.

Satiety: The sensation of fullness leading to the loss of desire to eat.

Sedentary: Inactive.

Senescence: The process of ageing. Senescence refers to the biological processes that are associated with advanced age.

Sertoli cells: Cells of the testes which are responsible for supporting spermatozoa as they differentiate from immature forms.

Shoulder dystocia: A complication of pregnancy, in which the shoulders of the baby cannot pass through the birth canal following delivery of the head. This can be life-threatening and often results in fractures of the clavicle and injury to the nerves which supply the shoulders and arms.

Single-locus mutation: Mutation of a single gene leading to disease consequences.

Single nucleotide polymorphism: Many genes exist in variant forms (alleles) which differ by the substitution of a single base pair. For example one allele could include the sequence TTCGAC, with a variant sequence TTTGAC. This difference is called a single nucleotide polymorphism (SNP). Some SNPs have been identified as having links to human disease states.

Skinfold thicknesses: Body composition can be estimated using a skinfold test in which a pinch of skin is precisely measured using calipers at standardized points on the body. This determines the subcutaneous fat layer thickness, which can then be included in equations that converted the measurements to an estimated body fat percentage. Typically measured sites are the triceps, sub-scapular, suprailiac and abdominal regions.

Spina bifida: A defect of the formation of the embryonic neural tube, which results in a lesion of the spinal cord. Spina bifida is one of the most common human birth defects.

Statins: Class of drugs which lower circulating cholesterol concentrations by inhibiting the enzyme, HMG-CoA reductase.

Steatorrhea: Production of non-solid, often foul-smelling faeces. Often an indicator of malabsorption of fats.

Stillbirth: The delivery of a dead baby.

Stools: Faeces.

Stroke: Cerebrovascular accident. Strokes may be haemorrhagic, in which blood leaks from blood vessels in the brain causing damage to local tissue, or thrombotic. Thrombotic strokes are caused by atherosclerosis in vessels supplying the brain. Blockage of vessels by clots starves the brain of oxygen and cause tissue damage.

Stroke volume: The volume of blood that is ejected in a single contraction of the left ventricle. It is a key determinant of the cardiac output.

Strontium ranelate: A drug used in the treatment of osteoporosis. It acts by stimulating the activity of osteoblasts and inhibiting action of osteoclasts.

Stunting: Growth-faltering in which the full stature (height) of a growing child is not achieved.

Subconjunctival haemorrhage: Damage to the blood vessels in the eye.

Subcutaneous fat: The layer of fat which lies beneath the skin.

Supplementation: Supplementation of the diet with a nutrient involves the consumption of that nutrient in a purified and artificial form, for example, a multivitamin pill, or a soluble fibre drink. Supplements usually deliver nutrients in high doses, for example, the equivalent of the requirement for a full day in a single dose.

Systematic review: A research approach in which a literature review is written to focus solely on a single question. The systematic review attempts to synthesize together the findings of all high-quality research evidence in the area, in an unbiased manner.

Telomere: A region of repetitive, non-coding DNA found at the end of a linear chromosome.

Teratogen: An agent that interferes with normal processes of development during embryonic or foetal life, and hence promotes congenital malformations.

Terpenoids: Plant compounds that provide the distinctive aromas found in cinnamon and ginger.

Testosterone: The principal androgenic hormone of mammals. Testosterone is a steroid hormone.

Thelarche: The first stage of breast development during puberty.

Thermogenesis: The process of endogenous heat production. Most thermogenesis is the product of metabolism within the liver, which maintains a constant body temperature. There are also components of thermogenesis that are activated by cold exposure (shivering and non-shivering thermogenesis) and by diet. Consumption of food generates heat associated with the digestion and metabolism of nutrients. Thermogenesis is an important component of total energy expenditure.

Thirst centre: Region of the hypothalamus which senses fluid balance and stimulates the desire to drink.

Total energy expenditure: The total energy utilized by an organism in a given period of time (usually measured over 24 h). The components of total energy expenditure in an adult are the resting metabolic rate, thermogenesis and physical activity.

Trabecular bone: Bone of low density comprising a lattice-type structure through which bone marrow, nerves and blood vessels pass. Also called cancellous or spongy bone.

Trans-fatty acids: Unsaturated fatty acids with double bonds in the trans-configuration as opposed to the cis arrangement of these isomers which is more usually seen in nature. Most trans-fatty acids in the human diet are the product of hydrogenation of vegetable oils in order to make them solidify.

Transformed cell: A cell which has become immortal (i.e. it has unlimited capacity to divide) through the mutation of a proto- or anti-oncogene.

Transit time: The time taken for components of food to pass from the mouth to the anus. This essentially measures the speed of digestion and elimination of waste products. Transit time can be measured through ingestion of a coloured marker such as carmine, which will appear in the stools.

Trauma: Physiological stress to the body. Trauma includes surgery, burns, infections, fractures and other injuries. All trauma events trigger a common metabolic response mediated by pro- and anti-inflammatory cytokines.

Trimester: A period of time relating to approximately one-third of pregnancy.

Tuberculosis (TB): An infectious disease caused by Mycobacterium tuberculosis. TB effects the lungs, and if untreated is fatal in approximately 50% of cases.

Tumour suppressor gene: A gene which encodes a protein product that inhibits cell division.

Ulcerative colitis: An inflammatory disease of the bowel in which ulcers develop within the colon. Ulcerative colitis is widely regarded as an autoimmune disease and is often treated by surgical removal of affected portions of bowel.

Umami: The specialized component of taste perception that detects monosodium glutamate.

Uracil misincorporation: DNA and RNA differ in their profile of bases. Whilst DNA contains thymine, in RNA this is replaced with uracil. The term 'uracil misincorporation' describes faulty DNA repair, in which a lack of thymine results in uracil being included within DNA strands. As this cannot be transcribed the affected genes are effectively mutated.

Vascular smooth muscle cells: Cells of the outer layers of arteries which provide the blood vessels with contractile properties.

Vegans: Individuals who follow an exclusively vegetarian diet, excluding all animal produce.

Vegetarians: Individuals who predominantly follow a diet that is of plant origin. There are different classes of vegetarian with varying dietary patterns. Vegans for example, exclude all animal produce, whilst lactoovo-vegetarians will include eggs and milk in their diet, but not eat meat.

Visceral fat: The fat that is stored around the organs of the peritoneal cavity.

Vital capacity: A marker of lung function. Vital capacity is the maximum volume of air that can be exhaled after maximum inhalation.

Waist circumference: The measurement of the waist circumference provides a proxy measure for the amount of fat stored within the abdomen. Men of healthy weight should have a waist circumference of less than 94 cm, whilst in women it should be less than 80 cm.

Waist–hip ratio: The waist circumference divided by the circumference measured around the hips provides a proxy measurement for body fatness. The adverse health consequences associated with overweight and obesity correlate closely with a waist hip ratio greater than in 0.9 men and 0.80 in women.

Wasting: Loss of weight due to utilization of fat and muscle reserves. In children wasting will manifest as a failure to increase weight during the period of growth.

Weaning: See Complementary feeding.

Xeroderma pigmentosa: An inherited disorder of DNA repair in which sensitivity to ultraviolet damage leads to early onset skin cancers.

CHAPTER 1

Introduction to lifespan nutrition

LEARNING OBJECTIVES

This chapter will enable the reader to:
- Describe what is meant by a lifespan approach to the study of nutrition and health
- Discuss the meaning of the term 'nutritional status' and describe how optimal nutrition requires a balance of nutrient supply and demand for nutrients in physiological and metabolic processes
- Show an awareness of the factors that contribute to undernutrition, including limited food supply and increased demands due to trauma or chronic illness
- Discuss global strategies for the prevention of malnutrition
- Understand that the biological response to food and nutrients is highly individual and is strongly dependent upon non-modifiable factors such as genetics, age and sex
- Describe how nutritional status is influenced by the stage of life due to the variation in specific factors controlling nutrient availability and requirements, as individuals develop from the fetal stage through to adulthood
- Show an appreciation of how anthropometry, dietary assessment, measurements of biomarkers and clinical examination can be used to study nutritional status in individuals and populations
- Describe approaches used in nutritional epidemiology to explore relationships between diet and disease
- Understand and interpret the findings of epidemiological studies and appreciate the power of systematic review and meta-analysis as a research tool
- Discuss the need for dietary standards in making assessments of the quality of diet or dietary provision, in individuals or populations
- Describe the variation in the basis and usage of dietary reference value systems in different countries

1.1 The lifespan approach to nutrition

The principal aim of this book is to explore relationships between nutrition and health and the contribution of nutrition-related factors to disease. In tackling this subject, there are many different approaches that could be taken, for example, considering diet and cardiovascular disease, nutrition and diabetes, obesity or immune function as separate and discrete entities, each worthy of their own chapter. The view of this author is that the final stages of life, that is, the elderly years, are effectively the products of events that occur through the full lifespan of an individual. Ageing is in actuality a continual, lifelong process of ongoing change and development from the moment of conception until the point of death. It is therefore inappropriate to consider how diet relates to chronic diseases that affect adults without allowance for how the earlier life experiences have shaped physiology. The lifespan approach that is used to organize the material in this book essentially asserts three main points:

1 All stages of life from the moment of conception through to the elderly years are associated with a series of specific requirements for nutrition.
2 The consequences of less than optimal nutrition at each stage of life will vary, according to the life stage affected.
3 The nature of nutrition-related factors at earlier stages of life will determine how individuals grow and develop. As a result, the relationship between diet and health in later stages of adult life, to some extent, depends upon events earlier in life. As a result, the nature of this relationship may be highly individual.

Although we tend to divide the lifespan into a series of distinct stages, such as infancy, adolescence, early

Nutrition, Health and Disease: A Lifespan Approach, Second Edition. Simon Langley-Evans.
© 2015 John Wiley & Sons, Ltd. Published 2015 by John Wiley & Sons, Ltd.
Companion website: www.wiley.com/go/langleyevans/lifespan

adulthood, middle age and older adulthood, few of these divisions have any real biological significance, and they are therefore simply markers of particular periods within a continuum. There are, however, key events within these life stages, such as weaning, the achievement of puberty or the menopause, which are significant milestones that mark profound physiological and endocrine changes and have implications for the nature of the nutrition and health relationship. On a continual basis, at each stage of life, individuals experience a series of biological challenges, such as infection, a change in the diet or exposure to carcinogens that threaten to disturb normal physiology and compromise health. Within a lifespan approach, it is implicit that the response of the system to each challenge will influence how the body responds at later life stages. Variation in the quality and quantity of nutrition is one of the major challenges to the maintenance of optimal physiological function and is also one of the main determinants of how the body responds to other insults.

In considering the contribution of nutrition-related factors to health and disease across the lifespan, it is necessary to evaluate the full range of influences upon quality and quantity of nutrition and upon physiological processes. This book therefore takes a broad approach and includes consideration of social or cultural influences on nutrition and health, the metabolic and biochemical basis of the diet–disease relationships and the influence of genetics and, where necessary, provides overviews of the main physiological and cellular processes that operate at each life stage. While the arbitrary distinctions of childhood, adolescence and adulthood have been used to divide the chapters, it is hoped that the reader will consider this work as a whole. For those requiring a primer in nutrition before engaging with specific chapters, the Appendix to the book describes the nutrients in simple terms. In this opening chapter, we consider some of the basic terms and definitions used in nutrition and lay the foundations for understanding more complex material in the following chapters.

1.2 The concept of balance

Balance is a term frequently used in nutrition, and, unfortunately, the precise meaning of the term may differ according to the context and the individual using it. It is common to hear the phrase 'a balanced diet', and, indeed, most health education literature that goes out to the general public urges the consumption of a diet that is 'balanced'. In this context, we refer to a diet that provides neither too much nor too little of the nutrients and other components of food that are required for normal functioning of the body. A balanced diet may also be viewed as a diet providing foods of a varied nature, in proportions such that consumption of foods rich in some nutrients does not limit intakes of foods rich in others.

1.2.1 A supply and demand model

There is another way of viewing the meaning of balance or a balanced diet, whereby the relationship between nutrient intake and function is the main consideration. A diet that is in balance is one where the supply of nutrients is equal to the requirement of the body for those nutrients. Essentially, balance could be viewed as equivalent to an economic market, in which supply of goods or services needs to be sufficient to meet demands for those goods or services. Figure 1.1 summarizes the supply and demand model of nutritional balance.

Whether or not the diet is in balance will be a key determinant of the *nutritional status* of an individual. Nutritional status describes the state of a person's health in relation to the nutrients in their diet and subsequently within their body. Good nutritional status would generally be associated with a dietary pattern that supplies nutrients at a level sufficient to meet requirements, without excessive storage. Poor nutritional status would generally (though not always) be associated with intakes that are insufficient to meet requirements.

The supply and demand model provides a useful framework for thinking about the relationship between diet and health. As shown in Figure 1.1, maintaining balance with respect to any given nutrient requires the supply of the nutrient to be equivalent to the overall demand for that nutrient. Demand comprises any physiological or metabolic process that utilizes the nutrient and may include use as an energy-releasing substrate, as an enzyme cofactor, as a structural component of tissues, as a substrate for the synthesis of macromolecules, as a transport element or as a component of cell–cell signalling apparatus. The supply side of the balance model comprises any means through which nutrients are made available to meet demand. This goes beyond delivery through food intake and includes stores of the nutrient that can be mobilized within the body and quantities of the nutrient that might be synthesized de novo (e.g. vitamin D is synthesized in the skin through the action of sunlight).

1.2.2 Overnutrition

When supply does not match demand for a nutrient, then the system is out of balance and this may have important consequences in terms of health and disease. Overnutrition (Figure 1.1) will generally arise because

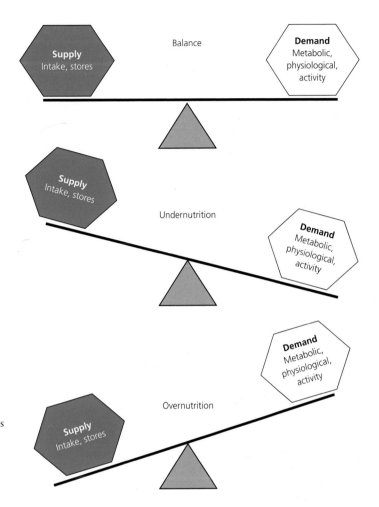

Figure 1.1 The concept of balance. The demands for nutrients comprise metabolic and physiological processes that utilize nutrients. Supply is determined by intakes of food, availability of nutrient stores and de novo production of nutrients.

the supply of a nutrient is excessive relative to demand. This is either because intake of foods containing that nutrient increases, because the individual consumes supplements of that nutrient or because demand for that nutrient declines with no equivalent adjustment occurring within the diet. The latter scenario particularly applies to the elderly, for whom energy requirements fall due to declining physical activity levels and resting metabolic rate (Rivlin, 2007). Commonly, intakes of energy that were appropriate in earlier adulthood will be maintained, resulting in excessive energy intake.

The consequences of overnutrition are generally not widely considered in the context of health and disease, unless the nutrient concerned is directly toxic or harmful when stored in high quantities. The obvious example here is, again, energy, where overnutrition will result in fat storage and obesity. For many nutrients, overnutrition within reasonable limits has no adverse effect as the excess material will either be stored or excreted. At megadoses, however, most nutrients have some capacity to cause harm. Accidental consumption of iron supplements or iron overload associated with inherited disorders is a cause of disease and death in children. At high doses, iron will impair oxidative phosphorylation and mitochondrial function, leading to cellular damage in the liver, heart, lungs and kidneys. Excess consumption of vitamin A has been linked to the development of birth defects in the unborn fetus (Martinez-Frias and Salvador, 1990). Vitamin D intoxication, for example, can arise due to overconsumption of supplements (Conti *et al.*, 2014) and leads to the formation of kidney stones and neurological damage.

Overnutrition for one nutrient can also have effects upon nutritional status with respect to other nutrients and can impact on physiological processes involving a broader range of nutrients. For example, regular consumption of iron supplements can impact upon absorption of other metals such as zinc and copper by competing for gastrointestinal transporters and hence promote undernutrition with respect to those trace elements. Having an excess of a particular nutrient within the body can also promote undernutrition with respect to another by increasing the demand associated with processing the excess. For example, a diet rich in the amino acid methionine will tend to increase circulating and tissue concentrations of homocysteine. The processing of this damaging intermediate increases the demand for B vitamins, folic acid, vitamin B6 and vitamin B12, which are all involved in pathways that convert homocysteine to less harmful forms (Lonn *et al.*, 2006; see Section "Folic acid and plasma homocysteine" of Chapter 8).

1.2.3 Undernutrition
Undernutrition arises when the supply of nutrient fails to meet demand. This can occur if intakes are poor or if demands are increased (Figure 1.1). In the short–medium term, low intakes are generally cushioned by the fact that the body has reserves of all nutrients that can be mobilized to meet demand. As such, for adults, it will usually require prolonged periods of low intake to have a significantly detrimental effect on nutritional status.

1.2.3.1 Increased demand
There are a number of situations that may arise to increase demand in such a way that undernutrition will arise if supply is not also increased accordingly. These include pregnancy, lactation and trauma. Trauma encompasses a wide range of physical insults to the body, including infection, bone fracture, burns, surgery and blood loss. Although diverse in nature, all of these physiological insults lead to the same metabolic response. This *acute phase response* (Table 1.1) is largely orchestrated by the cytokines including tumour necrosis

factor-α (TNF-α), interleukin-6 (IL-6) and interleukin-1 (IL-1) (Grimble, 2001). Their net effect is to increase demand for protein and energy and yet paradoxically they have an anorectic effect. Thus, demand increases and supply will be impaired, together leading to protein–energy malnutrition. While in many developing countries, we associate protein–energy malnutrition with starvation in children, in developed countries such as the United Kingdom, protein–energy malnutrition is most commonly noted in surgical patients and patients recovering from major injuries (Wild *et al.*, 2010).

1.2.3.2 The metabolic response to trauma
The human body is able to adapt rates of metabolism and the nature of metabolic processes to ensure survival in response to adverse circumstances. The metabolic response to adverse challenges will depend upon the nature of the challenge. Starvation leads to increased metabolic efficiency, which allows reserves of fat and protein to be utilized at a controlled rate that prolongs survival time and hence maximizes the chances of the starved individual regaining access to food. In contrast, the physiological response to trauma generates a hypermetabolic state in which reserves of fat and protein are rapidly mobilized in order to fend off infection and promote tissue repair (Table 1.1). Physiological stresses to the body, including infection, bone fracture, burns or other tissue injuries, elicit a common metabolic response regardless of their nature. Thus, a minor surgical procedure will produce the same pattern of metabolic response as a viral infection. It is the magnitude of the response that is variable, and this is largely determined by the severity of the trauma (Romijn, 2000).

The hypermetabolic response to trauma is driven by endocrine changes that promote the catabolism of protein and fat reserves. Following the initial physiological insult, there is an increase in circulating concentrations

Table 1.1 The acute phase inflammatory response to trauma or infection.

Acute phase response	Markers of the response
Metabolic change	Catabolism of protein, muscle wastage. Amino acids converted to glucose for energy or used to synthesize acute phase proteins. Catabolism of fat for energy
Fever	Body temperature rises to kill pathogens. Hypothalamic regulation of food intake disrupted, leading to loss of appetite
Hepatic protein synthesis	Acute phase proteins synthesized to combat infection (e.g. C-reactive protein, α1-proteinase inhibitor, caeruloplasmin). Liver reduces synthesis of other proteins, including transferrin and albumin
Sequestration of trace elements	Zinc and iron taken up by tissues to remove free elements that may be utilized by pathogens
Immune cell activation	B cells produce increased amounts of immunoglobulins. T cells release cytokines to orchestrate the inflammatory response
Cytokine production	Tumour necrosis factor-α and the interleukins 1, 2, 6, 8 and 10 work to produce a hypermetabolic state that favours production of substrates for immune function, but inhibits reproduction and spread of pathogens

of the catecholamines, cortisol and glucagon. Increased cortisol and glucagon serve to stimulate rates of gluconeogenesis and hepatic glucose output, thereby maintaining high concentrations of plasma glucose. The breakdown of protein to amino acids provides gluconeogenic substrates and also leads to greatly increased losses of nitrogen via the urine. Lipolysis is stimulated and circulating free fatty acid concentrations rise dramatically. These are used as energy substrates, along with glucose.

The response to trauma is essentially an inflammatory process, and, as such, the same metabolic drives are noted in individuals suffering from long-term inflammatory diseases including cancer and inflammatory bowel disease (Richardson and Davidson, 2003). The inflammatory response serves two basic functions. Firstly, it activates the immune system, raises body temperature and repartitions micronutrients in order to create a hostile environment for invading pathogens (Table 1.1). Secondly, it allocates nutrients towards processes that will contribute to repair and healing.

The inflammatory response is orchestrated by the pro-inflammatory cytokines (e.g. TNF-α, IL-1 and IL-6) and the anti-inflammatory cytokines (e.g. IL-10). Whenever injury or infection occurs, the pro-inflammatory species are released by monocytes, macrophages and T helper cells. The level of cytokines produced is closely related to the severity of the trauma (Lenz et al., 2007). The impact of pro-inflammatory cytokines is complex. On the one hand, they activate the immune system and protect the body from greater trauma. On the other, at the local level of any injury, they increase damage by stimulating the immune system to release damaging oxidants and other agents that indiscriminately destroy invading pathogens and the body's own cells. The production of pro-inflammatory cytokines therefore has to be counterbalanced as an excessive response can lead to death (Grimble, 2001). This is the role of the anti-inflammatory cytokines and some of the acute phase response proteins, several of which inhibit the proteinases released during inflammation and therefore limit the breakdown of host tissues.

In addition to stimulating proteolysis and lipolysis within muscle and adipose tissue, the cytokines have a number of actions that impact upon nutritional status. Firstly, they increase the basal metabolic rate. An element of creating a hostile environment for pathogens includes raising the core temperature of the body (fever). This greatly increases energy demands. The capacity to meet those demands through feeding is reduced as cytokines also act upon the gut and the centres of the hypothalamus that regulate appetite, effectively switching off the desire to eat. As can be seen in Table 1.2, the increased metabolic rate associated with

Table 1.2 The metabolic response to injury and infection increases requirements for energy and protein.

Nature and severity of trauma	Increase in energy requirement (x basal)	Increase in protein requirement (x basal)
Minor surgery or infection	1.1	1.0–1.5
Major surgery or moderate infection	1.3–1.4	1.5–2.3
Severe infection, multiple or head injuries	1.8	2.0–2.8
Burns (20% BSAB)	1.5	—
Burns (20–40% BSAB)	1.8	2.0–2.8*

*Dependent upon level of nitrogen losses in tissue exudates and age of patient. Children with burns have higher requirements. BSAB, body surface area burned.

the response to trauma greatly increases the demands of the body for both energy and protein. In severe cases, requirements can be doubled, even though the critically ill patient will be immobilized and not expending energy through physical activity. This can pose major challenges for clinicians managing such cases as the injured patient may be unable to feed normally, and due to the anorectic influences of pro-inflammatory cytokines, the capacity to ingest sufficient energy, protein and other nutrients is greatly reduced. Enteral or parenteral feeding is therefore a mainstay of managing major injuries.

With more severe trauma, the mobilization of reserves can produce marked changes in body composition. Muscle wasting may occur as the calcium-dependent calpains and ubiquitin–proteasome break down proteins rapidly to make amino acids available for gluconeogenesis and the synthesis of important antioxidants such as glutathione (Grimble, 2001). Body composition changes are beneficial to the injured patient as they primarily generate glucose. This is the optimal energy substrate for these circumstances, not least because it can be metabolized anaerobically to produce ATP in tissues where blood flow may be compromised and oxygen delivery impaired.

In the short term, the hypermetabolic response and the accompanying anorexia of illness are unlikely to impact significantly upon the nutritional status of an individual, although nutritional status prior to onset of trauma would be an important consideration. For example, the nutritional consequences of a fractured femur in a young, fit adult male may be dramatically different to those in a frail elderly woman. Prolonged periods of disease accompanied by inflammatory responses that drive hypermetabolism will promote states of protein–energy malnutrition, such as kwashiorkor, or can produce the emaciated state of cachexia. Cachexia is characterized by loss of weight, decline in appetite and muscle atrophy due to mobilization of muscle protein. It is generally associated with underlying chronic illnesses such as cancer, tuberculosis or untreated AIDS. Nutritional support (i.e. supplemental feeding) of chronically ill individuals or those who have suffered more acute trauma can limit the impact of the hypermetabolic response upon body composition and overall nutritional status. However, the catabolic metabolism cannot be reversed until the injury or illness is resolved, so the priority in these scenarios is limiting weight loss and loss of muscle mass, rather than achieving weight gain.

1.2.3.3 Compromised supply and deficiency

Clearly, there is a direct relationship between the supply of a nutrient to the body and the capacity of the body to carry out the physiological functions that depend upon the supply of that nutrient. As can be seen in Figure 1.2, the range of nutrient intakes over which optimal function is maintained is likely to be very broad, and there are a number of stages before functionality is lost. It is only when function can no longer be maintained that the term nutritional deficiency can be accurately used.

A nutrient deficiency arises when the supply of a nutrient through food intake is compromised to the extent that clinical or metabolic symptoms appear. The simplest example to think of here relates to iron deficiency anaemia in which low intakes of iron result in a failure to maintain effective concentrations of red blood cell haemoglobin, leading to compromised oxygen transport and hence the clinical symptoms of deficiency that include fatigue, irritability, dizziness, weakness and shortness of breath. Iron deficiency anaemia, like all deficiency disorders, reflects only the late stage of the process that begins with a failure of supply through intake to meet demands (Table 1.3). Once the body can no longer maintain function using nutrient supply directly from the diet, it will mobilize stores. In the case of iron, this will involve the release of iron bound to the protein, ferritin, to maintain haemoglobin concentrations. No change in function will occur at this stage, but the individual will now be in a state of greater vulnerability to deficiency. A further decline in supply through intake may not be matched through mobilization of stores, and so full deficiency becomes more likely. This situation in which intakes are sufficiently low that, although there are no signs of deficiency, biochemical indicators show that nutrition is subnormal is generally referred to as *marginal nutrition*, or subclinical malnutrition.

1.2.3.4 Malnutrition

Malnutrition describes the state where the level of nutrient supply has declined to the point of deficiency and normal physiological functions can no longer be maintained.

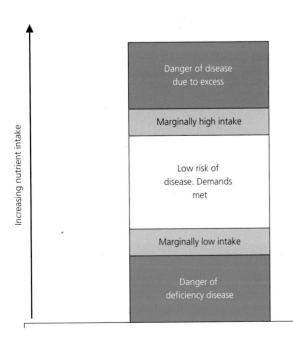

Increasing nutrient intake

Danger of disease due to excess

Marginally high intake

Low risk of disease. Demands met

Marginally low intake

Danger of deficiency disease

Figure 1.2 The association between nutrition and health. The requirements of the body for nutrients will be met by a broad range of intakes. Very low and very high intakes of any nutrient will be associated with ill health. The transition from intakes that are meeting demands and at which risk of disease is low to intakes that would be associated with disease is not abrupt.

Table 1.3 The three stages of iron deficiency.

Stage	Biochemical indicators and reference ranges
Normal iron status	Haemoglobin 14–18 g/dl (men) and 12–16 g/dl (women), serum ferritin 40–280 µg/l, transferrin saturation 31–60%
Depleted iron stores	Falling serum ferritin. Normal ranges for haemoglobin and transferrin saturation. Ferritin 13–20 µg/l
Iron deficiency	Transferrin saturation falls as transport of iron declines. Haemoglobin normal. Serum ferritin <12 µg/l. Transferrin saturation <16%
Iron deficiency anaemia	Haemoglobin synthesis cannot be maintained and declines to <13.5 g/dl (men) and <12 g/dl (women). Serum ferritin <10 µg/l. Transferrin saturation <15%

The manifestations of malnutrition will vary depending on the type of nutrient deficiencies involved and the stage of life of the malnourished individual. In adults, malnutrition is often observed as unintentional weight loss or as clinical signs of specific deficiency. In children, it is more likely to manifest as growth faltering, with the affected child being either underweight for their age (termed *wasted*) or of short stature for their age (termed *stunted*; see Section 6.2.2.1). Specific patterns of growth are indicative of different forms of protein–energy malnutrition. Wasting is associated with marasmus where a weight less than 60% of standard for age is used as a cut-off. Oedema with a weight less than 80% of standard for age is indicative of kwashiorkor.

From a clinical perspective, protein–energy malnutrition is the most serious undernutrition-related syndrome. Marasmus and kwashiorkor are the classical definitions of this form of malnutrition. Historically, marasmus was considered to be a pure energy deficiency and kwashiorkor to be protein deficiency, but it is now clear that the two are different manifestations of the same nutritional problems. Marasmic wasting is a sign of an effective physiological adaptation to long-term undernutrition. It is characterized by a depletion of fat reserves and muscle protein, along with adaptations to reduce energy expenditure. Children who become wasted in this way, if untreated, will generally die from infection as their immune functions cannot be maintained during the period of starvation. Kwashiorkor is a more rapid process, often triggered by infection alongside malnutrition. The metabolic changes with kwashiorkor are strikingly different to marasmus as the adaptation to starvation is ineffective. Fat accumulates in the liver, and expansion of extracellular fluid volume, driven by low serum albumin concentrations, leads to oedema. Micronutrient deficiencies often occur alongside protein–energy malnutrition and may partly explain why individuals with kwashiorkor, unlike those with marasmus, are unable to adapt successfully to malnutrition.

The causes of malnutrition are complex and are not simply related to a limited food intake. Where intake is reduced, this is often due to food insecurity associated with famine, poverty, war or natural disasters. Reduced food intake can also arise due to chronic illness leading to loss of appetite or feeding difficulties. Malnutrition will also arise from malabsorption of nutrients from the digestive tract. This, again, could be a consequence of chronic disease or be driven by infection of the tract. Losses of nutrients are an important consequence of repeated diarrhoeal infections in areas where there is no access to clean water and adequate sanitation. Malnutrition may also be driven by situations that increase the demand for nutrients including trauma (as described earlier), pregnancy and lactation, if those increased demands cannot be matched by intake.

Malnutrition is most common and most deadly in the developing countries, where it is the major cause of death in children. Stunting and wasting among malnourished children have long-term consequences too, as often the reduction in stature is not recovered, leading to reduced physical strength and capacity to work in adult life. As poverty is the most frequent cause of malnutrition, a self-perpetuating cycle can be established, as the stunted child becomes the adult with reduced earning capacity, whose children will live in poverty. Stunted, underweight women will also have children who are at risk due to lower weight at birth. Pregnancy is a time of high risk for malnutrition in women living in developing countries. Stunting is commonplace among women in South and Southeast Asia and is often accompanied by underweight. For example, in India and Bangladesh, up to 40% of women of childbearing age have a body mass index (BMI) of less than 18.5 kg/m^2 (Black *et al.*, 2008). Iron deficiency anaemia is endemic among pregnant women in developing countries, with prevalence of between 60 and 87% in the countries of southern Asia (Seshadri, 2001). Maternal and childhood malnutrition are believed to cause 3.1 million deaths among the under-fives every year (Black *et al.*, 2013).

Developed countries also have a burden of malnutrition among vulnerable groups. At greatest risk are the elderly, who may develop protein–energy malnutrition or micronutrient deficiencies due to specific medical conditions or through low intakes associated with frailty or loneliness (see Section 9.5.1). Surgical patients are at risk of protein–energy malnutrition as a result of the inflammatory response to trauma. As in the developing countries, poverty increases the risk of malnutrition among children and immigrant groups. There are many ways of targeting these at-risk groups, for example, monitoring the growth of infants or including regular weighing and nutritional assessments of hospital patients. Malnutrition is easily treated through appropriate nutritional support.

The prevention of malnutrition is a major public health priority on a global scale. While a lack of food security and the risk of protein–energy malnutrition remain a major issue for many populations, there have been a number of success stories in the battle to prevent clinically significant malnutrition. The basic approaches that can be used to prevent nutrient deficiency are diet diversification, supplementation of at-risk individuals and fortification. The basis for these approaches and their use in the attempt to eradicate vitamin A deficiency is described in Research Highlight 1.1. Similar strategies have been used to reduce the occurrence of iodine and iron deficiency diseases.

Iodine deficiency is an important issue for populations in all continents except Australasia. Availability of iodine is essentially limited by the iodine content of the soil and hence uptake by plants and animals. Iodine deficiency disorders, including cretinism and goitre, are a major manifestation of malnutrition, with approximately 740 million affected individuals worldwide. Fortification has been the cornerstone of the fight against iodine deficiency, with the Universal Salt Iodization (USI) programme providing iodized salt (20–40 mg iodine/kg salt) to 70% of households in affected areas. Where the iodized salt is consumed, marked improvements in iodine status of the population are rapidly noted (Sebotsa *et al.*, 2005). Although there are still significant numbers of individuals at risk of iodine deficiency disorders, due to lack of coverage of the USI programme, this fortification approach is widely considered to be a public health nutrition success for the World Health Organization (WHO).

1.2.4 Classical balance studies

Nutritional status with respect to a specific nutrient can be measured using balance studies. These have classically been used to determine requirements for some

Research Highlight 1.1 Strategies for combating vitamin A deficiency.

Vitamin A deficiency (VAD) is one of the most common forms of malnutrition on a global scale (West, 2003), with greatest prevalence in Africa, Central and South America and South and Southeast Asia. Subclinical VAD blights the lives of up to 200 million children every year and is a causal factor in up to half a million cases of childhood blindness and up to a million deaths of children under the age of 5 years. VAD is also responsible for stunted growth in children and may cause blindness in women with increased demands for vitamin A, due to pregnancy or lactation. In 1990, the World Health Organization pledged itself to the virtual elimination of VAD by the year 2000. The strategies used to achieve this goal provide useful examples of how all common nutrient deficiencies might be prevented at a population level. Three main approaches have been used to tackle VAD:

1 *Diet diversification*. For many populations in areas where VAD is common, the range of staple foods consumed is very limited. For example, rice is the basis of most meals for many in Southeast Asia. Rice is a poor vitamin A source. Diversification programmes include health education and promotion of consumption of a greater range of foodstuffs and the development of home gardening to provide vitamin A sources. Faber *et al.* (2002) showed that a home gardening programme in South Africa increased knowledge and awareness of VAD, improved availability of vitamin A sources and increased serum retinol concentrations in young children.

2 *Supplementation*. In most countries where VAD is common, children are now supplemented with vitamin A, using an oil capsule, two or three times a year, often coupling supplement doses with other public health activities such as immunizations. Berger *et al.* (2008) highlighted the major disadvantage of supplementation, which is that it fails to reach all those in need of supplements. For VAD, those most at risk are preschool children who have less access to school-based supplementation programmes. Often, the poor and those most in need of supplements are least likely to receive them. Supplementation is expensive, which may reduce efficacy of the approach in impoverished countries (Neidecker-Gonzales *et al.*, 2007).

3 *Fortification*. Fortification involves the addition of nutrients to staple foods at the point of their production, thereby increasing the amount of nutrient delivered to all consumers of that foodstuff. VAD in several countries has been tackled using this strategy. Red palm oil is widely available in many VAD-affected areas and is a rich source of β-carotene. In India and parts of Africa, the addition of this oil to other oils traditionally used in cooking, and to snacks, has been shown to effectively increase vitamin A intake by the general population (Sarojini *et al.*, 1999). Zagré *et al.* (2003) showed that introducing red palm oil to a population in Burkina Faso was highly effective in reducing occurrence of VAD. A similar approach involves increasing the vitamin A content of crops such as rice, either through genetic modification (e.g. 'golden rice') or traditional plant breeding (Mayer, 2007).

nutrients in humans. Essentially, the balance method involves the accurate measurement of nutrient intake for comparison with accurate measures of all possible outputs of that nutrient via the urine, faeces and other potential routes of loss (Figure 1.3). If there is a state of balance, that is, intake and output are at equilibrium, it can be assumed that the body is saturated with respect to that nutrient and has no need for either uptake or storage. This technique can be applied to almost any nutrient, and by repeating balance measures at different levels of intake, it is possible to determine estimates of requirements for specific nutrients. The balance model works on the assumption that in healthy individuals of stable weight, the body pool of a nutrient will remain constant. Day-to-day variation in intake can be compensated by equivalent variation in excretion. The highest level of intake at which balance can no longer be maintained will indicate the actual requirement of an individual for that nutrient.

Nitrogen balance studies were used to determine human requirements for protein (Millward *et al.*, 1997). Such studies involved experiments in which healthy subjects were recruited and allocated to consume dietary protein at specified levels of intake. After 4–6 days of habituation to these diets, urine and faeces were collected for determination of nitrogen losses over periods of 2–3 days. On this basis, it was possible to state dietary protein requirements for different stages of life as being the lowest level of protein intake that maintained nitrogen balance in healthy individuals, maintaining body weight and engaging in modest levels of physical activity. Nitrogen balance studies are problematic in several respects, including the fact that 24-h urine collections used in such studies are often incomplete, because studies may fail to allow sufficient time for subjects to

habituate to their experimental diet and because factors such as unobserved infection, stress or exercise may increase demand for protein. It has also been impossible to use balance studies to examine protein requirements for all age groups and in all health situations, so requirements for pregnant and lactating women and for children are based on balance studies in young adults and make estimates of allowances for tissue deposition, growth and milk synthesis and secretion.

1.2.5 Overall nutritional status

The diet delivers a multitude of components rather than single nutrients, and it is unlikely that any individual will have a diet that perfectly achieves balance for all of them. For example, an individual can be in balance for protein while consuming more energy than is required and insufficient iron to meet demand. Hence, it is often not appropriate to discuss overall nutritional status of an individual without consideration of nutritional status with respect to specific nutrients.

Whether considering the overall nutritional status of an individual, examining nutritional status with respect to a specific nutrient or investigating the nutritional status of a population, it is important to take into account a broad range of factors. It should be clear from the previous discussions that intake is just one component of the supply side of the balance model. Nutritional status is only partly determined by the food that is being consumed. Nutritional status also depends upon the activities and health status of the individuals concerned. Trauma and high levels of physical activity will increase demand, while a sedentary lifestyle will decrease demand. Most important though is the stage of life of the individuals under consideration. Physiological demands for nutrients vary to a wide degree, depending on age,

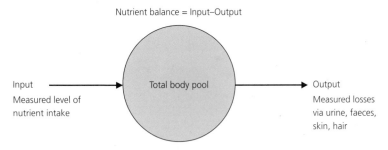

Nutrient balance = Input−Output

Input → Total body pool → Output

Measured level of nutrient intake

Measured losses via urine, faeces, skin, hair

Balance = 0 indicates that there is no net storage or loss of nutrient

Positive balance indicates that there is net deposition of nutrient to the body pool

Negative balance indicates that there is net loss of nutrient

Figure 1.3 Determining nutrient requirements using the balance method. Precise measurements of nutrient intake and of output by all possible routes enable determination of nutrient requirements. The highest level of intake at which balance can no longer be maintained will indicate the actual requirement of an individual for that nutrient.

body size and gender. The impact of variation within the diet upon health and well-being is largely, therefore, governed by age and sex.

1.3 The individual response to nutrition

The ingestion of food and nutrients is the beginning of a chain of events involving digestion and absorption, metabolic processing and physiological responses. For example, consumption of carbohydrate brings about an increase in blood glucose concentrations followed by insulin secretion and the uptake of glucose into cells and tissues for use in energy metabolism that will drive muscle contraction, thermogenesis and a host of other processes. Ingestion of sodium will result in haemodynamic changes that impact upon blood pressure and kidney function. The nature of the metabolic and physiological changes that occur following ingestion means that the response to nutrients plays a fundamental role in determining health and disease. All individuals have unique characteristics that shape the nature of the response to nutrition. This poses a problem in establishing guidelines for health nutrition as the desire is to provide general guidance on a 'one-size-fits-all' basis, but the reality is that some guidance will be inappropriate for a significant proportion of any population. Many factors will contribute to the individual response to nutrition (Figure 1.4), but genetic background and lifespan-related factors are of major significance.

1.3.1 Stage of the lifespan

Nutritional status is determined by the balance between the supply of nutrients and the demand for those nutrients in physiological and metabolic processes. So far in this chapter, we have seen that both sides of the supply–demand balance equation can be perturbed by a variety of different factors. Intake, for example, can be reduced in circumstances of poverty, while demand is elevated by physiological trauma. The main determinants of demand are, however, shaped by other factors such as the level of habitual physical activity (which will increase energy requirements), by gender, by body size and by age. It is this latter factor that provides the focus of this book.

The demand for nutrients to sustain function begins from the moment of conception. The embryonic and fetal stages of life are the least understood in terms of the precise requirements for nutrition, but it is clear that they are the life stages that are most vulnerable in the face of any imbalance. Demands for nutrients are high in order to sustain the rapid growth and the process of development from a single-celled zygote to a fully formed human infant. An optimal balance of nutrients is essential, but the nature of what is truly optimal is difficult to dissect out from the competing demands of the maternal system and the capacity of the maternal system to deliver nutrients to the fetus. The embryo and fetus represent a unique life stage from a nutritional perspective, as there are no nutrient reserves and there is a total dependence upon delivery of nutrients, initially by the yolk sac and later by the placenta. The consequences of undernutrition at this stage can be catastrophic, leading

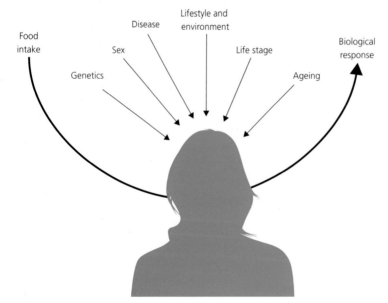

Food intake

Genetics

Sex

Disease

Lifestyle and environment

Life stage

Ageing

Biological response

Figure 1.4 The individual response to food is complex and determined by a range of modifiable and non-modifiable factors.

to miscarriage, failure of growth, premature birth, low weight at birth or birth defects (MRC Vitamin Study Group, 1991; Godfrey *et al.*, 1996; El-Bastawissi *et al.*, 2007). All of these are immediate threats to survival, but it is also becoming clear that less than optimal nutrition at this stage of life may also increase risk of disease later on in life (Langley-Evans, 2015).

After birth, the newborn infant has incredibly high nutrient demands that, in proportion to body weight, may be two to three times greater than those of an adult. These demands are again related to growth and the maturation of organ systems as in fetal life. Growth rates in the first year of life are more rapid than at any other time, and the maturation of organs such as the brain and lung continues for the first 3–8 years of life. Initially, the demands for nutrients are met by a single food source, milk, with reserves accrued from the mother towards the end of fetal life compensating for any shortfall in supply of micronutrients. In later infancy, there is the challenge of the transition to a mixed diet of solids (weaning), which is a key stage of physiological and metabolic development. The consequences of imbalances in nutrition can be severe. Infants are very vulnerable to protein–energy malnutrition and to micronutrient deficiencies, which will contribute to stunting of growth and other disorders. Iodine deficiency disorders and iron deficiency anaemia can both impact upon brain development, producing irreversible impairment of the capacity to learn. Obesity is now recognized as a major threat to the health of children in the developed countries. In this age group, it is not simply a product of excessive energy intake and low energy expenditure. Increasingly, we are seeing that the type or form of foods consumed at this time can influence long-term weight gain, with breastfed infants showing a lower propensity for obesity than those who are fed artificial formula milks (Arenz *et al.*, 2004; Bayol *et al.*, 2007).

Beyond infancy, nutrient demands begin to fall relative to body weight but still remain higher than seen in adulthood through the requirement for growth and maturation. These demands are at their greatest at the time of puberty when the adolescent growth spurt produces a dramatic increase in height and weight that is accompanied by a realignment of body composition. Proportions of body fat decline and patterns of fat deposition are altered in response to the metabolic influences of the sex hormones. Proportions of muscle increase and the skeleton increases in size and degree of mineralization. Nutrient supply must be of high quality to drive these processes, and in absolute terms (i.e. not considered in proportion to body size), the nutrient requirements of adolescence are the greatest of any life stage. However, adolescents normally have extensive nutrient stores and are therefore more tolerant of periods of undernutrition than preschool children (1–5 years).

The adult years have the lowest nutrient demands of any stage of life. As growth is complete, nutrients are required solely for the maintenance of physiological functions. The supply is well buffered through stores that protect those functions against adverse effects of undernutrition in the short term to medium term. In developed countries, and increasingly so in developing countries, the main nutritional threat is overweight and obesity, as it is difficult for adults to adjust energy intakes against declining physiological requirements and the usual fall in levels of physical activity that accompany ageing. Reducing energy intake, while maintaining adequate intakes (AI) of micronutrients, is a major challenge in elderly individuals. Chronic illnesses associated with ageing can promote undernutrition through increased nutrient demands, while limiting appetite and nutrient bioavailability.

For women, pregnancy and lactation represent special circumstances that may punctuate the adult years and increase demands for energy and nutrients. Nutrition is in itself an important determinant of fertility and the ability to reproduce (Hassan and Killick, 2004). In pregnancy, provision of nutrients must be increased for the growth and development of the fetus and to drive the deposition of maternal tissues. For example, there are requirements for an increase in size of the uterus, for the preparation of the breasts for lactation and for the formation of the placenta. To some extent, the mobilization of stores and adaptations that increase absorption of nutrients from the gut serve to meet these increased demands, but as described earlier, imbalances in nutrition may adversely impact upon the outcome of pregnancy. Lactation is incredibly demanding in terms of the energy, protein and micronutrient provision to the infant via the milk. As with pregnancy, not all of the increase in supply for this process depends upon increased maternal intakes, and in fact, women can successfully maintain lactation even with subclinical malnutrition. Adaptations that support and maintain breastfeeding may impact upon maternal health. For example, calcium requirements for lactation may be met by mobilization of bone mineral and, if not replaced once lactation has ceased, could influence later bone health. However, although nutritionally challenging, most evidence suggests that lactation is of benefit for maternal health and actually contributes to reduced risk of certain cancers and osteoporosis (Ritchie *et al.*, 1998; Danforth *et al.*, 2007).

Lifespan factors clearly impact upon nutritional status as they are a key determinant of both nutrient requirements and the processes that determine nutrient supply.

In studying relationships between diet, health and disease, one of the major challenges is to assess the quality of nutrition in individuals and at the population level. Tools used for these nutritional assessments will be described in the next section.

1.3.2 Genetics

Long-term disease states such as obesity, cancer or coronary heart disease are the products of a number of risk factors, working together, against a battery of protective factors. Disease is promoted by a poor diet, smoking, sedentary lifestyle and accumulated experiences across the lifespan. These factors all overlie the genetic background of the individual to determine how the body responds to nutrition and other environmental factors. The genotype of each individual comprises a complex set of traits that might be disease-promoting (susceptibility genes) or disease-suppressing (protective genes). For most disease states, more than one gene will be driving the components of risk.

Due to the complexity of the genetic determinants of physiological function, individuals will respond to nutritional signals in different ways. For example, some individuals will have a genetic make-up that promotes high energy expenditure. This enables them to maintain a healthy weight at a level of energy intake that is sufficient to promote obesity in other individuals, who may instead carry obesity-promoting genes.

Some of the risk of chronic disease is determined by single nucleotide polymorphisms (SNPs) (pronounced 'snips'), which are variants in the sequences of genes which control specific aspects of physiological and metabolic function (Joost *et al.*, 2007). SNPs are inherited sequences which differ from the most common sequence of a gene by just one base (e.g. a C replaced by a T; Figure 1.5). Such a change may generate a protein product of dramatically altered tertiary structure and impact significantly upon physiological function. SNPs are now well characterized as having interactions with components of the diet, and some detailed examples will be discussed in later chapters.

The C677T SNP in methylenetetrahydrofolate reductase (MTHFR) is one of the best studied examples of a genetic variant that impacts upon the variability of the individual response to diet. MTHFR is an enzyme that plays an important role in the metabolism of folates and effectively controls the availability of one-carbon donors in intermediary metabolism. Within the population, there will be three distinct populations based upon variants of C677T, namely, individuals carrying CC, CT or TT genotypes. For those carrying TT, circulating concentrations of the amino acid homocysteine will tend to be higher as activity of the enzyme is lower than with the CC variant (Figure 1.6). Hyperhomocysteinaemia is a known risk factor for cardiovascular disease, unless the diet delivers sufficient folate to offset this risk.

The contribution of a SNP to risk of disease should not be overestimated. Often, the influence of SNPs is miniscule compared to the impact of lifestyle factors. For example, a variant of the calpain-10 gene is associated

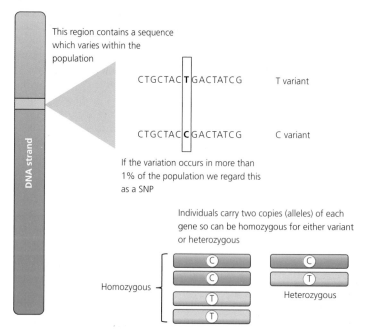

Figure 1.5 Single nucleotide polymorphisms (SNPs) arise when there are single base changes in the DNA sequence of a gene. As all individuals carry two copies of a gene, the polymorphism can result in individuals being homozygous or heterozygous for specific gene variants.

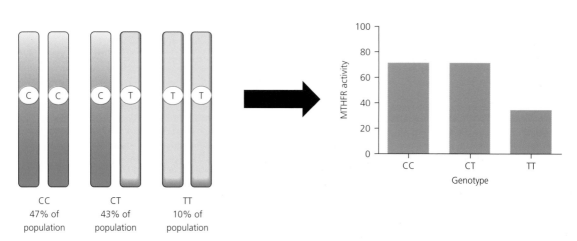

Figure 1.6 The CT677 SNP of methylenetetrahydrofolate reductase (MTHFR) influences the activity of the enzyme in tissues. This common variant of the gene can have significant impact on folate metabolism.

with a 20% increase in risk of type 2 diabetes, which is dwarfed by the 4- to 30-fold risk that is associated with obesity (Joost *et al.*, 2007). It should also be borne in mind that other genetically determined factors may modulate the influence of the SNP. In the case of the C677T polymorphism of MTHFR, the influence on disease risk varies between ethnic groups (Klerk *et al.*, 2002). Some SNPs may increase risk of one chronic disease yet protect against another. Cardiovascular disease-prone TT MTHFR variant-carrying individuals appear to have some protection against cancers of the large intestine (Joost *et al.*, 2007).

Understanding all of these processes is important. Throughout this book, you will encounter examples of uncertainty and variation in the effectiveness of nutritional interventions to prevent or manage disease. This is because the impact of diet upon physiological and metabolic processes will vary due to the genetic variation in the population and because even straightforward nutrient–gene interactions may generate opposing responses to nutrient signals under different circumstances. Some polymorphisms related to disease risk sometimes appear to have influences that are specific to gender, menopausal status or race. It is also the case that the expressed phenotype may be life stage specific. The Bsm1 SNP in the vitamin D receptor is strongly predictive of bone health and the response to calcium in children, but has no association with bone health in adults

(Ferrari *et al.*, 1998). It is therefore clear that the genotype can be an important determinant of disease risk. However, the instances of where it is the sole or major driver of risk are rare, and in most cases, genetic inheritance is just one of the many components that determine the overall risk profile for chronic disease. Research Highlight 1.2 describes one well-known gene polymorphism and its relationship to disease.

1.4 Assessment of nutritional status

The assessment of nutritional status is necessary in a variety of different settings. Working with individuals in a clinical setting, it may be necessary to assess dietary adequacy in order to plan the management of disease states, or to make clinical diagnoses. Public health nutritionists require data on dietary adequacy at a group level in order to make assessments of the contribution of nutritional factors to disease risk in the population and to develop public health policies or intervention strategies. Nutritional assessment is also a critical research tool used in determining the relationships between diet and disease. These situations, which rely on considerations of the likelihood of nutritional deficit or excess at the individual or population level, use tools that aim either to measure intakes of nutrients or the physiological manifestations of nutrient deficit or excess within the body.

Research Highlight 1.2 The ApoE gene and disease.

Cardiovascular disease is the product of disorders in a number of processes including inflammation, endothelial function, oxidant/antioxidant balance, macrophage function, lipid metabolism and cholesterol transport. Genotype variants and adverse nutrient–gene interactions related to any of these processes can therefore be regarded as candidates that may predispose an individual to atherosclerosis. Apolipoprotein E (ApoE) is one of the most widely studied of these candidate genes in the context of coronary heart disease. ApoE is a protein predominantly secreted by the liver, which plays a role in the overall regulation of lipoprotein metabolism. It is a key element of the system which clears chylomicrons and VLDL- and LDL-cholesterol from the circulation. ApoE is also produced by macrophages within atherosclerotic plaques, where it influences expression of adhesion molecules, proliferation of vascular smooth muscle cells and platelet aggregation (Jofre-Monseny et al., 2008).

There are several well-described SNPs of the ApoE gene, which give rise to different isoforms of the protein based around three basic alleles (E2, E3 and E4). This means that there are six possible genotypes in the population (E2E2, 1–2% of population; E2E3, 15% of population; E2E4, 1–2% of population; E3E3, 55% of population; E3E4, 25% of population; and E4E4, 1–2% of population).

The E4 allele has been associated with several disease outcomes. The strongest association is with Alzheimer's disease, where homozygous (E4/E4) individuals are more than 15 times more likely to develop the disease than those homozygous for the majority E3 allele (Jofre-Monseny et al., 2008). Homozygosity for E4 increases risk of atherosclerosis by 42%. The reason for this greater risk is unclear, but it may be attributable to defects of cholesterol transport, enhanced inflammatory responses or reduced antioxidant capacity (Kofler et al., 2012).

ApoE is of interest in terms of nutrition as the association of the E4 allele with cardiovascular disease risk appears to be modulated through interaction with other modifiable risk factors. Some studies show that individuals with the E4 genotype appear to derive greater benefit from reductions in intakes of total fat, saturated fats and cholesterol than those with a low genetic risk profile. In contrast, the positive LDL-cholesterol response to fish oil supplementation that is seen in individuals with an E2 or E3 genotype is totally negated by the E4 genotype (Olano-Martin et al., 2010). Individuals who carry E4 exhibit reductions in LDL-cholesterol concentrations with alcohol consumption, while those with the apparently protective E2 show the opposite response (Mukamal et al., 2004). The same is true for exercise which increases HDL-cholesterol concentrations in individuals with the E4 genotype (Corella et al., 2001). The ApoE genotype therefore provides an example of how genetic factors play a role in determining the biological response to nutrition. Genotypic variation is likely to contribute significantly to the diet–disease relationship in the 30% of the Caucasian population who carry the E4 allele.

Tools for nutritional assessment include anthropometric measures, dietary assessments, determination of biomarkers and clinical examination.

1.4.1 Anthropometric measures

Anthropometric methods make indirect measurements of the nutritional status of individuals and groups of individuals, as they are designed to estimate the composition of the body. Table 1.4 provides a summary of the commonly used anthropometric techniques. Many of these have been designed to estimate the lean or fat mass which are present within the body. Information about relative fatness or leanness can be a useful indicator of nutritional status since excess fat will highlight storage of energy consumed in excess, while declining fat stores and loss of muscle mass are indicative of malnutrition. Extremes within anthropometric measures, for example, the emaciation of cachexia or morbid obesity, are useful indicators of disease risk or progression in a clinical setting. In children, serial measures of height and weight can provide sensitive measures of growth and development that can be used to highlight and monitor nutritional problems. The most robust anthropometric measures are challenging as they require specialist equipment. As a result, most surveys and research projects that examine large groups of people use simply determined measures such as BMI (weight in kg divided by height in metres[2]). As shown in Figure 1.7, BMI is widely used as a measure of body fatness and to classify overweight and obesity, but it is a non-specific measure that can be misinterpreted (see Sections 6.4 and 8.4.1).

1.4.2 Estimating dietary intakes

Estimation of dietary intakes, either to determine intakes of specific macro- or micronutrients or to assess intakes of particular foods, is a mainstay of human nutrition research. A range of different methods are applied, depending on the level of detail required. All approaches are highly prone to measurement error.

1.4.2.1 Indirect measures

The least accurate measures of intake are those that make indirect estimates of the quantities of foodstuffs consumed by populations. These techniques are used to follow trends in consumption between national populations or within a national population over a period of time.

Food balance sheets are widely used by the United Nations Food and Agriculture Organization (FAO) to monitor the availability of foods, and hence nutrients,

Table 1.4 Anthropometric measures used to estimate body composition and nutritional status.

Technique	Component of body composition estimated	Limitations
Body mass index (weight/height²)	Weight relative to height	Does not distinguish between lean and fat mass. Does not measure the composition of the body
Skinfold thicknesses	Fat mass	Requires skill in measurement. Makes assumptions about the even distribution of fat in the subcutaneous layer
Waist circumference or waist/hip ratio	Fat distribution	A good indicator of abdominal fat deposition. Requires set protocols for measurement
Mid-upper arm circumference	Muscle mass	Prone to measurement error. Unsuitable for some groups (e.g. adolescents) with rapidly changing fat and muscle patterns. Good indicator of acute malnutrition
Bioimpedance	Fat mass	Influenced by hydration status of subjects
Underwater weighing	Body density, fat and lean mass	Requires subjects to undergo training for an unpleasant procedure. Underestimates fat mass in muscular individuals
Isotope dilution	Body water	Influenced by fluid intake of subject. Analytically difficult and expensive
Scanning techniques (NMR, computed tomography, DXA)	Proportions and distribution of lean and fat mass	Expensive, restricted access to scanners. Use ionizing radiation so unsuitable for children and pregnant women

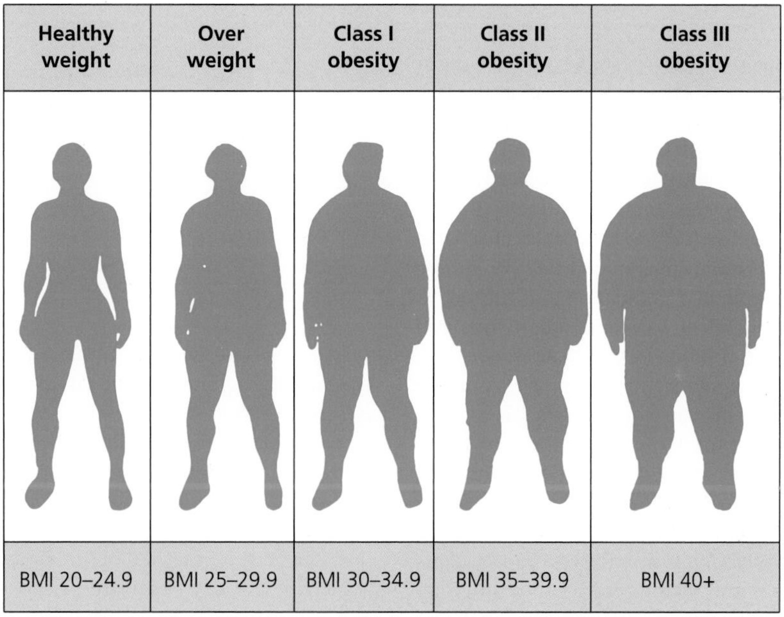

Healthy weight	Over weight	Class I obesity	Class II obesity	Class III obesity
BMI 20–24.9	BMI 25–29.9	BMI 30–34.9	BMI 35–39.9	BMI 40+

Figure 1.7 Body mass index (BMI) is commonly used to define and classify overweight and obesity.

within most nations of the world and are published on an annual basis. They allow temporal trends to be monitored easily and apply a standardized methodology on a global scale. A food balance sheet is essentially compiled from government records of the total production, imports and exports of specific foodstuffs. This allows the quantity of that foodstuff available to the population to be calculated (available food = production + imports − exports). Dividing that figure by the total number of people in the population allows the daily availability per capita to be estimated. Figure 1.8 shows data abstracted from the 2004 FAO food balance sheets, indicating how daily availability of protein from plant and animal sources varies with different regions of the world.

Food balance sheets are subject to considerable error due to assumptions that are made in their compilation. It will be assumed that the nutrient composition of a food will be the same regardless of where it is produced,

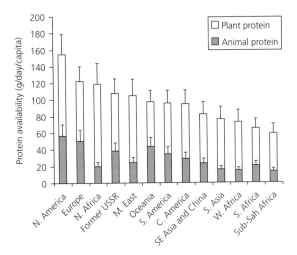

Figure 1.8 Availability of animal and plant protein by world region. Per capita availability of protein from plant and animal sources calculated from the 2004 FAO global food balance sheets.

which is clearly incorrect. For example, the selenium content of cereals from North America is considerably greater than in the same cereals from Europe as European soils are relatively impoverished in this mineral. The balance sheets also assume that all available food will be completely consumed by humans and do not allow for wastage or feeding to animals. It is also fallacious to assume that available food will be equally distributed to all people in a population and the sheets make no distinction between food available to men and women, to adults and children or to rich and poor.

Food accounts are a similar approach to estimating food availability, but instead of collecting data on a national scale, they are used to measure the food available to a household or an institution (e.g. a nursing home). By compiling an inventory of food stored at the start of a survey, monitoring food entering the setting (often measured by looking at invoices and receipts from food shopping) and taking into account any food grown in the setting, it is possible to calculate the food *available* per person over the period of the survey. As with the food balance sheet, this method does not allow accurate estimation of individual food intakes and does not allow for food wastage, but the food account can provide data on dietary patterns of families or similar groups at low cost and over an extended period of time.

1.4.2.2 Direct measures
Direct measures of nutrient intake collect data from individuals or groups of individuals and, in addition to their obvious application to clinical circumstances, are

Table 1.5 Advantages and disadvantages of dietary assessment methods.

Method	Advantages	Disadvantages
Dietary recall	Inexpensive; can be detailed; useful in clinical settings; can be repeated in the same individual; does not influence food intake	One recall seldom representative; relies on memory; intensive data entry; prone to under- and over-reporting; requires trained interviewer
Food frequency questionnaire	Can be self-administered; can use automated data entry; inexpensive for large population studies; represents usual intake over long periods of time	May not capture portion sizes; not useful for estimating absolute nutrient intake; subject must be literate; multiple foods may be covered by a single listed item; depends on memory
Food record	Does not depend on memory; data can be detailed and precise; captures intake over several days; can estimate nutrient intakes with good precision	Act of recording may alter diet; subject must be literate; intensive data entry; high burden on subject can lower response rates; prone to under- and over-reporting

well suited to research in human nutrition and epidemiology. Although more robust than the indirect estimates described earlier, all direct measures of intake are prone to bias and error and results must always be interpreted with caution. These methods may be particularly useful for studying individuals or populations in different settings and study types (Table 1.5).

1.4.2.2.1 Dietary recall methods
The dietary recall method is not only one of the best methods for examining nutrient intakes in a clinical setting, but it may also be used in research. One of the major disadvantages of the method is the need for a trained interviewer to spend a period of time with the patient or research subject to elicit detailed information on all food and drink consumed over a recent period of time (Table 1.5). An interview will explore all food and beverages consumed during that period and ask for descriptions of cooking methods, portion sizes, use of condiments and eating between meals. Most dietary recalls will be based upon intakes over the preceding

24h but in some cases may look at 48- or 72-h periods. Information obtained in this way can then be coded for detailed analysis of energy and nutrient intakes using appropriate nutritional analysis software or food tables. Dietary recall methods can generate detailed information on the types of food consumed and portion sizes. The use of photographic food atlases showing portion sizes for commonly consumed foods can enhance the quality of this quantitative information. Spending time interviewing a subject also makes it relatively easy to obtain recipes used in cooking and information about cooking techniques (e.g. use of oils in frying). Like all methods of estimating nutrient intake, the dietary recall is prone to inaccuracy due to under-reporting and over-reporting of food intake by certain groups of people. It is also dependent upon the memory of the subject and so loses accuracy when attempting to estimate habitual intakes.

1.4.2.2.2 Food record methods

Food records, or diaries, administered to subjects for completion in their own time are widely regarded as the most powerful tool for estimation of nutrient intakes. Subjects keep records for extended periods of time (usually 3–7 days) and note down all foods and beverages consumed at the time they are consumed. Portion sizes can be recorded in a number of different ways, with the subject most frequently either noting an estimated intake in simple household measures (e.g. 2 tablespoons of rice, 1 cup of sugar) or an intake estimated through comparison to a pictorial atlas of portion sizes. To improve the quality of the data, intake can be accurately determined by weighing the food on standardized scales, taking into account any wastage (a weighed food record). Frobisher and Maxwell (2003) found that in studying intakes of children aged 6–16, a food record with a photographic atlas of portion sizes gave a good level of agreement with weighed records. In some settings, it is possible for a researcher to do the weighing, thereby reducing influences upon the subject consuming the food. Inaccuracies in estimates of portion sizes are a major problem associated with food record methods, particularly with some subgroups in the population, and methods should be chosen that best serve the purpose of the dietary survey. Surveys of small groups of well-motivated people in a metabolic unit lend themselves well to weighed record methods, while in large surveys of free-living individuals, these are rarely practical.

Food records have a number of strengths compared to other methods of estimating intake. Complex data on meal patterns and eating habits can be obtained through study of food diaries, and this information can supplement estimates of nutrient intake. By obtaining records for periods of 5–7 days, the intakes of most micronutrients can be estimated with some degree of confidence (Table 1.5), in addition to energy and macronutrients. For some nutrients, it is suggested that records of 14 or more days may be required (Block, 1989). The major disadvantage of the food record approach is the reliance upon the subject to complete the record fully and accurately. Maintaining a food record is burdensome, and it is often noted that the degree of detail and hence accuracy will be greater in the first 2–3 days of a 7-day record compared to later days. The act of recording intake, especially if a weighed record is used, can change the eating behaviour of subjects and hence lead to an underestimate of habitual intakes.

Like other direct methods, the food record is prone to under-reporting and over-reporting of energy and nutrient intakes among certain subgroups in the population due to the tendency of individuals to report intakes that will reflect them in the best possible light to the researcher. Bazelmans et al. (2007) studied a group of elderly individuals, comparing self-reported intakes on a 24-h food record to estimates of likely energy intake based upon the subjects' basal metabolic rates calculated using the Schofield equation. It was found that approximately 20% of men and 25% of women significantly under-reported or over-reported their energy intakes. Subjects with a BMI under 25 kg/m² (i.e. in the ideal weight range) were most likely to over-report, while 13% of those with BMI in the overweight range and 27% of those with a BMI in the obese range were found to have under-reported their energy intake. Obese and overweight women are frequently found to under-report intakes in dietary surveys.

1.4.2.2.3 Food frequency questionnaire methods

Food frequency questionnaire methods involve the administration of food checklists to individuals, or groups of individuals, as a means of estimating their habitual intake of foods, or groups of foods. Subjects work through the checklist and, for each foodstuff, indicate their level of consumption (i.e. number of portions) on a daily, weekly or monthly basis (Figure 1.9). Semi-quantitative food frequency questionnaires also collect information on typical portion size.

Food frequency questionnaires can vary in their complexity and length. Often, a questionnaire will consist of 100–150 food items and will therefore allow for a comprehensive coverage of the dietary patterns of a subject. Some questionnaires are much shorter and may be focused upon a particular food group or the main sources of a specific type of nutrient. For example, Block and colleagues (1989) developed a questionnaire with

	Once per week	2–4 per week	5–6 per week	Daily	Once per month	Once per 3 months	Never
White bread	○	○	○	⦿	○	○	○
Brown bread	○	○	○	○	⦿	○	○
Wholemeal bread	○	⦿	○	○	○	○	○
Burger bun	⦿	○	○	○	○	○	○
Bagel	○	⦿	○	○	○	○	○
Pitta	○	○	○	○	○	⦿	○
Tortilla	⦿	○	○	○	○	○	○
Chapatti	○	○	○	○	○	○	⦿
Brioche	○	○	○	○	○	○	⦿

Figure 1.9 A food frequency questionnaire is used to estimate the habitual consumption of foodstuffs within the diet of an individual.

just 13 items in order to identify individuals who had high intakes of fat. This was used as a preliminary screening tool to select subjects for a more detailed investigation.

Food frequency questionnaires have many desirable attributes for researchers wishing to estimate intakes in large populations (Table 1.5). They are self-administered by the subject, are generally not time consuming and are unlikely to influence eating behaviours. Data entry can sometimes be automated, reducing the analytical burden for the researcher. Moreover, the food frequency questionnaire provides an estimate of habitual intake over a period of months or even years, as opposed to the snapshot obtained by looking at a food record representing just a few days. However, the food frequency questionnaire can be a weak tool when considering portion sizes and is therefore less effective for estimating micronutrient intakes than a food record. Food frequency questionnaires must also be valid for the population to be studied as the range of foods consumed will vary with age and various other social and demographic factors. For example, if attempting to survey nutrient intakes in a population with a wide ethnic diversity, the foods and food groups included on the questionnaire need to reflect that level of diversity. A questionnaire that fails to include staple foods consumed by particular ethnic groups will inevitably

underestimate their intake. For this reason, new food frequency questionnaires undergo extensive validation that includes comparing food frequency data with parallel analysis of dietary recalls and/or weighed food records in the same individuals.

1.4.3 Biomarkers of nutritional status

Biomarkers of nutritional status are measures of either the biological function of a nutrient or the nutrient itself in an individual or in samples taken from individuals. These measures can often provide the earliest indicator of a nutrient deficit as they register subnormal values ahead of any clinical symptoms. Biomarkers are therefore useful in monitoring the prevalence of nutrient deficiency, measuring the effectiveness of the treatment of deficiency and assessing preventive strategies. Given the huge difficulties of making accurate assessments of dietary intakes, as described earlier, biomarkers provide a useful means of validating dietary data and are often measured as adjuncts to dietary surveys. For example, in the UK National Diet and Nutrition Survey of preschool children (Gregory et al., 1995), measurements of circulating iron status were used to back up food record data collected on iron intakes. The doubly labelled water method (Koebnick et al., 2005) can be used to validate energy intakes estimated using dietary records or other means (Figure 1.10).

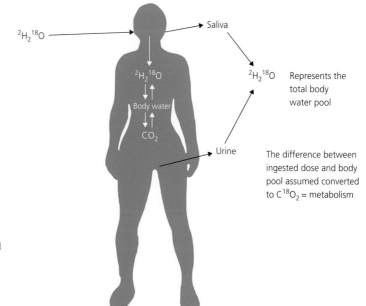

$^2H_2{}^{18}O$

Saliva

$^2H_2{}^{18}O$

Body water

CO_2

$^2H_2{}^{18}O$ Represents the total body water pool

Urine

The difference between ingested dose and body pool assumed converted to $C^{18}O_2$ = metabolism

Figure 1.10 The doubly labelled water method is a technique used to assess energy expenditure. Subjects consume water containing stable isotopes of hydrogen and oxygen. This water reaches equilibrium with the body water. Measures of the doubly labelled water in saliva and urine enable estimation of the loss of $^{18}O_2$ from body water. That loss can only occur through production of labelled carbon dioxide. Carbon dioxide production is a measure of metabolism.

Biomarkers of nutritional status are often regarded as being more objective than other indices. They include functional tests and measurements of nutrient concentration in easily obtained body fluids or other materials. The latter type of measurement can be a *static* test, which is performed on one occasion, or may be repeated at intervals to monitor change over time. The relative merits of these approaches will be discussed later in this section.

Functional tests measure biological processes that are dependent upon a specific nutrient. If that nutrient is present at suboptimal concentrations in the body, then it would be expected that the specific function would decline. The dark adaptation test is classic example of a functional test, which determines vitamin A status. The dark adaptation test measures visual acuity in dim light after exposure to a bright light that desensitizes the eye. The reformation of rhodopsin within the retina is dependent upon the generation of *cis*-retinol, and thus, the visual adaptation in the dark will be related to vitamin A status. Measurement of the excretion of xanthurenic acid is a functional test for vitamin B6 (pyridoxine) status. Xanthurenic acid is a breakdown product of tryptophan and kynurenine and is formed via pyridoxine-dependent reactions.

Non-functional measures of biomarkers typically involve direct measures of specific nutrients in simply obtained samples from individuals. These are most commonly samples of blood (plasma, serum or red cells) or urine but could include faeces, hair or, more rarely,

biopsy material from the adipose tissue or muscle. Static tests provide a snapshot of the nutrient concentration in the sample at a given point in time and could be misleading as they often provide an indicator of immediate intake rather than habitual intake. For example, plasma zinc concentrations will vary hugely from day to day, reflecting ongoing metabolic fluxes, and fall by up to 20% following a meal (King, 1990). Wherever possible, repeated tests should be taken to increase confidence in the measured biomarker, or tests should be performed in a sample that provides a stronger indicator of habitual intake. In the case of zinc, plasma measurements are of limited value as most zinc is held in functional forms within tissues and less than 1% of the total pool is in circulation. Red or white blood cell zinc concentrations could be used as a more robust biomarker, as could white cell metallothionein concentrations (metallothionein is a key zinc-binding protein). Hair zinc concentrations give a better intake of long-term status. Zinc is deposited in hair follicles slowly over time, and so using this sample source removes the influence of shorter-term fluctuations in status. Lakshmi Priya and Geetha (2011) measured zinc, selenium, magnesium, copper, lead and mercury in hair samples from children as part of a study to assess their putative role in autism. Similarly, the EURAMIC study (Kardinaal *et al.*, 1993) used measures of α-tocopherol and β-carotene in biopsies of adipose tissue to assess intakes of these vitamins. As fat-soluble vitamins are stored in this tissue, this gave an indicator of habitual intake over several weeks.

The levels of a measured biomarker are only useful in estimating nutritional status if there is a linear relationship between the measurement and intake. In addition to this, and the need to make measurements in a relevant sample, it is important to appreciate the non-dietary influences on the biomarker that could skew the interpretation of any measurement. Some measurements could be perturbed by the presence of disease or the use of medications to treat disease. For example, serum albumin concentration can be used as a marker of dietary protein intake, but is poor and non-specific. Serum albumin declines with low protein intakes and in clinical settings can provide a predictor of morbidity and mortality associated with protein–energy malnutrition. However, as described earlier in this chapter, serum albumin concentrations also fall with infection and inflammation, and in seriously ill patients, albumin could be administered as an element of any intravenous fluid infusion. Either situation would render albumin useless as a marker of nutritional status. Like any measure of nutritional status, biochemical indices can lack specificity and should ideally be used as part of a battery of tests based upon dietary assessments, biochemical measures, anthropometry and, if appropriate, clinical assessment.

1.4.4 Clinical examination

Performing a thorough physical examination and obtaining a detailed patient history are an effective method of determining symptoms associated with malnutrition in individuals. This approach can be most useful when dealing with children, where the paucity of nutrient stores can mean that clinical symptoms develop very quickly, as opposed to in adults where the symptoms are generally a sign of chronic malnutrition. Obtaining a patient history can highlight key points that are missed when assessing dietary intake or using anthropometric measures. Reported loss of appetite, loss of blood, occurrence of diarrhoea, steatorrhoea or nausea and vomiting may all be indicators of potential causes of malnutrition and should trigger further investigation. Physical examination can assess the degree of emaciation of a potentially malnourished individual. Careful assessment of the hair, skin, nails, eyes, lips, tongue and mouth can also highlight specific nutrient deficiencies. Bleaching of the hair is indicative of protein malnutrition, while cracking of the lips can suggest deficiency of B vitamins such as riboflavin. Pallor of the skin and spooning of the nails are clinical signs of iron deficiency. Evidence of rough spots on the conjunctiva of the eye will accompany early stages of vitamin A deficiency.

1.5 Nutritional epidemiology: Understanding diet–disease relationships

Epidemiology is the branch of medical science that studies the causes of health and disease in populations rather than in individuals. At the simplest level, epidemiology can be used to examine geographical and temporal trends in disease to determine initial clues to the causes of disease and then use more sophisticated techniques to examine those possible causes. Nutritional epidemiology focuses on nutrition and nutrition-related factors as both causal and preventative factors in disease. Understanding nutritional epidemiology is important as the findings from such work are used as the main evidence base to develop public health strategies, health education advice and government policy on nutrition. For example, international policies to combat iodine deficiency through USI would not be possible without robust epidemiology to show that the strategy would be both effective and safe.

Nutritional epidemiology studies focus on two key measurements: the exposure and the outcome. Exposure refers to a nutrition-related factor that may be related to disease. This could be a marker of body composition (e.g. BMI), a specific nutrient (e.g. folic acid), a dietary pattern (e.g. vegetarianism) or a food-related behaviour (e.g. alcohol consumption). The outcome is the disease of interest, which can be measured as confirmed diagnosis of ill health (morbidity), as risk factors for disease (e.g. raised blood pressure as a risk factor for heart disease) or as death from a disease (mortality).

1.5.1 Cause and effect

Establishing which foods and nutrients may be causally related to disease processes is a critical aim for nutritional epidemiology. Without knowledge of how nutrients and nutrition-related factors influence disease processes, it is impossible to design effective interventions that prevent disease or nutrition-based treatments for established disease. It can be relatively simple to identify associations or correlations between factors but less easy to determine which are biologically or clinically meaningful. It is always important to appreciate that correlation does not indicate causal relationship. For example, as shown in Figure 1.11, we might look for evidence that the amount of meat in the diet is related to risk of developing oesophageal cancer and in a simple sense could correlate the meat intakes of different populations with the occurrence of oesophageal cancer in those populations. One approach might be to find populations with low rates of cancer and populations with high rates of cancer and compare their meat

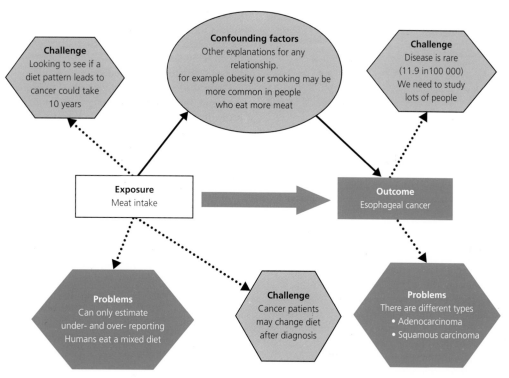

Figure 1.11 Measuring the relationship between a nutritional exposure and a disease outcome is complex, necessitating careful epidemiological designs. These designs must consider appropriate sampling in terms of size of population, length of study, measurement of diet and measurement of disease outcome.

intakes. The correlation we observe may be genuine or may be spurious, and much more information needs to be considered in designing a robust study to evaluate the relationship (e.g. the size of the sample needed, the method used to collect data on meat intake and the duration of the study) and interpreting the data obtained (considering alternative reasons for the correlation such as obesity or smoking habits).

1.5.2 Bias and confounding

Figure 1.11 shows the complexity of establishing a robust study for investigating a diet–disease relationship. Components of that figure such as sample size and who to sample, duration of study and consideration of the accuracy of measurement are all representatives of a phenomenon called bias, which can limit the usefulness of epidemiological studies. Studies which fail to control different types of bias, either at the point where the study is designed and initiated or during the analysis of the data, may draw spurious conclusions and be of no value in identifying diet–disease relationships.

Different types of bias may be present within a study, and bias is generally classified as 'selection bias',

'measurement bias' and 'confounding bias'. Selection bias refers to factors that relate to how the people involved in the study were recruited. It is rarely possible to assess diet and disease in a whole population, and so inevitably a smaller sample has to be assessed. We may, for example, be interested in the links between cancer and meat intake across the whole of the United Kingdom but cannot possibly examine all 60 million people in the population. Instead, a study is likely to consider a few thousand individuals to represent that whole population. Selection bias occurs when there is a difference in the relationship between the exposure (diet) and outcome (disease) between the people who took part in the study and those who did not. For example, there may be no relationship between meat and oesophageal cancer in young adults, but a strong relationship could be present in older adults. To avoid such bias, a wide age range should be sampled. Measurement bias (also called information bias) occurs when there are errors in the measurement of exposure or outcome that lead to misclassification of individuals. For example, if the method for measuring meat intake is inaccurate, individuals could be classed as high consumers when really they are

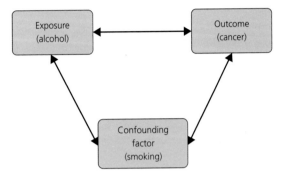

Figure 1.12 A confounding factor is an additional factor that may explain the relationship between an exposure and an outcome. The confounding factor is related to both outcome and exposure, but does not lie on the causal pathway between the two.

not. Measurement bias is a major problem for nutrition–disease studies as the methods for considering food intake are prone to misreporting by study participants (either deliberate or due to poor memory (specifically termed recall bias)) or differences in the measurement between interviewers. In the case of the meat–oesophageal cancer relationship (Figure 1.11), for example, considering oesophageal cancer as a single outcome as opposed to two different diseases would also lead to measurement bias. Adenocarcinoma may have a different relationship to meat intake than squamous cell carcinoma.

Confounding bias is another form of bias and describes the situation where a third factor explains the relationship between exposure and outcome. To be truly considered as a confounding factor, the additional factor must be related to both exposure and outcome but not lie on the causal pathway between the two. The classic example of confounding is shown in Figure 1.12 where the relationship between alcohol and cancer may be explained by the fact that tobacco smoking causes cancer and people who consume high amounts of alcohol are also more likely to be heavy smokers. Some epidemiological studies are able to limit confounding bias at the design stage (see the following text), but usually confounding is adjusted for when analysing data.

1.5.3 Quantifying the relationship between diet and disease

As will be outlined in the following text, there are a variety of approaches used in nutritional epidemiology to explore the relationships between diet and disease. Each of these approaches yields information which quantifies the impact of specific nutrition-related factors (dietary patterns, specific nutrient intakes, obesity)

upon disease outcomes (disease diagnosis, death) or risk factors for disease (blood pressure, elevated circulating biomarkers). Understanding the nature of these measured outcomes is critical for interpretation of the findings of epidemiological studies.

Some studies will yield relatively simple measures of outcome. For example, a study which measures blood pressure or elevated cholesterol concentrations in a group of people exposed to a factor and a group who are not will make a straightforward measure of whether the markers differ in the two groups of people. Considering differences in diagnosis or death, however, involves measures of 'risk' which are less familiar to those new to the subject.

One approach to quantifying risk is to provide data on prevalence or incidence rates (Table 1.6). These are essentially measures of the likelihood that individuals in a population will develop a disease (morbidity) or die from a disease (mortality), and an epidemiological study might, for example, compare the prevalence of cancer in meat eaters compared to non-meat eaters. Prevalence and incidence have different meanings. Prevalence is the measure of how likely an individual is to have a particular disease and is calculated as the number of cases in a population divided by the number of people in the population. So if in the United Kingdom there are 9600 cases of oesophageal cancer, then the prevalence is 9600 divided by 60 000 000, or 0.00016. This would be simplified to 16 per 100 000 population. Incidence describes the probability of a person being diagnosed with a disease during a given period of time, or in effect the number of newly diagnosed cases. For example, if over the course of 1 year there are 2500 new cases of oesophageal cancer diagnosed in the United Kingdom, the incidence would be 2500 divided by 60 000 000, or 0.000042. This simplifies to 4.2 new cases per 100 000 people per year.

A more commonly used approach to express the degree of risk associated with a nutrition-related factor is represented by odds ratios, relative risk and hazard ratios (Table 1.6). These are all variations on the same theme whereby risk is expressed as the likelihood in one group (e.g. meat eaters) relative to a reference group (e.g. non-meat eaters). This is generally easy to understand as an odds ratio of 10, indicating that people exposed to a particular factor are 10 times more likely to experience a disease event. An odds ratio of 0.2 means that people exposed to a particular factors are 80% $(1-0.2=0.8\times100=80\%)$ less likely to experience a disease event. However, all calculated ratios are estimates and as shown in Figure 1.13 must be interpreted with reference to the confidence intervals that are calculated. These give a measure of how reliable those estimates

Table 1.6 Definitions of key terms in epidemiology.

Term	Definition
Relative risk	An indicator of the risk of an event (e.g. disease) occurring in one group compared to another. It is the ratio of the probability* of an event occurring in an exposed group and the probability of an event occurring in a control group
Odds ratio	An indicator of the risk of an event (e.g. disease) occurring in one group compared to another. It is the ratio of the odds† of an event occurring in an exposed group and the odds of an event occurring in a control group
Hazard ratio	An indicator of the risk of an event (e.g. death) occurring in one group compared to another. It is calculated from the rates at which events occur over a period of time in the two groups
Incidence rate	Incidence measures the risk of developing a disease within a given measure of time (e.g. the number of new cases of cancer per year)
Prevalence rate	Prevalence measures the proportion of people within a population who have a particular disease. It is usually expressed as the number of affected people for a given population size (e.g. the number of cancer cases per 100 000 population)

*Probability is a measure of how likely an event is and is calculated as number of adverse outcome/total number of outcomes. It is usually expressed as a value from 0 to 1.
†Odds are also measures of how likely an event is but are calculated as probability of an event/1 minus the probability.

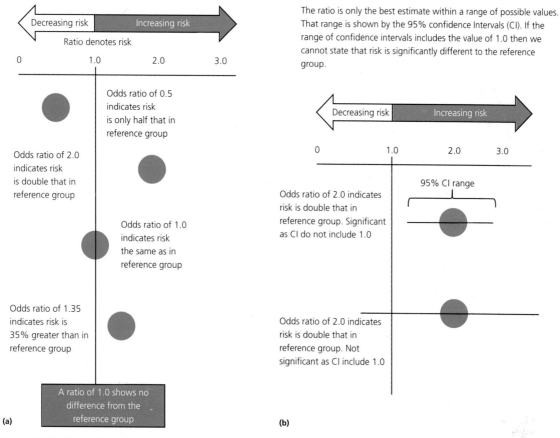

Figure 1.13 Understanding odds ratios. **a**) Odds ratio (OR) is a descriptor of the risk of event compared to a reference group. For the reference, the OR is set at 1.0. If OR is less than 1.0, that indicates decreased risk. If more than 1.0, it indicates increased risk. **b**) OR is an estimate of risk and the quality of that estimate will depend upon methodological factors and biological variation. The range of possible values for OR is represented by 95% confidence intervals. These are used to distinguish between OR estimates that show a significant relationship between exposure and risk and those which do not.

are. There are important differences between odds ratios, hazard ratios and relative risk ratios, and they are all calculated in different ways (Table 1.6). As a result, they are not interchangeable terms and they are often used with specific study types. Odds ratios are calculated in most case–control studies, while relative risk is more often used in much larger cohort studies or with randomized controlled trials (RCTs).

1.5.4 Study designs in nutritional epidemiology

There are a number of different approaches that can be taken to explore diet–disease relationships in human populations, and these vary in their capacity to determine causality of relationships (Table 1.7). Figure 1.14 shows a hierarchy of research designs that has the study designs with the lowest methodological quality (animal studies and *in vitro* studies, ecological studies) at the bottom and the highest methodological quality (RCTs and meta-analyses) at the top. Data from all studies needs to be interpreted with this hierarchy in mind. Work performed in animals must always be viewed through the lens of species differences between animals and humans. Studies of large populations of free-living individuals (cohort studies) will inevitably be subject to unaccounted-for confounding factors and other bias, which can only be eliminated though an RCT.

Table 1.7 Study designs in nutritional epidemiology.

Study design	Approach taken
Ecological study	Nutritional exposures and disease outcomes are considered in populations that are grouped by geographical area or time period. Only population averages and not individual data are analysed
Cross-sectional study	A descriptive study which measures nutritional exposure and disease outcome in a single population at a specific point in time
Case–control study	A study which compares nutritional exposures in a population with a specific disease to a similar reference population without disease
Cohort study	An observational study which follows a population over a period of time. This allows nutritional exposure measured at the beginning (baseline) to be related to disease that develops over the course of the study. Follow-up from baseline may be over many years
Randomized controlled trial	An experimental study in which a randomly selected group of people are administered nutrients, foodstuffs or other interventions focused on nutrition and are compared to a matched control group over a period of follow-up

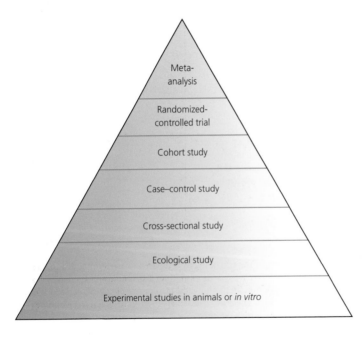

Figure 1.14 Hierarchy of evidence in nutrition–disease studies. Experiments in animals or *in vitro* have the lowest methodological quality, while randomized controlled trials and meta-analyses are of highest quality.

1.5.4.1 Ecological studies

An ecological study is an observational study which seeks to compare the general characteristics of whole populations in order to determine the factors which explain variation in disease risk between those populations (Table 1.7). For example, there may be gross differences in coronary heart disease death among the countries of Europe, and we may wish to determine whether those differences arise due to variation in diet. Alternatively, we may wish to determine why rates of coronary heart disease death in one location in 2012 are much lower than in 1992. To approach these questions, data about outcome will generally be extracted from government or international databases, and data about exposure will be collected from national diet and nutrition surveys or international sources such as the FAO food balance sheets. Importantly, this is summary data about large groups of people rather than data that has been collected on individuals (Figure 1.15). This data is then used to examine simple correlations between exposures and outcomes.

Ecological studies are ideal for examining new ideas and developing hypotheses that can be explored using approaches with greater methodological quality and

capacity for determining causality. They have many weaknesses, however, not least the fact that the findings generated from group data are not necessarily applicable to individuals in a population (this is termed the ecological fallacy). The way in which data is collected leads to numerous problems, for example, the data on dietary exposure may have been collected in different ways in different countries (heterogeneity of exposure) and may not be truly comparable. The exposure and outcome may not have even been determined in exactly the same populations (e.g. data on diet in 1992 was collected in England, Wales and Scotland, but data on heart disease was collected in the whole United Kingdom – England, Wales, Northern Ireland and Scotland). Ecological studies are also highly prone to uncontrollable confounding factors.

1.5.4.2 Cross-sectional studies

A cross-sectional study is an observational study in which the exposure and outcome are measured simultaneously in a group of individuals (Figure 1.15). The cross-sectional study will then attempt to relate disease outcomes to current dietary factors (Table 1.7). This can be a quick and inexpensive approach to examine simple

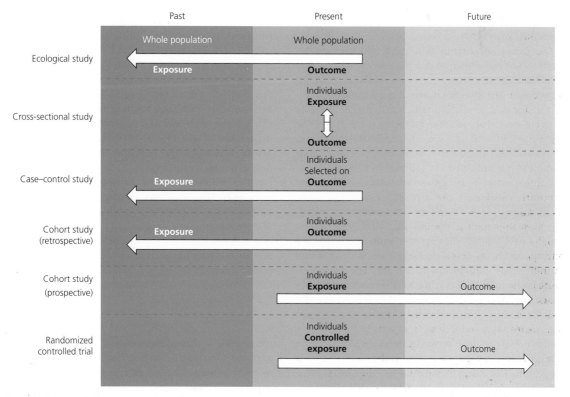

Figure 1.15 Research designs in epidemiology.

diet–disease relationships. For example, it could very quickly show a relationship between BMI and energy intake. However, it is not possible to state with any certainty whether a relationship is causal. Is high energy intake a cause of high BMI, or do people of high BMI consume more energy to meet a greater demand? Another problem of the cross-sectional study is that the individuals who have a disease may change their behaviour because of the disease and hence mask the relationship. Subjects with high blood pressure, for example, may be advised by their doctors to reduce salt intake, thereby hiding a simple relationship between salt and blood pressure.

1.5.4.3 Case–control studies

Case–control studies are observational studies which deliberately sample a group of people who are confirmed to have a disease of interest (cases) for comparison with a group of people without the disease (controls; Table 1.7). The exposure of the two groups to dietary factors in the past will then be compared to see if risk of disease can be related to those factors (Figure 1.15). For example, a group of people with high blood pressure can be compared to a group with normal blood pressure by considering salt intakes over the preceding 10 years. This approach could address the question of whether long-term, habitual salt intake is a causal factor in development of high blood pressure.

The case–control study is a quick and inexpensive approach to epidemiology as a relatively small number of subjects are required. This is because the selection of people with the disease ensures a good representation of the diseased population which may not be possible with a cohort study (see the following text). When the disease of interest is rare, the case–control design becomes especially powerful as it draws together a population that is unlikely to be sampled in a cohort study. The case–control study can also consider more than one exposure variable in the diet. There are significant problems with case–control designs however, of which the most important is the fact that while outcome is usually well defined, the exposure must be established retrospectively. As described earlier, assessment of diet in individuals is problematic, and this becomes even more prone to recall bias when looking back over many years. The other major problem is the recruitment of a suitable control group. Matching closely to the cases (e.g. similar ages, same sex) is important for reducing confounding bias. The control group should also come from the same geographical area as the cases so that it represents the same population as the cases were recruited from. Often, they are patients with other conditions who are recruited from the same clinics and hospitals as the cases. Good studies will carefully examine the health of the controls to ensure that they do not have the disease of interest (undiagnosed cases). Poor selection of controls can greatly undermine the quality of a case–control study.

1.5.4.4 Cohort studies

Cohort studies are also referred to as longitudinal studies as they seek to study a large group of people over a period of time (Figure 1.15). They identify exposures in a population and then by following the cohort over time identify outcomes as they occur and compare the incidence of disease in exposed individuals with unexposed individuals (Table 1.7). The Framingham Heart Study, for example, recruited 5209 men and women aged 30–62 in the town of Framingham, Massachusetts, in 1948. These subjects have been examined every 2 years since the inception of the study, allowing determination of the major cardiovascular risk factors that predict heart disease morbidity and mortality (blood pressure, blood cholesterol, obesity, diabetes, physical inactivity).

Cohort studies may report findings from *prospective* cohorts or *retrospective* cohorts. A prospective cohort is generally recruited for a specific purpose and collects baseline data and conducts follow-up measurements at intervals over several years before reporting final outcomes. A retrospective cohort will generally involve collecting disease outcome data in a large group of people and then tracing back events by collecting historical records that provide the exposure data. For example, a prospective cohort to examine the relationship between diet and cancer would recruit a population, characterize their diet and follow for a period to see if occurrence of cancer was related to diet many years before. A retrospective cohort would look at a population of people, including people with and without cancer, and look back to see if the diets of subjects from 10 to 20 years earlier differed among cancer sufferers and those without cancer. Retrospective cohorts are generally smaller and less expensive to study than prospective cohorts but are more prone to confounding bias due to the passing of time and incomplete historical record-keeping.

1.5.4.5 RCTs

RCTs are generally regarded as the gold-standard method for an epidemiological study (Table 1.7). RCTs are essentially clinical experiments in which individuals are randomly assigned to be a control (no treatment) or to receive some form of intervention as a controlled exposure (Figure 1.15). In nutritional epidemiology, that intervention will generally be the administration of a supplemental nutrient (e.g. antioxidant, essential fatty acid) or a behavioural intervention related to food intake or weight control (e.g. increased physical activity, adoption of a meat-free diet).

The nature of the RCT design means that it can provide strong evidence of cause and effect. If control and intervention groups are carefully matched for key characteristics, there will generally be no issue of confounding, and as the experimenters have control over the exposure, there are few issues of bias in the measurement of that exposure. Problems can arise due to non-compliance with the protocol. Participants may, for example, not take supplements as directed. RCTs in nutrition are, however, often less effective than similar studies where the treatments are drugs (clinical trials). This is because often the diet–disease relationships can be quite weak and take years to develop. It is generally not feasible to carry out a supplementation trial over many years due to expense, because the subjects may become disaffected and drop out (e.g. the consumption of fish oil capsules causes bad breath and so cannot be tolerated for more than a few months) and because the nature of the intervention may become apparent to the control group prompting them to change their diet and behaviour in a way that detracts from the analysis (e.g. although not allocated to receive a folate supplement, the controls may consume more natural sources in the belief it will be healthier). While drug trials can be easily blinded so that the participants and researchers are not aware of allocation to control or test groups, this is sometimes not possible within a nutrition trial (e.g. exercise intervention cannot be disguised as something else). Thus, the intervention can introduce behavioural changes among participants, which can distort study findings.

1.5.4.6 Systematic review and meta-analysis

Systematic review is an approach to research that makes use of existing evidence to address a specific research question. In the same way as a laboratory experiment, clinical trial or single epidemiological study, the systematic review will use rigorous methodology to ensure that the quality of the finished review is reliable and robust. Systematic reviews synthesize the findings of all available research on a particular topic in an unbiased manner and produce an impartial summary of the findings, which fully considers flaws and gaps in the evidence base. This is an extremely powerful tool for evaluating the balance of evidence, particularly in areas where there is apparent controversy and uncertainty. The use of explicit, systematic methods in reviews limits bias (systematic errors) and reduces chance effects. This provides more reliable results upon which to draw conclusions, as these can be based on the totality of the available

evidence rather than the elements that suit the bias of a narrative review. Systematic reviews use modern electronic database searches to access all published works related to a research question. These works and any material obtained from other sources (e.g. direct communication with experts in the field to obtain unpublished material) comprise the data that is subsequently analysed.

Systematic reviews are often combined with the analytical technique called meta-analysis. Meta-analysis enables researchers to exploit greater statistical power by effectively combining the results of several studies to generate a larger and robust sample. This enables inconsistency between studies to be both quantified and overcome and more precise measures of risk to be calculated. An example of the power of meta-analysis to resolve contentious issues is shown in Research Highlight 1.3. Other chapters of this book will make frequent reference to meta-analysis.

The 2007 World Cancer Research Fund Expert Report detailed a systematic review of the evidence on salt and stomach cancer, which included data from 3 cohort studies, 21 case–control studies and 12 ecological studies. This systematic review was able to generate a meta-analysis that included data from two of the cohorts and

Research Highlight 1.3 The power of meta-analysis.

> For many years, there has been a concern about the use of salt as a preservative and flavouring for foods. High consumption of salted foods and the addition of salt to food at table are well known to have an adverse impact upon blood pressure, but there is also interest in the relationship between salt and stomach cancer as populations where salt-pickling and preserving is a cornerstone of the preparation of staple foods have been noted to have high prevalence of this disease.
>
> The literature on salt and stomach cancer is, however, highly conflicting. The cohort study of Tsugane et al. (2004) found that there was a significantly increased risk of cancer with high salt consumption, but that this relationship was only seen in men and not women. Other cohort studies examined the relationship and found that there was no significant association between cancer risk and salt intake (Van den Brandt et al., 2003). Case–control studies offer a wide range of data with some studies confirming the negative association between salt and cancer (Nazario et al., 1993), some finding no association (Setiawan et al., 2000) and at least one study finding that a high salt intake decreased risk of stomach cancer (Muñoz et al., 2001). With this range of conflicting evidence, a systematic review of the literature is the only realistic way of resolving the question and generating a clear picture of the nature of the relationship between salt and cancer.

nine of the case–control studies (WCRF, 2007). Using the combined data sets, the expert group found that there were a small but significant relationship apparent in the cohort studies (relative risk 1.08, 95% CI 1.00–1.17) and a close to significant relationship apparent in the case–control studies (relative risk 1.01, 95% CI 0.99–1.04). On this basis, the reviewers were able to conclude that there is a probable causal relationship between high salt intake and stomach cancer. Without a robust, unbiased review process and well-conducted meta-analysis, this conclusion would have been impossible to reach.

1.6 Dietary reference values

Dietary reference values (DRVs) are standards that are set by the health departments of governments in a number of countries around the world. DRVs are guidelines that can be used to define the composition of diets that will maintain good health. There are many complex systems of DRVs used in different countries. These vary according to national health priorities and policies; predominant health status, socio-economic status, body mass and rates of growth; and local factors, for example, the composition of foods or other lifestyle influences, that determine the absorption and hence bioavailability of nutrients (Pavlovic *et al.*, 2007).

DRVs are used in a variety of different ways. While some systems, such as those developed for the United Kingdom, are generally intended to be used only with populations or subgroups within populations, others (e.g. the US Dietary Reference Intakes) are widely used in providing dietary guidance for individuals. On a population level, the DRVs are useful yardsticks with which to assess the adequacy of the diet of a population and hence protect individuals within that population against the adverse consequences of either deficiency or excess. By using DRVs as standard measures against which dietary survey data can be compared, it is possible to estimate the prevalence of risk of deficiency for specific nutrients within a population.

In some countries, there are regular surveys of national dietary patterns among age- and gender-specific groups, for example, the UK National Diet and Nutrition Surveys (Bates *et al.*, 2014) or the US National Health and Nutrition Examination Surveys (Centers for Disease Control, 2014). Findings from such surveys are compared to the DRVs in order to highlight potential nutrient deficiencies. In other countries, food supply data at the national level, such as the food balance sheets collected by the FAO, can be used to crudely estimate the average

per capita availability of energy and the macronutrients and compared to international standards. Although such data are prone to error, as described earlier, they can be used for tracking trends in the food supply and determining availability of micronutrient-rich foods. By comparison of such data with DRVs, it is possible to uncover evidence of gross inadequacies in the quality of the diet across whole populations (but not subgroups such as children or the elderly). Standards for nutrient provision based upon DRVs can also be used in the planning of food supplies to regions (e.g. in humanitarian aid) or in menu planning for caterers in hospitals, schools or other institutional settings. Many of the food labelling schemes used in supermarkets are based upon published DRVs for specific nutrients.

1.6.1 The UK DRV system

In 1979, the United Kingdom set a series of DRVs termed the recommended daily amounts (RDAs). In 1991, a new series of DRVs were published to replace these RDA values, as they were considered to be prone to misunderstanding and misuse. The term 'recommended' wrongly suggests a level of intake that an individual must consume on a daily basis in order to avoid adverse consequences. The new system of DRVs produced by the Committee on Medical Aspects of Food Policy (COMA) (DoH, 1991) therefore dropped the word recommended and was developed to indicate different levels of intake that would be suitable for healthy populations, broken down by age and gender.

In setting the DRVs, the COMA reviewed research for each macro- and micronutrient in order to determine the levels of intake that are necessary to maintain normal health and physiological function. In considering the available evidence, the key issues to be explored for each nutrient were as follows: (1) What level of intake is necessary to maintain circulating or tissue concentrations within normal ranges? (2) What level of intake is necessary to avoid clinical deficiency in individuals or in populations? (3) What level of intake has been established as being effective in treating clinical deficiency? (4) What level of intake has been shown to maintain normality in a biomarker of adequacy?

As shown in Figure 1.16, the relationship between nutrient intake and disease risk is not linear. At low levels of intake, the probability of adverse consequences (deficiency disease, loss of physiological function) is elevated. With rising intakes, the probability of such consequences declines to zero as intakes provide the requirements of most of the individuals in a population. At higher intakes, the probability of adverse consequences associated with overnutrition begins to rise. In

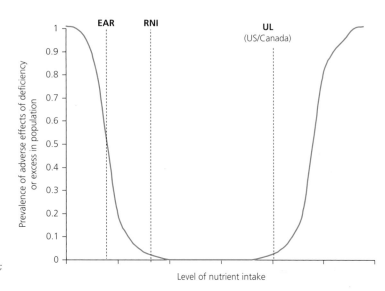

Figure 1.16 The association between risk of nutrition-related risk and level of nutrient intake. EAR, estimated average requirement; RNI, reference nutrient intake; UL, tolerable upper limit.

developing a set of DRVs appropriate for a population like the United Kingdom, in which the economic wealth of the population makes overnutrition more likely than undernutrition, this continuum between risk and intake must be recognized.

In common with the United States and other countries (see the following text), the UK DRVs were developed to map onto the expected distribution of nutrient requirements in a population. As shown in Figure 1.17, this would usually be expected to follow a normal distribution, which actually relates to the left-hand side of the distribution of risk plotted against intake (Figure 1.17). In this context, the mean value (midpoint) in a normal distribution would represent a level of nutrient intake at which the requirements of 50% of the people in a population would be met. Within the UK DRV system, this point is termed the estimated average requirement (EAR). When a population is consuming a nutrient at a level close to the EAR, it can be assumed that for 50% of people, this will be sufficient, but that for up to 50%, nutritional status would be compromised.

The other DRVs are set at points that are two standard deviations either side of the mean. The reference nutrient intake (RNI) is the upper value and within the normal distribution would represent a level of intake that should meet the requirements of 97.5% of the population. When a population is consuming a nutrient at a level close to the RNI, it can be assumed that for most individuals, this intake will be sufficient or will exceed true requirements, but that for the 2.5% of individuals with extremely high requirements, nutritional status would be compromised. The lower reference nutrient intake (LRNI) lies at the lower end of the normal distribution and represents a

level of intake that would meet the requirements of just 2.5% of the population. If a population was consuming a nutrient at a level close to the LRNI, it could be assumed that for most individuals, this will be insufficient and that deficiency disease would be rife.

For some nutrients (e.g. pantothenic acid, biotin and molybdenum), the COMA had insufficient data to be able to derive estimates of requirements but recognized the biological importance of these compounds in the diet. In the absence of extensive information, the safe intake was set. This is an upper level (UL) of intake set at a point likely to prevent deficiency and avoid toxicity. Safe intakes are of greatest importance to vulnerable groups in the population such as infants and children (DoH, 1991).

The DRVs are published as a comprehensive series of tables (DoH, 1999), which, for most nutrients, provide reference values for males and females separately and for different age groups (typically 0–12 months, 1–3 years, 4–6 years, 7–10 years, 11–14 years, 15–18 years, 19–50 years and 50+ years). To reflect increased demands for nutrients during pregnancy and lactation, some tables show additional increments of intake for pregnant and breastfeeding women. For micronutrients and trace elements, published values include all three terms (LRNI, EAR and RNI). With respect to protein, only EAR and RNI values were determined. Given that excess energy consumption is a driver of obesity and related disorders, it is undesirable to set reference values at an upper point such as the RNI, as a population that consumed energy at that level would be expected to have a high prevalence of related adverse effects such as obesity. DRV tables for energy therefore include only

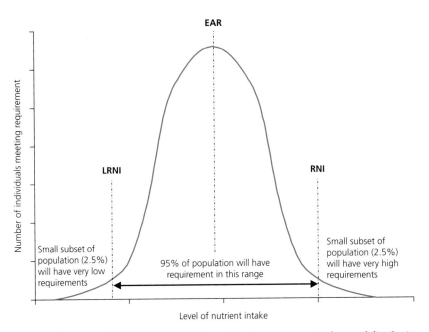

Figure 1.17 The normal distribution as a basis for DRVs. UK DRVs are based upon an assumed normal distribution of individuals' nutrient requirements and level of nutrient intake. The estimated average requirement (EAR) is set at the centre (mean) of the distribution. The lower reference nutrient intake (LRNI) and reference nutrient intake (RNI) values are placed two standard deviations below and above the mean, respectively. The nutrient requirements of all but 5% of the population should therefore be met by levels of intake between these two values.

the EAR value and include modifiers to allow for levels of physical activity.

Humans have a requirement for essential fatty acids, and children can develop clinical deficiency of linoleic acid. There are DRVs that indicate minimum intakes of essential fatty acids, but as low intakes of the majority of lipids are not associated with adverse health effects, the three main DRV terms are not applied to fats and carbohydrates. Instead, the COMA set population average guidelines for consumption of saturated, monounsaturated and polyunsaturated fats based on percentage of dietary energy provided by those sources. These guidelines represent maximum intakes in the light of the established risk of cardiovascular disease with high-fat intakes (see Chapter 8, Guidelines for healthy nutrition). This element of the UK DRV system differs from other components as it firmly indicates guidelines for individuals to follow rather than appropriate ranges for healthy populations (Whitehead, 1992). In the same way, the COMA set guidance values for sugars and complex carbohydrates based on percentages of dietary energy intake. Population averages are designed to encourage lower intakes of non-milk extrinsic (free) sugars and fats, while increasing intakes of starch and non-starch polysaccharides. Population averages for

carbohydrate are likely to be revised following the 2014 report of the UK Scientific Advisory Committee on Nutrition (SACN, 2014) which proposed reductions in guidelines for free sugars (no more than 5% of dietary energy per day) and an increase for dietary fibre (25 g/day for adults).

In the United Kingdom, the DRVs are not intended to be guidelines for individuals. It is generally considered a fruitless activity to make estimates of nutrient intakes for individuals, given problems with obtaining accurate data on food intake and because it is impossible to estimate what the true requirements for any individual are likely to be. In making assessments of dietary intakes of groups within a population, the RNI is considered to be the most important benchmark for comparison. The nearer the average intake of a group within a survey is to the RNI, the less likely it is that any individual within that group will have an inadequate intake. However, the LRNI value provides a better indicator of the likely risk of widespread deficiency, whether clinical or subclinical. The nearer the average intake of the group is to the LRNI, the greater is the probability that some individuals within that group are not consuming that nutrient at a level adequate to meet their requirements.

An example of the DRVs in use is provided by the study of Cowin and colleagues (2000). This group assessed the nutrient intakes of 1026 18-month-old infants living in the southwest of England using a 3-day unweighed dietary record. By comparing recorded intakes with the RNI values for micronutrients, the survey concluded that intakes of most nutrients were adequate in this population group. However, for iron and vitamin D, it was noted that mean intakes were considerably below the RNI, suggesting that these nutrients could be a cause for concern in this population group. Indeed, for iron, where the LRNI is 3.7 mg/day for infants, it was noteworthy that the 2.5% of the population with the lowest intakes (i.e. the group who might be expected to be meeting their requirements despite low intake) consumed only 2.4 (girls) to 2.7 (boys) mg/day, figures well below the LRNI. Data of this kind can be the start point for further studies that identify the causes of deficiency and for formulating appropriate interventions and dietary recommendations (Cowin *et al.*, 2001).

Although not intended for use with individuals, the DRVs could still be used in a clinical setting. When working with healthy individuals, assessments of dietary intakes that indicate intakes below or close to the LRNI could indicate a dietary problem and might be a stimulus for a more in-depth assessment of biochemical or clinical indicators of nutritional status. In planning a diet for an individual, the delivery of nutrients at the level of the RNI would be a basic priority to ensure optimal health.

1.6.2 DRVs in other countries

The UK system described earlier is just one example of DRVs defined with the purpose of guiding the provision of healthy nutrition on a population-wide scale. Many other countries use similar systems that have also been derived to map against the normal distribution of nutrient intakes against provision of nutrient demands. This approach is generally applicable for Westernized countries where the nutrition-related health concerns are usually focused on the consequences of nutrient excess rather than nutrient deficiency. Table 1.8 summarizes the dietary reference terms used in North America, Australia and New Zealand.

Among the countries of the European Union (EU), there is considerable variation in the terminology used to describe DRVs and in the precise nature of recommendations made for particular population groups, most particularly children. There are suggestions that the European countries should harmonize their DRV systems (Pavlovic *et al.*, 2007) and that in the course of generating a common system, a further

Table 1.8 Definitions of dietary reference value terms used in the United Kingdom, North America and Oceania.

Region	Dietary reference terms	Definition
United Kingdom	LRNI	*Lower reference nutrient intake*
	RNI	*Reference nutrient intake*
	EAR	*Estimated average requirement*
	Safe intake	
United States/Canada	EAR	*Estimated average requirement*
	RDA	*Recommended daily allowance*
	AI	*Adequate intake*
	UL	*Tolerable upper limit*
Australia/NZ	EAR	*Estimated average requirement*
	RDI	*Recommended daily intake*
	AI	*Adequate intake*
	EER	*Estimated energy requirement*
	UL	*Upper level of intake*

review of the evidence could be conducted to determine whether regional variation reflecting health status and other local issues is necessary or desirable. The EU Scientific Committee on Food defined three levels of DRVs: average requirement, population reference intake and lowest threshold intake. In general intent, these terms map against the UK EAR, RNI and LRNI values. In 2010, the European Food Safety Authority set some simple references for nutrient intakes, which included references for consumption of total carbohydrates, sugars, fibre, fats and water (EFSA, 2010).

As in the United Kingdom, the countries of North America reviewed their existing reference values, originally set in 1941, and replaced them with a new comprehensive format in the early 1990s (Kennedy and Meyers, 2005). In Canada and the United States, the EAR and RDA terms are exact equivalents of the UK EAR and RNI terms but are used in a different manner to that seen in the United Kingdom. EAR is a term that would be used to estimate the prevalence of inadequate intakes in a population, but RDA is a term specifically intended for use with individuals. A habitual intake below this level would be associated with increased risk of dietary inadequacy. In population surveys, however, comparing mean intakes to the RDA would tend to overestimate the likely prevalence of deficiency, as it is a figure set at a level where the requirements of 97.5% of the population are being met. This means that a significant proportion of the population is likely to be exceeding requirement (Kennedy and Meyers, 2005). For example, if the RDA for iron intake in children is 11.2 mg/day and the mean intake for a population is found to be 8.4 mg/day, it should not be assumed that deficiency will have a high prevalence. The majority of children in the population may be consuming well below the RDA value and still be achieving requirement. This could also be seen as a problem with the UK RNI. The tolerable UL term is defined as the highest average daily nutrient intake level that is unlikely to result in adverse health effects for almost all individuals in a population. Effectively, individuals could use this as a guide to limit their intake, and at the population level, it provides a benchmark against which estimates can be made of the likelihood of problems related to overnutrition. The AI term is similar to the UK safe intake in that it is used only where there is insufficient data to determine the EAR for a particular nutrient.

In Australia and New Zealand, the system of DRVs is broadly similar to that used in North America, except a fifth term (EER) is defined for energy. The EER comprises two separate terms. The estimated energy requirement for maintenance (EERM) is the energy intake that is estimated to maintain balance in healthy individuals or populations at a given level of physical activity and body size. The desirable estimated energy requirement (DEER) is the level of energy intake that should maintain energy balance in healthy individuals or populations of a defined gender, age, weight, height and level of physical activity, consistent with optimal health. Although complex, this is an important distinction as the EERM represents an actual energy requirement of an individual or group of individuals, while the DEER allows calculation of energy references that can be used to guide weight loss in a clinical situation (National Health and Medical Research Council of Australia, 2006).

In less affluent countries where there is a high burden of malnutrition-related disease, the priorities of governments are different, and DRVs are set at levels that are more appropriate for a setting where maintaining and monitoring food security are the main applications of the figures. Often, the values used in these situations are obtained from the FAO and focus heavily on setting levels of intake that will provide the basic requirements of most of the population and therefore avoid widespread clinical nutrient deficiency.

SUMMARY

- Nutritional balance depends upon the supply of nutrients being able to meet the physiological and metabolic demand for nutrients to be used as structural components or as substrates and cofactors for metabolism. Undernutrition or overnutrition arises through disturbance of this balance.
- Undernutrition can result from either a decrease in intake or an increase in the demand for nutrients. Increased demands are often a consequence of physiological insult or stressors, including trauma, pregnancy and lactation.
- Prolonged undernutrition can lead to micronutrient deficiency or malnutrition, which are common among infants and women in developing countries and among the elderly and poor in developed nations.
- The way in which the body responds to food and nutrients is strongly influenced by genetic factors. Single nucleotide polymorphisms result in common gene variants that can influence diet–disease relationships. This means that more individualized approaches to dietary guidelines may be more effective than general population guidelines.
- Stage of life is one of the most important determinants of nutritional status, as the nature of demands for nutrients and the way in which those demands are met undergo profound changes over the human lifespan.
- Nutritional status can be assessed by using anthropometric methods, by using different methods of measuring intake, through clinical examination or by measuring specific biomarkers. All methods are limited in their scope and are prone to inaccuracy.
- Exploring relationships between diet and disease relies on well-designed epidemiological studies. Simple ecological and cross-sectional studies can provide clues to diet–disease associations, but more robust cohort studies and randomized controlled trials are necessary to confirm causal relationships.
- DRVs are standards for nutrient intake, which are set by governments. They are widely used as the basis of nutrition-related advice and interventions. They can be used as research tools, as guidance for meal planners and caterers and for the monitoring of food security at a national level.

References

Arenz, S., Rückerl, R., Koletzko, B. and von Kries, R. (2004) Breast-feeding and childhood obesity—a systematic review. *International Journal of Obesity*, **28**, 1247–1256.

Bates, B., Lennox, A., Prentice, A. *et al.* (2014) National Diet and Nutrition Survey: Results from Years 1-4 (combined) of the Rolling Programme (2008/2009 – 2011/12), *Public Health England*, London.

Bayol, S.A., Farrington, S.J. and Stickland, N.C. (2007) A maternal 'junk food' diet in pregnancy and lactation promotes an exacerbated taste for 'junk food' and a greater propensity for obesity in rat offspring. *British Journal of Nutrition*, **98**, 843–851.

Bazelmans, C., Matthys, C., De Henauw, S. *et al.* (2007) Predictors of misreporting in an elderly population: the 'Quality of life after 65' study. *Public Health Nutrition*, **10**, 185–191.

Berger, S.G., de Pee, S., Bloem, M.W. *et al.* (2008) Malnutrition and morbidity among children not reached by the national vitamin A capsule programme in urban slum areas of Indonesia. *Public Health*, **122**, 371–378.

Black, R.E., Allen, L.H., Bhutta, Z.A. *et al.* (2008) Maternal and child undernutrition: global and regional exposures and health consequences. *Lancet*, **371**, 243–260.

Black, R.E., Victora, C.G., Walker, S.P. *et al.* (2013) Maternal and child undernutrition and overweight in low-income and middle-income countries. *Lancet*, **382**, 427–451.

Block, G. (1989) Human dietary assessment: methods and issues. *Preventive Medicine*, **18**, 653–660.

Block, G., Clifford, C., Naughtton, M.D. *et al.* (1989) A brief dietary screen for high fat intake. *Journal of Nutrition Education*, **21**, 199–207.

Centers for Disease Control (CDC) (2014) *National Health and Nutrition Examination Survey*, http://www.cdc.gov/nchs/nhanes.htm (accessed July 2014).

Conti, G., Chirico, V., Lacquaniti, A. *et al.* (2014) Vitamin D intoxication in two brothers: be careful with dietary supplements. *Journal of Pediatric Endocrinology & Metabolism*, **27** (7–8), 763–767.

Corella, D., Guillén, M., Sáiz, C. *et al.* (2001) Environmental factors modulate the effect of the APOE genetic polymorphism on plasma lipid concentrations: ecogenetic studies in a Mediterranean Spanish population. *Metabolism*, **50**, 936–944.

Cowin, I., Emmett, P. and ALSPAC Study Team (2000) Diet in a group of 18-month-old children in South West England, and comparison with the results of a national survey. *Journal of Human Nutrition and Dietetics*, **13**, 87–100.

Cowin, I., Emond, A., Emmett, P. *et al.* (2001) Association between composition of the diet and haemoglobin and ferritin levels in 18-month-old children. *European Journal of Clinical Nutrition*, **55**, 278–286.

Danforth, K.N., Tworoger, S.S., Hecht, J.L. *et al.* (2007) Breastfeeding and risk of ovarian cancer in two prospective cohorts. *Cancer Causes and Control*, **18**, 517–523.

Department of Health (DoH) (1991) *Dietary Reference Values for Energy and Nutrients for the United Kingdom*, Stationery Office, London.

Department of Health (DoH) (1999) *Dietary Reference Values for Energy and Nutrients for the United Kingdom*, Stationery Office, London.

El-Bastawissi, A.Y., Peters, R., Sasseen, K. *et al.* (2007) Effect of the Washington Special Supplemental Nutrition Program for Women, Infants and Children (WIC) on pregnancy outcomes. *Maternal and Child Health Journal*, **11**, 611–621.

European Food Safety Authority (EFSA) (2010) *Dietary Reference Values and Dietary Guidelines*, http://www.efsa.europa.eu/en/topics/topic/drv.htm (accessed July 2014).

Faber, M., Phungula, M.A., Venter, S.L. *et al.* (2002) Home gardens focusing on the production of yellow and dark-green leafy vegetables increase the serum retinol concentrations of 2–5-y-old children in South Africa. *American Journal of Clinical Nutrition*, **76**, 1048–1054.

Ferrari, S.L., Rizzoli, R., Slosman, D.O. and Bonjour, J.P. (1998) Do dietary calcium and age explain the controversy surrounding the relationship between bone mineral density and vitamin D receptor gene polymorphisms? *Journal of Bone and Mineral Research*, **13**, 363–370.

Frobisher, C. and Maxwell, S.M. (2003) The estimation of food portion sizes: a comparison between using descriptions of portion sizes and a photographic food atlas by children and adults. *Journal of Human Nutrition and Dietetics*, **16**, 181–188.

Godfrey, K., Robinson, S., Barker, D.J. *et al.* (1996) Maternal nutrition in early and late pregnancy in relation to placental and fetal growth. *British Medical Journal*, **312**, 410–414.

Gregory, J.R., Collins, D.L., Davies, P.S.W. *et al.* (1995) *National Diet and Nutrition Survey: Children Aged 1 1/2 to 4 1/2 Years. Volume 1: Report of the Diet and Nutrition Survey*, HMSO, London.

Grimble, R.F. (2001) Stress proteins in disease: metabolism on a knife edge. *Clinical Nutrition*, **20**, 469–476.

Hassan, M.A. and Killick, S.R. (2004) Negative lifestyle is associated with a significant reduction in fecundity. *Fertility and Sterility*, **81**, 384–392.

Jofre-Monseny, L., Minihane, A.M. and Rimbach, G. (2008) Impact of apoE genotype on oxidative stress, inflammation and disease risk. *Molecular Nutrition and Food Research*, **52**, 131–145.

Joost, H.G., Gibney, M.J., Cashman, K.D. *et al.* (2007) Personalised nutrition: status and perspectives. *British Journal of Nutrition*, **98**, 26–31.

Kardinaal, A.F., Kok, F.J., Ringstad, J. *et al.* (1993) Antioxidants in adipose tissue and risk of myocardial infarction: the EURAMIC study. *Lancet*, **342**, 1379–1384.

Kennedy, E. and Meyers, L. (2005) Dietary reference intakes: development and uses for assessment of micronutrient status of women–a global perspective. *American Journal of Clinical Nutrition*, **81**, 1194S–1197S.

King, J.C. (1990) Assessment of zinc status. *Journal of Nutrition*, **120** (Suppl. 11), 1474–1479.

Klerk, M., Verhoef, P., Clarke, R. *et al.* (2002) MTHFR 677C→T polymorphism and risk of coronary heart disease: a meta-analysis. *Journal of the American Medical Association*, **288**, 2023–2031.

Koebnick, C., Wagner, K., Thielecke, F. *et al.* (2005) An easy-to-use semi-quantitative food record validated for energy intake by using doubly labelled water technique. *European Journal of Clinical Nutrition*, **59**, 989–995.

Kofler, B.M., Miles, E.A., Curtis, P. *et al.* (2012) Apolipoprotein E genotype and the cardiovascular disease risk phenotype: impact of sex and adiposity (the FINGEN study). *Atherosclerosis*, **221**, 467–470.

Langley-Evans, S.C. (2015) Nutrition in early life and the programming of adult disease: a review. *Journal of Human Nutrition and Dietetics*, **28** (Suppl. 1), 1–14.

Lakshmi Priya, M.D. and Geetha, A. (2011) Level of trace elements (copper, zinc, magnesium and selenium) and toxic elements (lead and mercury) in the hair and nail of children with autism. *Biological Trace Elements Research*, **142**, 148–158.

Lenz, A., Franklin, G.A. and Cheadle, W.G. (2007) Systemic inflammation after trauma. *Injury*, **38**, 1336–1345.

Lonn, E., Yusuf, S., Arnold, M.J. *et al.* (2006) Homocysteine lowering with folic acid and B vitamins in vascular disease. *New England Journal of Medicine*, **354**, 1567–1577.

Martinez-Frias, M.L. and Salvador, J. (1990) Epidemiological aspects of prenatal exposure to high doses of vitamin A in Spain. *European Journal of Epidemiology*, **6**, 118–123.

Mayer, J.E. (2007) Delivering golden rice to developing countries. *Journal of AOAC International*, **90**, 1445–1449.

Millward, D.J., Fereday, A., Gibson, N. and Pacy, P.J. (1997) Aging, protein requirements, and protein turnover. *American Journal of Clinical Nutrition*, **66**, 774–786.

MRC Vitamin Study Group (1991) Prevention of neural tube defects: results of the Medical Research Council Vitamin Study. MRC Vitamin Study Research Group. *Lancet*, **338**, 131–137.

Mukamal, K.J., Cushman, M., Mittleman, M.A. *et al.* (2004) Alcohol consumption and inflammatory markers in older adults: the Cardiovascular Health Study. *Atherosclerosis*, **173**, 79–87.

Muñoz, N., Plummer, M., Vivas, J. *et al.* (2001) A case-control study of gastric cancer in Venezuela. *International Journal of Cancer*, **93**, 417–423.

National Health and Medical Research Council of Australia (2006) *Nutrient Reference Values for Australia and New Zealand*, http://www.nrv.gov.au/Energy.aspx (accessed 18 February 2008).

Nazario, C.M., Szklo, M., Diamond, E. *et al.* (1993) Salt and gastric cancer: a case-control study in Puerto Rico. *International Journal of Epidemiology*, **22**, 790–797.

Neidecker-Gonzales, O., Nestel, P. and Bouis, H. (2007) Estimating the global costs of vitamin A capsule supplementation: a review of the literature. *Food and Nutrition Bulletin*, **28**, 307–316.

Olano-Martin, E., Anil, E., Caslake, M.J. *et al.* (2010) Contribution of apolipoprotein E genotype and docosahexaenoic acid to the LDL-cholesterol response to fish oil. *Atherosclerosis*, **209**, 104–110.

Pavlovic, M., Prentice, A., Thorsdottir, I. *et al.* (2007) Challenges in harmonizing energy and nutrient recommendations in Europe. *Annals of Nutrition and Metabolism*, **51**, 108–114.

Richardson, R.A. and Davidson, H.I. (2003) Nutritional demands in acute and chronic illness. *Proceedings of the Nutrition Society*, **62**, 777–781.

Ritchie, L.D., Fung, E.B., Halloran, B.P. *et al.* (1998) A longitudinal study of calcium homeostasis during human pregnancy and lactation and after resumption of menses. *American Journal of Clinical Nutrition*, **67**, 693–701.

Rivlin, R.S. (2007) Keeping the young-elderly healthy: is it too late to improve our health through nutrition? *American Journal of Clinical Nutrition*, **86**, 1572S–1576S.

Romijn, J.A. (2000) Substrate metabolism in the metabolic response to injury. *Proceedings of the Nutrition Society*, **59**, 447–449.

Sarojini, G., Nirmala, G. and Geetha, R. (1999) Introduction of red palm oil into the 'ready to eat' used supplementary feeding programme through ICDS. *Indian Journal of Public Health*, **43**, 125–131.

Scientific Advisory Committee on Nutrition (SACN) (2014) *Carbohydrates and Health Report*, http://www.sacn.gov.uk/pdfs/draft_sacn_carbohydrates_and_health_report_consultation.pdf (accessed July 2014).

Sebotsa, M.L., Dannhauser, A., Jooste, P.L. and Joubert, G. (2005) Iodine status as determined by urinary iodine excretion in Lesotho two years after introducing legislation on universal salt iodization. *Nutrition*, **21**, 20–24.

Seshadri, S. (2001) Prevalence of micronutrient deficiency particularly of iron, zinc and folic acid in pregnant women in South East Asia. *British Journal of Nutrition*, **85** (Suppl. 2), S87–S92.

Setiawan, V.W., Zhang, Z.F., Yu, G.P. *et al.* (2000) GSTT1 and GSTM1 null genotypes and the risk of gastric cancer: a case-control study in a Chinese population. *Cancer Epidemiology Biomarkers and Prevention*, **9**, 73–80.

Tsugane, S., Sasazuki, S., Kobayashi, M. and Sasaki, S. (2004) Salt and salted food intake and subsequent risk of gastric cancer among middle-aged Japanese men and women. *British Journal of Cancer*, **90**, 128–234.

van den Brandt, P.A., Botterweck, A.A. and Goldbohm, R.A. (2003) Salt intake, cured meat consumption, refrigerator use and stomach cancer incidence: a prospective cohort study (Netherlands). *Cancer Causes and Control*, **14**, 427–438.

West, K.P. (2003) Vitamin A deficiency disorders in children and women. *Food and Nutrition Bulletin*, **24** (Suppl. 4), S78–S90.

Whitehead, R.G. (1992) Dietary reference values. *Proceedings of the Nutrition Society*, **51**, 29–34.

Wild, T., Rahbarnia, A., Kellner, M. *et al.* (2010) Basics in nutrition and wound healing. *Nutrition*, **26**, 862–866.

World Cancer Research Fund (WCRF) (2007) *Food, Nutrition, Physical Activity, and the Prevention of Cancer: A Global Perspective*, WCRF/AICR, Washington, DC.

Zagré, N.M., Delpeuch, F., Traissac, P. and Delisle, H. (2003) Red palm oil as a source of vitamin A for mothers and children: impact of a pilot project in Burkina Faso. *Public Health Nutrition*, **6**, 733–742.

Additional reading

If you would like to find out more about the material discussed in this chapter, the following sources may be of interest.

Department of Health (DoH) (1991) *Dietary Reference Values of Food Energy and Nutrients for the United Kingdom: Report of the Panel on Dietary Reference Values of the Committee on Medical Aspects of Food*, Stationery Office, London.

Institute of Medicine (US) (2001) *Dietary Reference Intakes: Applications in Dietary Assessment*, National Academies Press, Washington, DC.

Kok, F., Bouwman, L. and Desiere, F. (2004) *Personalised Nutrition*, CRC Press, Boca Raton, FL.

Kaput, J. and Rodriguez, R.L. (2006) *Nutritional Genomics*, Wiley-Blackwell, Hoboken, NJ.

Lee, R.D. and Nieman, D.C. (2012) *Nutritional Assessment*, McGraw-Hill, New York.

Margetts, B.M. and Nelson, M. (1997) *Design Concepts in Nutritional Epidemiology*, Oxford Medical Publications, Oxford/New York.

CHAPTER 2

Before life begins

LEARNING OBJECTIVES

This chapter will enable the reader to:
- Describe how trends in modern healthcare have made it both possible and desirable to change diet and lifestyle in preparation for pregnancy
- Show an understanding of the endocrine control of both female and male reproductive functions
- Discuss the contribution of body fatness to initiation and maintenance of normal reproductive cycling in women
- Critically review the evidence that commonly consumed agents such as alcohol and caffeine may have an adverse effect on female fertility
- Discuss the possible contribution of antioxidant nutrients to optimal fertility in men and women
- Show an understanding of dietary factors and non-nutrient components of food that may have an adverse impact on male fertility
- Describe the importance of reducing intake of vitamin A and increasing intake of folic acid, for reducing risk of embryonic malformation in the earliest stages of pregnancy

2.1 Introduction

The twentieth century saw a profound change in the manner in which human reproductive health and function was managed. Medicalization of the process of childbirth and the management of pregnancy transformed human reproduction. In the early part of the century, death rates among newborn infants in the United Kingdom were as high as 150–200 per 1000 births, and pregnancy-related complications were the major cause of death among young women, with death rates of 5–6 per 1000 births (Office for National Statistics, 1997). Improved medical care, hygiene, diet and housing conditions have brought death rates among infants down to 4–6 per 1000 births, and maternal deaths are now very rare events (<0.1 per 1000 births). As shown in Figure 2.1, maternal and neonatal deaths are falling, but remain high in developing countries.

These changes have also transformed the priorities for researchers and health professionals working in the field of human reproduction. With less emphasis on the avoidance of catastrophic pregnancy outcomes, it is now of prime importance to promote good health in pregnant women and to ensure achievement of the optimal maternal environment for the development of the baby. In terms of nutrition, it is becoming clear that many of the important changes that women should consider making to their diets need to be implemented before conception. In most Western countries, the majority (60%) of pregnancies are planned and this allows scope for optimizing nutrition. Attaining optimal body weights, avoiding potentially harmful substances and increasing intakes of nutrients that are of greatest importance to fetal development are all most effective when achieved while planning a pregnancy.

Nutrition may also be of major importance in achieving conception for many couples. Nutritional status, and in particular female body fatness, plays a role in determining fertility. This chapter will primarily set out the key nutrition-related issues that impact upon the ability of men and women to conceive a child. Estimates of infertility rates vary considerably between developed and developing countries, but globally 12% of women seeking to conceive cannot do so within 12 months, with higher prevalence in Central and Eastern Europe, Central and South Asia and North Africa (Mascarenhas *et al.*, 2012).

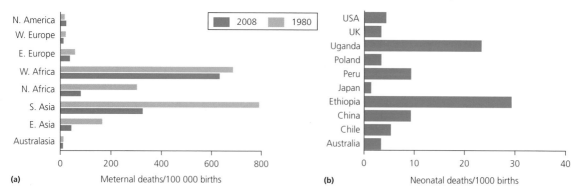

Figure 2.1 Maternal and neonatal mortality. **a)** Maternal mortality declined in most regions of the world between 1980 and 2008, but remains markedly higher in the developing countries. **b)** There is considerable global variation in neonatal mortality, with highest mortality in the African nations (figures shown for 2009–2013 in selected countries).
Data sources: UN, World Bank and Hogan *et al.* (2010).

Twelve per cent of US women of childbearing age report having undergone fertility treatment and 1% of all US babies are born following assisted reproductive treatments. In parts of Europe, this figure is as high as 3%. Consistent with the changing priorities in relation to how reproduction is managed in developed countries, the chapter will also consider the dietary changes that women should consider ahead of conception in order to optimize their nutrient reserves for pregnancy and minimize the likelihood of embryonic exposure to harmful agents in the first few weeks of life.

2.2 Nutrition and female fertility

2.2.1 Determinants of fertility and infertility

Female fertility is primarily determined by factors that are seemingly unrelated to nutritional status. Whereas men generally retain some degree of fertility throughout their adult lives, women have a fixed reproductive span that runs from menarche (the onset of reproductive cycling) to menopause (when reproductive cycling ends). Infertility or subfertility in women can arise due to problems with the endocrine regulation of reproductive system function or due to other medical conditions that impair reproductive capacity. These medical conditions include infections of the reproductive tract, ovarian disease, trauma to the reproductive organs, endometriosis and polycystic ovary syndrome (PCOS). Although these reproductive events appear to be determined by age and ill health, it is becoming clear that nutritional status can have some impact on the timing of menarche, and hence duration of reproductive span, and upon the maintenance of normal reproductive cycling.

2.2.1.1 The endocrine control of female reproduction

The endocrine regulation of female reproductive function is extremely complex, and this text will attempt to give only a simple overview. Within the ovaries, women have primary follicles containing immature oocytes which are present from the time of birth. The hormones involved in the regulation of the menstrual cycle function to facilitate the maturation of a small number of these oocytes, the release of a single mature ovum in each cycle and the preparation of the uterine lining for the implantation of a fertilized egg. The menstrual cycle comprises two distinct phases, with follicle and egg maturation occurring in the follicular phase. After ovulation, the cycle enters the luteal phase, in which the corpus luteum (remnants of the follicle which released the mature ovum at ovulation) acts as the main controller of the uterine environment. It can either promote the maintenance of a suitable environment for implantation or pregnancy, or in the absence of fertilization, it can degenerate and promote the sloughing of the uterine lining and hence menstrual bleeding.

The endocrine factors that regulate the menstrual cycle are shown in Figure 2.2. The hypothalamus is the central integrator of the cycle, acting through production of gonadotrophin-releasing hormone (GnRH). This stimulates the production of two hormones from the anterior pituitary. Follicle-stimulating hormone (FSH) acts on the ovaries to stimulate the maturation of the follicles and to drive the production of oestrogens. Oestrogens also stimulate follicular development and act upon the uterus to build up the endometrial lining. During the follicular phase, oestrogen concentrations tend to be low, but this is still sufficient to lower the production of FSH from the anterior pituitary and GnRH from the hypothalamus,

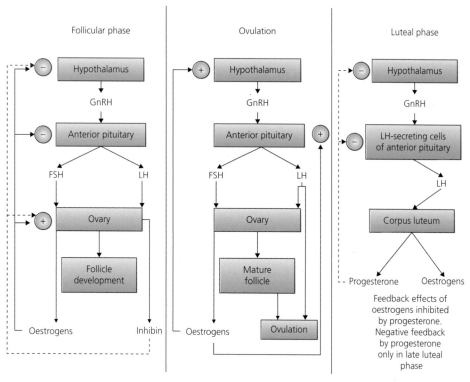

Figure 2.2 The endocrine control of female reproductive function. The menstrual cycle lasts for an average of 28 days. This can be divided into a distinct follicular phase (days 1–13) during which oestrogen, LH and FSH stimulate follicular development. Ovulation driven by high concentrations of LH and oestrogen occurs on day 14. The luteal phase (days 15–28) is driven by hormone production from the corpus luteum, which produces high concentrations of progesterone and oestrogen to prepare the uterine lining for implantation of a fertilized embryo. In the absence of fertilization, feedback inhibition of progesterone promotes the degeneration of the corpus luteum and menstrual bleeding.

through a negative feedback mechanism. The other anterior pituitary hormone produced in response to GnRH secretion is luteinizing hormone (LH). The ovaries are a target for LH where, like FSH, it stimulates follicular development. The ovaries also produce the hormone inhibin in response to LH, and this selectively inhibits the secretion of FSH (Figure 2.2). This, together with the effects of oestrogen, means that LH concentrations tend to rise towards the midpoint in the cycle, while FSH concentrations tend to fall.

While effects of oestrogen upon the hypothalamus and anterior pituitary involve negative feedback, oestrogens exert positive feedback effects on the ovaries to generate more oestrogen (Figure 2.2). This means that by the midpoint in the menstrual cycle, oestrogen concentrations spike dramatically. Rising levels of oestrogens have a paradoxical effect upon the hypothalamus and anterior pituitary and now start to *stimulate* secretion of LH and to a lesser extent FSH. The resultant surge in LH is the trigger for ovulation. The mature follicle ruptures and

releases the ovum. At the same time, the corpus luteum is formed and the cycle now enters the luteal phase.

During the luteal phase, the key anterior pituitary factor is LH, which stimulates the corpus luteum to produce initially low levels of oestrogens and progesterone. The concentrations of these sex steroids rise gradually, and progesterone in particular reaches a very high concentration. This inhibits the further production of GnRH and hence LH and FSH and thereby prevents the maturation of further follicles should a pregnancy occur (Figure 2.2). If there is no pregnancy, the corpus luteum degenerates as LH is no longer produced to maintain it and hence production of progesterone and oestrogen ends.

2.2.1.2 Disordered reproductive cycling
Disordered menstrual cycling can arise for a number of reasons. Stress, excessive or intense exercise, smoking, ovarian or uterine disease, use of certain medications and treatments such as chemotherapy, drug abuse, illness and emotional traumas have all been shown to

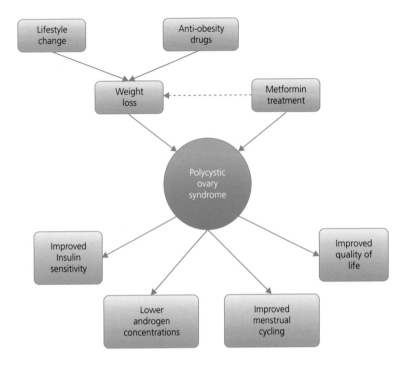

Figure 2.3 Polycystic ovary syndrome (PCOS) is alleviated by weight loss. Approximately 50% of women with PCOS are overweight and obese. PCOS symptoms can be reduced by weight loss, achieved through increased physical activity and dietary change or by treatment with metformin. Metformin is an anti-diabetic drug, which acts by suppressing hepatic gluconeogenesis.

impact upon hypothalamic and ovarian production of hormones. Any problems with secretion of LH, FSH or oestrogens will impact upon the normal reproductive cycle, with several possible outcomes. In some women, menstrual cycles cease entirely (amenorrhoea), or the cycle may become excessively long, perhaps lasting for 45–90 days instead of the usual 28 (oligorrhoea). If there is insufficient production of LH or oestrogen, then there may be an absence of ovulation (anovulation). As will become clear in later sections, poor nutritional status is a major cause of menstrual cycle disorders and hence an important factor in unexplained (idiopathic) infertility in women.

2.2.1.3 PCOS

PCOS is one of the more common medical causes of female subfertility and infertility. Women with PCOS develop clusters of immature follicles within the ovaries, all of which fail to develop and eventually form fluid-filled cysts. Generally, women with PCOS will either be anovulatory or will have infrequent periods and oligorrhoea. One of the features of the syndrome is the production of high concentrations of male sex hormones (androgens), which can often manifest physically as excess facial or chest hair growth (hirsutism), loss of head hair and acne. In addition to producing abnormally high levels of testosterone, women with PCOS generally overproduce LH.

Obesity, and therefore nutritional status, is a major determinant of risk of PCOS, although it has also been related to a family history of the condition. There is a high prevalence of obesity among women with PCOS (Pasquali *et al.*, 2006), and abdominal fat deposition appears to confer particularly high risk. Women with central obesity of this nature tend to develop insulin resistance, which is characterized by excessively high levels of circulating insulin. Insulin inhibits synthesis of sex hormone binding globulin in the liver. This protein plays a key role in controlling the access of sex hormones to their target tissues, and in the absence of sex hormone binding globulin, concentrations of free androgens rise. Obesity also favours increased synthesis of androgens and other mechanisms operating in adipose tissue serve to drive hyperandrogenaemia.

Weight loss in women with PCOS is effective in restoring normal endocrine functions and reproductive cycling (Figure 2.3). Pasquali *et al.* (2006) reported that a 12-month period of dieting to promote significant weight loss in women with PCOS significantly improved symptoms (partial restoration of menstrual cycles, reduction in hirsutism) and that these changes were associated with markedly lower circulating insulin concentrations, improved insulin sensitivity and lower testosterone concentrations. Several studies have examined the optimal weight loss strategy for treatment of PCOS. Moran and colleagues (2012) conducted a systematic review to evaluate the impact of these approaches. High-protein diets promote satiety and therefore reduce overall energy intake and, importantly, produce less variation in insulin secretion after a meal. These diets produce positive psychological effects in women with PCOS and improve compliance with lifestyle change (Galletly et al., 2007; Moran et al., 2012). Marsh and Brand-Miller (2005), however, suggest that high-protein diets may actually worsen insulin resistance and are no more effective than high-carbohydrate diets in promoting improvement of reproductive functions through weight loss. Although there is some evidence that low-glycaemic index diets (rich in complex carbohydrate) result in greater improvements in reproductive function, weight loss through caloric restriction remains the most important approach to managing PCOS, regardless of the overall dietary composition (Moran et al., 2012).

2.2.2 Importance of body fat

Body fatness is a major factor determining the span of reproductive life in women and, as illustrated by the example of PCOS, determines some of the risk of developing menstrual cycle disturbances. It was noted several decades ago that young women who partake in high-intensity sport or dance activities tend to exhibit delayed menarche and will later be at greater risk of amenorrhoea or anovulation. Amenorrhoea is also observed in women who are excessively thin, or who undergo extreme weight loss, either as a result of eating disorders (e.g. anorexia nervosa) or through other restrictive dietary practices. Weight loss equivalent to around 10–15% of normal weight for height in women is associated with menstrual cycle abnormalities. Obesity is also associated with amenorrhoea. Together, these observations suggest that both too much and too little body fat can have an adverse impact on female fertility (Frisch, 1987).

Young women at the present time are significantly taller and heavier than their counterparts in earlier centuries, and with this change in growth, they are attaining greater proportions of body fat at earlier ages. This secular trend is associated with a trend for menarche to occur at an earlier age. In the nineteenth century, the average age for first menses was between 17 and 18 years old. By the 1920s, this had declined to 14 years and by the 1990s was between 12 and 13 years. In developed countries, a steady decline in age at menarche was observed across the twentieth century with girls initiating menstruation approximately 15 months earlier in the 1990s than in the 1920s. The proportion of girls entering puberty before age 10, which was extremely rare in the 1940s, was approximately 2% in 1990. The main contributor to the decline in age at menarche is believed to be increased body fatness in the population. Chang-Mo et al. (2012) reported that in a Korean population, menarche before 12 years of age was up to seven-fold more likely in girls who were taller, heavier and of greater body mass index (BMI) at ages 8 and 9. Girls who matured early were approximately 5 kg heavier than girls who reached menarche after 12 years and had a greater percentage body fat at age 13.

The growth spurt during adolescence is obviously associated with a significant increase in both height and weight but is also a time when body composition undergoes major changes. In girls, there is a relative increase in the proportion of body fat, which increases from around 5 kg in total to 11 kg. Lean body mass increases to a much lesser extent. Frisch et al. (1973) studied adolescent girls and found that on attainment of stable reproductive cycling, all had approximately 22% body fat, regardless of their absolute height or weight. These studies identified this proportion of body fat as being the minimum required to maintain stable menstrual cycling, and hence women restricting diet to promote weight loss and women engaged in intense physical activity develop amenorrhoea and other cycle problems as they fall below this fat threshold. There is a difference between menarche and attainment of stable and regular cycles, and the minimum threshold of body fat required to trigger menarche is lower, at 17% of body weight (Frisch, 1987).

There are therefore minimal levels of body fat required to support reproductive function in women. It is easy to see how such a system has evolved in humans. Body fat is essentially a store of metabolizable energy and provides a metabolic indicator of the nutritional environment and fitness of a woman to support a pregnancy and later breastfeed an infant. Mechanisms that prevent conception during times of famine would have been a considerable survival advantage to early humans. Allal et al. (2004) showed that in developing countries such as the Gambia, delayed reproductive maturity and hence a later first pregnancy allow women to grow to a greater height. Greater maternal stature is associated with reduced infant death.

2.2.3 Role of leptin

There is a simple hormonal signal that links the body fatness of women to the hypothalamic–pituitary–ovarian axis that ultimately governs their fertility. Leptin is one of a group of peptide hormones, termed adipokines, produced from adipose tissue. Other adipokines, including resistin and adiponectin, have been suggested to play a role in controlling fertility. Adiponectin, for example, appears to play a role in follicle maturation and preparation of the uterus for implantation. While the role of

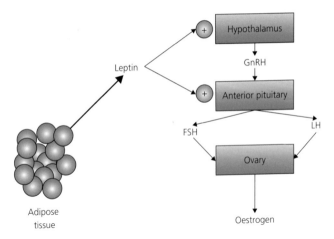

Figure 2.4 Adipose tissue-derived leptin and the hypothalamic–pituitary–ovarian axis. Leptin from adipose tissue promotes production of GnRH, FSH and LH and therefore has a stimulatory effect on the hypothalamic–pituitary–ovarian axis.

leptin in regulating menstrual cycle function is well established, effects of other adipose tissue-derived hormones upon human reproductive function have not been clearly demonstrated (Mitchell *et al.*, 2005). Leptin is the product of the *ob* gene which is only expressed in adipose tissue. As a result, plasma concentrations of leptin are closely correlated with the overall level of body fat. Leptin is a satiety hormone, which acts at the hypothalamus to suppress appetite and increase energy expenditure through thermogenesis. Satiety effects are mediated indirectly as leptin, within the arcuate nucleus of the hypothalamus, stimulates release of further satiety-inducing peptides, including neuropeptide Y (NPY) and agouti-related peptide (AGRP).

The first clues for a role of leptin in controlling fertility came from studies of a range of genetically obese rodents. The *ob/ob* mouse produces a defective leptin that is unable to bind the leptin receptors, while the *db/db* mouse and *fa/fa* rat have defective receptors which do not fully mediate the effects of leptin on binding. All of these rodent strains exhibit problems with fertility. The female *ob/ob* mouse is totally infertile as it never achieves puberty and cannot produce mature follicles. These mice have abnormal levels of FSH and GnRH in circulation. Similarly, the female *fa/fa* rat is rarely fertile, having a suppressed LH surge and lower FSH secretion, preventing normal ovulation.

In humans, changes in leptin concentrations occur around the time of puberty, but only in girls. As a result, women have higher leptin concentrations (normal range 5–20 ng/ml) than are seen in men, at all ages. This reflects their higher proportions of body fat at any given weight or height. Leptin concentrations in women also vary according to stage of the menstrual cycle (Goumenou *et al.*, 2003), which suggests that there are relationships between leptin secretion and the reproductive hormones. Sustaining normal ovulatory cycles depends on a minimum level of leptin (~3 ng/ml), and women who are anovulatory have lower concentrations than women with normal cycles, while amenorrhoeic women have still lower concentrations. Leptin also explains the relationship between body fatness and age at menarche, as a threshold of 12 ng/ml leptin is required to initiate cycling.

Figure 2.4 shows how leptin influences the hypothalamic–pituitary–ovarian axis. Leptin receptors are present in key nuclei of the hypothalamus and in the anterior pituitary, and it therefore directly influences the secretion of GnRH, LH and FSH. In the absence of leptin, the normal pulsatile secretion of all of these factors is lost (Goumenou *et al.*, 2003). The *ob/ob* mouse, lacking leptin, is analogous to the excessively thin woman, and both will have fertility problems for the same reasons.

Given the stimulatory role of leptin upon the reproductive axis, the negative effects of excess body fat appear to be paradoxical. Obese individuals typically exhibit very high concentrations of leptin. The explanation for the negative effect on fertility is provided by the concept of leptin resistance. The effects of leptin within the brain are mediated through its binding to two different forms of the leptin receptor. The short-form receptor, Ob-Ra, has a transport role and carries leptin across the blood–brain barrier, thereby providing access to the hypothalamic tissues. The long-form Ob-Rb receptor is membrane bound and mediates the physiological effects of leptin via several signal transduction mechanisms, as shown in Figure 2.5. One of these mechanisms is the Janus kinase (JAK)–signal transducer and activator of transcription 3 (STAT3) pathway. Binding of leptin stimulates phosphorylation of STAT3 and hence gene transcription to mediate cellular responses. Leptin resistance involves impairment of both Ob-Ra and Ob-Rb functions (El-Haschimi *et al.*, 2000). Impaired Ob-Ra function is poorly understood but clearly reduces the amount of leptin reaching target sites. Leptin

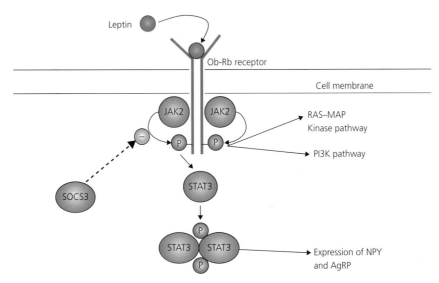

Figure 2.5 Leptin receptor signalling cascade. Binding of leptin to the membrane bound Ob-Rb receptor activates multiple signalling pathways, including the phosphoinositol 3 kinase (PI3K) pathway and the RAS–MAP kinase pathway. Binding of leptin activates JAK2, which phosphorylates STAT3. Formation of phosphorylated STAT3 complexes drives activation of transcription of target genes including NPY and AgRP. Leptin resistance develops through leptin up-regulation of the expression of suppressor of the cytokine signalling-3 (SOCS3), which inhibits the JAK2–STAT3 pathway.

up-regulates expression of suppressor of the cytokine signalling-3 (SOCS3), which is an inhibitor of the JAK–STAT3 pathway. Thus, the very high concentrations of leptin associated with obesity will suppress leptin action in the hypothalamus and remove the stimulatory effect of the hormone on the hypothalamic–pituitary–ovarian axis, leading to disordered reproductive cycling. The *fa/fa* rat, which has leptin receptor defects, provides an analogy to the obese woman, and their reproductive cycle defects are similar.

2.2.4 Antioxidant nutrients

A free radical is any molecule that has unpaired electrons, and as such, these molecules are highly reactive and short lived. Free radicals and associated oxidants formed from oxygen within biological systems are termed reactive oxygen species (ROS). These include the superoxide (O_2^-) and hydroxyl (OH·) radicals, hydrogen peroxide, nitric oxide (NO) and lipid hydroperoxides (Halliwell, 1999). As will be seen in later chapters, the reactive nature of ROS gives them the capacity to cause widespread cellular and tissue damage that is associated with the development and progression of many disease states. Exposure to ROS is an unavoidable feature of life in oxygen, as they are mainly formed as a by-product of mitochondrial respiration. Other important sources of ROS in biological systems are shown in Table 2.1. ROS have the capacity to damage all components of cells, as they will react with all types of macromolecules (Figure 2.6). Thus,

they damage proteins (e.g. protein–protein cross-linking), nucleic acids (e.g. DNA strand scission) and phospholipids in membranes (lipid peroxidation).

Life in oxygen is only possible due to the presence of antioxidant species that have the capacity to neutralize ROS (Table 2.1). Most aspects of antioxidant protection are to some extent influenced by the diet and nutritional status. The antioxidant enzymes generally have metal ions at their active sites (e.g. CuZn superoxide dismutase), and scavenging antioxidants such as ascorbate, ß-carotene and vitamin E are all obtained directly through the diet. These scavenging species must be constantly replenished as interaction with ROS leads to their destruction.

Oxidative stress, the situation where ROS activity is not fully buffered by the presence of antioxidants, is a known feature of normal reproductive function in women. ROS play a key role in several aspects of the menstrual cycle, including follicle maturation, ovulation, development of the endometrium for implantation and synthesis of progesterone by the corpus luteum (Ruder *et al.*, 2009). While ovulation will not occur without ROS, excess production or inadequate antioxidant status is associated with poor fertility. Endometriosis is a condition in which the tissue that lines the uterus grows in areas outside the reproductive tract, causing pain, irregular bleeding and subfertility. Excessive oxidative stress, and in particular overproduction of NO, is believed to contribute to the condition (Agarwal *et al.*,

Table 2.1 Reactive oxygen species and antioxidants in biological systems.

Reactive oxygen species		Antioxidants		
Free radicals	Non-radicals	Enzymes	Scavengers	Ion binding proteins
Superoxide, O_2^-	Hydrogen peroxide H_2O_2	Superoxide dismutase	Ascorbate	Albumin
Hydroxyl radical, OH	Ozone O_3	Catalase	Polyphenols	Ferritin
Peroxyl radical, RO_2	Hypochlorous acid HOCl	Glutathione peroxidase	α-Tocopherol	Transferrin
Alkoxyl radical, RO	Hypobromous acid HOBr		β-Carotene	Caeruloplasmin
Nitric oxide, NO			Lutein	

Reactive oxygen species are either generated endogenously through processes such as respiration and the respiratory burst of immune cells or can be derived from exogenous sources (pollutants, drugs, food contaminants). Enzymatic antioxidants are present in most cells and some forms occur in circulation. Scavenging antioxidants are generally derived from the diet and are found in body fluids and the cytosol of most cells. Ion binding proteins are transtport proteins that provide antioxidant protection by removing free iron and copper ions, which can generate free radical species when they react with oxygen.

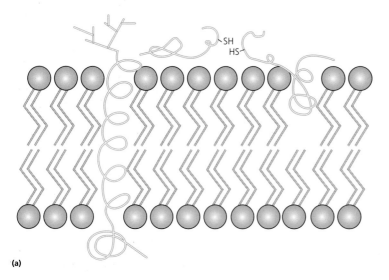

(a)

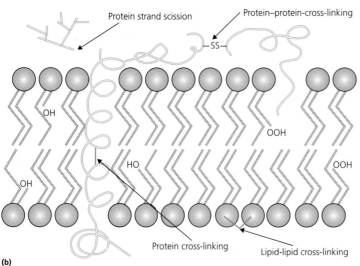

(b)

Figure 2.6 ROS are damaging within biological systems. **a)** A section of membrane in a mammalian cell comprises the phospholipid bilayer with a transmembrane protein and cell surface proteins. **b)** After interaction with a reactive oxygen species, the section of membrane is heavily damaged due to the chain reactions established by the oxidation of macromolecules. Oxidative damage to the lipid bilayer (lipid peroxidation) will impact upon membrane properties such as permeability. Damage to proteins will alter conformation and impact upon receptor, signalling, transport and enzyme functions.

2005). In the process of *in vitro* fertilization (IVF), excess ROS damages embryos and reduces success of the procedure, so antioxidants are routinely added to the media used for fertilizing the egg.

To ensure that antioxidant stress is controlled, the reproductive system is rich in antioxidants. Follicular fluid is rich in scavenging antioxidants and the endometrium expresses superoxide dismutase as part of the normal response to progesterone (Ebisch *et al.*, 2007). Follicular fluid may be especially important (Ruder *et al.*, 2009) with reports that successful oocyte retrieval and embryo transfer in assisted reproduction are related to the total antioxidant capacity of follicular fluid. Melatonin and α-tocopherol may play a role in the protection of the oocyte from oxidative stress and, *in vitro*, melatonin has been shown to enhance oocyte maturation and improve IVF outcomes in women with PCOS.

Subfertility is generally the product of inadequate gamete production or quality, or a hostile environment for fertilization or implantation. A role for antioxidants in optimizing these aspects of female reproductive health has been suggested by virtue of the importance of controlled oxidative processes in menstrual cycle function. Polak *et al.* (2001) observed that in women with idiopathic infertility, activity of ROS was higher and antioxidant capacity was lower in peritoneal fluid than in fertile women. If peritoneal fluid is accepted as a proxy for the environment in the fallopian tubes where fertilization will occur, this may suggest infertility stems from oxidative damage to sperm, preventing fertilization. Sperm are highly vulnerable to oxidative damage (Agarwal *et al.*, 2005). As a result, many trials have been conducted to evaluate the impact of antioxidant supplementation upon female fertility. These have generally proved inconclusive. Showell *et al.* (2013) conducted a systematic review and meta-analysis of 28 trials and found that oral antioxidant supplements had no significant benefits for women's reproductive health.

2.2.5 Caffeine and alcohol

In many parts of the world, it is part of the normal culture to consume alcohol and/or caffeine in the form of beverages. These widely consumed agents are known to be highly active substances that are capable of exerting toxic effects at high levels and major metabolic and physiological responses at low to moderate levels of consumption. Both alcohol and caffeine consumption have been linked to problems with female fertility and indeed may interact with each other in lowering the chances of conception. The impact of alcohol is explained in Research Highlight 2.1.

Caffeine is pharmacologically active, acting as a central nervous system stimulant. It is consumed in a variety of forms, principally tea and coffee but also as an additive to soft drinks and in some over-the-counter medicines. Several animal studies have shown that caffeine can have adverse reproductive effects and that it is potentially hazardous to the early embryo. However, in humans, it is more difficult to interpret the findings of studies that relate caffeine intake to reproductive function and to develop a credible explanation of how it could reduce fertility. Certainly, caffeine can deplete the body of certain micronutrients through either inhibition of absorption (e.g. iron and zinc) or through increasing losses (e.g. calcium and thiamin), but these nutrients have no clear role in determining female fertility.

First concerns over caffeine and female fertility arose when Olsen (1991) reported that subfecundity was associated with very high intakes (eight or more cups per day) of coffee. However, this negative effect on fertility (OR 1.35; 95% CI, 1.02–1.48) was noted only for women who also smoked. The study has been criticized on the basis that it took no account of reproductive disorders, or key factors such as the frequency of sexual intercourse, which would clearly determine odds of conception. The findings of Olsen are, however, largely backed up by most other studies that have considered the effects of very high caffeine consumption. Bolúmar *et al.* (1997) studied 3187 women from five European countries and were able to allow for all sources of caffeine (although coffee was the chief source), major confounding factors and for the regional and cultural variations in how coffee is prepared and brewed. Women who consumed more than 500 mg caffeine/day (in excess of five cups) had a longer average waiting time to pregnancy on cessation of contraceptive use (8.9 months compared to 6.5 months in women who consumed <100 mg caffeine/day). High caffeine consumption (more than 500 mg/day) increased odds of subfecundity by 45% compared to women consuming 100 mg/day or less. The effect was stronger in smokers (56% greater risk) than in non-smokers (38% greater risk).

Hassan and Killick (2004) reported similar findings from a study of 2112 UK women. Tea and coffee consumption was a determinant of risk of subfecundity but only when consumed at high levels. Seven or more cups per day increased risk by 70% (95% CI, 1.1–2.7) after adjusting for alcohol intake, BMI, contraceptive use and frequency of intercourse. Women who consume excessive amounts of coffee also tend to consume more alcohol. Hakim and colleagues (1998) found that the two factors together contributed to reduced fertility and that lowest conception rates were associated with highest intakes of alcoholic beverages and coffee. In contrast, Hatch and colleagues (2012) reported that consumption of caffeine from all sources, and specifically coffee

Research Highlight 2.1 Complex relationship between alcohol and fertility in women.

The consumption of alcohol has been widely reported to impair fertility in women. A standard unit of alcohol in a beverage is approximately 12 g of ethanol, which equates to a small measure of spirits, or a half pint of beer. Studies that consider the relationship between alcohol consumption and fertility tend to be cross-sectional cohort studies that examine the impact of consumption on fertility endpoints in a large group of women. In this way, it is possible to determine odds ratios as an indicator of infertility risk. This can be examined as a dose–response relationship, comparing risk against units of alcohol consumption.

Most reports suggest that alcohol consumption increases risk of infertility as reviewed by Barbieri (2001). Moderate alcohol consumption (4–7 units/week) was noted by Grodstein et al. (1994) to increase risk of ovulatory infertility, OR 1.3 (95% CI, 1.0–1.7), and of endometriosis, OR 1.6 (95% CI, 1.1–2.3). However, not all studies back up this viewpoint. Hassan and Killick (2004) reported that while heavy alcohol consumption by males (>20 units/week) increased the risk that a couple would be subfecund, OR 2.2 (95% CI, 1.1–4.4), alcohol intake of women had no impact on the outcome.

One explanation for this discrepancy may be that alcohol is consumed in different forms and in the process may deliver other compounds, including antioxidant flavonoids found in red wine, that might also influence fertility. Juhl and colleagues (2003) studied a cohort of 39 612 women, comprising 35% of all pregnant women in Denmark at the time of the study, and evaluated the impact of alcohol from different sources on the time taken to conceive a child after cessation of contraception. The consumption of beer by women had no effect on risk of delayed conception (more than 12 months to conceive). Wine at all levels of intake resulted in a shorter time to conception and reduced risk of delayed conception, OR 0.71 (95% CI, 0.58–0.88). Spirits at moderate intakes (2–7 units/week) also reduced risk of delayed conception, OR 0.56 (95% CI, 0.41–0.77), but at higher intakes impaired fertility, OR 2.40 (95% CI, 1.00–5.73). Although allowance was made in this study for confounding factors, the authors could not exclude the possibility that these findings reflect other characteristics of the women. Wine drinkers tend to also consume a more balanced diet of healthier foods.

Effects of alcohol are often confounded by tobacco smoking behaviour, and some studies suggest that the two factors interact with genetic influences. Taylor and colleagues (2011) reported reduced fertility in women who smoked and consumed at least one alcoholic drink per day. This adverse effect was only present in women who had a 'slow' phenotype for N-acetyltransferase 2, an enzyme that metabolizes components of tobacco smoke. The relationship between alcohol consumption and fertility in women is therefore highly complex and is strongly influenced by social status and other characteristics of women.

(comparing >300 mg/day with <100 mg/day), had no impact upon time to conception in women who were planning a pregnancy. Although the evidence is inconclusive, current advice is that women who wish to become pregnant should reduce intake of both alcohol and caffeine, with six cups of tea per day, three cups of coffee per day and one to two units of alcohol per week suggested as sensible limits.

2.3 Nutrition and male fertility

2.3.1 Determinants of fertility and infertility

While the origins of infertility in women are often complex and difficult to define, male fertility is readily assessed through simple measures of sperm production and quality. In general terms, the fertility of men depends on the quantity of sperm produced (defined either as sperm concentration per millilitre of ejaculate or as total numbers of sperm produced per ejaculation) or the characteristics of the sperm produced. The latter can be measured in terms of sperm motility (the capacity of the sperm to swim) and sperm morphology (assessments of the proportion of sperm cells with a normal healthy structure).

The process of sperm production is termed spermatogenesis, and this takes place in the seminiferous tubules

within the male reproductive tract. These tubules contain two specific cell types that drive the process. Germ cells are the cells that have the capacity to develop into sperm cells. These cells are supported by Sertoli cells which surround the germ cells, providing a protective barrier, and secrete nutrients and hormones. Spermatogenesis begins with the most primitive stage of germ cells which are termed spermatogonia. As shown in Figure 2.7, these cells go through rounds of mitotic and meiotic divisions before undergoing differentiation to produce mature sperm cells with specialized tail, mid- and head sections that can perform the required swimming and fertilization functions.

Spermatogenesis begins in males at around the time of puberty and will then continue throughout the adult lifespan. The process is regulated by a variety of hormonal factors which are produced by the hypothalamic–pituitary–gonadal axis (Figure 2.8). The hypothalamus produces GnRH in a pulsatile manner, with concentrations peaking every 90 min. Thus, a new batch of sperm cells can be produced every hour and a half throughout adult life. GnRH acts on the anterior pituitary to stimulate production of LH and FSH, each of which has different functions. LH acts directly on the Leydig cells of the testis to stimulate production of the main androgenic steroid, testosterone. In this context, testosterone is responsible for the stimulation of spermatogenesis, but this hormone is critical to male reproduction in other

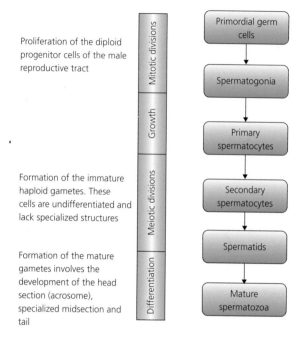

Proliferation of the diploid progenitor cells of the male reproductive tract

Formation of the immature haploid gametes. These cells are undifferentiated and lack specialized structures

Formation of the mature gametes involves the development of the head section (acrosome), specialized midsection and tail

Figure 2.7 Endocrine control of male reproductive function. In males, pulsatile hypothalamic production of GnRH stimulates the release of FSH and LH which stimulate the production of testosterone and the development of mature sperm in the testes. Testis-derived inhibin-B and testosterone have negative feedback effects in the anterior pituitary and hypothalamus and thereby regulate the hypothalamic–pituitary–testicular axis.

ways, as it initiates puberty, stimulates the male sex drive and promotes the development of the male secondary sexual characteristics. Testosterone stimulates spermatogenesis through action on the Sertoli cells. These cells are also a target for FSH which has the same function. This endocrine axis is subject to negative feedback regulation at two key points. Testosterone negatively feedbacks on production of both GnRH and LH, while FSH secretion is directly controlled by the production of inhibin-B from the Sertoli cells. As Sertoli cells require both FSH and testosterone stimulation to maintain spermatogenesis, inhibin-B effectively limits sperm production by reducing FSH production.

The male reproductive system may be particularly vulnerable to adverse effects of poor nutrition or environmental exposures by virtue of the way in which it develops and functions. The repeated production of new sperm over rapid intervals throughout adult life means that short-term influences on spermatogenesis may become important in determining fertility. Fetal life and early infancy may, however, represent more important points in life when food-borne influences may have the greatest impact on later fertility.

Initially, both male and female embryos develop a common ductal system, termed the Mullerian duct, that will ultimately go on to form the reproductive system. In males, early formation of Sertoli cells results in the production of anti-Mullerian hormone, causing the Wolffian

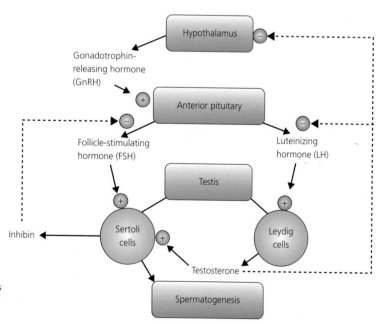

Figure 2.8 The formation of mature sperm. Sperm production in the male reproductive tract consists of mitotic and meiotic divisions followed by a differentiation phase in which sperm acquire their specialized structures.

duct to develop. This eventually forms the male reproductive organs. Masculinization of the reproductive
tissues also depends on production of testosterone and
its binding to the androgen receptor. There are many
defects of this process that have been identified, which
in the most extreme cases will lead to ambiguous genitalia, intersex and infertility (Sharpe, 1999). Development
of male fertility therefore depends heavily on Sertoli cell
numbers and function, which peak at around 1 year of
age. Earlier in the chapter, it was stated that a high
proportion of female subfertility and infertility can be
attributed to specific medical conditions. There are also
conditions which affect the male reproductive tract that
can impact upon fertility, of which the most important
are hypospadias and cryptorchidism. These appear to be
the product of adverse influences on early life development (Sharpe, 1999).

Hypospadias is a defect in which the opening of the
urethra is misplaced and may be at any point along the
shaft of the penis. This is one of the most common birth
defects of the male genitalia, occurring in as many as
1 in 125 boys. Like hypospadias, cryptorchidism is a
defect associated with early development of the reproductive tract. Cryptorchidism refers to a failure of the
testes to descend from the abdomen into the scrotum.
This occurs in approximately 3% of babies, but will
resolve in the majority, leaving around 1% of mature
adults with the condition. Both of these conditions can
reduce male fertility (e.g. around 10% of men with
cryptorchidism will be subfertile), and there is some evidence that the incidence of these conditions and other
defects of the reproductive tract (e.g. testicular cancers)
is on the increase (Sharpe, 1999). On a global scale, the
numbers of reported hypospadias increased by almost
threefold between 1950 and 1980 and by a further
twofold from 1980 to 2005. In the United States, 1% of
baby boys born in 2005 had hypospadias, compared to
0.4% in 1968. Cryptorchidism cases doubled between
1960 and 2002.

It is estimated that problems with male fertility explain
around 40% of subfecundity in couples attempting to
conceive a child. Initial reports from the United States of
a steady decline in sperm counts in the second half of
the twentieth century raised concerns that male fertility
may be declining in developed countries. Other reports
suggested that the European average sperm count in the
1940s and 1950s was around 170 million cells/ml, but
this had declined to 60 million cells/ml by 1990 (Sharpe
and Irvine, 2004). The assertion that male fertility is falling has been disputed by many researchers, as surveys
conducted across five decades may fail to use equivalent
methodologies and populations. However, methodological differences do not fully explain the observations

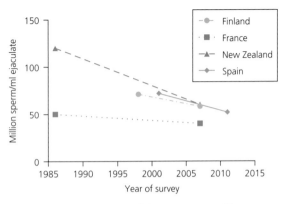

Figure 2.9 Contemporary trends in sperm counts. The
assertion that sperm counts fell sharply between the 1940s
and 1990s has been widely disputed. However, data from
recent surveys using robust methodologies often indicate a
progressive decline over a more recent period.
Data sources: Shine *et al.* (2008); Jørgensen *et al.* (2011);
Geoffroy-Siraudin *et al.* (2012); Mendiola *et al.* (2013).

as more recent surveys, using robust methodologies, in
a number of developed countries indicate small but
significant declines in sperm counts over the last two to
three decades (Figure 2.9). This clearly raises the question of why this has occurred and here attention must
shift to the environmental changes that have occurred
in Western populations over the same period. While
there are a number of environmental factors that may
be of importance, one of the main changes from the
1950s to the end of the twentieth century was the
industrialization of food production and the profound
change to the type of diet consumed by the population.
As developing countries go through improvements in
their economies and alongside this adopt a more westernized diet, sperm counts appear to fall accordingly.

2.3.2 Obesity

Obesity is a major problem for all Western countries,
and the rising trends in overweight and obesity largely
mirror the time period over which male fertility has
been in decline. Rates of overweight and obesity have
roughly doubled every 10 years over the last few decades, and in the United Kingdom, like most of Europe,
overweight (defined as BMI over 25 kg/m^2) is now seen
in two-thirds of men over the age of 15 (WHO, 2013).
In 2010, 26% of British men were defined as obese
(BMI over 30 kg/m^2). Over a third of US men are classified as obese (Ogden *et al.*, 2013).

BMI appears to be strongly associated with indices
of sperm quantity and quality. Underweight men have
low circulating testosterone concentrations and consequently fail to maintain normal spermatogenesis. Several

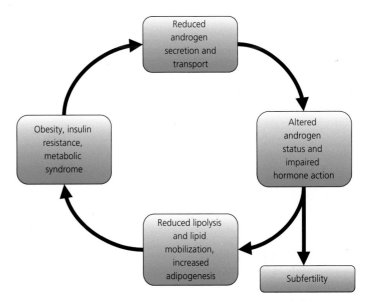

Figure 2.10 The relationship between male obesity and subfertility. Obesity and insulin resistance are a cause of infertility as they interfere with the normal secretion and transport of androgens. As androgens are activators of lipolysis, further adiposity is stimulated by impaired action of the androgens.

studies similarly show that overweight lowers sperm counts. Reports suggest that subfertile men are three times more likely to be obese than men with normal fertility (Magnusdottir *et al.*, 2005). A number of studies have reported that obese men produce lower sperm concentrations than men of ideal BMI. Sermondade *et al.* (2013) found that men of BMI 30–35 kg/m² were 31% more likely to have a sperm count below 40 million cells/ml ejaculate than men of BMI 20–25. Morbidly obese men (BMI > 35 kg/m²) were twice as likely to have lower sperm counts. Sperm samples from overweight and obese men have also been reported to show more evidence of oxidative damage.

Obesity has important effects on the endocrine control of spermatogenesis. Men with excess body fat have lower circulating testosterone concentrations and also produce lower quantities of sex hormone binding proteins which play a key role in the transport of testosterone to the gonads. The lowering of testosterone appears to be driven by a reduced secretion of LH in response to GnRH pulses. As shown in Figure 2.10, there is a cyclical relationship between obesity and sex hormone production in men, as while excess body fat lowers testosterone production, the lower androgen stimulation of the adipose tissue reduces lipolysis and hence promotes further fat deposition. Obesity in men is also associated with a lower production of inhibin-B. While this might initially be thought to promote spermatogenesis by reducing negative feedback on FSH production (see Figure 2.8), lower inhibin-B production is likely to be indicative of lower Sertoli cell numbers and hence reduced capacity for spermatogenesis.

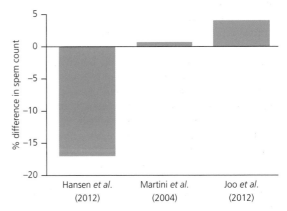

Figure 2.11 The impact of alcohol intake on sperm count is minimal. Moderate intake of alcohol is not associated with adverse effects upon sperm counts. Hansen *et al.* (2012) compared men consuming 96 units of alcohol or more with non-consumers. Martini *et al.* (2004) considered any alcohol consumption against non-consumption, and Joo *et al.* (2012) evaluated the effect of >33 g alcohol/day against <6.4 g/day. None of the studies found a statistically significant effect.

2.3.3 Alcohol

Excess consumption of alcohol has been linked to subfertility in males, in studies of both humans and animals. Studies that compare fertile and subfertile men indicate that alcohol consumption is generally higher in the subfertile population, but as shown in Figure 2.11, there is little evidence that moderate alcohol consumption has a direct effect upon sperm production. Excessive alcohol intakes impair the hypothalamic–pituitary–testicular axis and Sertoli cell functions and are associated with lower total sperm counts, semen volume, sperm motility and increased numbers of sperm with abnormal morphology (Emanuele and Emanuele, 2001). The full mechanism that drives this process is not well established in humans, but studies of animals indicate that chronically high alcohol intakes lower testosterone production and that ethanol may be directly toxic to testicular tissues. Certainly, the increased numbers of sperm with abnormal morphology associated with excess alcohol may be suggestive of a spermatotoxic effect.

2.3.4 Zinc

Zinc is an essential micronutrient required for the production of a wide range of enzymes, receptors and structural proteins. Zinc is an active site component of over 200 different metalloenzymes and is chiefly involved in stabilization of protein structures, synthesis of DNA and RNA, formation of chromatin, protein synthesis, digestive processes (notably the pancreatic enzymes), antioxidant defences (cofactor for superoxide dismutase) and oxygen transport.

Zinc is postulated to play a role in several components of male reproductive function, and zinc deficiency in some parts of the Middle East has been classically linked to delayed sexual maturation in adolescent boys. The testes have a very high zinc content compared to other organs and tissues, and zinc concentrations are particularly high in the seminal fluid produced by the prostate gland. Data on the role of zinc in maintaining fertility in human males is sparse. There are reports, however, that men with low sperm counts (<20 million cells/ml) have reduced seminal zinc concentrations compared to normospermic individuals (Fuse et al., 1999) and seminal zinc concentration is positively correlated with sperm quality. It has been suggested that a small proportion of idiopathic infertility in men may be explained by poor zinc status. Intervention studies that have considered the impact of zinc supplementation on fertility suggest some improvements in sperm counts, motility and morphology and increased testosterone concentrations. In the study of Wong and colleagues (2002), administration of 66 mg/day zinc sulphate over 6 months had no impact on indices of sperm quality or quantity in fertile men, but in subfertile men increased numbers of sperm with normal motility and morphology by 74%. Despite this major increase, the mean sperm counts in these subfertile men remained below the 20 million cells/ml that the World Health Organization (WHO) use as the cut-off to define subfertility.

2.3.5 Antioxidant nutrients

Free radicals and other ROS were discussed in the context of female fertility earlier in this chapter. While ROS are generally perceived as having negative, tissue-damaging effects in biological systems, it is important to realize that endogenously generated ROS also play a number of important physiological roles. The manufacture of sperm is one such role, and ROS produced within immature sperm cells are important in the production of the tail sheath that encloses the mitochondria of the midsection, which will ultimately generate ATP and provide the motile function of the sperm cells. ROS are also important in the functions of spermatozoa during fertilization and are generated to promote attachment to oocytes and to generate the acrosome reaction, which allows the sperm to penetrate the zona pellucida layer of the oocyte.

As ROS are critical for normal sperm functions, mature sperm cells are less protected with antioxidants than most other cell types, although the immature cells are rich in the antioxidant enzymes superoxide dismutase, glutathione peroxidase (GPx) and catalase. Mature cells are vulnerable to damage by ROS, which will principally cause fragmentation of DNA, the primary morphological abnormality noted in subfertile men. Immature sperm cells are vulnerable as they are producing ROS for differentiation and are present in a membrane-rich tissue. Biological membranes are rich in polyunsaturated fatty acids, which are a major target for ROS-mediated damage. There is clearly a delicate balance between oxidative and antioxidant processes in sperm cells and their associated support tissues.

On the basis of this, it is widely asserted that increasing antioxidant intakes, particularly through supplements, will improve fertility, especially in subfertile men. Although there are biologically plausible mechanisms that could explain any beneficial effect of antioxidants, there is a dearth of strong evidence to suggest that antioxidant therapy is truly effective or necessary (Showell et al., 2011). A number of studies have compared subfertile men with healthy, normospermic donors and reported that subfertile men have higher concentrations of ROS and lower concentrations of antioxidant nutrients in semen samples (Moustafa et al., 2004). Other studies have shown that the addition of antioxidants, for example, glutathione or α-tocopherol to culture media used in artificial reproductive technologies, boosts conception rates by increasing the motility of spermatozoa (Ozawa et al., 2006).

There are few studies that have considered the impact of antioxidant intakes within a normal diet upon indices of male fertility. Eskenazi and colleagues (2005) assessed intakes of vitamins A, C and E, along with zinc and selenium using food frequency questionnaires in fertile men. The intakes of these nutrients were then considered in relation to indices of semen quality. While zinc and selenium intakes were not associated with markers of fertility, higher vitamin C, ß-carotene and α-tocopherol intakes were all associated with greater semen quality. Considering all three antioxidant nutrients together, it was shown that higher intakes increased sperm concentrations and numbers of motile sperm cells. Similarly, a small cross-sectional study by Schmid *et al.* (2012) reported that higher intakes of vitamin C, vitamin E, folate and zinc were associated with less oxidative damage to sperm, but only in men over 44 years of age.

Studies of supplementation generally use very high doses of single antioxidant nutrients, and their findings are largely inconclusive. The lack of clear effects may be a product of poor study design or adverse responses to high local concentrations of antioxidant compounds, many of which have a paradoxical pro-oxidant activity in excess. Menezo *et al.* (2007), for example, reported that while multivitamin supplements reduced DNA fragmentation in sperm from subfertile men, the high ascorbic acid dose appeared to promote sperm chromatin decondensation, a process that should normally occur only after fertilization of an oocyte. Tremellen *et al.* (2007) reported improved success in ICSI following oral administration of a mixed supplement of folic acid, selenium, zinc and antioxidants. Ross *et al.* (2010) performed a systematic review of the literature to assess the efficacy of antioxidant supplements in improving sperm parameters and the ability to conceive a child in infertile men. They concluded that although more adequately powered trials of antioxidants are needed, there is sufficient evidence to support the use of oral antioxidants to improve sperm quality and pregnancy rates.

2.3.6 Selenium

It is well established from animal studies that selenium is a key nutrient for the maintenance of male fertility. Selenium deficiency in animals or the knockout of key genes in mice that lead to production of selenoproteins leads to lower sperm production and poor sperm motility. Selenium appears to be particularly important in the formation of the tail piece in mammalian sperm. As described previously, this is a process that involves the generation of ROS and a balance between oxidative and antioxidative processes is critical in normal differentiation of the spermatids. Selenium is a cofactor for the antioxidant enzyme GPx, and in sperm, the GPX4 isoform appears particularly important in tail formation (Beckett and Arthur, 2005). Although there is clear evidence that many subfertile men with sperm defects have abnormalities of GPX4 in their sperm, it is unlikely that in most cases this is due to limiting intakes of selenium in the diet.

In populations where selenium intakes are low (e.g. Scotland), there is no strong evidence of lower fertility. A detailed study of men whose selenium status was controlled for a period of 120 days while living on a metabolic unit (Hawkes and Turek, 2001) suggested that while a high-selenium diet produced large increases in seminal selenium concentrations, sperm motility actually decreased. This suggests that the common recommendation to consume rich sources of selenium, for example, Brazil nuts, for men preparing for fatherhood may be ineffective.

2.3.7 Phytoestrogens and environmental oestrogens

In developed countries, populations are constantly exposed to a range of chemical agents that have endocrine-disrupting properties. Endocrine disruptors are agents that interfere with normal hormonal functions within the body, either by having a direct hormonal effect or by opposing the actions of endogenous hormones (anti-hormones). Human exposure to endocrine disruptors comes from a wide range of different sources (Table 2.2), most of which are unavoidable due to their presence in the food chain, atmosphere and water supply.

Endocrine disruptors are known from studies of the impact of human activity on wildlife to be particularly potent within the reproductive organs. For example, tributyltin, an antifouling agent used on ships, was found to be an anti-hormone blocking production of oestrogen and masculinizing shellfish. The excretion of oestrogen metabolites in urine from women using certain oral contraceptives has been blamed for the feminization of male fish found around sewage outlets. Clear examples of effects of endocrine disruptors on human male fertility

Table 2.2 Environmental sources of human exposure to endocrine-disrupting chemicals.

Source	Examples	Putative effects
Atmosphere (inhalation)	Polyaromatic hydrocarbons	Suppress oestrogen metabolism
Cosmetics	Parabens (in shampoos, perfumes, deodorants)	Oestrogen mimics
	Phthalates	Suppress testosterone synthesis
	Nitromusks	Inhibit hypothalamic–gonadotrophic axis
Food chain	Plasticizers (phthalates)	Suppress testosterone synthesis
	Polyaromatic hydrocarbons	Suppress oestrogen metabolism
	Pesticides and fungicides	Oestrogenic and anti-androgenic effects
Water supply	Atrazine (herbicide)	Oestrogen mimic
	17β-Oestradiol	Oestrogenic effect

are more difficult to demonstrate, but there are a number of agents that have been proposed as potentially harmful. These are described in the following.

2.3.7.1 Phthalates

Phthalates are a class of chemicals used to make plastics. They are widely used in the production of cosmetics, toys and all manner of goods that require flexible plastics. Phthalates are known to adversely affect the male reproductive system in animals, inducing both hypospadias and cryptorchidism and leading to reduced testosterone production and sperm counts (Sharpe and Irvine, 2004). Exposure to phthalates during human fetal development has been linked to feminization of baby boys, and this has led to widespread concern at the potential for these agents to enter formula milk consumed by infants during the critical phase of reproductive development. However, levels of phthalates in formula milks have been shown to be low and are now monitored. Studies show that phthalates also appear in breast milk, as they are excreted following maternal exposure. There is also some evidence of associations between phthalate exposure and fertility in mature men. The mode of phthalate action is simply to inhibit testosterone production. Measurements of phthalate metabolites have proved to be inversely proportional to sperm counts (Sharpe and Irvine, 2004).

2.3.7.2 Phytoestrogens

Phytoestrogens are plant-derived compounds that have a weak oestrogenic activity by virtue of a similar molecular structure to oestrogens (Figure 2.12). Within the human diet, they are ingested either in the form of lignans, which are present in vegetable matter, or as soya-derived isoflavones, which include genistein and daidzein. Intakes of isoflavones within the diet vary immensely both within and between different populations. Average intakes for omnivores in the United Kingdom are around 1 mg/day, while vegetarians have much higher intakes at

around 7–8 mg/day. In Japan and Southeast Asia, soya is consumed as a staple food, for example, as tempeh or tofu, and intakes are around 25–100 mg/day.

The oestrogenic effects of phytoestrogens have a number of positive effects upon health in women, which will be dealt with elsewhere in this book. There have been concerns over their impact upon male reproductive health, particularly as within a Western diet soya is becoming very widely used as an ingredient in processed foods and as a meat substitute. These concerns arise primarily from studies of animals suggesting that phytoestrogens may have effects on both young, developing males but not mature individuals. Several studies have shown in rats and mice that comparing offspring of pregnant animals fed diets containing soya to those fed a soya-free diet reveals differences in testicular weight, circulating FSH and capacity to successfully mate with females. Atanassova and colleagues (2000) found that adverse effects of genistein on indices of fertility in male rats were at their greatest when it was administered during puberty. In contrast, Tan *et al.* (2006) studied the impact of feeding soy formula milk to baby marmosets and found no gross effects upon their reproductive organs in later life.

In humans, dietary phytoestrogens appear to have pronounced effects on endocrine markers in women, but not in men. There is no evidence that in Asian countries where intakes are high, fertility is impaired. This may in part be due to the low prevalence of obesity in such populations. Trials that have considered the impact of high-dose isoflavone consumption in men indicate that there is little risk to reproductive health. Six weeks of consumption of flax seed had no effect on plasma testosterone or sex hormone binding globulin (Shultz *et al.*, 1991), and the study of Mitchell *et al.* (2001) found no effect of 40 mg/day isoflavones on sex hormone concentrations, testicular volume or indices of semen quantity or quality. A critical review by Messina (2010) concluded that soybean isoflavones have no feminizing

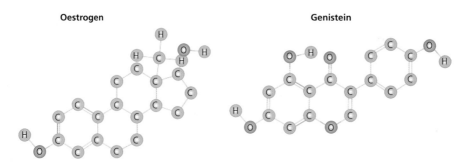

Figure 2.12 The structures of oestrogen and phytoestrogens. Phytoestrogens such as genistein and daidzein (the principal soya isoflavones) have a similar chemical structure to oestrogens, allowing binding to the oestrogen receptors.

effects upon adult men, with no significant impact on fertility. However, Xia *et al.* (2013) reported that in a population of over 1000 Chinese men, the odds of infertility were increased in those in the highest quintile of daidzein excretion (>260 μg/g creatinine; 2.5-fold risk of low sperm count, 2-fold risk of low sperm motility).

While data on exposure of older men to phytoestrogens does not consistently support the evidence of risk inferred from animal studies, an impact of phytoestrogen exposure during infancy cannot be excluded. Early life exposure to isoflavones through sources other than soy milk formula in infancy is difficult to evaluate, but there is some data suggesting an association with reproductive abnormalities. A study of the ALSPAC cohort, a large longitudinal study of pregnancy and childhood in the Bristol area of the United Kingdom, suggested that vegetarian mothers were almost five times more likely to have baby boys with hypospadias than omnivorous mothers (North and Golding, 2000). This may be attributed either to the high phytoestrogen content of the maternal diet or to greater ingestion of pesticides and other contaminants on fruit and vegetable matter. There are no data available on fertility rates or markers of semen quality from individuals exposed to high levels of phytoestrogen in fetal life or infancy.

2.3.7.3 Pesticides

A huge range of organic pesticides are present within the environment, and many of these are known to have endocrine-disrupting properties. Of greatest concern are those which have the potential to enter the food chain as contaminants. Vinclozolin is an example of a pesticide that has been linked to male fertility problems in animals (Gray *et al.*, 1999). Vinclozolin is a fungicide used in the production of oil seed rape, peas and fruits such as grapes.

Studies of this agent in rats and other species show that, at doses that may be consumed by humans, it can feminize males and damage their reproductive capacity. As with phthalates, the early stages of fetal development appear to be a sensitive period for exposure. Although there is no clear evidence of harmful effects in humans, approvals for use of this agent on strawberries, tomatoes, lettuce and raspberries were withdrawn by the UK and European Commission in the 1990s.

The impact of pesticide exposure upon fertility might best be evaluated by considering the effects of occupational exposure in farmers, the individuals who actually make direct use of these chemicals during food production. Organic farmers, who produce food without use of chemical fertilizers and pesticides, make an interesting reference group. A number of studies (Table 2.3) have compared sperm counts in organic farmers with other groups of workers and have found that the organic farmers tend to have higher sperm concentrations. However, such studies may be flawed as they fail to take into account the other occupational exposures experienced by the non-farming group. The study of Juhler and colleagues (1999) avoided this problem by comparing 14 indices of sperm quantity and quality in a group of organic compared to conventional farmers. No differences in any of the indices were noted, suggesting that agricultural chemical exposure did not impact on fertility. The lack of clear risk associated with direct use of agricultural chemicals (Table 2.3) would suggest that the much lesser exposure experienced by the majority of men via the food chain is unlikely to be harmful to fertility. However, it is important to note that there are no robust studies that have considered the impact of exposure to pesticide contaminants in food during the first year of life, or fetal development.

Table 2.3 Organic food, pesticide exposure and semen quality.

Study reference	Comparison	Outcomes
Abell *et al.* (1994)	Organic farmers compared to printers, electricians and metalworkers	Sperm counts higher in organic farmers (100 vs 55 million cells/ml)
Jensen *et al.* (1996)	Organic food association members compared to airline workers	Sperm counts higher in organic group (99 vs 48 million cells/ml)
Larsen *et al.* (1999)	Organic farmers compared to traditional farmers	No difference in sperm count, motility or morphology
Juhler *et al.* (1999)	Organic farmers compared to traditional farmers, considering consumption of organic produce	No differences in 14 different indices of male fertility
Kenkel *et al.* (2001)	Traditional farmers and low chemical-exposure risk occupations	Farmers at higher risk (OR 2.13) for reduced sperm count
De Fleurian *et al.* (2009)	Pesticide use among men of varied occupations	No significant risk associated with pesticide use OR for abnormal semen 3.6 (0.8–15.8)
Hossain *et al.* (2010)	Farmers with low or high exposure to pesticides	Lower sperm count with high exposure (21 vs 55 million cells/ml). Less motile sperm

2.4 Preparation for pregnancy

2.4.1 Why prepare for pregnancy?

With modern healthcare and an increasing emphasis on maintaining and promoting health, rather than treating disease, provision of advice and care during the preconceptual period is becoming more commonplace in developed countries. The main aim of any work in this area will be to maximize the health of both prospective parents, and this will maximize their fertility (as described previously) and minimize the potential for the early embryo to be exposed to potentially harmful agents. To achieve this aim, it is necessary to address the controllable risk factors for adverse pregnancy outcomes while parents are still planning a pregnancy (Table 2.4). Clearly, not all such factors are directly related to nutrition, but social, environmental and behavioural elements are all interlinked and impact upon individuals' attitudes, choices and opportunities in relation to lifestyle and diet.

In addition to maximizing fertility, it is important to eliminate the potential for an early embryo to be exposed to factors that could exert harmful effects should a conception occur. To this end, the preparatory phase before conception should ideally involve lifestyle changes for both men and women. Although women are preparing and providing the environment in which the fetus will develop, their chances of success in making lifestyle changes will be considerably greater if they do so in partnership. Men are therefore responsible for much more than maximizing their own fertility and should cooperate with women in maintaining a healthy body weight, in ensuring that immunizations against infections that might harm the fetus (e.g. Rubella) are up to date and in reducing exposures to alcohol and tobacco smoke. From a dietary point of view, there are two important changes that should be made to minimize risk of birth defects. These are increasing intakes of folic acid and reducing exposure to high doses of vitamin A, both of which are described in more detail in the following.

2.4.2 Maternal weight management

In addition to adverse effects upon female fertility, maternal overweight and excessive weight gain in pregnancy is a major risk factor for poor pregnancy outcomes, as will be described in Chapter 3. Weight during pregnancy and the rate of weight gain during pregnancy are closely linked to weight prior to pregnancy, and pre-pregnancy weight is strongly associated with risk of gestational diabetes and hypertensive complications in pregnancy (Li *et al.*, 2013) and may also predict the health of children in later life (Hinkle *et al.*, 2013). The recommendations on pregnancy weight gain made by the US Institute of Medicine (2009) are stratified by pre-pregnancy BMI (see Section 3.4.2.1), reflecting the important contribution of weight prior to conception upon pregnancy outcomes.

Although lower weight gain in pregnancy is advised for overweight or obese women, weight loss is not advised during pregnancy, as this may limit provision of nutrients to the developing fetus. Weight loss advice is instead targeted at women prior to conception. In 2010, the UK National Institute for Health and Clinical Excellence issued a guideline that health professionals should identify women with BMI over 30 kg/m^2 prior to pregnancy and advise a 5–10% weight loss prior to conception (NICE, 2010). This guidance aims to improve conception rates and reduce pregnancy complications.

2.4.3 Vitamin A and liver

Vitamin A is one of the essential nutrients in the diet, but intake should be restricted during pregnancy due to a well-established association with birth defects. In the diet, vitamin A is available in two forms, the first being animal-derived retinol and the second plant-derived carotenoids. Due to this diversity of sources, vitamin A intakes are generally described in terms of retinol activity equivalents (RAE) with one RAE being equivalent to 1 µg retinol or 6 µg ß-carotene. Generally, intakes of vitamin A are measured as mg retinol equivalents or international units (IU, with one RAE equivalent to 3.3 IU). Once within the body, vitamin A undergoes extensive metabolism as shown in Figure 2.13 and in addition to mediating some of the classically defined

Table 2.4 Factors that impact on parental health during the periconceptual period.

Controllable factors		Examples
Environmental factors:	the influence of home and workplace	Hygiene, sanitation, occupational chemical exposure
Lifestyle factors:	the health choices and behaviours of the parents	Smoking, alcohol, diet, exercise
Uncontrollable factors		**Examples**
Social factors:	the circumstances in which the parents live	Family income Access to healthcare, education
Physiological factors:	the underlying health circumstances of the parents	Genetic disorders, age, obstetric disorders, infection

Adapted from Langley-Evans (2004).

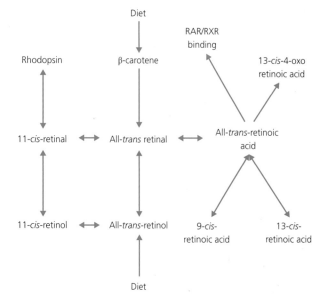

Figure 2.13 The metabolism of vitamin A. Dietary sources of vitamin A deliver preformed retinol (from animal sources) or ß-carotene. Retinol from the diet or formed within the liver is used to generate rhodopsin in the retina and is converted to retinoic acid which modulates gene expression via the RAR/RXR receptors. Retinoic acid can be metabolized to a number of intermediates that are known to have teratogenic properties in animals and humans.

functions, such as formation of rhodopsin within the retina, is an important regulator of gene expression through the retinoic acid and retinoid X receptors.

Vitamin A first was shown to be a teratogen in studies of animals. The administration of high doses of retinol and all-trans retinoic acid during pregnancy induced abnormalities in almost all tissues of fetal mice, rats, hamsters, rabbits and non-human primates (Soprano and Soprano, 1995). The demonstration that the same effects occur in humans has generally relied on the observation of the adverse effects of certain pharmacological agents. Retinoid derivatives are widely used in the treatment of skin conditions such as severe acne. Pregnant women who used products containing 12-*cis*-retinoic acid had babies with craniofacial abnormalities such as cleft lip, with heart defects and with abnormalities of the central nervous system. Such products are therefore contraindicated in women who are pregnant or considering having a child.

There are very few recorded cases in which overconsumption of dietary vitamin A can be firmly attributed as the cause of birth defects in humans. However, where this is the case (Soprano and Soprano, 1995), the defects generated tend to be highly variable and to occur across multiple organ systems, including the heart. Martinez-Frias and Salvador (1990) compared Spanish women who had given birth to babies with congenital malformations (cases) with women whose babies were normally developed (controls). The overwhelming majority of cases were unrelated to vitamin A teratogenicity, but among women who had taken megadose supplements of vitamin A, there were

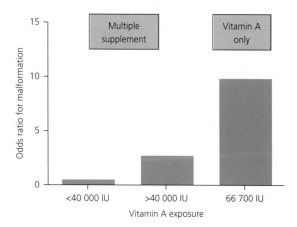

Figure 2.14 Vitamin A supplementation and fetal malformations. The relationship between vitamin A supplementation and fetal malformations was explored in a population of Spanish women. The data shows odds of malformations associated with vitamin A in a multivitamin supplement, higher levels of vitamin A in a multivitamin supplement and megadose supplements of vitamin A alone. *Data source:* Martinez-Frias and Salvador (1990).

significant associations between consumption and malformations. As shown in Figure 2.14, at doses below 40 000 IU, there was no increased risk, but over 40 000, the odds of malformation were increased 2.7-fold. The greatest risk was associated with consumption of vitamin A alone, at doses of over 60 000 IU. Further studies have gone on to suggest that vitamin A doses of only 10 000–25 000 IU may be harmful during embryonic and fetal development. As a result, pregnant women, or those planning a pregnancy, should avoid vitamin A containing supplements. Typical multivitamins available over-the-counter contain approximately 8000–9000 IU. Although the Martinez-Frias study suffers from the generic problems associated with case–control studies (choice of control group can be problematic, study cannot firmly demonstrate causal relationships, exposure to nutrient has to be done retrospectively and may be inaccurate), together with the data from animal and pharmacological studies, it appears that excessive levels of vitamin A consumption do play a causal role in development of fetal abnormalities.

Liver is a major source of preformed retinol within the diet, and a 100 g portion of beef liver may deliver 32 000 IU vitamin A in a single meal. The vitamin A content of liver has increased since the 1980s due to intensive farming, and so the associated risk in modern times is likely to be greater than in the past, when pregnant women were actively encouraged to eat liver as a source of iron. In particular, liver appears to increase circulating concentrations of two of the most teratogenic isomers of retinoic acid, namely, 13-*cis*-retinoic acid and 13-*cis*-4-oxo-retinoic acid. Arnhold *et al.* (1996) showed that feeding male volunteers fried turkey liver significantly elevated concentrations of all metabolites of retinol within a short period of time. Similarly, Hartmann *et al.* (2005) found that feeding non-pregnant women 120 000 IU vitamin A in a liver meal greatly increased plasma 13-*cis*-retinoic acid and 13-*cis*-4-oxo-retinoic acid concentrations. Clearly, with these observations, alongside the studies of Martinez-Frias and Salvador (1990), caution is appropriate and liver should be avoided by women planning a pregnancy. An important consideration is that consumption of liver appears to increase circulating retinoic acid metabolites in women, to a much greater extent than consumption of a vitamin A supplement of equivalent dosage (van Vliet *et al.*, 2001).

2.4.4 Folic acid and neural tube defects

Neural tube defects (NTDs) are among the most common fetal abnormalities observed in Western populations. These conditions, of which the most significant are spina bifida and anencephaly, currently affect 0.3 births in every 1000 in the United Kingdom, representing around 150–200 cases every year. However, the true number of NTDs is considerably higher (~4 cases per 1000 births) and most affected fetuses are terminated after diagnosis with antenatal ultrasound scans.

Spina bifida and anencephaly are different manifestations of the same developmental problem. During normal development, the embryonic neural tube, which will go on to become the brain and the spinal cord, undergoes a process of folding and closing to form an enclosed neural canal. This closure of the neural tube will normally occur in the fourth week of gestation, a time which is generally too early for the mother to be aware of her pregnancy. Failure of the neural tube to close results in permanent disability, the severity of which depends on the location of the tube lesion. A lesion high up along the neural tube will result in anencephaly, a condition in which the cerebral arches of the brain will be absent. Babies with anencephaly will inevitably die, either during gestation or within a few hours of birth. Lesions lower down the neural tube will result in spina bifida. As the spinal cord is not fully encased in bone, it is vulnerable to injury and damaged spinal nerves and cord are associated with paralysis, incontinence and in some cases delayed cognitive development and learning disabilities.

As shown in Research Highlight 2.2, low maternal intake of folic acid is one of several risk factors for NTDs. The demands of the fetus for folate around the time of the closure of the neural tube are high as folates are important cofactors for the synthesis of purine nucleotides and thymidylate which are required for cell division. If folate is a limiting nucleotide at this time, then neural tube closure may be irreversibly compromised. The link between folic acid and NTDs was firmly established through intervention trials using varying doses of folic acid in combination with other micronutrients (Laurence *et al.*, 1981; Czeizel and Dudas, 1992). The MRC Vitamin Study Group (1991) performed a randomized, double-blind trial of 1817 women in 33 centres, across 7 countries. All women had a previous history of a pregnancy with NTD and were randomized to either a placebo group; a group given a supplement of folic acid alone (4 mg/day); a group provided with a supplement containing vitamins A, D, B1, B2, B6 and C and nicotinamide; or a fourth group provided with the same multivitamin supplement plus folate. Supplementation to 12 weeks of gestation produced the greatest beneficial effect when folate was given alone (72% reduction in NTD risk). Folate as an element of a multivitamin supplement was effective, but less so than as a single nutrient.

On the basis of the MRC study and the work of Czeizel and Dudas (1992), it is clear that increasing dietary supply of folic acid will reduce the risk of a pregnancy being affected by an NTD. Accordingly, the RNI for folic acid increases during pregnancy from 200 to 600 mg/day. However, as neural tube closure is an early event in embryonic development, any increase in maternal supply has to occur prior to conception to ensure risk is minimal. To this end, there are two strategies that can be used to protect the population: supplementation and fortification.

Research Highlight 2.2 Risk factors for neural tube defects.

The risk of a neural tube defect (NTD)-affected pregnancy is multifactorial (Agopian *et al.*, 2013), with greater risk associated with a family history of such defects, particular ethnic backgrounds, obesity, poorly controlled diabetes before pregnancy, gestational diabetes, low intakes of folate, use of anticonvulsant drugs for epilepsy and maternal hyperthermia (e.g. use of saunas). The role of genetics is considerable, and women who have previously had an NTD-affected pregnancy are at 100-fold greater risk in subsequent pregnancies. A number of genetic susceptibilities have been identified which include some of the enzymes involved in folic acid metabolism, genes associated with glucose homeostasis and insulin resistance (Lupo *et al.*, 2012). The genetic risk predictors are complex as multiple genotypes may interact within the mother and between mother and fetus to determine how the neural tube develops.

The major avoidable risk factors are obesity and folate intake. The impact of obesity is considerable and may be linked to the metabolic impact of excess body fatness upon glucose homeostasis. Gao *et al.* (2013) reported OR of 2.45 for NTD associated with overweight and a systematic review of 39 articles by Stothard *et al.* (2009) found that risk of all NTD was increased by 1.87-fold (95% CI, 1.62–2.15) in obese women (OR for spina bifida 2.24 (0.86–2.69)). Risk was shown to be considerably higher in women with two features of the metabolic syndrome (Ray *et al.*, 2007) or in women with excessive sugar intakes prior to conception.

Obesity may also modify risk of NTD through changes in folate metabolism, transport and storage. Benefits of folate supplementation are only seen in women of normal weight and are absent in overweight or obese groups (Wang *et al.*, 2013). Tinker *et al.* (2012) reported that in women with higher BMI, serum folate concentrations were lower than in women of ideal BMI, while red cell folate concentrations were elevated. This suggested that obesity may impact upon the distribution and availability of folate to the developing embryo. On this basis, recommendations for folic acid supplementation might need to be different for women of greater BMI. However, there is also evidence that the relationship between obesity and NTD risk is independent of any influence of folate. By comparing the prevalence of NTD in obese women in the United States prior to and after the introduction of mandatory fortification of grains with folic acid, Ray *et al.* (2005) showed that the risk associated with obesity increased after the folate status of the population had improved. This would indicate that folate-independent mechanisms increase NTD risk in overweight women.

2.4.4.1 Supplementation with folic acid

Supplementation with folic acid prior to conception and in the early stages of pregnancy is the approach to NTD prevention in most European countries. In 1992, the UK Chief Medical Officer first announced a firm recommendation that women who are considering pregnancy should take a 400 µg/day supplement of folic acid for 3 months prior to conception and for the first 12 weeks of pregnancy, in order to reduce risk of NTD. This strategy was devised with the intention that it would cover the period of neural tube closure (often occurring before a woman knows she is pregnant) and reduce risk by approximately half. Supplementation was considered necessary as achieving 400 µg/day extra intake through diet alone would require impossible increases in consumption of fruits and vegetables. Women with a prior history of NTD were advised to take a 4 mg/day supplement, the dose noted to be effective in the MRC Vitamin Study Group trial.

As shown in Figure 2.15, the impact of folic acid supplementation in the United Kingdom upon NTD prevalence was modest, with a decline that was barely distinguishable from a general downward trend associated with improved antenatal screening and other factors. This limited success highlights the main difficulty with supplementation on a population-wide scale, which is providing the necessary health education and awareness campaigns to ensure a high level of compliance.

Younger women, women of lower educational achievement and women who smoke are the population groups that are least likely to use folate supplements (Langley-Evans and Langley-Evans, 2001). Moreover, with 40% of pregnancies reported to be unplanned, the impact of periconceptual supplementation is inevitably reduced.

2.4.4.2 Fortification with folic acid

As described previously, the major problem with a prevention strategy based on supplementation is that full coverage of all of the at-risk population can never be achieved. In the United Kingdom, it was found that even after many years to allow for training of health professionals and promotion of supplementation through health education, the policy did not achieve the expected reduction in risk. The alternative to supplementation, which depends upon individuals making an active decision to change dietary behaviour, is fortification of staple foods that are widely consumed by the target population.

Fortification of wheat flours has been adopted worldwide as a public health nutrition strategy in over 50 countries including Canada (1998, addition of 150 µg folate/100 g grain), Chile (1998, 220 µg folate/100 g grain), Costa Rica (180 µg folate/100 g grain) and South Africa (2003, 150 µg folate/100 g grain). The level of fortification varies between countries to reflect national trends in consumption of wheat products. Fortification

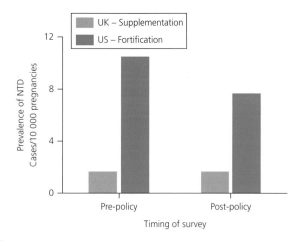

Figure 2.15 US fortification with folic acid has been more effective than supplementation in the United Kingdom in the prevention of neural tube defects. In 1992, the United Kingdom introduced guidelines recommending supplementation with folic acid in preparation for pregnancy to reduce NTD risk. The United States introduced mandatory fortification of grains with folic acid in 1998. UK data corresponds to 1990 (pre-policy) and 1999 (post-policy) and shows a decline of 2%. US data corresponds to 1995–1996 (pre-policy) and 1999–2000 (post-policy) and shows a decline of 27%.
Data sources: CDC (2004); Morris and Wald (1999).

with folate became mandatory in the United States in 1998 (140 μg folate/100 g grain) and as shown in Figure 2.15 proved highly effective in reducing the prevalence of NTDs. Pfeiffer and colleagues (2005) examined the impact of this policy on folate status in the US population and found that fortification reduced the prevalence of low serum folate concentrations dramatically, with benefits observed in all ethnic groups, in both sexes and in people of all ages. Between 1995, when a period of optional fortification began, and 2002, intakes of folate in the US population doubled. The prevalence of spina bifida declined by 36% among Hispanic women (the highest-risk group in the United States) and 34% among the white population (Williams *et al.*, 2005).

Fortification through wheat flours may not reach all women of childbearing age, and so other fortified products are required to achieve full coverage in the population. In the United States, although NTD levels declined sharply among Hispanic women, this group remained at higher risk than other ethnic groups. The staple for this population is corn masa flour which is not fortified. It is estimated that inclusion of this product in the fortification programme could achieve further reductions in NTD among Hispanics (Tinker *et al.*, 2013).

Where fortification of staple foods with folate has been introduced, there are reports of benefits to the wider adult population in terms of cardiovascular health and cancer risk (See Section 8.4.4.3.4). This shows a reach for this policy that extends beyond the intended target group. However, governments in a number of countries including the United Kingdom, Germany, Ireland and the Netherlands have been reluctant to implement fortification despite recommendations from expert committees (SACN, 2006) to do so. There are two key concerns about the adverse consequences of folate overconsumption that have led to this caution.

Firstly, there have been reports that following introduction of fortification in North America, or with supplementation at 400 μg/day folic acid, there was an increase in risk of colorectal and breast cancer (Charles *et al.*, 2004; Mason *et al.*, 2007). This may be because some tumours remain in a pre-malignant state for long periods in individuals with poor folate status, becoming malignant only when intake increases and availability of nucleotide precursors meets demand for tumour cell division. The other concern is that improving folate status in elderly people may mask the haematological symptoms of vitamin B12 deficiency, increasing the risk of pernicious anaemia. The experience from the United States, however, is that folate fortification had no impact on the prevalence of low B12 status in the elderly population. Intakes of folic acid up to 1 mg/day are not associated with delayed diagnosis of vitamin B12 deficiency (SACN, 2006). Consumption in countries with fortification tends to be well below that level (e.g. median intake in post-fortification United States is around 450 μg/day). Less than 5% of elderly US adults consume more than 1 mg/day, and this is achieved only through supplementation.

> **SUMMARY**
>
> - Reduced risk of infant and maternal deaths during pregnancy has shifted priorities of medical care towards optimizing parental health in order to maximize fertility and reduce risk of fetal abnormalities.
> - In women, the key determinant of fertility is a healthy body weight. Low levels of body fat or excessive adiposity disrupt the actions of leptin upon the hypothalamic–pituitary–ovarian axis and prevent normal reproductive cycling.
> - Consumption of caffeine and alcohol appears to have a negative impact on female fertility. Antioxidant nutrients are important in assisted reproduction, but there is limited evidence of benefits for natural fertility in women.
> - Male fertility appears to be decreasing and the prevalence of abnormalities of the male reproductive

tract is increasing. This may be associated with increased exposure to endocrine disruptors in the food chain and environment. Obesity reduces male fertility due to reductions in androgen synthesis and transport.

- Zinc and selenium are key nutrients associated with male fertility. Suggested relationships of indices of fertility with increased intakes of antioxidant nutrients are of interest but, as yet, inconclusive.

- Vitamin A is a teratogen associated with central nervous system and heart defects in the human embryo. Women considering pregnancy should avoid rich sources of vitamin A, such as liver, and vitamin A supplements.

- Optimizing maternal weight prior to conception is regarded as a means of reducing the risk of adverse outcomes for mothers and children during pregnancy, as well as enhancing fertility.

- Folic acid protects the embryo from neural tube defects during the first few weeks of development. In many parts of the world, public health strategy has been based on prevention of these defects through supplementation of women who are planning a pregnancy. Fortification is a more effective strategy, but in many countries has not been adopted due to concerns about detriment to some groups in the population.

References

Abell, A., Ernst, E. and Bonde, J.P. (1994) High sperm density among members of organic farmers' association. *Lancet*, **343**, 1498.

Agarwal, A., Gupta, S. and Sharma, R.K. (2005) Role of oxidative stress in female reproduction. *Reproductive Biology and Endocrinology*, **3**, 28–48.

Agopian, A.J., Tinker, S.C., Lupo, P.J. *et al.* (2013) Proportion of neural tube defects attributable to known risk factors. *Birth Defects Research A Clinical and Molecular Teratology*, **97**, 42–46.

Allal, N., Sear, R., Prentice, A.M. and Mace, R. (2004) An evolutionary model of stature, age at first birth and reproductive success in Gambian women. *Proceedings Biological Sciences*, **271**, 465–470.

Arnhold, T., Tzimas, G., Wittfoht, W. *et al.* (1996) Identification of 9-cis-retinoic acid, 9,13-di-cis-retinoic acid, and 14-hydroxy-4,14-retro-retinol in human plasma after liver consumption. *Life Science*, **59**, PL169–PL177.

Atanassova, N., McKinnell, C., Turner, K.J. *et al.* (2000) Comparative effects of neonatal exposure of male rats to potent and weak (environmental) estrogens on spermatogenesis at puberty and the relationship to adult testis size and fertility: evidence for stimulatory effects of low estrogen levels. *Endocrinology*, **141**, 3898–3907.

Barbieri, R.L. (2001) The initial fertility consultation: recommendations concerning cigarette smoking, body mass index, and alcohol and caffeine consumption. *American Journal of Obstetrics and Gynecology*, **185**, 1168–1173.

Beckett, G.J. and Arthur, J.R. (2005) Selenium and endocrine systems. *Journal of Endocrinology*, **184**, 455–465.

Bolúmar, F., Olsen, J., Rebagliato, M. and Bisanti, L. (1997) Caffeine intake and delayed conception: a European multi-center study on infertility and subfecundity. European Study Group on Infertility Subfecundity. *American Journal of Epidemiology*, **145**, 324–334.

Centers for Disease Control (CDC) (2004) *Spina Bifida and Anencephaly Before and After Folic Acid Mandate – United States, 1995–1996 and 1999–2000*, http://www.cdc.gov/mmwr/preview/mmwrhtml/mm5317a3.htm (accessed 4 January 2015).

Chang-Mo, O., In-Hwan, O., Kyung-Sik, C. *et al.* (2012) Relationship between body mass index and early menarche of adolescent girls in Seoul. *Journal of Preventive Medicine and Public Health*, **45**, 227–234.

Charles, D., Ness, A.R., Campbell, D. *et al.* (2004) Taking folate in pregnancy and risk of maternal breast cancer. *British Medical Journal*, **329**, 1375–1376.

Czeizel, A.E. and Dudas, I. (1992) Prevention of the first occurrence of neural-tube defects by periconceptional vitamin supplementation. *New England Journal of Medicine*, **327**, 1832–1835.

De Fleurian, G., Perrin, J., Ecochard, R. *et al.* (2009) Occupational exposures obtained by questionnaire in clinical practice and their association with semen quality. *Journal of Andrology*, **30**, 566–579.

Ebisch, I.M., Thomas, C.M., Peters, W.H. *et al.* (2007) The importance of folate, zinc and antioxidants in the pathogenesis and prevention of subfertility. *Human Reproduction Update*, **13**, 163–174.

El-Haschimi, K., Pierroz, D.D., Hileman, S.M. *et al.* (2000) Two defects contribute to hypothalamic leptin resistance in mice with diet-induced obesity. *Journal of Clinical Investigation*, **105**, 1827–1832.

Emanuele, M.A. and Emanuele, N. (2001) Alcohol and the male reproductive system. *Alcohol Research and Health*, **25**, 282–287.

Eskenazi, B., Kidd, S.A., Marks, A.R. *et al.* (2005) Antioxidant intake is associated with semen quality in healthy men. *Human Reproduction*, **20**, 1006–1012.

Frisch, R.E. (1987) Body fat, menarche, fitness and fertility. *Human Reproduction*, **2**, 521–533.

Frisch, R.E., Revelle, R. and Cook, S. (1973) Components of weight at menarche and the initiation of the adolescent growth spurt in girls: estimated total water, llean body weight and fat. *Human Biology*, **45**, 469–483.

Fuse, H., Kazama, T., Ohta, S. and Fujiuchi, Y. (1999) Relationship between zinc concentrations in seminal plasma and various sperm parameters. *International Urology and Nephrology*, **31**, 401–408.

Galletly, C., Moran, L., Noakes, M. *et al.* (2007) Psychological benefits of a high-protein, low-carbohydrate diet in obese women with polycystic ovary syndrome-A pilot study. *Appetite*, **49**, 590–593.

Gao, L.J., Wang, Z.P., Lu, Q.B. *et al.* (2013) Maternal overweight and obesity and the risk of neural tube defects: a case-control study in China. *Birth Defects Research A Clinical and Molecular Teratology*, **97**, 161–165.

Geoffroy-Siraudin, C., Loundou, A.D., Romain, F. *et al.* (2012) Decline of semen quality among 10 932 males consulting for couple infertility over a 20-year period in Marseille, France. *Asian Journal of Andrology*, **14**, 584–590.

Goumenou, A.G., Matalliotakis, I.M., Koumantakis, G.E. and Panidis, D.K. (2003) The role of leptin in fertility. *European Journal of Obstetrics Gynecology and Reproductive Biology*, **106**, 118–124.

Gray, L.E., Ostby, J., Monosson, E. and Kelce, W.R. (1999) Environmental antiandrogens: low doses of the fungicide vinclozolin alter sexual differentiation of the male rat. *Toxicology and Industrial Health*, **15**, 48–64.

Grodstein, F., Goldman, M.B. and Cramer, D.W. (1994) Infertility in women and moderate alcohol use. *American Journal of Public Health*, **84**, 1429–1432.

Hakim, R.B., Gray, R.H. and Zacur, H. (1998) Alcohol and caffeine consumption and decreased fertility. *Fertility and Sterility*, **70**, 632–637.

Halliwell, B. (1999) Antioxidant defence mechanisms: from the beginning to the end (of the beginning). *Free Radical Research*, **31**, 261–272.

Hansen, M.L., Thulstrup, A.M., Bonde, J.P. *et al.* (2012) Does last week's alcohol intake affect semen quality or reproductive hormones? A cross-sectional study among healthy young Danish men. *Reproductive Toxicology*, **34**, 457–462.

Hartmann, S., Brors, O., Bock, J. *et al.* (2005) Exposure to retinoic acids in non-pregnant women following high vitamin A intake with a liver meal. *International Journal of Vitamin and Nutrition Research*, **75**, 187–194.

Hassan, M.A. and Killick, S.R. (2004) Negative lifestyle is associated with a significant reduction in fecundity. *Fertility and Sterility*, **81**, 384–392.

Hatch, E.E., Wise, L.A., Mikkelsen, E.M. *et al.* (2012) Caffeinated beverage and soda consumption and time to pregnancy. *Epidemiology*, **23**, 393–401.

Hawkes, W.C. and Turek, P.J. (2001) Effects of dietary selenium on sperm motility in healthy men. *Journal of Andrology*, **22**, 764–772.

Hinkle, S.N., Sharma, A.J., Kim, S.Y. and Schieve, L.A. (2013) Maternal prepregnancy weight status and associations with children's development and disabilities at kindergarten. *International Journal of Obesity*, **37**, 1344–1351.

Hogan, M.C., Foreman, K.J., Naghavi, M. *et al.* (2010) Maternal mortality for 181 countries, 1980–2008: a systematic analysis of progress towards Millennium Development Goal 5. *Lancet*, **375**, 1609–1623.

Hossain, F., Ali, O., D'Souza, U.J. and Naing, D.K. (2010) Effects of pesticide use on semen quality among farmers in rural areas of Sabah, Malaysia. *Journal of Occupational Health*, **52**, 353–360.

Institute of Medicine (2009) *Weight Gain During Pregnancy: Reexamining the Guidelines*, National Academies Press, Washington, DC.

Jensen, T.K., Giwercman, A., Carlsen, E. *et al.* (1996) Semen quality among members of organic food associations in Zealand, Denmark. *Lancet*, **347**, 1844.

Joo, K.J., Kwon, Y.W., Myung, S.C. and Kim, T.H. (2012) The effects of smoking and alcohol intake on sperm quality: light and transmission electron microscopy findings. *Journal of Internal Medical Research*, **40**, 2327–2335.

Jørgensen, N., Vierula, M., Jacobsen, R. *et al.* (2011) Recent adverse trends in semen quality and testis cancer incidence among Finnish men. *International Journal of Andrology*, **34**, e37–e48.

Juhl, M., Olsen, J., Andersen, A.M. and Gronbaek, M. (2003) Intake of wine, beer and spirits and waiting time to pregnancy. *Human Reproduction*, **18**, 1967–1971.

Juhler, R.K., Larsen, S.B., Meyer, O. *et al.* (1999) Human semen quality in relation to dietary pesticide exposure and organic diet. *Archives of Environmental Contamination and Toxicology*, **37**, 415–423.

Kenkel, S., Rolf, C. and Nieschlag, E. (2001) Occupational risks for male fertility: an analysis of patients attending a tertiary referral centre. *International Journal of Andrology*, **24**, 318–326.

Langley-Evans, S.C. (2004) Before life begins: preconceptual influences on child health, in *Biology of Child Health/Aspects of Biological Development in Childhood* (eds S. Neill and H. Knowles), Macmillan Palgrave, Basingstoke, pp. 1–21.

Langley-Evans, S.C. and Langley-Evans, A.J. (2001) Use of folic acid supplements in the first trimester of pregnancy. *Journal of the Royal Society for the Promotion of Health*, **122**, 181–186.

Larsen, S.B., Spano, M., Giwercman, A. and Bonde, J.P. (1999) Semen quality and sex hormones among organic and traditional Danish farmers. ASCLEPIOS Study Group. *Occupational and Environmental Medicine*, **56**, 139–144.

Laurence, K.M., James, N., Miller, M.H. *et al.* (1981) Double-blind randomised controlled trial of folate treatment before conception to prevent recurrence of neural-tube defects. *British Medical Journal*, **282**, 1509–1511.

Li, N., Liu, E., Guo, J. *et al.* (2013) Maternal prepregnancy body mass index and gestational weight gain on pregnancy outcomes. *PLoS One*, **8**, e82310.

Lupo, P.J., Canfield, M.A., Chapa, C. *et al.* (2012) Diabetes and obesity-related genes and the risk of neural tube defects in the national birth defects prevention study. *American Journal of Epidemiology*, **176**, 1101–1109.

Magnusdottir, E.V., Thorsteinsson, T., Thorsteinsdottir, S. *et al.* (2005) Persistent organochlorines, sedentary occupation, obesity and human male subfertility. *Human Reproduction*, **20**, 208–215.

Marsh, K. and Brand-Miller, J. (2005) The optimal diet for women with polycystic ovary syndrome? *British Journal of Nutrition*, **94**, 154–165.

Martinez-Frias, M.L. and Salvador, J. (1990) Epidemiological aspects of prenatal exposure to high doses of vitamin A in Spain. *European Journal of Epidemiology*, **6**, 118–123.

Martini, A.C., Molina, R.I., Estofán, D. *et al.* (2004) Effects of alcohol and cigarette consumption on human seminal quality. *Fertility and Sterility*, **82**, 374–377.

Mascarenhas, M.N., Flaxman, S.R., Boerma, T. *et al.* (2012) National, Regional, and Global Trends in Infertility Prevalence Since 1990: a Systematic Analysis of 277 Health Surveys. *PLoS Medicine*, **9**, e1001356.

Mason, J.B., Dickstein, A., Jacques, P.F. *et al.* (2007) A temporal association between folic acid fortification and an increase in colorectal cancer rates may be illuminating important biological principles: a hypothesis. *Cancer Epidemiology Biomarkers and Prevention*, **16**, 1325–1329.

Mendiola, J., Jørgensen, N., Mínguez-Alarcón, L. *et al.* (2013) Sperm counts may have declined in young university students in Southern Spain. *Andrology*, **1**, 408–413.

Menezo, Y.J., Hazout, A., Panteix, G. *et al.* (2007) Antioxidants to reduce sperm DNA fragmentation: an unexpected adverse effect. *Reproductive Biomedicine Online*, **14**, 418–421.

Overall, pregnancy is an anabolic state and hormones produced by the placenta ensure that nutrients are metabolized in a manner that allows maintenance of maternal homeostasis, provides support for the growth of the placenta and foetus and prepares the maternal system for later lactation (King, 2000). Many of the adaptations that are necessary to maintain a successful pregnancy occur at a very early stage of gestation. Although growth of the foetus is limited in the first trimester, as described earlier, this is the period where implantation occurs and the placenta becomes established. The maternal cardiovascular, renal and respiratory systems undergo major change, early in pregnancy, to be able to support placental perfusion and delivery of oxygen and nutrients that will drive the later growth of the foetus.

3.2.1 Maternal weight gain and body composition changes

Weight gain in pregnancy can be highly variable, but typically will be of the order of 12.5 kg. Most of this weight gain occurs during the second half of gestation. As shown in Figure 3.1, only a third of the weight gain is due to the growth of the foetus and most of the increase is attributable to maternal changes. Some of the changes to maternal weight are explained by altered cardiovascular and renal functions, which serve to increase the blood volume and drive retention of water in the interstitial compartment. There are also major increases in the size of the uterus as the pregnancy proceeds, and the breasts can increase in size by up to 0.5 kg. This latter change appears to be an adaptation to ensure that the breasts are ready for lactation after the birth of the baby. Women also deposit large reserves of fat, typically in the abdomen, thighs and back. These reserves start to be mobilized in later stages

of pregnancy to drive foetal growth and also act as an energy source for later lactation.

As will be described later in this chapter, maternal weight gain is an important predictor of pregnancy outcome. Insufficient or excessive weight gains are associated with poor outcomes for both mother and foetus. Desirable weight gains are therefore in a range that optimizes maternal survival, reduces complications in pregnancy and labour and gives the greatest foetal growth and protection from morbidity and mortality (Butte and King, 2005; Institute of Medicine, 2009). It is suggested that the optimal range of maternal weight gain is dependent upon maternal body mass index (BMI) prior to pregnancy. As shown in Table 3.2, women who are underweight prior to pregnancy should aim for a greater degree of weight gain, while the overweight may need to control weight gain to some degree.

3.2.2 Blood volume expansion and cardiovascular changes

During pregnancy, there is a need for the maternal cardiovascular system to adapt in order to supply enlarged organs and maintain the perfusion of the placenta. This ensures an adequate exchange of materials with the foetal compartment. Placentation necessitates an increase in the overall volume of blood within the maternal system and this is achieved through a repartitioning of water between the intracellular and extracellular compartments. Overall, body water increases by 1.5 l (pre-pregnant body water volume is 2.6 l) within the first 20 weeks of pregnancy and continues to rise throughout gestation. The volume of water held in cells (intracellular fluid) is unchanged, and the increased fluid volume is partitioned between the interstitial spaces and the blood plasma.

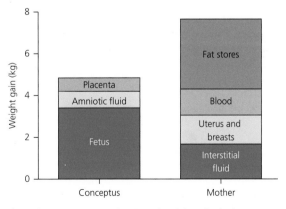

Figure 3.1 Components of maternal weight gain during pregnancy.

Table 3.2 Optimal weight gain for women in pregnancy is dependent upon their pre-pregnancy BMI.

BMI at conception (kg/m²)	Optimal maternal weight gain (kg)
<18.5	13–18
18.5–24.9	11–16
25–29.9	7–11
>30	5–9

Data Source: Institute of Medicine (2009). Reproduced with permission of The National Academies Press.
Optimal weight gain ranges are those associated with favourable pregnancy outcomes for mother and foetus and which lead to birth weight between 3.1 and 3.6 kg.

Increased blood plasma volume has a number of important consequences. Firstly, the fluid expansion enables the delivery of the increased workload required of the heart during pregnancy. The heart needs to deliver more oxygen to tissues than pre-pregnancy, and the increased vascularization of the uterus and placenta require a greater cardiac output. The heart increases in volume by approximately 20% during pregnancy and this enables a greater stroke volume (the amount of blood pumped from the ventricles with each contraction). The pulse rate increases, typically rising from 70 in the non-pregnant state to 85 by late pregnancy. The combination of raised heart rate and stroke volume increases cardiac output by 40%. Cardiac output is an important contributor to blood pressure, but the latter remains largely unchanged, as the peripheral resistance to blood flow is reduced.

The other main consequence of increased plasma volume is a change in the composition of the blood. Overall, the plasma volume increases by 40–50% over the course of pregnancy and this results in a reduction in the concentrations of many plasma proteins, most notably albumin. In order to meet the increased demand for oxygen transport, there is greater production of red blood cells and as a result the total amount of haemoglobin in circulation increases (Figure 3.2). However, as the 20% increase in red cell volume achieved by full-term gestation is considerably less than the increase in blood volume, the number of red cells per millilitre blood and overall haemoglobin concentration fall, as gestation advances. This makes diagnosis of iron deficiency anaemia more challenging in pregnancy as the

stage of gestation has to be considered. For example, a haemoglobin concentration of 10.5 g/dl would be indicative of anaemia in a non-pregnant woman, and in a woman at 20 weeks gestation, but would be considered within normal ranges at 30 weeks.

3.2.3 Renal changes

Modifications in the function of kidneys are among the earliest physiological responses to pregnancy. The purpose of these adaptations is to support the cardiovascular changes, modify maternal fluid balance and increase capacity for excretion of metabolic waste. Tubular reabsorption of water and electrolytes is increased during pregnancy, and although pregnant women experience more frequent micturition due to the pressure of the uterus upon the bladder, the actual daily volume of urine produced is only 80% of that seen in non-pregnant women. Chapman *et al.* (1998) observed that blood flow through the maternal kidneys, and hence the glomerular filtration rate, was significantly increased by 6 weeks gestation and that renal function reached the maximum for pregnancy by as early as 8–12 weeks. Increased renal blood flow and reduced arterial resistance in the kidneys are important mechanisms through which maternal cardiac output can be increased without producing dangerous increases in blood pressure.

3.2.4 Respiratory changes

A number of changes take place to improve maternal gaseous exchange. These adaptations ensure that the maternal blood is enriched with oxygen and is effectively cleared of carbon dioxide. This maximizes concentration gradients across the placental membranes and aids delivery of oxygen and removal of carbon dioxide from the foetal system. The maternal diaphragm takes on a greater range of movement and the ribs flare outwards. This means that during early–mid pregnancy, there is a greater tidal movement of air during each breath and effectively more fresh air is inhaled and more used air exhaled with each breath. As pregnancy proceeds, the mass of the uterus and foetus press upon the diaphragm and limit this tidal movement, but respiratory efficiency is maintained by a more rapid rate of breathing.

The efficient removal of carbon dioxide from the maternal blood is of importance for the nutrition of the foetus as well as for gaseous exchange across the placenta. Carbon dioxide is transported in the blood as bicarbonate ions (HCO_3^-). With less of this anion in circulation, there is a reduced requirement for appropriate cations (Na^+, K^+ and Ca^{2+}) to be in circulation and these are therefore available for transfer to the foetus for growth and skeletal mineralization. Maternal

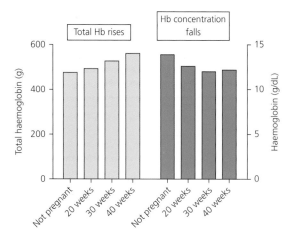

Figure 3.2 Changes in iron status during pregnancy. The total amount of haemoglobin in circulation (▢) increases, but due to rising plasma volume, the haemoglobin concentration (▦) decreases.

blood concentrations of cations therefore fall from around 155 m.equiv/l pre-pregnancy to 147 m.equiv/l in mid-gestation.

3.2.5 Gastrointestinal changes

The maternal gastrointestinal tract is influenced by the high prevailing concentrations of progesterone and oestrogen. These produce adaptations that increase the capacity of the gut to absorb nutrients and hence increase availability for incorporation into maternal or foetal structures and stores. In the stomach, the secretion of gastric juices is reduced, but gastric emptying is slowed. This means that ingested food is churned within the stomach for a longer period and is more effectively pulped. This improves digestion lower down the tract. The motility of both the small and large intestines is reduced, and this exposes food materials to digestive enzymes for longer time and also increases the duration of time during which nutrients can be absorbed and water recovered.

3.2.6 Metabolic adaptations

Demands for energy and protein are increased during pregnancy and these increased demands are partly met through adaptations in the metabolism of macronutrients. There is an accretion of approximately 0.5 kg of protein during pregnancy, around half of which is deposited in the conceptus (foetus and placenta). As described in the preceding section, pregnancy is associated with decreased gastrointestinal motility and this improves the absorption of amino acids from ingested food. Absorbed amino acids are transported to the liver, where normally they would be used in protein synthesis, or deaminated so that any excess is excreted via the urine in the form of urea. During pregnancy, the enzymes responsible for deamination are inhibited by hCG first and later by placental growth hormone. This means that more amino acids enter the maternal circulation and these can be used for expansion of maternal tissues and the placenta, or exported to the foetal compartment.

The hormonal changes that accompany pregnancy serve to create a state of insulin resistance. By the second and third trimesters, pregnant women secrete 2–2.5-fold more insulin than in the non-pregnant state (Barbour, 2003). Despite this, the disposal of glucose in the skeletal muscle and liver is suppressed and as a result the circulating glucose concentration remains high, ensuring the supply to the foetal tissues. The mechanisms through which the insulin resistance of pregnancy develops are not fully understood. As shown in Figure 3.3, normal glucose uptake by tissues such as skeletal muscle is dependent upon the translocation of the GLUT4 glucose transporter to the cell membrane following insulin binding to the insulin receptor. The insulin signal to GLUT4 depends upon the binding of phosphorylated insulin receptor substrate 1 (IRS-1) to phosphatidylinositol 3 kinase (PI3-K). Formation of the IRS-1–PI3-K complex is the key event that activates GLUT4 translocation. In pregnancy, it is apparent that the formation of this complex is inhibited and this essentially limits glucose uptake by maternal tissues (Barbour, 2003).

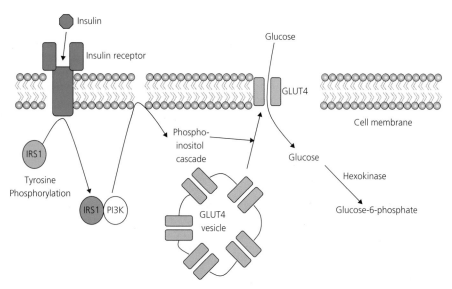

Figure 3.3 The role of GLUT4 in glucose transport. GLUT4 translocation is a key step in the movement of glucose across cell membranes. In pregnancy, the formation of IRS-1–PI3-K complexes is inhibited, leading to insulin resistance.

In addition to these metabolic adaptations that promote maximum availability of energy substrates to support the pregnancy, there are behavioural adaptations that similarly make more energy available to the developing foetus. It is generally reported that pregnant women alter their profile of food choices and consume smaller portions of food on a more frequent basis. This helps to maintain raised blood glucose throughout the day. Furthermore, as pregnancy advances, most women reduce the levels of physical activity and this reduces overall energy expenditure (King, 2000).

3.3 Nutrient requirements in pregnancy

It should be clear from the preceding sections that pregnancy is a time of major remodelling of maternal tissues, deposition of new tissue in the uterus and in the form of the placenta and of considerable metabolic change. As a result, maternal demands for all nutrients would be expected to increase markedly. It is, however, becoming clear that in normal pregnancy, the same suite of adaptations that leads to increased nutrient demand also optimizes bioavailability and utilization of nutrients. As a result, major changes to maternal intake are generally unwarranted.

3.3.1 Energy, protein and lipids
Pregnancy considerably increases the maternal demand for energy in order to drive the growth of the foetus and placenta, the deposition of fat reserves for lactation and the expansion of maternal tissues. The increase in maternal body size in itself will increase the basal metabolic rate (BMR) and will increase the amount of energy required for physical activity. Estimates of the total energy cost of pregnancy vary greatly, but in general most studies support the early work of Hytten and Leitch (1971) who estimated that the increase in basal metabolism (30 000 kcal, 126 MJ) and the extra requirement associated with increasing body size (40 000 kcal, 167 MJ) totalled 70 000 kcal (293 MJ) over the whole gestation period. This equates to an extra requirement of 250 kcal/day (1.04 MJ/day).

Studies of pregnant women in developed countries show that this energy demand is not met by increased intakes of energy. Durnin (1991) reported that women typically did not increase intake at all until the third trimester, and even then, increases were only of the order of 100 kcal/day (0.42 MJ/day). Despite an apparent shortfall of energy intake, the women had normal pregnancy outcomes. This and other studies strongly suggested that pregnancy is associated with adaptive responses to conserve energy.

Conservation of energy may involve reductions of either basal metabolism or physical activity (King, 2000). Prentice and Goldberg (2000) suggested that there is wide variation in the metabolic response to pregnancy. While most women increase BMR as would be expected with increasing tissue mass, some women actually exhibit a decrease during early gestation. This form of energy conserving response is most common among women who are undernourished, with limited fat stores and high demands for physical activity to ensure survival (e.g. women depending on subsistence agriculture in developing countries). In developed countries where the food supply is secure, most energy conservation is likely to occur through reduction in overall levels of physical activity or improved efficiency of movement (Durnin, 1991). A number of studies have shown that pregnant women perform a similar range of activities to nonpregnant women, but generally avoid more strenuous tasks (King, 2000). Given the greater body mass in pregnancy, any weight-bearing activity should involve greater energy expenditure. However, where weight-bearing exercise is unavoidable, some pregnant women appear to reduce the pace or intensity of the activity (e.g. walking more slowly while carrying a load).

It is clear that the control of energy balance in pregnancy is subject to a diverse range of influences and there is a high level of inter-individual variation. This is explained by the fact that energy requirements and processes that match intake to expenditure are influenced by rates of maternal weight gain, foetal growth rates, maternal lifestyle and activity levels, maternal body composition and genetic factors (King, 2000). In the United Kingdom, COMA suggested an additional increment of 200 kcal/day (0.84 MJ/day) to be added to the EAR (Department of Health, 1999). This assumed an average pregnancy weight gain of 12.5 kg and a foetus of average weight at birth. Women who are underweight prior to pregnancy and those who are unable to reduce physical activity may require greater increases in energy intake. In the United States, the RDA for pregnancy includes an increment of 300 kcal/day, targeted at the second and third trimesters.

There are undoubtedly major requirements for protein during pregnancy. Growth of the foetus, placenta, and maternal tissues all require protein deposition. However, there are no recommendations for major changes to maternal intakes in developed countries. In the United Kingdom, the Reference Nutrient Intake (RNI) increment for pregnancy is a mere 6 g/day, while in the United States, an RDA increment of 10 g/day is advised (Millward, 1999). With intakes of protein in developed countries ranging from 60 to 110 g/day, there seems no need for dietary change to meet the demands for protein. However, women in developing countries and women from poor backgrounds may struggle to obtain dietary protein requirements. As will be described in Chapter 4, this may be associated with long-term disease risk in their offspring.

The dietary supply of essential fatty acids may become important during pregnancy. These lipids give rise to the n-6 and n-3 series of fatty acids, which have major biological functions (Figure 3.4). The long-chain polyunsaturated fatty acids (LCPUFAs) from these series give rise to the pro- and anti-inflammatory eicosanoids and hence modulate cell-signalling pathways. LCPUFAs are also involved in the regulation of gene expression through their interaction with transcription factors (Wainwright, 2002). In humans, LCPUFAs are heavily concentrated in the brain and retina, where they account for approximately 35% of the total fatty acid profile. The foetal and neonatal brain has particularly high demand for arachidonic acid (n-6 series) and docosahexaenoic acid (DHA, n-3) series. While these can be synthesized de novo from the essential dietary fatty acids, as shown in Figure 3.4, in the foetal brain the activity of these pathways is low. There is consequently

a dependence upon their transfer across the placenta from the maternal circulation. The accrual of DHA, in particular, in the foetal brain and retina occurs largely during the third trimester. DHA is incorporated into phosphatidylethanolamine and phosphatidylserine in these tissues (Innis, 2005).

Transfer of LCPUFAs from mother to foetus appears to occur at a rate that is closely correlated with maternal intake. Maternal concentrations are predictive of arachadonic acid and DHA concentrations in umbilical cord plasma and red cells at birth (Connor et al., 1996). The best sources of LCPUFAs in the diet are oily fish, eggs, meat and certain seed oils. Maintaining an adequate supply to the foetus appears to be critical to neurodevelopment as maternal intakes are predictive of brain fatty acid composition and size in the foetus (Wainwright, 2002). Depletion of DHA has been associated with reduced visual function and learning defects in children. Intervention using supplements of cod liver oil and other n-3 containing sources has suggested that maternal supplementation from the start of the second trimester may improve visual-evoked potentials and performance on tests of intelligence and achievement in infants (Jensen, 2006).

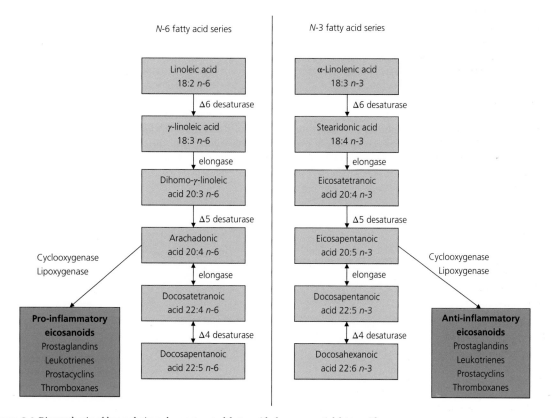

Figure 3.4 Biosynthesis of long-chain polyunsaturated fatty acids from essential fatty acids.

A number of observational studies have suggested that low maternal intakes of LCPUFAs may be associated with adverse outcomes of pregnancy. High intakes of *n*-3 fatty acids have been proposed to extend gestation, increase weight at birth, and reduce risk of premature delivery (Jensen, 2006). This raises the possibility that pregnant women might be recommended to consume supplements of these lipids. For some groups of women, this could be more important than for others. Vegetarian or vegan mothers, for example, consume a pattern of diet that strongly favours the generation of *n*-6 series fatty acids over the *n*-3 series (Sanders, 1999). Englund-Ögge *et al.* (2011) considered dietary patterns associated with premature labour in a large cohort of Norwegian women. A 'traditional' dietary pattern that included fish carried a lower risk of prematurity than a western diet. The randomized controlled trial of Carlson *et al.* (2013) found that 600 mg/day DHA supplementation over the second half of gestation was associated with longer gestation, greater birth weight and an 87% reduction in risk of delivery before 34 weeks gestation. Balanced against the desire to boost availability of substrates for foetal brain growth are concerns about the contamination of fish oils with mercury and other potentially teratogenic agents. Moreover, some studies have suggested that fish oil supplementation may increase maternal bleeding and risk of post-partum haemorrhage (Jensen, 2006). The supplementation study of Carlson *et al.* (2013) found no evidence of adverse effects of DHA for mothers or babies.

3.3.2 Micronutrients

3.3.2.1 Iron

Maternal requirements for iron during pregnancy are high, with the foetus taking up as much as 400 mg over full gestation, with up to 175 mg accumulating in the placenta (Whittaker *et al.*, 1991). With further allowances for maternal production of red blood cells and blood losses during delivery, an extra 430–1000 mg are required in a normal pregnancy. To some extent, these requirements are delivered through savings associated with the cessation of menstrual cycling, but women still require an extra 1 mg/day in the first trimester, rising to 6 mg/day in late gestation (Figure 3.5). Little adjustment to the diet is generally required, as absorption of iron across the gut increases markedly from 7.6% of ingested iron in the first trimester to 37.4% by 36 weeks gestation.

Poor maternal iron status is a recognized risk factor for preterm delivery, low birth weight and neonatal death, particularly in the developing countries. Iron deficiency anaemia is highly prevalent in many populations and in some parts of the world more than half of pregnant women will be affected. The timing of onset of iron deficiency anaemia is important in predicting outcome. Klebanoff and colleagues (1991) showed that there was no association between third trimester anaemia and preterm delivery, but risk was increased by almost twofold in women with anaemia between 13 and 26 weeks gestation. This is in keeping with the fact that iron deficiency exerts its influence on pregnancy outcomes through impact upon the maternal plasma volume expansion, which is at a critical phase in the second trimester of pregnancy.

Elevated haemoglobin (>14.5 g/l) is also predictive of adverse pregnancy outcomes (more preterm delivery, more low birth weight and greater risk of foetal death) suggesting that the relationship between iron status and pregnancy outcomes is U-shaped (Scholl and Reilly, 2000). Raised haemoglobin is indicative of a failure to increase plasma volume and the ensuing hypovolemia results in cardiac output and placental perfusion being suboptimal.

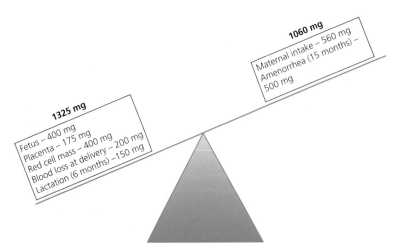

Figure 3.5 Contributors to maternal iron status during pregnancy. Replenishment of iron stores will be less in women who do recommence menstruation sooner (not breastfeeding) but may be aided by improved absorption of dietary iron in the third trimester of pregnancy.

In developing countries, iron supplementation may be an important element of antenatal care that could significantly reduce the risk of perinatal death. Many studies have shown that iron supplements, either in isolation or when combined with other nutrients such as folic acid, can increase average birth weights and significantly reduce the prevalence of low birth weight (Mishra *et al.*, 2005). There is some concern, however, that giving iron alone could lead to other micronutrient deficiencies, for example, zinc and copper, by competing for gastrointestinal uptake. Some studies suggest that optimal supplementation strategies should include a wider range of micronutrients (Zagré *et al.*, 2007).

Among better nourished women from industrialized countries, the benefits of routine iron supplementation are questionable, and in many nations (e.g. the United Kingdom), this practice has been abandoned. Given that iron supplements lead to constipation and other gastrointestinal symptoms, and are expensive when administered on a population-wide scale, it is reasoned that supplementation should be reserved for women with greater need, for example, those with multiple pregnancies, or women with iron deficiency anaemia. Even among this latter group, the benefits of iron supplementation are unclear. Certainly, iron status is improved by supplementation (Scholl and Reilly, 2000), but there is little evidence that the intervention will prevent preterm birth or reduce the likelihood of low birth weight. Most trials to assess the efficacy of supplementation are hampered by the fact that they only recruit women with pre-existing iron deficiency anaemia. As anaemia is generally diagnosed only after the plasma volume expansion has been largely completed, it is unlikely that intervention will have any impact upon adverse outcomes related to impaired cardiovascular adaptations to pregnancy.

3.3.2.2 Calcium and other minerals

The foetus accumulates large quantities of most minerals during late gestation. The foetal skeleton deposits calcium, magnesium and phosphorus in the last trimester of pregnancy, and high uptakes of zinc, copper and other trace metals are also noted. In some countries, notably the United States, these increased demands associated with pregnancy have prompted the inclusion of pregnancy increments over and above the published RDA values. In the United Kingdom, however, there are no extra allowances for pregnancy, as it is assumed that maternal adaptations are capable of providing sufficient mineral to maintain foetal demands.

Pregnancy is associated with improved absorption of most micronutrients from the digestive tract due to the increased gastrointestinal transit times. Increased absorption and the mobilization of minerals from stores in the maternal skeleton ensure the foetal supply. In the case of magnesium, for example, the foetus accumulates an average of 8 mg/day over the full gestation. To meet this demand, with an average absorption of 50% of dietary magnesium, and to meet the demand for magnesium from the placenta and other maternal structures, pregnancy increases overall demand by 26 mg/day (Department of Health, 1999). Given that average intakes are in the range 200–280 mg/day, this is a small extra demand that should be easily met by release from the skeleton where 60% of magnesium is stored.

The same principle applies to calcium, phosphorus, copper and zinc. Demand for zinc is considerable in late gestation at 5.6–14 mg/day, which is in excess of normal ranges of intake. However, zinc supplementation studies have shown little or no benefit for pregnant women and their babies. Similarly, studies of pregnant women with mild–moderate zinc deficiency show that there are no adverse consequences. It is therefore assumed that the increased requirement is met by mobilizing stores (Department of Health, 1999).

The only circumstances in which mineral nutrition may become problematic in pregnancy are when the mother is still at her growing stage. Adolescent pregnancy is a risk factor for many adverse outcomes of pregnancy, and much of the risk is associated with competition for nutrients between the growing foetus and the maternal system. Antenatal mineral supplementation may therefore be appropriate for this age group.

Iodine is an essential nutrient for foetal development, where it is particularly important in the development of the central nervous system during the first trimester of pregnancy. Severe maternal iodine deficiency is associated with foetal death or with cretinism in the affected baby. In countries such as the United Kingdom, where iodine deficiency is extremely rare, the extra 25 µg/day iodine required during pregnancy is comfortably delivered by dietary sources. However, in countries where iodine status tends to be poor, pregnancy is a time when careful intervention should be implemented. Most countries where iodine deficiency disorders are a problem have implemented fortification schemes, such as the highly successful Universal Salt Iodization (USI) program. USI adds iodine to salt used in food production and for home consumption and has coverage in over 120 countries. The World Health Organization has estimated that 68% of the five billion people who live in countries where iodine deficiency disorders occur have access to iodized salt at an average cost of US$0.05 per year.

Several studies have suggested that fortification programs such as USI either fail to reach a significant number of pregnant women, particularly in developing countries, or lack the capacity to produce sufficient increases in iodine status in pregnant women. The World Health Organization states that urinary iodine excretion of 100–199 µg/l is indicative of healthy iodine status in non-pregnant adults, and that this should increase to 150–249 µg/l in pregnant women. Routine fortification at a high level increases the risk of hyperthyroidism, particularly in the elderly, and so the level of iodine added to salt has to be carefully monitored and controlled at a local level to reduce adverse effects. Thus demands for pregnancy may not be met. Jaiswal and colleagues (2014) however reported that iodine fortification in India was sufficient to meet requirements of pregnant women. Interestingly widespread iodine deficiency tends to be a feature of the more developed countries. Marchioni *et al.* (2008) reported that 92% of women in a sample of Italian pregnancies had inadequate (median 80 µg/l) iodine status, despite a program of salt iodination. A study of over 2000 pregnant women in Spain found that 80% had urinary iodine below 150 µg/l in the first trimester, with 54% below healthy iodine status in the second trimester (Aguayo *et al.*, 2013). Analysis by the US NHANES surveys (2005/06 and 2009/10) found a median urinary iodine concentration of 129 µg/l indicating widespread inadequate iodine status among pregnant women (Caldwell *et al.*, 2013).

3.3.2.3 Vitamin D

Pregnant women have increased requirements for vitamin D, by virtue of the increased mobilization of calcium for transfer across the placenta to drive growth of the foetal skeleton. Pregnancy is associated with changes in the metabolism of vitamin D. Concentrations of the biologically active form, 1,25-dihyroxy vitamin D_3 (1,25-dihydroxycholecalciferol, Figure 3.6), are increased, while circulating 25-hydroxy vitamin D_3 (25-hydroxycholecalciferol) decreases. Pregnant women show a marked seasonal variation in vitamin D status in climates where sunlight is markedly lower in the winter months, and as a result, their babies are at greater risk of defects associated with calcium metabolism and dental problems associated with vitamin D deficiency (Department of Health, 1999). Javaid *et al.* (2006) reported that vitamin D insufficiency was relatively common (31%) in a population of otherwise well-nourished pregnant British women. Eighteen percent of these women were classified as vitamin D deficient. Interestingly, after adjustment for appropriate confounding factors, the mothers' 25-hydroxycholecalciferol concentrations were predictive of their children's bone mass at 9 years of age. This supports the idea that maternal vitamin D status is of major importance in foetal skeletal development. Prevalence of vitamin D insufficiency is high even in regions with strong sunlight exposure. Bener *et al.* (2013) reported that 48% of a sample of pregnant women in Doha were insufficient, and in South Carolina

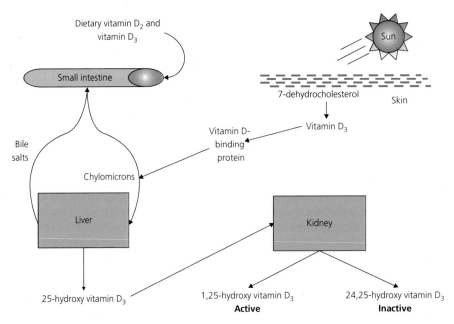

Figure 3.6 Metabolism of vitamin D.

(one of the sunny southern states of the United States) (Hamilton *et al.*, 2010), 85% of pregnant women were vitamin D deficient or insufficient. In common with similar recommendations in other countries, women in the United Kingdom are advised to either increase their intake of vitamin D–fortified foods or to consume a supplement of 10 μg/day. Poor vitamin D status is associated with adverse outcomes of pregnancy, including preterm delivery, pre-eclampsia (PE) and gestational diabetes mellitus (GDM) (Wei *et al.*, 2013).

3.4 Diet in relation to pregnancy outcomes

Human gestation is long and has evolved to maximize the growth of the brain and produce an infant that is well developed and relatively mature when compared to many other mammalian species. The long gestation brings with it an extended period during which the developing infant is vulnerable to adverse factors that impact upon the mother. Many of these adverse factors can compromise the pregnancy by imposing physiological and metabolic stressors upon a maternal system that is already operating outside normal functional limits. Although modern medical care has drastically reduced the impact of an adverse environment upon maternal and foetal health, pregnancy remains a hazardous process. Nutrition-related factors play an important role in determining the outcomes of pregnancy.

3.4.1 Miscarriage and stillbirth

Miscarriage, also termed spontaneous abortion, is defined as the natural end of pregnancy at a stage of foetal development prior to the foetus being capable of survival. With modern medical technology, foetuses of 23–24 weeks gestation may be considered viable, so miscarriage refers to loss of pregnancy prior to this stage. Later in pregnancy, the foetus may die either prior to delivery or during the delivery. The former case is termed late foetal death, while the latter is referred to as stillbirth. The death of a baby within the first 28 days after delivery is termed neonatal death.

There are a number of indicators that nutrition-related factors are predictive of miscarriage or later loss of the foetus. Miscarriages occur in approximately 15% of pregnancies and their causes are generally unexplained. The major risk factors for miscarriage in the first trimester of pregnancy are a previous history of miscarriage, assisted conception, being an older woman, alcohol consumption, and having a low BMI prior to pregnancy (Maconochie *et al.*, 2007). Women with a pre-pregnancy BMI below 18.5 kg/m² (i.e. underweight)

have been reported to have between 24 and 72% greater risk of miscarriage than women with a BMI of 18.5–24.9 kg/m² going into pregnancy (Helgstrand and Andersen, 2005). It is suggested that this risk may be associated with lower circulating leptin concentrations. Leptin plays a key role in the regulation of ovarian function and is also involved in promoting angiogenesis, which is an important process in the implantation of the embryo and development of the placenta.

Overweight or obesity does not appear to have an impact upon the risk of miscarriage in women who conceive naturally (Maconochie *et al.*, 2007), but in women undergoing assisted reproduction, it may increase the risk of early spontaneous abortion by up to fourfold (Yu *et al.*, 2006). Women with polycystic ovary syndrome find conception difficult. Among such women, obesity increases the risk of miscarriage by 25–37%. Wang and colleagues (2002) showed that among women undergoing fertility treatment, both overweight (BMI 25–29.9 kg/m²) and obesity (BMI 30 kg/m²) significantly increased the risk of miscarriage. Risk increased in proportion to BMI, such that women with BMI in excess of 35 kg/m² had a 2.19-fold greater risk of losing their pregnancies. Obesity also increases the risk of later foetal death and has been shown to increase occurrence of both stillbirth and neonatal death by more than twofold (Yu *et al.*, 2006).

Alcohol is often identified as a risk factor for miscarriage, and pregnant women are advised to avoid alcohol completely or to reduce intake to one or two units per week. Hannigan and Armant (2005) suggest that alcohol is a particular cause of spontaneous abortion later in pregnancy and that rates of miscarriage are up to threefold higher in heavy drinkers compared to non-drinkers. Despite this concern, it appears that moderate amounts of alcohol consumption (<14 units/week) do not increase the risk of miscarriage significantly (Maconochie *et al.*, 2007).

Several studies have identified caffeine as a potential risk factor for miscarriage, and although the data are not clear-cut and the area is controversial, the Department of Health in the United Kingdom has recommended that pregnant women reduce intake to no more than 300 mg/day. This is equivalent to approximately three mugs of instant coffee. Weng and colleagues (2008) studied a population of over 1000 women and found that consumption of caffeine at a level above 200 mg/day from any source (coffee or other beverages containing caffeine) increased the odds of miscarriage by 2.23 (95% CI 1.34–3.69). Women consuming caffeine at lower levels were not at any significant risk of miscarriage when compared to non-consumers.

Some degree of protection against miscarriage may be obtained through appropriate dietary advice and change at the start of pregnancy. Kramer and Kakuma (2003) performed a systematic review of the literature to explore the influence of nutritional advice to pregnant women, and supplemental energy and protein during pregnancy, upon pregnancy outcomes. They did not report any significant effects of advice or supplements upon risk of miscarriage but found that nutritional advice and balanced supplements of energy and protein reduced the occurrence of both stillbirth and neonatal death. There is a conflicting literature on the effects of vitamin supplementation upon risk of miscarriage. Maconochie and colleagues (2007) found that women who took micronutrient supplements, notably those containing folic acid or iron, reduced the risk of first trimester miscarriage by as much as 47%. Similarly, women who consumed fresh fruit and vegetables on a daily basis were half as likely to suffer a miscarriage as women who did not consume these foods daily. In contrast Nohr *et al.* (2014) found that women who consumed multivitamin supplements in the periconceptual period were at greater risk (OR 1.29, 95% CI 1.12–1.48) of losing their pregnancy. This risk was not seen with supplements of folic acid, which in the US Nurses Health Study (Gaskins *et al.*, 2014) decreased risk of miscarriage by 20%. The meta-analysis of Rumbold *et al.* (2011) which included 28 studies of vitamin supplementation during pregnancy found no significant risk or benefits with respect to miscarriage and stillbirth.

3.4.2 Premature labour

Babies who are born prior to 37 weeks gestation are termed premature or preterm. Preterm delivery is the main cause of perinatal death and neonatal morbidity in developed countries. It is also associated with significant levels of disability among children. As such, premature birth is associated with a major human cost and also has a significant economic impact upon health services, due to the expense of neonatal intensive care.

Intrauterine growth retardation leading to a small-for-gestational age (SGA) baby is commonly associated with preterm delivery. There are many other known risk factors for premature labour, including maternal infection, psychological trauma of the mother and maternal smoking (Table 3.3), but around one-third of cases are of no known cause. Lifestyle factors including nutrition-related factors and excessive physical activity are believed to contribute to some of these cases.

3.4.2.1 Pre-pregnancy BMI and pregnancy weight gain

Maternal BMI is a major indicator of risk for a number of adverse outcomes of pregnancy, including preterm birth. Overweight and obesity are of greatest concern

(Figure 3.7), but underweight is also a risk factor for poor outcomes. In the United Kingdom, it is estimated that the prevalence of obesity among women of child-bearing age increased from 12 to 20% between 1993 and 2010 (Public Health England, 2014) and 5% of pregnancies (38 478 per year) were associated with morbid obesity (BMI > 35 kg/m^2; CMACE, 2010). There are around 1500 UK pregnancies per year where maternal BMI exceeds 50 kg/m^2 (Figure 3.8). The American College of Obstetrics and Gynecology (2013) estimated that more than half of US pregnant women were overweight or obese. In contrast less than 2% of US women aged 19–39 are underweight (BMI < 18.5 kg/m^2; Fryar *et al.*, 2010). It is widely recognized that among severely obese pregnant women, interventions to control weight gain may be important in preventing major complications of pregnancy and improving pregnancy outcomes (Research Highlight 3.1).

Studies of the relationship between pre-pregnancy BMI and weight gain in pregnancy suggest that risk of preterm delivery may be increased at either extreme of their ranges. Obesity and overweight are widely regarded as risk factors for preterm delivery. The association with risk of preterm delivery in these cases appears to be a result of the increased prevalence of complications of pregnancy that stems from the greater blood pressures and relative insulin resistance that accompany obesity. These are more likely to necessitate

Table 3.3 Risk factors for preterm delivery.

Risk factors	Explanation of risks
Multiple births	Twins and other multiple pregnancies are often delivered early for medical management
Premature rupture of membranes	Delivery necessary to avoid infection
Obstetric emergencies	Maternal bleeding, placental abruption or other placental problems require delivery of baby
Cervical incompetence	The weight of the uterus in late pregnancy may not be supported by the cervix, leading to delivery
Pre-eclampsia	Delivery is the only option to prevent maternal and foetal death
Maternal age	Mothers under the age of 15 or older than 35 are at greater risk of preterm delivery
Stress	Only extremely traumatic psychological stressors will cause premature labour

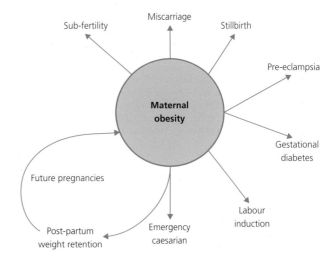

Figure 3.7 Obesity in pregnancy is a risk factor for adverse outcomes.

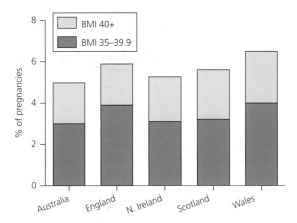

Figure 3.8 Prevalence of morbid obesity (BMI > 35 kg/m²) in pregnancy.
Data Source: CMACE (2010) and McIntyre *et al.* (2012).

medical intervention and premature induction of labour. A study of the very large Danish National Birth cohort (100 000 women, studied between 1996 and 2002) showed that a pre-pregnancy BMI in the obese range (over 30 kg/m²) significantly increased the risk of both induced and spontaneous preterm birth by approximately 50% (Nohr *et al.*, 2007). This risk was enhanced by excessive weight gain during pregnancy (more than 676 g/week). However, a study of a cohort that included only women screened to exclude those with GDM found that there was no association of overweight or obesity with preterm birth (Jensen *et al.*, 2003).

Maternal underweight has been shown in some studies to increase the risk of preterm birth to the same extent as obesity. The study of Nohr *et al.* (2007) showed a 40% increase in risk comparing women with a pre-pregnancy BMI of less than 18.5 kg/m² to those with a BMI between 18.5 and 24.9 kg/m². Lower weight gain in pregnancy was also associated with greater risk. Other studies are consistent with this finding, but often report a lower degree of risk (Sebire *et al.*, 2001). The risk associated with underweight and poor maternal weight gain is almost certainly attributable to maternal undernutrition and a lack of sufficient reserve of energy and other nutrients to meet demands for foetal growth. Merlino and colleagues (2006) demonstrated, in a small cohort of women, that underweight women were at greater risk of preterm delivery when in their second pregnancy rather than their first pregnancy. This risk was greatly increased if weight loss corresponding to 5 BMI units (kg/m²) had occurred between first and second pregnancies. Although this is indicative of a role for undernutrition in promoting preterm birth, studies that have considered iron deficiency anaemia (Scholl and Reilly, 2000) or the impact of protein and energy status (Kramer and Kakuma, 2003) have not identified a clear and unequivocal role for specific nutrients.

3.4.2.2 Alcohol and caffeine consumption

Alcohol consumption during pregnancy has a number of adverse impacts, of which the most important are the foetal alcohol syndrome (FAS, see Section 3.8.3) and alcohol-related birth defects (ARBD). These are consequences of alcohol consumption at excessive levels, with women engaging in either regular binge drinking (more than four alcoholic drinks in a session) or chronic daily alcohol use. It is clear from studies of such women that alcohol has an impact upon gestation length, with somewhere between 25 and 50% of FAS-associated pregnancies ending in preterm birth (Hannigan and Armant, 2005).

Research Highlight 3.1 The management of weight in pregnancy.

Maternal obesity during pregnancy increases the risk of adverse pregnancy outcomes including miscarriage, gestational diabetes and hypertensive disorders (CMACE, 2010; Li *et al.*, 2013; Sommer *et al.*, 2014) and is a significant risk factor for maternal and foetal death (CMACE, 2010). Where they exist, guidelines for maternal weight gain are generally based on the US Institute of Medicine (2009) recommended ranges, with obese mothers advised to gain 5–9 kg across pregnancy, compared to the 12.5–16 kg recommendation for women of healthy weight, or they emphasise the importance of managing weight before conception or after delivery (National Institute of Health and Clinical Excellence, 2010). Weight loss is not advised during pregnancy as it may pose a risk to foetal nutrition and development.

Although the need to manage weight among overweight and obese pregnant women is recognised, there is little evidence that effective strategies are in place to ensure that weight gain is not excessive or to prevent pregnancy complications. This is surprising as the antenatal period puts women into greater contact with health professionals and is therefore an ideal time for health education. Mothers are generally open and more readily motivated to make lifestyle changes that could benefit the health of themselves and their baby (Ritchie *et al.*, 2010; Wilkinson and McIntyre, 2012; May *et al.*, 2014; Wilkinson *et al.*, 2015). Some studies have evaluated the impact of antenatal diet, exercise or weight management programmes upon pregnancy outcomes, but generally yield inconsistent results. Thornton and colleagues (2009) found that monitoring the food intake of obese women was associated with lower gestational weight gain and lower prevalence of gestational hypertension. Shirazian *et al.* (2010) reported that a lifestyle modification in obese pregnant women reduced weight gain but had no effect on adverse pregnancy outcomes such as pre-eclampsia. The meta-analysis of Thangaratinam *et al.* (2012) found that weight management interventions in pregnancy reduced the risk of pre-eclampsia but had no impact upon other obstetric outcomes. There are also a number of ongoing studies evaluating intervention strategies, such as the LIMIT trial in Australia (Dodd *et al.*, 2011) and the UK UPBEAT study (Poston *et al.*, 2013). LIMIT has reported that a researcher-led diet and physical activity intervention did not achieve lower gestational weight gain or improved maternal outcomes (Dodd *et al.*, 2014). In contrast, the UK Bumps and Beyond intervention (McGiveron *et al.*, 2015) showed that an intensive midwife and health educator-led programme greatly reduced pregnancy weight gain in morbidly obese women and achieved a 90–95% decrease in hypertensive disorders of pregnancy. This programme led to antenatal weight loss in some women, but this was not associated with any adverse outcomes for mothers and babies.

The impact of lower levels of alcohol use is less understood, particularly because factors such as low socioeconomic status tend to confound possible associations between alcohol in pregnancy and preterm delivery. Some studies have suggested that even low consumption of alcohol during the final trimester of pregnancy may increase the risk of preterm delivery by as much as threefold (Lundsberg *et al.*, 2007), whereas others have shown that occasional consumption or even daily consumption in small quantities carries no associated risk (Jaddoe *et al.*, 2007). In the Danish National Birth Cohort (Rasmussen *et al.*, 2014), a maternal dietary pattern that included alcohol was not associated with preterm birth. Patra *et al.* (2011) performed a meta-analysis of 36 case–control and cohort studies and found no impact of moderate alcohol consumption on either risk of preterm birth or low birth weight. No dose-dependent effect of alcohol was noted until intakes exceeded 36 g alcohol per day (4.5 units/day), and in fact, up to 18 g/day there was a slightly lower risk of preterm delivery.

Caffeine is a widely consumed stimulant, which may be consumed by pregnant women in the form of beverages (e.g. coffee, tea and soft drinks) or as over-the-counter medications. Although there has been sufficient concern that this may be a risk factor for preterm birth to prompt advice for women to control intake, the evidence base suggests that beyond the early stages of pregnancy, the risk is negligible (Research Highlight 3.2).

3.4.2.3 Oral health

The risk of preterm delivery increases in all situations where an inflammatory response is mounted within the maternal system. The pro-inflammatory cytokines and prostaglandins that are released in response to infection promote the premature rupture of the amniotic and chorionic membranes. This may lead to the spontaneous initiation of premature labour or prompt the need for a medically induced preterm delivery.

Periodontitis is an oral health problem and represents one of the most common chronic disease states on a global scale. Milder forms of periodontitis are noted in 50% of the population at some stage of life and more advanced destructive periodontitis is noted in 5–10% of people. Periodontitis is essentially an inflammation of the gums, which in mild cases manifests as gingivitis. In the more advanced form, the disease results in destruction of gum tissue and underlying bone, leading to tooth loss. Periodontitis is the result of infection of the gum tissues by anaerobic bacterial species such as *Porphyromonas gingivalis*. This infection results in activation and recruitment of neutrophils to the gums. The subsequent release of reactive oxygen species causes local host tissue injury and the associated inflammatory response has systemic effects (Sculley and Langley-Evans, 2003). Periodontitis-related inflammation has been linked to development of other conditions, including coronary heart disease (Beck *et al.*, 1996).

Research Highlight 3.2 Advice to reduce caffeine intake in pregnancy.

Caffeine is widely reported as being hazardous in pregnancy, if consumed in large quantities. In the United Kingdom, women are advised to restrict intake to 300 mg/day or less, from all sources, in order to avoid risk of miscarriage in early pregnancy or preterm delivery later in gestation. Associations between caffeine and miscarriage risk are well established, but the relationship with preterm birth is controversial.

The idea that caffeine may be a risk factor for preterm labour is plausible, since caffeine is known to cross the placental barrier to act in foetal tissues, increases maternal catecholamine production and diminishes placental blood flow. Moreover, in pregnancy, the metabolism of caffeine is inhibited, producing a more protracted response to any given dose. Coffee is the main source of caffeine in the diet. Although most women become averse to coffee and reduce intake during their pregnancy, it is still consumed to some extent by 70–80% of pregnant women.

The perceived risk of preterm delivery associated with caffeine stems largely from the fact that it appears to impair foetal growth. Martin and Bracken (1987) reported that the risk of a low birth–weight baby was increased by 4.6-fold in women consuming caffeine in high quantities. Foetal growth retardation is a recognized risk factor for preterm delivery, but very few studies have unequivocally shown that women consuming caffeine, particularly in coffee, have greater risk of premature labour. Eskenazi *et al.* (1999) reported odds of preterm delivery of 2.3 (95% CI 1.3–4.0) comparing high coffee consumption to non-consumption. Other studies have highlighted moderate caffeine consumption in the second trimester as a risk factor (Pastore and Savitz, 1995). However, many of these earlier studies may be misleading as they either relied on mothers recall of caffeine consumption, retrospectively, or failed to adjust for confounding factors. More recent studies indicate that restricting to no more than 300 mg/day is appropriate as consumption below this level has no effect upon the length of gestation or birth weight (Jarosz *et al.*, 2012), whilst more than 300 mg/day may lead to more small-for-dates pregnancies (Hoyt *et al.*, 2014).

Caffeine consumption tends to be greater in women who smoke tobacco, and smoking is itself an important risk factor for both low birth weight and preterm delivery. Studies that robustly adjust for smoking habit, and which have collected data on caffeine consumption prospectively, tend to show that there is no risk of preterm labour associated with caffeine intakes, even as high as 400 mg/day (Peacock *et al.*, 1995; Chiaffarino *et al.*, 2002; Clausson *et al.*, 2002). The view that caffeine is a hazardous substance for pregnant women may therefore be unmerited, once pregnancy is well established and beyond the vulnerable first trimester. Jahanfar and Jaafar (2013) reported that replacing caffeinated coffee with decaffeinated coffee in the second or third trimester had no effect on gestation length. A meta-analysis of 15 cohort and 7 case–control studies found no association between caffeine consumption at any stage of pregnancy and preterm birth (Maslova *et al.*, 2010).

Systemic activation of the immune system and elevated concentrations of inflammatory agents may be a trigger for preterm delivery in pregnant women. Unravelling the true contribution of periodontitis to risk is problematic as the condition is far more common in cigarette smokers than non-smokers. Smoking is in itself a risk factor for preterm delivery and other complications of pregnancy. Pitiphat *et al.* (2008) reported that, after robust adjustment for smoking, women with periodontal disease were more likely to have a baby that was born prematurely, or at full term but SGA (OR 2.26, 95% CI 1.05–4.85). As shown in Figure 3.9, periodontitis has also been identified as a risk factor for PE. The meta-analysis of Sgolastra *et al.* (2013) suggested a more than doubled risk of PE in women with periodontitis, but low methodological quality of the papers reviewed weakened the strength of the observation. Periodontitis may also be associated with intrauterine growth restriction and low birth weight (Kumar *et al.*, 2013), but these observations are not seen in all studies (Abati *et al.*, 2013) and appear to be very population specific. Further evidence favouring a contribution of periodontitis to risk comes from some small intervention studies, which have shown that effective treatment of periodontal disease during

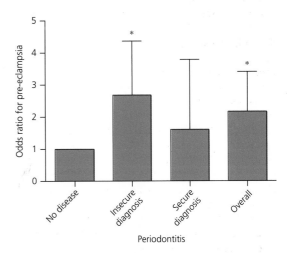

Figure 3.9 Periodontal disease may be a risk factor for pre-eclampsia. Meta-analysis of 15 studies shows a significant risk, but this is mostly attributed to studies where the diagnosis of periodontitis was not robust. Data are shown as odds ratio ± 95% confidence interval. *Significantly different ($P < 0.05$). Sgolastra *et al.* (2013). Reproduced with permission from Sgolastra *et al.*

pregnancy can reduce the risk of preterm delivery and the delivery of SGA infants (López *et al.*, 2002; Jeffcoat *et al.*, 2003).

The mechanisms to explain the associations between periodontal disease and pregnancy complications are not well understood. There are two favoured possibilities which involve either direct interaction between the oral pathogens, or their products, with the foetal placental unit, or effects of pro-inflammatory cytokines upon the foetal-placental unit Sanz and Kornman, 2013). Individuals with periodontal disease have high circulating concentrations of tumour necrosis factor-alpha and prostaglandin E2 which could promote placental dysfunction.

3.4.3 Hypertensive disorders of pregnancy

Rising blood pressure is a common feature of pregnancy and reflects the changing renal function, requirement to maintain placental perfusion and alterations in fluid balance. In some women, the increased blood pressure crosses the threshold of systolic pressure over 140 mmHg and diastolic pressure over 90 mmHg at which hypertension is clinically diagnosed. When hypertension has onset in the latter part of pregnancy, this is termed gestational hypertension. If hypertension has an onset in the first 6 weeks of pregnancy and persists throughout gestation, it is termed chronic hypertension of pregnancy. Neither of these conditions is of major significance in terms of maternal or foetal health.

In contrast, PE is an extremely dangerous condition that threatens the lives of both mother and foetus. PE occurs in 2–7% of pregnancies (Poston, 2006) and is characterized by the development of hypertension after 20 weeks gestation and urinary excretion in excess of 300 mg protein/24 h. In some cases, blood pressure may not rise above the 140/90 mmHg threshold for hypertension diagnosis but will rise sharply (more than 30 mmHg) over a few weeks. Although not used as diagnostic criteria for PE, affected women will also develop severe oedema and metabolic disturbances. PE is a progressive condition that cannot be reversed or controlled. Without intervention, women are at risk of developing eclampsia. Eclampsia is the end stage of the PE disorder and is characterized by maternal seizures and coma due to oedema of the brain. Eclampsia can result in multiple organ failure, renal collapse, abruption of the placenta and death of both mother and baby. In the medical management of PE, in developed countries, the usual protocol is to monitor progress closely and deliver the baby preterm. This is the only way to bring the maternal disease to an end. As a result, PE is the major cause of preterm birth (accounting for around 25% of cases).

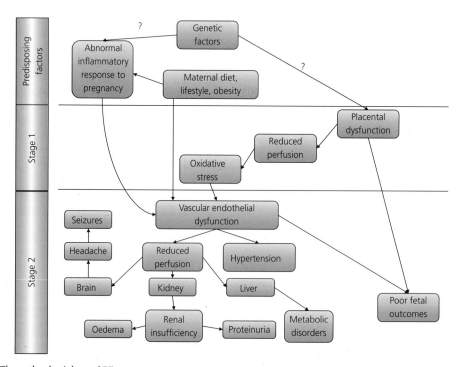

Figure 3.10 The pathophysiology of PE.

3.4.3.1 The aetiology of PE

The primary cause of PE is defective placentation (Poston, 2006). Histological examination of placental tissue from affected pregnancies suggests that there is a partial failure of the invasion of the uterine lining during the early stages of placental formation and as a result the formation of the maternal spiral arteries is incomplete. Blood flow through the placenta is reduced and the capacity to maintain normal perfusion of the organ is impaired. PE is generally regarded as being a two-stage process (see Figure 3.10) and this placental defect represents the first stage (Roberts and Gammill, 2005).

The second stage in the development of PE is the appearance of the maternal disorders. The impaired perfusion of the placenta is believed to result in the release of factors that impact upon vascular endothelial cell function throughout the maternal system. It is argued that one of the key drivers of this dysfunction could be oxidative injury in the placental tissue (Poston, 2006). With reduced placental perfusion, the placental tissue is likely to undergo periods of hypoxia followed by improved blood flow and renewed delivery of oxygen. This hypoxia–reperfusion process will result in the release of free radicals and other reactive oxygen species, causing placental injury. In response to this injury, the placenta will release pro-inflammatory cytokines and activate cells of the immune system. In effect, a systemic inflammatory response is initiated.

The inflammatory response is the main driver of the maternal disorders associated with PE. Primarily, it generates maternal vascular endothelial dysfunction and the main consequences of this are hypertension and a reduction of the blood flow to major organs, including the brain, kidney and liver (Figure 3.10). In the liver, the inflammatory response is responsible for metabolic changes that are remarkably similar to those that are known to occur in cardiovascular disease (Roberts and Gammill, 2005). Indeed, PE is often compared to a speeded up form of atherosclerosis, specifically impacting upon the placenta. Proinflammatory cytokines are antagonists of insulin action and as a result PE is associated with insulin resistance. Maternal circulating free fatty acid and triglyceride concentrations rise, as does low-density lipoprotein cholesterol, while high-density lipoprotein concentrations decrease. Uric acid concentrations in maternal circulation are also reported to increase dramatically with PE and this may be related to declining renal function (Pereira *et al.*, 2014). Hyperuricaemia was shown by Zhou *et al.* (2012) to be a strong predictor of PE (OR 1.99, 95% CI 1.16–3.40), but as it also is predictive of GDM, it may not be seen as a specific biomarker of risk. However, when detected in women with gestational hypertension, it is a strong predictor of progression to PE (Wu *et al.*, 2012). It has been suggested that hyperuricaemia may play a causal role in the development of PE as it occurs in PE before the onset of renal dysfunction and could promote oxidative stress, inflammation and endothelial cell dysfunction (Roberts *et al.*, 2005).

The true determinants of the risk that a woman may develop PE are unknown. It is clear that not all women with placental dysfunction go on to develop PE, which suggests that the presence of other factors is necessary to move from stage 1 to stage 2. Some of the risks may be genetically determined, and certainly women with a previous history of PE are at increased risk. Although the heritability of PE is estimated from twin studies to be 55% (Williams and Broughton-Pipkin, 2011), no universally accepted susceptibility genes have been identified. Lifestyle factors including diet have therefore been a major focus in research aimed at the prevention of PE.

3.4.3.2 Nutrition-related factors and PE

While it is suspected that dietary factors may be important in determining the risk of PE, there is no convincing research that implicates any one specific nutrient (Roberts *et al.*, 2003). Historically, it has been believed that variation in macronutrient intake was an important factor, but contributions of low-protein diets, high intakes of *n*-6 fatty acids or low intakes of *n*-3 fatty acids have largely been excluded.

A number of micronutrients have also been suggested to play a role in development of PE, largely on the basis that women afflicted by the disease manifest abnormalities of biomarkers of mineral status. For example, it is observed that women with PE have low serum concentrations of zinc, calcium and iron (Kim *et al.*, 2012). Many of these changes are now considered to be a consequence of the PE rather than the cause. Iron represents a primary example of this, in that women with PE manifest reduced serum ferritin and transferrin, both being suggestive of low iron status. However, both of these proteins are involved in the inflammatory response and it is more likely that changes associated with PE are explained by this role than it is that iron deficiency contributes to disease risk. Magnesium status has been shown to be poor in women with PE, suggesting a potential role in the disease. However, trials have shown that magnesium supplementation have not provided any benefits in pregnant women (Roberts *et al.*, 2003).

There is a stronger case for calcium playing a causal role in PE. It is noted that women with PE excrete less calcium in their urine than is normal for pregnancy, and supplementation trials have shown that using very high doses of calcium (1.5–2.0 g/day) reduces the prevalence of hypertension in pregnant women by as much as 50% but appears to reduce the risk of PE only in the small subset of women with very poor calcium status going into pregnancy. Hofmeyr *et al.* (2010) performed a systematic review and meta-analysis that was able to evaluate the effects of calcium supplements in women in different categories of PE risk and at different levels of habitual intake. The strength of the evidence of benefit to women with poor calcium status was such that the World Health Organization (2011) issued guidelines stating that women living in areas with habitually low calcium intakes should take a daily supplement of 1.5–2.0 g/day calcium to prevent PE. There are a number of concerns about this advice, however, as high dose calcium will impede absorption of iron, are costly, bulky and may have a negative impact upon post-natal bone mineralization (Von Dadelszen *et al.*, 2012). A review of the evidence regarding lower dose (<1 g/day) calcium supplementation demonstrated that this would also significantly reduce PE risk (RR 0.38 95% CI 0.28–0.52; Hofmeyr *et al.*, 2014). There is an extensive literature describing the involvement of antioxidant nutrients in PE. This is described in detail in Research Highlight 3.3.

Pre-pregnancy BMI is the main nutrition-related predictor of PE risk. Studies suggest that women who are underweight going into pregnancy are at lower risk, while, in general, obese women have substantially elevated risk (Sebire *et al.*, 2001). Jensen and colleagues (2003) reported that women with a BMI over 30 kg/m^2 were at 3.8-fold greater risk than those with a pre-pregnancy BMI between 18.5 and 24.9 kg/m^2. Weight gain in pregnancy is also critical. An intervention which targeted women with BMI over 35 kg/m^2 showed that limiting weight gain below 5 kg reduced the risk of PE by 95% (McGiveron *et al.*, 2015). Studies that have assessed the impact of PE in one pregnancy upon risk in subsequent pregnancies suggest that gaining weight between confinements adds to risk. An increase in BMI of 3 kg/m^2 doubles the risk of PE, even in women of normal weight. Weight loss decreases risk (Walsh, 2007).

The association between PE and obesity is most likely explained by the fact that obesity creates a pro-inflammatory state, with adipose tissue expressing a number of cytokines. Obesity is also associated with insulin resistance and endothelial dysfunction, independently of pregnancy. Thus, for obese women, there is a low-grade inflammatory response due to excess adiposity, superimposed upon the low-grade inflammation that occurs in normal pregnancy (Poston, 2006). This may

Research Highlight 3.3 Antioxidant nutrients and pre-eclampsia.

Oxidative processes appear to play a key role in the development of pre-eclampsia (PE). PE arises due to defective placentation and reactive oxygen species drive this by promoting inflammation, activating apoptosis and generating anti-angiogenic factors that inhibit the formation of new blood vessels and the formation of maternal spiral arteries within the placenta (Poston *et al.*, 2011).

Due to the apparent role of oxidative stress in the development of PE, a number of studies have focused on the potential use of antioxidant vitamin supplements as a strategy for prevention of the disease. One of the first was a small-scale intervention using a combined vitamin C (1000 mg/day) and vitamin E (400 IU/day) supplement, which suggested that antioxidant supplementation could reduce the risk of PE by 76% (Chappell *et al.*, 1999). This formed the basis of a large-scale, multicentred randomized placebo-controlled trial involving women at high risk of PE. However, with this trial there was no reduction in the incidence of PE and, alarmingly, the antioxidant supplement increased the risk of low birth weight by 15% (Poston *et al.*, 2006). Most other studies similarly show that supplements of vitamins C and E similarly fail to impact upon PE risk (Villar *et al.*, 2009; Bastani *et al.*, 2011; Weissgerber *et al.*, 2013).

The lack of effect of supplementation with the antioxidant vitamins has been explained on the basis of inappropriate supplementation strategy (Poston *et al.*, 2011) including dose and timing. The possibility that supplementation is generally too late to influence PE was in part explored by Roberts *et al.* (2010) who administered vitamins C and E from the ninth week of gestation. As with the studies which began supplementation at a later stage (usually early in the second trimester), there was no reduction in PE risk. Other studies have considered a broader range of antioxidant nutrients with mixed findings. Parrish and colleagues (2013) randomized women to receive placebo or a phytonutrient supplement (powdered concentrate of fruit and vegetable juices) but found no evidence of any impact upon PE. A small trial of supplementation with a mixed cocktail of antioxidants reported that supplementation reduced PE by 88% (Wibowo *et al.*, 2012). As this supplement was provided with milk, it may be that the benefits were due to provision of other nutrients, most notably calcium, rather than a specific antioxidant effect.

Overall there would appear to be no evidence to suggest that antioxidant nutrients can prevent PE in high-risk women. This does not mean, however, that antioxidants play no role in determining risk. High-risk women may develop PE due to strong drivers that are not influenced by antioxidants, whilst lower-risk women may experience benefits that have not been explored by the existing literature. Maintaining good intakes of antioxidant nutrients prior to pregnancy may ensure that the very early stages of placentation are protected.

make the progression from stage 1 of PE (placental dysfunction) to fully symptomatic PE, a significantly greater probability.

3.4.4 Abnormal labour

The duration of normal labour, from the first onset of contractions to delivery of the baby, can vary tremendously in length from just a few minutes to 2 or 3 days. On average, women experience labour between 4 and 8 h. Labour has three stages. In the first stage, contractions result in cervical dilatation, thereby opening up the birth canal for the passage of the infant. This first stage is the most protracted element of the labour. In the second stage, the baby moves through the vagina and is born. The third stage of labour is the delivery of the placenta. Risk of foetal or neonatal death is increased in protracted labour, particularly if the labour fails to progress once full cervical dilatation has occurred. In modern medical management of labour, a failure for labour to progress will result in intervention to protect the health of mother and baby. The most extreme intervention is caesarean section, but other interventions that may be used in the second stage include the use of forceps or ventouse to deliver the baby (instrumented delivery). For most women, labour begins spontaneously, but if there is no onset of labour beyond 42 weeks gestation, it is normal for medical staff to artificially induce labour, either using hormone administration or through artificially rupturing membranes. This reduces the risk of adverse maternal health outcomes.

Interventions in labour are not closely related to maternal nutritional status, but it is clear that maternal BMI is a predictor of these outcomes. As shown in Figure 3.11, a survey of pregnancy outcomes in Lincoln, UK, found that women with a BMI in the obese range were significantly more likely to require caesarean delivery. There is also evidence that obese women are more likely to have labour-induced, ventouse or forceps deliveries and have longer hospital stays after delivery (Morgan et al., 2014). The development of complications may vary according to the stage of labour and depend on a woman's previous reproductive history. Labour complications (induction, caesarean, epidural anaesthesia) associated with obesity in a first pregnancy may be absent in subsequent pregnancies (O'Dwyer et al., 2013). As GDM (see Section 3.8.1) is often seen in obese women, there is a greater prevalence of babies being large-for-gestational age (LGA). This contributes to the greater need for medical intervention and also increases the prevalence of shoulder dystocia in babies born to obese mothers.

In contrast, women who are underweight appear to have lower risk of labour complications than women with BMI in the ideal range. BMI less than 20 kg/m² is associated with less frequent induction of labour, fewer instrumented deliveries and lower risk of emergency caesarean (Sebire et al., 2001). Post-partum haemorrhage (PPH) is one of the most serious maternal complications of labour and is the major cause of maternal mortality. Between 5 and 12% of women experiencing normal vaginal delivery will experience PPH. In developed countries, medical management means that the death rate is low (<10 cases per million births), but in the developing world, PPH accounts for around 125 000 maternal deaths every year. PPH is more common in obese women, but being underweight reduces the risk.

3.5 Nausea and vomiting of pregnancy

3.5.1 Nausea and vomiting of pregnancy as a normal physiological process

Nausea and vomiting of pregnancy (NVP) is a commonly reported symptom associated with early pregnancy. Most studies estimate that the prevalence of NVP is somewhere between 60 and 80%, with generally higher rates of occurrence in westernized countries than in developing countries (Furneaux et al., 2001). Given the high prevalence, NVP is widely regarded as a normal, but unpleasant feature of pregnancy. It usually manifests somewhere between 2 and 6 weeks after conception, and for many women it is the first sign that make them feel that they have conceived. Generally, the peak in NVP symptoms occurs between 10 and 12 weeks gestation and for most women, the condition disappears by 20 weeks. For some women, NVP continues throughout the pregnancy.

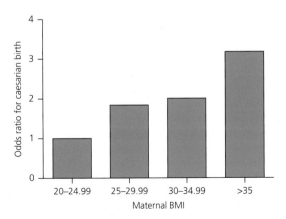

Figure 3.11 Risk of caesarean birth is greater in women who are overweight or obese.
Data Source: Langley-Evans *et al.*, unpublished observations.

NVP is colloquially known as 'morning sickness', but this is a misnomer. Although most women will experience nausea or vomiting in the early morning, there are also peak times for symptoms at other points in the day, and episodes are often triggered by exposure to cooking odours or the preparation and consumption of meals. NVP is for many women a debilitating issue that can cause major interference with the pursuit of normal day-to-day activities. NVP may vary greatly in severity (Coad *et al.*, 2002). In mild cases, there may be nothing more than the sensation of nausea. Moderate cases may suffer some episodes of vomiting, but in severe NVP, women may struggle to retain the meals that they have consumed. The most extreme manifestation of NVP is hyperemesis gravidarum (HG), which will be discussed in the next section. NVP is more common in some groups of women, most notably those having their first baby, women with multiple pregnancies, those of greater BMI, non-smokers and women with a family history of NVP.

The causes of NVP are not fully understood, but most evidence suggests that the symptoms arise as a consequence of the major endocrine changes that accompany the early stages of pregnancy. Oestrogen and progesterone concentrations are high at this stage and both may contribute to the development of NVP (Coad *et al.*, 2002). Progesterone is a modulator of muscle tone in the gastrointestinal tract and may promote gastric reflux by causing a reduction in the patency of the oesophageal sphincter. The mode of action of oestrogen is unclear, but it is noted that women who have a nauseous reaction to oral contraceptives based upon oestrogens are highly likely to develop NVP.

hCG is produced in early pregnancy and plays a key role in the implantation of the embryo and establishment of the placenta. Many lines of circumstantial evidence point to hCG as an important driver of NVP in the first trimester. Firstly, there is a close temporal association between hCG secretion and NVP symptoms (Figure 3.12). The onset of NVP for most women coincides with the first appearance of hCG, and the peak in hCG concentrations in maternal circulation falls around 9–12 weeks, shortly preceding maximum symptoms of NVP. Women with the most severe NVP are found to have elevated concentrations of hCG compared to asymptomatic women, and correlations have been shown between hCG concentrations and the severity of NVP (Furneaux *et al.*, 2001). hCG has a critical role in the establishment of pregnancy, and disturbances in the secretion of this hormone are associated with adverse pregnancy outcomes. Women who underproduce hCG are more likely to suffer spontaneous abortion in early pregnancy and have a greater risk of ectopic pregnancy. Extremely high hCG is also predictive of poor

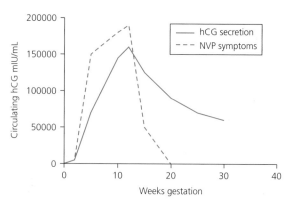

Figure 3.12 The temporal association between symptoms of nausea and vomiting in pregnancy and concentrations of hCG.

outcomes, including foetal death, premature birth and lower weight at birth.

As mentioned earlier, NVP symptoms are the norm rather than the exception for pregnant women in westernized countries. The very high prevalence of a condition that is so debilitating, and in rare cases lethal, to women in early pregnancy, has prompted some researchers to propose that it serves some function that increases the chances of reproductive success. One view is that NVP serves to change patterns of maternal intake and that this prompts the ingestion of foods that are optimal for the development of the placenta (Coad *et al.*, 2002). Most women with NVP quickly learn that, unlike most nausea, these symptoms are alleviated or suppressed by the regular consumption of foods that are rich in complex carbohydrates. An alternative view expressed by Flaxman and Sherman (2000) is that NVP has evolved as a defence mechanism to protect the early embryo from maternal ingestion of food-borne pathogens or toxins. The peak period for NVP corresponds to maximum vulnerability of the foetus or embryo to abortifacients, infected foodstuffs or teratogens. NVP leads most women to avoid ingestion of caffeine containing beverages, meats, fatty foods, burnt food or spicy food. It is argued that many of these foodstuffs would have represented a major risk for pregnant women in the early history of humankind.

There is a wealth of data to support either theory of the origins of NVP, as clearly women who exhibit mild to moderate symptoms are at reduced risk of a number of poor pregnancy outcomes. Czeizel and Puhó (2004) observed that women reporting that they had suffered from NVP had longer gestation periods and had a lower prevalence of premature delivery. This finding confirms observations of a cohort of 300 British women (Figure 3.13), where an absence of NVP was associated

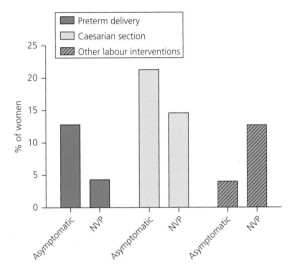

Figure 3.13 NVP is associated with reduced risk of preterm delivery. Three hundred pregnant women were questioned about symptoms of NVP in the first trimester of pregnancy and the outcome of pregnancy was followed up. Women who reported no NVP symptoms were significantly more likely to give birth prior to 37 weeks gestation.
Data Source: Langley-Evans and Langley-Evans, unpublished observations.

with a 3.26-fold (95% CI 1.19–8.91) greater risk of premature delivery and slightly increased risk of caesarean delivery. Within this study, it was apparent that NVP had no major impact upon women's actual consumption of nutrients in the first trimester of pregnancy. The only significant difference was that NVP sufferers consumed less alcohol (an important teratogen) than women who were asymptomatic. Maconochie and colleagues (2007) reviewed the major risk factors for spontaneous abortion in the first trimester of pregnancy, using a large UK population. Nausea was found to be the most important of a number of factors associated with reduced risk of miscarriage. Women with NVP within the first 12 weeks of pregnancy were 70% less likely than asymptomatic women to lose their pregnancy, and those with the most severe symptoms were 93% less likely. A systematic review of 10 papers considering NVP and pregnancy outcomes found favourable effects of NVP on risk of miscarriages, congenital abnormalities and premature delivery (Koren *et al.*, 2014).

3.5.2 Hyperemesis gravidarum

The severity of NVP symptoms varies enormously between women, but only rarely does the extent of those symptoms become so great that there is a threat to the health of the pregnant woman or her child. HG lies at the extreme end of the NVP spectrum and may in fact have completely different causes. HG is characterized by intractable nausea and vomiting, which results in metabolic disturbances, ketosis, dehydration, reduction in maternal blood volume and loss of around 5% of the pre-pregnancy body weight (Figure 3.14). Like NVP, the onset of HG is usually between 4 and 10 weeks gestation and the condition resolves for most women by 20 weeks (Verberg *et al.*, 2005). For 10% of women with HG, the condition will continue for the whole of their pregnancy. HG is relatively uncommon and occurs in 0.3–1.5% of pregnancies (Bailit, 2005; Dodds *et al.*, 2006). Women who suffer from HG in their first pregnancy are at very high risk of developing the same degree of nausea and vomiting in subsequent pregnancies. Trogstad *et al.* (2005) found that odds of recurrence were as high as 26-fold. The risk of HG in a second pregnancy appeared to reduce if the second child had a different father to the first. This suggests an involvement of paternal genes in the development of HG and may give some clues to the aetiology of the problem.

The severity of HG symptoms will generally result in hospitalization for appropriate treatment using vitamin supplements and intravenous infusion of fluids and electrolytes. Before the introduction of this therapy, HG was a cause of maternal death for around 16 in every 100 000 pregnancies. Most HG cases are successfully treated through fluid infusion, and if this does not lead to recovery, women are treated with antiemetic drugs. For around 2% of women with HG, there is no response to treatment and it becomes necessary to terminate the pregnancy (Verberg *et al.*, 2005).

Although, with treatment, the impact of HG on maternal health can be greatly reduced, there may be greater risks for the foetus in an HG-complicated pregnancy. Tan and colleagues (2007) reported that the severity of HG as measured by biomarkers of maternal fluid and electrolyte status was a determinant of pregnancy outcomes. More severe symptoms were associated with a greater prevalence of GDM, more intervention during labour and more emergency procedures. Bailit (2005) found that HG was associated with shorter gestation, a greater prevalence of SGA and greater risk of foetal death. Within the same study, it was shown that babies born prematurely (24–30 weeks) were at greater risk of death if born to women with HG. Examination of birth records from over two million pregnancies in Norway (Vandraas *et al.*, 2013) found a greater risk of perinatal death (OR 1.27) associated with HG, along with lower birth weight (21.4 g smaller). HG affected pregnancies were, however, significantly less likely to end in very preterm birth. In contrast the much smaller Norwegian Mother and Child cohort (Vikanes *et al.*, 2013) found no relationship between HG and any birth outcomes.

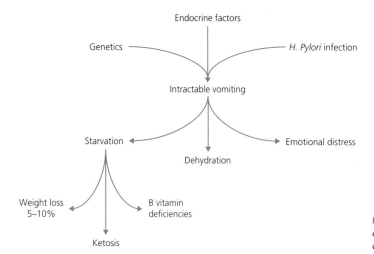

Figure 3.14 Hyperemesis gravidarum is a serious condition of unknown origin. It results in severe dehydration and reduced food intake.

Failure to gain weight and less effective perfusion of the placenta due to reduced blood volume expansion are the most likely routes through which risk of adverse pregnancy outcomes are associated with HG. Certainly, there is very limited evidence that HG has a major effect upon maternal nutritional status. There are reports of numerous deficiencies of vitamins and minerals. These have been attributed to raised demands of pregnancy, reduced food intakes and greater nutrient losses. However, the only consistent findings relate to thiamine and vitamin K (Verberg *et al.*, 2005).

3.6 Cravings and aversions

Just as nausea and vomiting are common symptoms experienced by pregnant women, the majority of women in the first trimester report changes in preferences for certain foodstuffs. These changes are often aversive, with women rejecting foods or beverages that might have been staples within their diet prior to pregnancy. Food cravings are strong desires to consume particular food items, which may not have been major elements of the pre-pregnancy diet. Surveys of the prevalence of food aversions and cravings suggest that between 50 and 60% of women will experience these changes to their eating and drinking behaviours (Furneaux *et al.*, 2001; Bayley *et al.*, 2002).

Aversions reported by pregnant women are most commonly to caffeine-based drinks, red and white meats, fish and eggs. Furneaux and colleagues (2001) observed that two-thirds of pregnant women among a sample of 300 reported aversion to coffee, with 54% developing an aversion to tea. Other foods rejected by this sample of women included spicy foods and foods that were fatty or greasy. Cravings in early pregnancy are often for foods with a high sugar content, with sweets, chocolate and cakes being widely favoured, along with fruit and fruit juices.

The reasons why women develop cravings and aversions in pregnancy are not well understood. Some researchers have suggested that taste and aroma perception is altered by the hormonal changes that accompany early pregnancy and that this produces a preference for sweet foods over bitter foods and a dislike of the smell of foods high in fat (Coad *et al.*, 2002). There are also some suggestions that cravings and aversions have no biological foundation and are instead the products of cultural expectations. One proposal that has received considerable attention and popular support is that cravings and aversions are an element of the broader spectrum of NVP and contribute to foetal defence during embryonic development (Flaxman and Sherman, 2000). It is suggested that NVP symptoms lead to taste aversion learning, in which women are conditioned to avoid foods that are associated with bouts of nausea or vomiting (Bayley *et al.*, 2002). Within an evolutionary perspective, this conditioned behaviour would lead to rejection of the foods most likely to carry toxins or pathogens that might threaten foetal survival.

Support for this idea is partly provided by evidence that women suffering from NVP are more likely to report food aversions than those who do not. Bayley and colleagues (2002) noted that women whose NVP was moderate to severe were more likely to report food aversions and suffered aversions to a greater range of foods than women whose NVP was mild or absent. Importantly, the onset of food aversions appeared to coincide with the onset of NVP symptoms. In contrast, cravings were no more common in women with NVP than in those without and tended to begin much earlier in pregnancy and several weeks ahead of any NVP symptoms. These findings are not supported by all studies (Furneaux *et al.*, 2001), and in contrast to the study by Bayley *et al.* (2002), Coad and colleagues (2002) reported that women with NVP were more likely to have both food aversions and cravings than those who were asymptomatic. Weigel *et al.* (2011) found that women suffering with NVP symptoms were more likely to report increased odour sensitivity and aversions to foods and were more likely to crave for fruit. The roots of cravings and aversions may be different, however, and cravings are often reported to occur in women whose NVP begins very early in pregnancy. The high-carbohydrate foods that are most commonly craved often appear to be of benefit in suppressing or controlling feelings of nausea. A study of nearly 52 000 women in the Norwegian Mother and Child Cohort (Chortatos *et al.*, 2013) found that NVP was associated with higher intakes of carbohydrates and sugary drinks. Whilst the simplest interpretation of this is that women choose these foods to control symptoms, the authors could not discount the possibility that high consumption of these foods may be a cause of NVP.

3.6.1 Pica

Pica represents an extreme form of craving behaviour, which in addition to being noted in pregnancy is associated with mental illness and some micronutrient deficiencies, including iron deficiency anaemia. Pica is the ingestion of substances that have no nutritive value and pica behaviours include the consumption of clay or soil, ice, laundry starch or other substances such as soap or chalk (Table 3.4). Pica in pregnancy appears to be a behaviour that is most commonly associated with women of low socioeconomic status, often including those from ethnic minority groups. Mikkelsen *et al.* (2006) noted that among a large (over 70 000) well-nourished Danish population with relatively low

numbers of ethnic minorities, pica was a rare behaviour that was reported by just 0.7% of women. This was in stark contrast to figures quoted for the United States, where pica is commonplace (30–50%) in migrant women of African origin or African Americans. Indeed, such is the demand for material among such women, some US stores stock clay for human consumption (Stokes, 2006). Rainville (1998) found a high prevalence of pica among deprived, mostly African-American women in Texas. Pica occurred in 77% of pregnant women with the most common substances consumed being ice or the frost from freezers and refrigerators. Although commonplace, there was no evidence that the pica behaviours had any negative effect upon the outcome of pregnancy. However, the women with pica had lower haemoglobin concentrations at delivery than those without pica. While this US study could not with confidence identify iron deficiency as a cause or consequence of pica, due to confounding influences of maternal smoking and educational achievement, other studies show pica and iron deficiency are closely associated. Pica was noted in around 20% of pregnant women in an Argentine study (López *et al.*, 2007), with women reported as consuming ice or dirt. As with Rainville (1998), birth weight and anthropometry among infants were not compromised by pica, but markers of iron status were greatly reduced in the women with pica.

Associations of this nature have lent some support to the concept that pica develops as a response to nutrient deficiency. Consumption of clay, for example, could be seen as a means of ingesting the minerals present in the clay matrix. Malnutrition could thus be a trigger for pica, explaining the higher prevalence in women from deprived backgrounds. However, studies using clay slurries in artificial models of the digestive tract show that clay, for example, would tend to exacerbate malnutrition as iron, zinc and copper become bound to the clay matrix, especially under acid conditions (Stokes, 2006). Geophagia could therefore promote malnutrition rather than be a corrective behaviour. In developing countries, soil and clay are likely to carry pathogenic organisms that may cause harm to pregnant women. Young *et al.* (2007) examined infection with nematodes in an African population of pregnant women. Pica was common in these women and the main behaviours were consumption of clay (7% of women), ice (21%), uncooked rice (55%) and unripe mangoes (84%). Although there was no clear difference in risk of infection when comparing women with geophagia with those showing no pica, there was a tendency for greater levels of hookworm infection in clay eaters. Hookworm infection is an important cause of iron deficiency anaemia in African countries.

Table 3.4 Pica behaviours.

Pica behaviours	Items that are consumed
Amylophagia	Laundry starch
Coniophagia	Dust
Geophagia*	Clay, dirt, soil
Lithophagia	Small stones, grit
Pagophagia*	Ice
Trichophagia	Hair and wool

*Pagophagia and geophagia are most frequently reported by pregnant women.

It seems unlikely then that pica develops to replace nutrient losses or address deficiency. It is possible that these behaviours may help women deal with nausea and vomiting, but far more likely that pica is a cultural phenomenon. This could explain the very high occurrence in women of African origin (Stokes, 2006). As described above, there is no clear evidence of pica causing harm to infants. The potential for harm is clearly present though. Pica, particularly where consumption of clay or soil is involved, has the potential to introduce pathogens or toxins, such as lead, to the body. There are also reports of pica as a cause of GDM. Jackson and Martin (2000) reported two cases of pregnant women with uncontrolled diabetes in a home setting, which spontaneously reversed without treatment on admission to hospital. On investigation, it emerged that these women were consuming large quantities of laundry starch (corn starch) each day.

3.7 Gastrointestinal disturbances in pregnancy

As described earlier in this chapter, the gastrointestinal tract undergoes a number of functional changes during pregnancy, largely under the influence of progesterone. These changes serve to slow down transit times and hence maximize the absorption of nutrients and reabsorption of water from the tract. A combination of these effects of steroid hormones on the tract and the physical expansion of the uterus, baby and placenta as pregnancy progresses can produce a series of minor symptoms of the gastrointestinal tract. These cause discomfort to many pregnant women but only rarely impact upon pregnancy outcomes.

Heartburn (dyspepsia) is a symptom that afflicts many women early in gestation due to declining competency of the oesophageal sphincter. In later gestation, the pressure of the uterus upon the stomach can limit the total stomach capacity and also drive gastric reflux. The period of rapid late gestation foetal growth, where demands for nutrients and fluids are at their greatest, therefore corresponds to the time of lowest stomach capacity, so at this time women need to consume smaller but more frequent meals.

Constipation is also a common symptom of later gestation, impacting upon around a quarter of pregnancies (Bradley *et al.*, 2007). This is largely a consequence of the slow transit of faecal material through the colon and the highly efficient reabsorption of water. Dry compacted faecal material becomes harder to pass and this can also increase the risk of haemorrhoids, which are

another complaint associated with pregnancy. Certain factors increase the likelihood of constipation, including low intakes of water, low fibre diets, reduced physical activity and the prescribing of iron supplements to combat iron deficiency anaemia.

3.8 High-risk pregnancies

A number of pregnancies may be considered to be at higher than normal risk and merit close monitoring and possible medical intervention in order to ensure a successful outcome. Women may be identified as being at high risk on the basis of pre-existing medical conditions (e.g. type 1 and type 2 diabetes), socioeconomic status and lifestyle factors. Maternal factors that are associated with greater risk include pre-pregnancy underweight or obesity, low socioeconomic status, a history of eating disorders, HIV infection and alcohol or other substance abuse.

Maternal age is also a major indicator of risk. Women over the age of 35 are at greater risk of PE, preterm delivery, placenta previa and caesarean section. Consequently, foetal and maternal mortality rates are higher in these older women. The reasons underlying this greater risk are not fully understood but could be related to a greater level of obesity, pre-existing hypertension and insulin resistance in this population. Risk associated with pregnancy also increases markedly in adolescent mothers. Adolescents are at greater risk of iron deficiency anaemia, preterm delivery and having babies that are SGA. This partly relates to their often poor dietary behaviours but is mostly explained by the fact that they are still growing themselves. Girls continue to grow for between 4 and 7 years beyond menarche, with the phase of maximum adolescent growth occurring between the ages of 11 and 13. Pregnancy before the age of 14 will therefore be complicated by competition between mother and foetus for energy and nutrients. As a result, adolescent mothers are unable to lay down sufficient fat reserves in early pregnancy to drive foetal growth in the third trimester, resulting in foetal growth retardation. For similar reasons, women with short intervals between pregnancy are perceived as being at higher risk, as their capacity to replenish nutrient reserves between confinements is limited.

3.8.1 Gestational diabetes

GDM is a syndrome of insulin resistance that develops during pregnancy. In the past, it was referred to as latent diabetes, in reference to the fact that it most likely represents a state in which the metabolic stress of pregnancy causes an existing pre-diabetic state to progress to a symptomatic state. As already mentioned in this chapter, pregnancy is a state in which the mother becomes increasingly insulin resistant. This produces a metabolic scenario in which post-prandial plasma glucose concentrations are elevated, and on fasting, there is greater mobilization of triglycerides, free fatty acids and ketones (Carpenter, 2007). This ensures substrate supply to the placenta and foetus. In 2–3% of pregnancies, these metabolic changes lead to GDM. There is a greater likelihood of GDM being more common in women who are obese, have a family history of diabetes or have other factors that predispose to type 2 diabetes.

In most cases, GDM is a transient state that resolves with the end of pregnancy. However, women suffering from GDM are more likely to develop type 2 diabetes at a later date and around 50% of women with GDM will also develop the condition in subsequent pregnancies (Reader, 2007). GDM is associated with a number of adverse pregnancy outcomes and, in particular, is closely related to the hypertensive disorders of pregnancy (e.g. PE). These associations suggest a common aetiology that relates to inflammatory processes associated with insulin resistance and excess adiposity (Carpenter, 2007).

GDM has a number of negative impacts upon foetal and infant health. One of the most significant of these is macrosomia or 'large baby syndrome'. Babies are defined as being LGA if they weigh over 4.5 kg at birth, regardless of gestational age. LGA is more common in pregnancies associated with GDM. It makes an operative delivery more likely as the large baby is unable to progress through the birth canal without sustaining significant injury such as shoulder dystocia, subconjunctival haemorrhage or fractures (Hadden, 2008). GDM promotes macrosomia of the foetus through spillover of glucose from mother to foetus, across the placenta (Figure 3.15).

Infants whose mothers have GDM may also suffer a period of hypoglycaemia after birth due to the steep fall in glucose input once out of the uterus. GDM is also associated with foetal hypocalcaemia. High prevailing insulin and insulin-like growth factor 1 concentrations in response to high glucose concentrations drive calcium into bone. The GDM-affected foetus tends to have high bone mineral mass, but low circulating calcium, and in extreme cases, this can lead to convulsions after birth. In addition to these immediate hazards, there is a growing body of evidence that suggests that the foetus exposed to GDM is more likely to be obese and to develop type 2 diabetes later in life (Hussain *et al.*, 2007).

Women with GDM require careful monitoring and nutritional management to limit the risk of adverse pregnancy outcomes. Therapies aim to control blood glucose concentrations, without the use of insulin injection. Management is therefore focused around control of carbohydrate intake, while maintaining appropriate rates of weight gain and intakes of other nutrients. Prospective studies from the United States and Australia have shown that such approaches are effective in limiting the need for more robust medical intervention and reducing the risk of serious perinatal complications

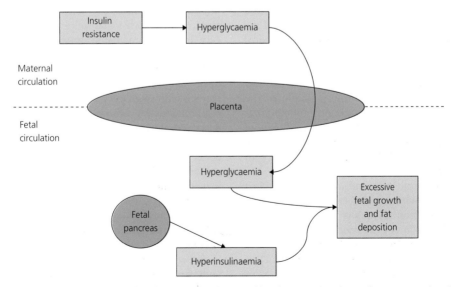

Figure 3.15 GDM is a condition of maternal insulin resistance. Maternal insulin resistance drives glucose across the placenta to the foetal tissues. The ensuing increase in foetal insulin secretion drives excessive foetal growth and leads to LGA.

(Reader, 2007). Physical activity is an important element of the management of GDM. There is evidence that increasing activity before pregnancy and maintaining this during gestation can reduce risk. Care should be taken to monitor blood glucose before and after exercise, and pregnant women should avoid periods of vigorous activity in excess of 15–30 min.

3.8.2 Multiple pregnancies

Multiple pregnancies (twins, triplets, quadruplets or greater) are associated with significantly greater risks for a number of adverse maternal and foetal outcomes of pregnancy. Naturally occurring multiparity is relatively uncommon, with around 1 in 80 natural conceptions resulting in twin pregnancy, 1 in 80^2 (64 000) resulting in triplets and 1 in 80^3 (512 000) leading to quadruplets. However, the numbers of multiple pregnancies have increased markedly since the 1980s due to the greater use of assisted reproductive technologies (Brown and Carlson, 2000). Often techniques such as in vitro fertilization result in the implantation of two or three fertilized embryos to maximize the chances of a successful outcome. As the majority of women undergoing assisted reproduction are older (>35 years), the combination of multiparity and greater age has a particularly marked impact upon their risk profile.

Multiple pregnancies carry significant risk for both mother and babies (Rosello-Soberon et al., 2005). There are greater risks of maternal and neonatal mortalities arising from increased risk of preterm delivery, increased prevalence of preeclampsia, gestational diabetes and post-partum haemorrhage (Rao et al., 2004). Much of the risk of preterm delivery is related to intrauterine growth retardation, with 50% of twins and 90% of triplets being SGA. The combination of SGA and prematurity is a particularly high risk for neonatal death (Brown and Carlson, 2000).

As with other outcomes of pregnancy, maternal BMI pre-pregnancy and weight gain during gestation are the strongest predictors of the outcome of multiple pregnancy. Weight before pregnancy is a key determinant of pregnancy weight gain and availability of maternal reserves to drive the extra foetal growth. Women with twin pregnancies who are obese are significantly less likely to have preterm birth and infants of low birth weight than those who are underweight before pregnancy (Rosello-Soberon et al., 2005). Yeh and Shelton (2007) showed that in twin-bearing women with BMI 29 kg/m², birth weights were up to 170 g greater than in women with BMI <19.8 kg/m² before conception. This study found that achieving a weight gain in excess of 25 kg across pregnancy could increase the birth weights of twins by up to 500 g and furthermore reduced the risk

of being born before 36 weeks gestation and of SGA. This was emphasized by the study of Flidel-Rimon et al. (2005) who showed that in women expecting triplets, achieving a weight gain in excess of 16.2 kg over the first 24 weeks of gestation significantly reduced the risk of SGA, irrespective of the pre-pregnancy BMI. For triplet pregnancies, having a higher pre-pregnancy BMI, even if in the overweight or obese range, reduces the risk of negative pregnancy outcomes.

Final achieved birth weight in multiple pregnancies is most closely related to weight gain in the first trimester, with the period 20–28 weeks gestation also being of great importance (Luke, 2005). It is suggested that to minimize risk associated with multiparity, the early phase of pregnancy should be targeted with appropriate advice to maximize weight maternal gain. Just as with singleton pregnancies, weight gain should be greater in women of lower BMI and reduced in women who are obese. However, proposed gains are considerably greater than for singleton pregnancies. Underweight women carrying twins should aim to gain 22–28 kg over the first 28 weeks of pregnancy, at a rate of 0.5–0.8 kg/week in the first trimester (Luke, 2005). Recommended gains are 17–25, 14–23 and 11–19 kg for women in normal weight, overweight and obese BMI ranges respectively (Rasmussen et al., 2009). Higher gains are desirable in multiple pregnancies as preterm delivery is far more likely, so the period of intrauterine growth is shorter. Maximizing weight at delivery greatly reduces the risk of morbidity and mortality in preterm infants. In all pregnancies, the function of the placenta declines in late gestation. In multiple pregnancies, the decline in function is more rapid. It is suggested that more rapid maternal weight gain in early pregnancy helps to establish a more robust placentation (Luke, 2005).

Women with multiple pregnancies are assumed to have significantly greater energy requirements than women with singleton pregnancies, based purely upon requirements to achieve the optimal weight gains described above. Although there are several recommendations published, there is a lack of robust evidence base available to support any nutritional guidance for multiple pregnancies (Ballard et al., 2011). Brown and Carlson (2000) have suggested that over a full pregnancy, the extra energy requirement for a twin pregnancy would be equivalent to 150 kcal/day, on top of the enhanced requirement for pregnancy. Goodnight and Newman (2009) suggest a greater increment, with a recommendation of 40–45 kcal/kg body weight/day. This is the equivalent of 3150 kcal/day for a 70 kg woman and is well above the 1940 kcal/day (2140 kcal/day in the third trimester) for a singleton pregnancy. Luke (2005) suggests that energy intakes should be 3000 kcal/day for obese mothers with twin pregnancies and 4000 kcal/day for underweight mothers.

Pregnant women, in general, begin gestation with normal insulin secretion and sensitivity, but as pregnancy proceeds develop an exaggerated insulin response to feeding. Insulin concentrations in late pregnancy can be more than three times greater in late pregnancy than in the non-pregnant state. Pregnant women are therefore insulin resistant and this metabolic adaptation helps to shunt substrates across the placenta to the foetus (Butte, 2000). This is enhanced in multiple pregnancy, and as a result, maternal glucose concentrations tend to be low and glycogen stores deplete very rapidly. Development of ketosis as metabolism switches to the utilization of fat, as will occur rapidly during periods of fasting in such women, is predictive of poor pregnancy outcomes (Luke, 2005) and so women with multiple pregnancies are advised to consume food frequently (three meals plus three snacks daily).

In keeping with the extra demand for foetal growth and deposition of maternal tissue to support that growth, micronutrient requirements for multiple pregnancy will be greater than with a singleton pregnancy. Iron status for example will be markedly impacted by the needs of multiple foetuses, possibly additional placentation and the greater maternal blood volume expansion. It is suggested that requirements may be 1.8-fold higher than in a singleton pregnancy (Rosello-Soberon *et al.*, 2005). The US Institute of Medicine has made recommendations relating to intakes of a number of micronutrients in women with multiple pregnancies (Table 3.5), which are over and above the standard recommendations for antenatal supplements. These recommendations are not matched by equivalent advice in other countries. The potential benefits and hazards associated with supplementation with minerals and folate have not been well defined and it may be more appropriate for women to meet the increased need for these nutrients by consuming more nutrient-dense foods. There is some evidence that essential fatty acid concentrations are reduced in multiparous women, suggesting that there may be increased demands for these nutrients. Increased intakes of eggs, fatty fish and oils may therefore be appropriate.

3.8.3 Foetal alcohol spectrum disorders

This chapter has already highlighted the risks associated with alcohol consumption in pregnancy, in relation to miscarriage and preterm birth. Extremes of alcohol consumption, for example, where pregnant woman is an alcoholic, are associated with a range of foetal abnormalities that are collectively known as the foetal alcohol spectrum disorders (FASD). FASD is defined as arising when a child has confirmed exposure to maternal alcohol consumption, craniofacial abnormalities, pre- and post-natal growth retardation and neurocognitive defects (Figure 3.16). The related disorders are FAS, partial FAS, ARBD, and alcohol-related neurodevelopmental disorder (ARND), in which some of the features of FASD may be absent, or specific elements may be more pronounced. For example, in FAS, the confirmed exposure to maternal drinking is often absent, while in ARND, the neurocognitive defects are the most pronounced manifestation (Mukherjee *et al.*, 2006).

The prevalence of these disorders is difficult to estimate as affected children can be undiagnosed until they reach school age. Estimates for FAS vary widely, but 1–3 affected births per 1000 appear reasonable (Hannigan and Armant, 2005). Prevalence rises to 60 per 1000 births for pregnancies where the mother is a confirmed alcoholic. For ARND and partial FAS, the prevalence is likely to be higher and is possibly as much as 30 cases per 1000 births.

Alcohol is able to freely cross the placenta by diffusion. This means that foetal tissues are effectively exposed to the same concentrations as the maternal tissues. However, the foetal system is unable to metabolize alcohol as effectively and so effects are prolonged. When alcohol exposure occurs during critical periods of organ development in the first and second trimesters of pregnancy, there can be major impacts on organ growth and morphogenesis. The central nervous system is most vulnerable to effects of alcohol and it is believed that as much as 20% of all mental retardation in developed countries could be related to FASD. Affected children are born with microcephaly (small head), functional deficits (e.g. loss of hearing), and go on to have lower

Table 3.5 US Institute of Medicine recommendations for micronutrient supplementation in multiple pregnancy.

Micronutrients	Recommended supplement dose*
Iron	30 mg/day
Zinc	15 mg/day
Calcium	250 mg/day
Copper	2 mg/day
Folate	300 µg/day
Vitamin B6	2 mg/day
Vitamin C	50 mg/day
Vitamin D	5 µg/day

*To be introduced after week 12 gestation.

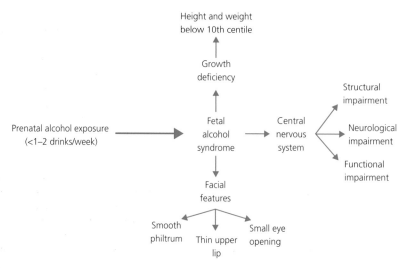

Figure 3.16 The characteristics of fetal alcohol syndrome.

IQ, learning difficulties, language deficits and social and behavioural problems that often lead to disrupted schooling and alcohol and drug abuse problems (Mukherjee *et al.*, 2006). The heart and kidneys are also major targets for ARBD.

The impacts of FASD upon affected children appear to be long lasting and certainly extend into adulthood. FASD is associated with criminal behaviour in adolescence (Momino *et al.*, 2012) and affected individuals have impaired immunity, impaired metabolic function and increased risk of cancer in adulthood (Mead and Sarkar, 2014). In adulthood, it is clear that while some craniofacial abnormalities are resolved, stunted height and microcephaly are not and adults with FAS show a high prevalence of moderate-to-severe mental retardation (Spohr *et al.*, 2007). There is emerging evidence that alcohol exposure during foetal development impacts upon the epigenome, changing DNA and histone marks in a heritable manner. In this way maternal drinking may impact upon more than one generation. Kvigne *et al.* (2008) reported that the grandchildren of women who had abused alcohol in pregnancy were at greater risk of FASD. Given the potentially devastating effect of excessive alcohol consumption in pregnancy, it is alarming to note the growth of binge-drinking cultures among young women in countries such as the United Kingdom. Cessation of drinking should be a priority for women considering pregnancy, as the greatest effects of alcohol may occur during embryogenesis and may precede confirmation of conception.

SUMMARY

- Pregnancy is accompanied by major maternal adaptations that support the development of the placenta and allow foetal growth and development. These adaptations, and the growth of the foetus, greatly increase the demand for energy and nutrients.
- Changes to maternal physiology, behaviour and the mobilization of pre-pregnancy stores are often sufficient to meet requirements for nutrients without changes to intake.
- Optimal maternal weight gain in pregnancy is a key determinant of pregnancy outcome. Advised weight gains vary depending upon pre-pregnancy BMI.
- Nutrition-related factors are predictive of a number of adverse pregnancy outcomes, including miscarriage and stillbirth, gestational diabetes, preterm delivery and the hypertensive disorders of pregnancy.
- Maternal obesity is a major risk factor for most of the adverse pregnancy outcomes.
- Nausea and vomiting of pregnancy is a normal feature of the early stages of most pregnancies. These symptoms may be protective and are associated with a lower risk of early miscarriage.
- Hyperemesis gravidarum is the most extreme form of nausea and vomiting in pregnancy. This condition requires robust intervention as it is associated with greater risk of both maternal foetal death.
- Excessive alcohol consumption in pregnancy is associated with neurocognitive and other congenital disorders in the foetus. These abnormalities are collectively termed the Foetal Alcohol Spectrum Disorders.

References

Abati, S., Villa, A., Cetin, I. *et al.* (2013) Lack of association between maternal periodontal status and adverse pregnancy outcomes: a multicentric epidemiologic study. *Journal of Maternal Fetal and Neonatal Medicine*, **26**, 369–372.

Aguayo, A., Grau, G., Vela, A. *et al.* (2013) Urinary iodine and thyroid function in a population of healthy pregnant women in the North of Spain. *Journal of Trace Elements in Medicine and Biology*, **27**, 302–306.

American College of Obstetrics and Gynecology (2013) *Obesity in Pregnancy*, https://www.acog.org/Resources_And_Publications/Committee_Opinions/Committee_on_Obstetric_Practice/Obesity_in_Pregnancy (last accessed June 2014).

Bailit, J.L. (2005) Hyperemesis gravidarum: epidemiologic findings from a large cohort. *American Journal of Obstetrics and Gynecology*, **193**, 811–814.

Ballard, C.K., Bricker, L., Reed, K. *et al.* (2011) *Nutritional advice for improving outcomes in multiple pregnancies.* Cochrane Database of Systematic Reviews, CD008867.

Barbour, L.A. (2003) New concepts in insulin resistance of pregnancy and gestational diabetes: long-term implications for mother and offspring. *Journal of Obstetrics and Gynaecology*, **23**, 545–549.

Bastani, P., Hamdi, K., Abasalizadeh, F. *et al.* (2011) Effects of vitamin E supplementation on some pregnancy health indices: a randomized clinical trial. *International Journal of General Medicine*, **4**, 461–464.

Bayley, T.M., Dye, L., Jones, S. *et al.* (2002) Food cravings and aversions during pregnancy: relationships with nausea and vomiting. *Appetite*, **38**, 45–51.

Beck, J., Garcia, R., Heiss, G. *et al.* (1996) Periodontal disease and cardiovascular disease. *Journal of Periodontitis*, **67**, 1123–1137.

Bener, A., Al-Hamaq, A.O. and Saleh, N.M. (2013) Association between vitamin D insufficiency and adverse pregnancy outcome: global comparisons. *International Journal Womens Health*, **5**, 523–531.

Bradley, C.S., Kennedy, C.M., Turcea, A.M. *et al.* (2007) Constipation in pregnancy: prevalence, symptoms, and risk factors. *Obstetrics and Gynaecology*, **110**, 1351–1357.

Brown, J.E. and Carlson, M. (2000) Nutrition and multifetal pregnancy. *Journal of the American Dietetic Association*, **100**, 343–348.

Butte, N.F. (2000) Carbohydrate and lipid metabolism in pregnancy: normal compared with gestational diabetes mellitus. *American Journal of Clinical Nutrition*, **71**, 1256S–1261S.

Butte, N.F. and King, J.C. (2005) Energy requirements during pregnancy and lactation. *Public Health Nutrition*, **8**, 1010–1027.

Caldwell, K.L., Pan, Y., Mortensen, M.E. *et al.* (2013) Iodine status in pregnant women in the National Children's Study and in U.S. women (15–44 years), National Health and Nutrition Examination Survey 2005–2010. *Thyroid*, **23**, 927–937.

Carlson, S.E., Colombo, J., Gajewski, B.J. *et al.* (2013) DHA supplementation and pregnancy outcomes. *American Journal of Clinical Nutrition*, **97**, 808–815.

Carpenter, M.W. (2007) Gestational diabetes, pregnancy hypertension, and late vascular disease. *Diabetes Care*, **30** (Suppl 2), S246–S250.

Chapman, A.B., Abraham, W.T., Zamudio, S. *et al.* (1998) Temporal relationships between hormonal and hemodynamic changes in early human pregnancy. *Kidney International*, **54**, 2056–2063.

Chappell, L.C., Seed, P.T., Briley, A.L. *et al.* (1999) Effect of antioxidants on the occurrence of pre-eclampsia in women at increased risk: a randomised trial. *Lancet*, **354**, 810–816.

Chiaffarino, F., Parazzini, F., Chatenoud, L. *et al.* (2002) Coffee drinking and risk of preterm birth. *European Journal of Clinical Nutrition*, **60**, 610–613.

Chortatos, A1., Haugen, M., Iversen, P.O. *et al.* (2013) Nausea and vomiting in pregnancy: associations with maternal gestational diet and lifestyle factors in the Norwegian Mother and Child Cohort Study. *British Journal of Obstetrics and Gynaecology*, **120**, 1642–1653.

Clausson, B., Granath, F., Ekbom, A. *et al.* (2002) Effect of caffeine exposure during pregnancy on birth weight and gestational age. *American Journal of Epidemiology*, **155**, 429–436.

CMACE (2010) *Maternal Obesity in the UK*, http://www.hqip.org.uk/assets/NCAPOP-Library/CMACE-Reports/10.-December-2010-Maternal-Obesity-in-the-UK-Findings-from-a-national-project-2008-2010.pdf (last accessed June 2014).

Coad, J., Al-Rasasi, B. and Morgan, J. (2002) Nutrient insult in early pregnancy. *Proceedings of the Nutrition Society*, **61**, 51–59.

Connor, W.E., Lowensohn, R. and Hatcher, L. (1996) Increased docosahexaenoic acid levels in human newborn infants by administration of sardines and fish oil during pregnancy. *Lipids*, **31**, S183–S187.

Czeizel, A.E. and Puhó, E. (2004) Association between severe nausea and vomiting in pregnancy and lower rate of preterm births. *Paediatric and Perinatal Epidemiology*, **18**, 253–259.

Department of Health (1999) *Dietary Reference Values for Energy and Nutrients for the United Kingdom*, Stationary Office, London.

Dodd, J.M., Turnbull, D.A., McPhee, A.J. *et al.* (2011) Limiting weight gain in overweight and obese women during pregnancy to improve health outcomes: the LIMIT randomised controlled trial. *BMC Pregnancy and Childbirth*, **11**, 79.

Dodd, J.M., Turnbull, D., McPhee, A.J. *et al.* (2014) Antenatal lifestyle advice for women who are overweight or obese: LIMIT randomised trial. *British Medical Journal*, **348**, g1285.

Dodds, L., Fell, D.B., Joseph, K.S. *et al.* (2006) Outcomes of pregnancies complicated by hyperemesis gravidarum. *Obstetrics and Gynecology*, **107**, 285–292.

Durnin, J.V. (1991) Energy requirements of pregnancy. *Diabetes*, **40** (Suppl 2), 152–156.

Englund-Ögge, L., Brantsæter, A.L., Sengpiel, V. *et al.* (2011) Maternal dietary patterns and preterm delivery: results from large prospective cohort study. *British Medical Journal*, **348**, g1446.

Eskenazi, B., Stapleton, A.L., Kharrazi, M. *et al.* (1999) Associations between maternal decaffeinated and caffeinated coffee consumption and fetal growth and gestational duration. *Epidemiology*, **10**, 242–249.

Flaxman, S.M. and Sherman, P.W. (2000) Morning sickness: a mechanism for protecting mother and embryo. *Quarterly Review of Biology*, **75**, 113–148.

Flidel-Rimon, O., Rhea, D.J., Keith, L.G. *et al.* (2005) Early adequate maternal weight gain is associated with fewer small for gestational age triplets. *Journal of Perinatal Medicine*, **33**, 379–382.

Fryar, C.D., Carroll, M.D. and Ogden, C.L. (2010) *Prevalence of Overweight, Obesity, and Extreme Obesity among Adults: United States, Trends 1960–1962 Through 2009–2010*, http://www.cdc.gov/nchs/data/hestat/obesity_adult_09_10/obesity_adult_09_10.htm (last accessed June 2014).

Furneaux, E.C., Langley-Evans, A.J. and Langley-Evans, S.C. (2001) Nausea and vomiting of pregnancy: endocrine basis and contribution to pregnancy outcome. *Obstetric and Gynecological Surveys*, **56**, 775–782.

Gaskins, A.J., Rich-Edwards, J.W., Hauser, R. *et al.* (2014) Maternal prepregnancy folate intake and risk of spontaneous abortion and stillbirth. *Obstetrics and Gynecology*, **124**, 23–31.

Goodnight, W. and Newman, R. (2009) Optimal nutrition for improved twin pregnancy outcome. *Obstetrics and Gynecology*, **114**, 1121–1134.

Hadden, D.R. (2008) Prediabetes and the big baby. *Diabetic Medicine*, **25**, 1–10.

Hamilton, S.A., McNeil, R., Hollis, B.W. *et al.* (2010) Profound vitamin D deficiency in a diverse group of women during pregnancy living in a sun-rich environment at latitude 32°N. *International Journal of Endocrinology*, **2010**, 917428.

Hannigan, J.H. and Armant, D.R. (2005) Alcohol in pregnancy and neonatal outcome. *Seminars in Neonatology*, **5**, 243–254.

Helgstrand, S. and Andersen, A.M. (2005) Maternal underweight and the risk of spontaneous abortion. *Acta Obstetrica et Gynecologica Scandinavica*, **84**, 1197–1201.

Hofmeyr, G.J., Lawrie, T.A., Atallah, A.N. *et al.* (2010) *Calcium supplementation during pregnancy for preventing hypertensive disorders and related problems. Cochrane Database of Systematic Reviews*, CD001059.

Hofmeyr, G., Belizán, J. and von Dadelszen, P. (2014) Low-dose calcium supplementation for preventing pre-eclampsia: a systematic review and commentary. *British Journal of Obstetrics and Gynaecology*, **8**, 951–957.

Hoyt, A.T., Browne, M., Richardson, S. *et al.* (2014) Maternal caffeine consumption and small for gestational age births: results from a population-based case-control study. *Maternal and Child Health Journal*, **18**, 1540–1551.

Hussain, A., Claussen, B., Ramachandran, A. *et al.* (2007) Prevention of type 2 diabetes: a review. *Diabetes Research and Clinical Practice*, **76**, 317–326.

Hytten, F.E. and Leitch, I. (1971) *The Physiology of Human Pregnancy*, Blackwell, Oxford.

Innis, S.M. (2005) Essential fatty acid transfer and fetal development. *Placenta*, **26** (Suppl A), S70–S75.

Institute of Medicine (2009) *Weight Gain During Pregnancy: Reexamining the Guidelines*, National Academies Press, Washington, D.C.

Jackson, W.C. and Martin, J.P. (2000) Amylophagia presenting as gestational diabetes. *Archives of Family Medicine*, **9**, 649–652.

Jaddoe, V.W., Bakker, R., Hofman, A. *et al.* (2007) Moderate alcohol consumption during pregnancy and the risk of low birth weight and preterm birth. The generation R study. *Annals of Epidemiology*, **17**, 834–840.

Jahanfar, S. and Jaafar, S.H. (2013) *Effects of restricted caffeine intake by mother on fetal, neonatal and pregnancy outcome. Cochrane Database of Systematic Reviews*, CD006965.

Jaiswal, N., Melse-Boonstra, A., Sharma, S.K. *et al.* (2014) *The iodized salt programme in Bangalore, India provides adequate* iodine intakes in pregnant women and more-than-adequate iodine intakes in their children. *Public Health Nutrition* In Press.

Jarosz, M., Wierzejska, R. and Siuba, M. (2012) Maternal caffeine intake and its effect on pregnancy outcomes. *European Journal of Obstetrics Gynecology and Reproductive Biology*, **160**, 156–160.

Javaid, M.K., Crozier, S.R., Harvey, N.C. *et al.* (2006) Maternal vitamin D status during pregnancy and childhood bone mass at age 9 years: a longitudinal study. *Lancet*, **367**, 36–43.

Jeffcoat, M.K., Hauth, J.C., Geurs, N.C. *et al.* (2003) Periodontal disease and preterm birth: results of a pilot intervention study. *Journal of Periodontology*, **74**, 1214–1218.

Jensen, C.L. (2006) Effects of n-3 fatty acids during pregnancy and lactation. *American Journal of Clinical Nutrition*, **83**, 1452S–1457S.

Jensen, D.M., Damm, P., Sørensen, B. *et al.* (2003) Pregnancy outcome and prepregnancy body mass index in 2459 glucose-tolerant Danish women. *American Journal of Obstetrics and Gynecology*, **189**, 239–244.

Kim, J., Kim, Y.J., Lee, R. *et al.* (2012) Serum levels of zinc, calcium, and iron are associated with the risk of preeclampsia in pregnant women. *Nutrition Research*, **32**, 764–769.

King, J.C. (2000) Physiology of pregnancy and nutrient metabolism. *American Journal of Clinical Nutrition*, **71**, 1218S–1225S.

Klebanoff, M.A., Shiono, P.H., Selby, J.V. *et al.* (1991) Anemia and spontaneous preterm birth. *American Journal of Obstetrics and Gynecology*, **164**, 59–63.

Koren, G., Madjunkova, S. and Maltepe, C. (2014) The protective effects of nausea and vomiting of pregnancy against adverse fetal outcome—a systematic review. *Reproductive Toxicology*, **47C**, 77–80.

Kramer, M.S. and Kakuma, R. (2003) *Energy and protein intake in pregnancy. Cochrane Database Systematic Reviews*, CD000032.

Kumar, A., Basra, M., Begum, N. *et al.* (2013) Association of maternal periodontal health with adverse pregnancy outcome. *Journal of Obstetric and Gynaecological Research*, **39**, 40–45.

Kvigne, V.L., Leonardson, G.R., Borzelleca, J. *et al.* (2008) Characteristics of grandmothers who have grandchildren with fetal alcohol syndrome or incomplete fetal alcohol syndrome. *Maternal and Child Health Journal*, **12**, 760–765.

Li, N., Liu, E., Guo, J. *et al.* (2013) Maternal prepregnancy body mass index and gestational weight gain on pregnancy outcomes. *PLoS One*, **8**, e82310.

López, N.J., Smith, P.C. and Gutierrez, J. (2002) Periodontal therapy may reduce the risk of preterm low birth weight in women with periodontal disease: a randomized controlled trial. *Journal of Periodontology*, **73**, 911–924.

López, L.B., Langini, S.H. and Pita dePortela, M.L. (2007) Maternal iron status and neonatal outcomes in women with pica during pregnancy. *International Journal of Gynaecology and Obstetrics*, **98**, 151–152.

Luke, B. (2005) Nutrition and multiple gestation. *Seminars in Perinatology*, **29**, 349–354.

Lundsberg, L.S., Bracken, M.B. and Saftlas, A.F. (2007) Low-to-moderate gestational alcohol use and intrauterine growth retardation, low birthweight, and preterm delivery. *Annals of Epidemiology*, **7**, 498–508.

Maconochie, N., Doyle, P., Prior, S. *et al.* (2007) Risk factors for first trimester miscarriage—results from a UK-population-based case-control study. *British Journal of Obstetrics and Gynaecology*, **114**, 170–186.

Marchioni, E., Fumarola, A., Calvanese, A. *et al.* (2008) Iodine deficiency in pregnant women residing in an area with adequate iodine intake. *Nutrition*, **24**, 458–461.

Martin, T.R. and Bracken, M.B. (1987) The association between low birth weight and caffeine consumption during pregnancy. *American Journal of Epidemiology*, **126**, 813–821.

Maslova, E., Bhattacharya, S., Lin, S.W. *et al.* (2010) Caffeine consumption during pregnancy and risk of preterm birth: a meta-analysis. *American Journal of Clinical Nutrition*, **92**, 1120–1132.

May, L., Suminski, R., Berry, A. *et al.* (2014) Diet and pregnancy: health-care providers and patient behaviors. *Journal of Perinatal Education*, **23**, 50–56.

McGiveron, A., Foster, S., Pearce, J. *et al.* (2015) Limiting antenatal weight gain improves maternal health outcomes in severely obese pregnant women: findings of a pragmatic evaluation of a midwife-led intervention. *Journal of Human Nutrition and Dietetics*, **28** Suppl 1, 29–37.

McIntyre, H.D., Gibbons, K.S., Flenady, V.J., and Callaway, L.K. (2012) Overweight and obesity in Australian mothers: epidemic or endemic? *Medical Journal of Australia*, **196**, 184–188.

Mead, E.A. and Sarkar, D.K. (2014) Fetal alcohol spectrum disorders and their transmission through genetic and epigenetic mechanisms. *Frontiers in Genetics*, **5**, 154.

Merlino, A., Laffineuse, L., Collin, M. *et al.* (2006) Impact of weight loss between pregnancies on recurrent preterm birth. *American Journal of Obstetrics and Gynecology*, **195**, 818–821.

Mikkelsen, T.B., Andersen, A.M. and Olsen, S.F. (2006) Pica in pregnancy in a privileged population: myth or reality. *Acta Obstetrica et Gynecologica Scandinavica*, **85**, 1265–1266.

Millward, D.J. (1999) Optimal intakes of protein in the human diet. *Proceedings of the Nutrition Society*, **58**, 403–413.

Mishra, V., Thapa, S., Retherford, R.D. *et al.* (2005) Effect of iron supplementation during pregnancy on birthweight: evidence from Zimbabwe. *Food and Nutrition Bulletin*, **26**, 338–347.

Momino, W., Félix, T.M., Abeche, A.M. *et al.* (2012) Maternal drinking behavior and fetal alcohol spectrum disorders in adolescents with criminal behavior in southern Brazil. *Genetics and Molecular Biology*, **35** (4 Suppl), 960–965.

Morgan, K.L., Rahman, M.A., Hill, R.A. *et al.* (2014) Physical activity and excess weight in pregnancy have independent and unique effects on delivery and perinatal outcomes. *PLoS One*, **9**, e94532.

Mukherjee, R.A., Hollins, S. and Turk, J. (2006) Fetal alcohol spectrum disorder: an overview. *Journal of the Royal Society of Medicine*, **99**, 298–302.

National Institute for Health and Clinical Excellence; NICE (2010) *Dietary Interventions and Physical Activity Interventions for Weight Management Before, During and After Pregnancy. Public Health Guidance PH27*, http://publications.nice.org.uk/weight-management-before-during-and-after-pregnancy-ph27 (last accessed June 2014).

Nohr, E.A., Bech, B.H., Vaeth, M. *et al.* (2007) Obesity, gestational weight gain and preterm birth: a study within the Danish National Birth Cohort. *Paediatric and Perinatal Epidemiology*, **21**, 5–14.

Nohr, E.A., Olsen, J., Bech, B.H. *et al.* (2014) Periconceptional intake of vitamins and fetal death: a cohort study on multivitamins and folate. *International Journal of Epidemiology*, **43**, 174–184.

O'Dwyer, V., O'Kelly, S., Monaghan, B. *et al.* (2013) Maternal obesity and induction of labor. *Acta Obstetrics Gynecology Scandinavia*, **92**, 1414–1418.

Parrish, M.R., Martin, J.N., Jr, Lamarca, B.B. *et al.* (2013) Randomized, placebo controlled, double blind trial evaluating early pregnancy phytonutrient supplementation in the prevention of preeclampsia. *Journal of Perinatology*, **33**, 593–599.

Pastore, L.M. and Savitz, D.A. (1995) Case-control study of caffeinated beverages and preterm delivery. *American Journal of Epidemiology*, **141**, 61–69.

Patra, J., Bakker, R., Irving, H. *et al.* (2011) Dose-response relationship between alcohol consumption before and during pregnancy and the risks of low birthweight, preterm birth and small for gestational age (SGA)—a systematic review and meta-analyses. *British Journal of Obstetrics and Gynecology*, **118**, 1411–1421.

Peacock, J.L., Bland, J.M. and Anderson, H.R. (1995) Preterm delivery: effects of socioeconomic factors, psychological stress, smoking, alcohol, and caffeine. *British Medical Journal*, **311**, 531–535.

Pereira, K.N., Knoppka, C.K. and da Silva, J.E. (2014) Association between uric acid and severity of pre-eclampsia. *Clinical Laboratory*, **60** (2), 309–314.

Pitiphat, W., Joshipura, K.J., Gillman, M.W. *et al.* (2008) Maternal periodontitis and adverse pregnancy outcomes. *Community Dentistry and Oral Epidemiology*, **36**, 3–11.

Poston, L. (2006) Endothelial dysfunction in pre-eclampsia. *Pharmacological Reports*, **58** (Suppl), 69–74.

Poston, L., Briley, A.L., Seed, P.T. *et al.* (2006) Vitamins in Pre-eclampsia (VIP) trial consortium. Vitamin C and vitamin E in pregnant women at risk for pre-eclampsia (VIP trial): randomised placebo-controlled trial. *Lancet*, **367**, 1145–1154.

Poston, L., Igosheva, N., Mistry, H.D. *et al.* (2011) Role of oxidative stress and antioxidant supplementation in pregnancy disorders. *American Journal of Clinical Nutrition*, **94** (6 Suppl), 1980S–1985S.

Poston, L., Briley, A.L., Barr, S. *et al.* (2013) Developing a complex intervention for diet and activity behaviour change in obese pregnant women (the UPBEAT trial); assessment of behavioural change and process evaluation in a pilot randomised controlled trial. *BMC Pregnancy Childbirth*, **13**, 148.

Prentice, A.M. and Goldberg, G.R. (2000) Energy adaptations in human pregnancy: limits and long-term consequences. *American Journal of Clinical Nutrition*, **71**, 1226S–1232S.

Public Health England (2014) *Maternal Obesity*, http://www.noo.org.uk/NOO_about_obesity/maternal_obesity (last accessed June 2014).

Rainville, A.J. (1998) Pica practices of pregnant women are associated with lower maternal hemoglobin level at delivery. *Journal of the American Dietetic Association*, **98**, 293–296.

Rao, A.K., Cheng, Y.W. and Caughey, A.B. (2004) Perinatal complications among different Asian-American subgroups. *American Journal of Obstetrics and Gynecology*, **194**, e39–41.

Rasmussen, K.M., Catalano, P.M. and Yaktine, A.L. (2009) New guidelines for weight gain during pregnancy: what obstetrician/gynecologists should know. *Current Opinion in Obstetrics & Gynecology*, **21** (6), 521–526.

Rasmussen, M.A., Maslova, E., Halldorsson, T.I. *et al.* (2014) Characterization of dietary patterns in the Danish national birth cohort in relation to preterm birth. *PLoS One*, **9**, e93644.

Reader, D.M. (2007) Medical nutrition therapy and lifestyle interventions. *Diabetes Care*, **30** (Suppl 2), S188–S193.

Ritchie, L.D., Whaley, S.E., Spector, P. *et al.* (2010) Favorable impact of nutrition education on California WIC families. *Journal of Nutrition Education and Behaviour*, **42**, S2–S10.

Roberts, J.M. and Gammill, H.S. (2005) Preeclampsia: recent insights. *Hypertension*, **46**, 1243–1249.

Roberts, J.M., Balk, J.L., Bodnar, L.M. *et al.* (2003) Nutrient involvement in preeclampsia. *Journal of Nutrition*, **133**, 1684S–1692S.

Roberts, J.M., Bodnar, L.M., Lain, K.Y. *et al.* (2005) Uric acid is as important as proteinuria in identifying fetal risk in women with gestational hypertension. *Hypertension*, **46**, 1263–1269.

Roberts, J.M., Myatt, L., Spong, C.Y. *et al.* (2010) Vitamins C and E to prevent complications of pregnancy-associated hypertension. *New England Journal of Medicine*, **362**, 1282–1291.

Roselló-Soberón, M.E., Fuentes-Chaparro, L. and Casanueva, E. (2005) Twin pregnancies: eating for three? Maternal nutrition update. *Nutrition Reviews*, **63**, 295–302.

Rumbold, A., Middleton, P., Pan, N. *et al.* (2011) *Vitamin supplementation for preventing miscarriage. Cochrane Database of Systematic Reviews*, CD004073.

Sanders, T.A. (1999) Essential fatty acid requirements of vegetarians in pregnancy, lactation, and infancy. *American Journal of Clinical Nutrition*, **70**, 555S–559S.

Sanz, M. and Kornman, K. (2013) Periodontitis and adverse pregnancy outcomes: consensus report of the Joint EFP/AAP Workshop on Periodontitis and Systemic Diseases. *Journal of Periodontology*, **84** (4 Suppl), S164–169.

Scholl, T.O. and Reilly, T. (2000) Anemia, iron and pregnancy outcome. *Journal of Nutrition*, **130**, 443S–447S.

Sculley, D.V. and Langley-Evans, S.C. (2003) Periodontal disease is associated with lower antioxidant capacity in whole saliva and evidence of increased protein oxidation. *Clinical Science*, **105**, 167–172.

Sebire, N.J., Jolly, M., Harris, J. *et al.* (2001) Is maternal underweight really a risk factor for adverse pregnancy outcome? A population-based study in London. *British Journal of Obstetrics and Gynaecology*, **108**, 61–66.

Sgolastra, F., Petrucci, A., Severino, M. *et al.* (2013) Relationship between periodontitis and pre-eclampsia: a meta-analysis. *PLoS One*, **8**, e71387.

Shirazian, T., Monteith, S., Friedman, F. *et al.* (2010) Lifestyle modification program decreases pregnancy weight gain in obese women. *American Journal of Perinatology*, **27** (5), 411–414.

Sommer, C., Mørkrid, K., Jenum, A.K. *et al.* (2014) Weight gain, total fat gain and regional fat gain during pregnancy and the association with gestational diabetes: a population-based cohort study. *International Journal of Obesity*, **38**, 76–81.

Spohr, H.L., Willms, J. and Steinhausen, H.C. (2007) Fetal alcohol spectrum disorders in young adulthood. *Journal of Pediatrics*, **150**, 175–179.

Stokes, T. (2006) The earth eaters. *Nature*, **444**, 543–544.

Tan, P.C., Jacob, R., Quek, K.F. *et al.* (2007) Pregnancy outcome in hyperemesis gravidarum and the effect of laboratory clinical indicators of hyperemesis severity. *Journal of Obstetrics and Gynaecology Research*, **33**, 457–464.

Thangaratinam, S., Rogozinska, E., Jolly, K. *et al.* (2012) Effects of interventions in pregnancy on maternal weight and obstetric outcomes: meta-analysis of randomised evidence. *British Medical Journal*, **344**, e2088.

Thornton, Y.S., Smarkola, C., Kopacz, S.M. *et al.* (2009) Perinatal outcomes in nutritionally monitored obese pregnant women: a randomized clinical trial. *Journal of the National Medical Association*, **101**, 69–577.

Trogstad, L.I., Stoltenberg, C., Magnus, P. *et al.* (2005) Recurrence risk in hyperemesis gravidarum. *British Journal of Obstetrics and Gynaecology*, **112**, 1641–1645.

Vandraas, K.F., Vikanes, A.V., Vangen, S. *et al.* (2013) Hyperemesis gravidarum and birth outcomes-a population-based cohort study of 2.2 million births in the Norwegian Birth Registry. *British Journal of Obstetrics and Gynaecology*, **120**, 1654–1660.

Verberg, M.F., Gillott, D.J., Al-Fardan, N. *et al.* (2005) Hyperemesis gravidarum, a literature review. *Human Reproduction Update*, **11**, 527–539.

Vikanes, Å.V., Støer, N.C., Magnus, P. *et al.* (2013) Hyperemesis gravidarum and pregnancy outcomes in the Norwegian Mother and Child Cohort—a cohort study. *BMC Pregnancy and Childbirth*, **13**, 169.

Villar, J., Purwar, M., Merialdi, M. *et al.* (2009) World Health Organisation multicentre randomised trial of supplementation with vitamins C and E among pregnant women at high risk for pre-eclampsia in populations of low nutritional status from developing countries. *British Journal of Obstetrics and Gynaecology*, **116**, 780–788.

von Dadelszen, P., Firoz, T., Donnay, F. *et al.* (2012) Preeclampsia in low and middle income countries-health services lessons learned from the PRE-EMPT (PRE-eclampsia-eclampsia monitoring, prevention and treatment) project. *Journal of Obstetrics and Gynaecology Canada*, **34**, 917–926.

Wainwright, P.E. (2002) Dietary essential fatty acids and brain function: a developmental perspective on mechanisms. *Proceedings of the Nutrition Society*, **61**, 61–69.

Walsh, S.W. (2007) Obesity: a risk factor for preeclampsia. *Trends in Endocrinology and Metabolism*, **18**, 365–370.

Wang, J.X., Davies, M.J. and Norman, R.J. (2002) Obesity increases the risk of spontaneous abortion during infertility treatment. *Obesity Research*, **10**, 551–554.

Wei, S.Q., Qi, H.P., Luo, Z.C. *et al.* (2013) Maternal vitamin D status and adverse pregnancy outcomes: a systematic review and meta-analysis. *Journal of Maternal Fetal and Neonatal Medicine*, **26**, 889–899.

Weigel, M.M., Coe, K., Castro, N.P. *et al.* (2011) Food aversions and cravings during early pregnancy: association with nausea and vomiting. *Ecology of Food and Nutrition*, **50**, 197–214.

Weissgerber, T.L., Gandley, R.E., Roberts, J.M. *et al.* (2013) Haptoglobin phenotype, pre-eclampsia, and response to supplementation with vitamins C and E in pregnant women with type-1 diabetes. *British Journal of Obstetrics and Gynecology*, **120**, 1192–1199.

Weng, X., Odouli, R. and Li, D.K. (2008) Maternal caffeine consumption during pregnancy and the risk of miscarriage: a prospective cohort study. *American Journal of Obstetrics and Gynecology*, **198**, e1–e8.

Whittaker, P.G., Lind, T. and Williams, J.G. (1991) Iron absorption during normal human pregnancy: a study using stable isotopes. *British Journal of Nutrition*, **65**, 457–463.

Wibowo, N., Purwosunu, Y., Sekizawa, A. *et al.* (2012) Antioxidant supplementation in pregnant women with low antioxidant status. *Journal of Obstetric and Gynaecological Research*, **38**, 1152–1161.

Wilkinson, S.A. and McIntyre, H.D. (2012) Evaluation of the 'healthy start to pregnancy' early antenatal health promotion workshop: a randomized controlled trial. *BMC Pregnancy and Childbirth*, **12**, 131.

Wilkinson, S.A., van der Pligt, P., Gibbons, K.S. *et al.* (2015) Trial for reducing weight retention in New Mums: a randomised controlled trial evaluating a low intensity, postpartum weight management programme. *Journal of Human Nutrition and Dietetics*, **28** Suppl 1, 15–28.

Williams, P.J. and Broughton Pipkin, F. (2011) The genetics of pre-eclampsia and other hypertensive disorders of pregnancy. *Best Practice in Research in Clinical Obstetrics and Gynaecology*, **25**, 405–417.

World Health Organization (2011) *Recommendations for the Prevention and Treatment of Pre-eclampsia and Eclampsia*, http://whqlibdoc.who.int/publications/2011/9789241548335_eng.pdf (last accessed June 2014).

Wu, Y., Xiong, X., Fraser, W.D. *et al.* (2012) Association of uric acid with progression to preeclampsia and development of adverse conditions in gestational hypertensive pregnancies. *American Journal of Hypertension*, **25**, 711–717.

Yeh, J. and Shelton, J.A. (2007) Association of pre-pregnancy maternal body mass and maternal weight gain to newborn outcomes in twin pregnancies. *Acta Obstetrica et Gynecologica Scandinavica*, **86**, 1051–1057.

Young, S.L., Goodman, D., Farag, T.H. *et al.* (2007) Geophagia is not associated with Trichuris or hookworm transmission in Zanzibar, Tanzania. *Transactions of the Royal Society of Tropical Medicine*, **101**, 766–772.

Yu, C.K.H., Teoh, T.G. and Robinson, S. (2006) Obesity in pregnancy. *British Journal of Obstetrics and Gynaecology*, **113**, 1117–1125.

Zagré, N.M., Desplats, G., Adou, P. *et al.* (2007) Prenatal multiple micronutrient supplementation has greater impact on birthweight than supplementation with iron and folic acid: a cluster-randomized, double-blind, controlled programmatic study in rural Niger. *Food and Nutrition Bulletin*, **28**, 317–327.

Zhou, J., Zhao, X., Wang, Z. *et al.* (2012) Combination of lipids and uric acid in mid-second trimester can be used to predict adverse pregnancy outcomes. *Journal of Maternal Fetal and Neonatal Medicine*, **25**, 2633–2638.

Additional reading

If you would like to find out more about the material discussed in this chapter, the following sources may be of interest.

Lammi-Keefe, C.J., Couch, S.C. and Philipson, E. (eds) (2008) *Handbook of Nutrition and Pregnancy*, Springer, Totowa.

Symonds, M.E. and Ramsay, M.M. (eds) (2010) *Maternal-Fetal Nutrition During Pregnancy and Lactation*, Cambridge University Press, Cambridge, UK.

CHAPTER 4
Fetal nutrition and disease in later life

LEARNING OBJECTIVES

This chapter will enable the reader to:
- Understand the adaptive nature of fetal development and the capacity of the fetal organs and tissues to respond to changes in the maternal environment
- Define what is meant by the terms fetal or nutritional programming and outline the basis of the Developmental Origins of Health and Disease hypothesis
- Describe the association between risk factors operating in fetal life and disease during adulthood
- Discuss the epidemiological evidence that suggests that maternal nutrition during pregnancy may programme the risk of major disease later in life
- Demonstrate an awareness of the limitations of epidemiology as a tool for exploring nutritional programming of disease
- Give an overview of the evidence obtained from experimental models that shows the biological plausibility of the nutritional programming concept
- Discuss the candidate mechanisms that have been proposed to explain how maternal undernutrition might programme disease in the developing fetus
- Show an awareness of the epigenetic mechanisms through which gene expression is regulated and describe how these processes might define the functions of cells, tissues and organs
- Discuss the ways in which variation in the individual response to food arises beyond the genetic level
- Discuss the potential application of understanding of nutritional programming in designing future public health interventions or personalized nutrition strategies to prevent coronary heart disease, obesity and type 2 diabetes

4.1 Introduction

Chapter 3 outlined the importance of nutrition during pregnancy from the perspective of maintaining the health of the pregnant woman and ensuring the safe delivery of her infant. It is now clear that nutrition during pregnancy is also important in determining the long-term health and well-being of the developing fetus. This concept lies at the core of the idea that health and disease and the individual response to food at all stages of life are the product of cumulative experiences across the lifespan. This chapter will focus upon the evidence that early life under- or overnutrition can exert powerful effects, termed 'programming', upon the development of organs and systems, and that these programming effects are an important risk factor for disease. The chapter will review some of the proposed mechanisms that link nutrition during fetal life to diseases such as coronary heart disease and diabetes in the older adult.

4.2 The developmental origins of adult disease

4.2.1 The concept of programming

The term programming describes the process through which exposure to environmental stimuli or insults during critical phases of development brings about permanent changes to the physiology or metabolism of the organism. A dramatic example of programming at work is provided by the mechanisms that determine sex in crocodilians. Alligators and crocodiles lack sex chromosomes. Their eggs are laid into heaped mounds within which exists a temperature gradient. At most temperatures within the nest, the embryos will develop into females, while within a very specific range of 4–5°C, the embryos are programmed to become males. These effects are seen because the temperature of the egg determines the expression of genes responsible for the synthesis of the sex steroids, which then govern the physiological

Nutrition, Health and Disease: A Lifespan Approach, Second Edition. Simon Langley-Evans.
© 2015 John Wiley & Sons, Ltd. Published 2015 by John Wiley & Sons, Ltd.
Companion website: www.wiley.com/go/langleyevans/lifespan

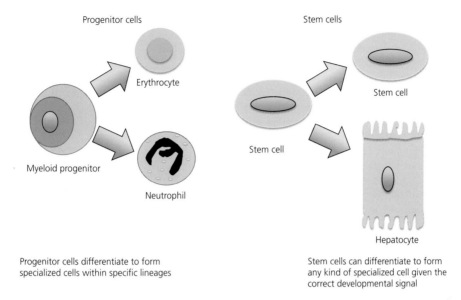

Progenitor cells

Stem cells

Erythrocyte

Stem cell

Myeloid progenitor

Stem cell

Neutrophil

Stem cell

Hepatocyte

Progenitor cells differentiate to form specialized cells within specific lineages

Stem cells can differentiate to form any kind of specialized cell given the correct developmental signal

Figure 4.1 Progenitor cells and stem cells have the property of plasticity whereby growth factor or cytokine signals can trigger a differentiation response or cell division. The fates of progenitor cells are limited to specific lineages of cells within a tissue or system, but embryonic stem cells are pluripotent and in response to cues during development can give rise to any cell type.

development of these reptiles. This is clearly a programming response under the definition provided earlier, since the stimulus is temperature, the critical phase of development lies within the embryonic period and the effect of the exposure is permanent.

Within mammalian systems, programming is a feature of the plasticity of cell lines during embryonic and fetal life. Plasticity refers to the ability of cells and tissues to adapt their differentiation and maturation programmes in response to their current environment. In some types of cell, this adaptive capacity remains present throughout life but in most cases is a feature of the embryonic and fetal stages. The developing organism has populations of progenitor cells that have the capacity to differentiate into mature cell types (Figure 4.1). Progenitors can only develop into target cells related to their particular lineage and may remain present in adult tissues in order to enable tissue repair. In contrast, stem cells are able to either replicate themselves or develop into a range of different cell types in response to growth factor or cytokine signals. Their plasticity enables them to form variable cell types in response to the prevailing environment. Embryonic stem cells are termed *pluripotent* as their plasticity confers the capacity to differentiate into any cell type. These cells are present only in embryonic and fetal life. These are the critical developmental phases that are of greatest interest in the context of nutrition and human health and disease.

The capacity to programme mammalian systems through early life stimuli can be demonstrated just as

dramatically as the example of temperature-dependent sex determination in reptiles. Treatment of newborn female rats with testosterone in the first few days of life impacts upon their lifelong reproductive function. Regions of the hypothalamus that control the reproductive axis and archetypal female reproductive behaviours are remodelled to resemble the male brain and the female rats are rendered sterile (Arai and Gorski, 1968). The critical period in which this androgenizing treatment is effective is relatively short, but the effects are permanent.

There is also evidence that programming by the environment is a normal feature of human physiology. The Japanese military made the discovery during the Second World War that the number of sweat glands in humans is set soon after birth and cannot then be further adjusted. Individuals born in cooler climates activate a smaller number of sweat glands than individuals born in warmer climates. Thus, the response to the prevailing environment during the early postnatal period brings about permanent changes to physiology that allow the individual born in a warm climate to be optimally adapted for life in that climate. The individual from a cold climate will cope less well with the heat.

4.2.2 Fetal programming and human disease

4.2.2.1 Fetal growth

The capacity of the developing mammal to respond to environmental cues or physiological insults in the manner described earlier suggests something profound and unexpected about the nature of development. For decades, we have believed that development is essentially a gene-led process and that activation and switching off of the expression of genes, in well-ordered sequences, brings about the normal growth and development of organisms, from the fertilized egg to the adult offspring. The concepts of developmental plasticity and programming would suggest that the environment can change the profile of genes that are expressed at any given stage of development and, in the case of adult stem cells, throughout life. In other words, the genes do not necessarily lead the process of development and instead can follow the signals from the mother that indicate the availability of nutrients, the presence of stressors and the need to adapt accordingly.

The impact of the environment upon apparently genetically determined processes could be simply observed by looking at the effects of maternal factors upon fetal growth. The growth trajectory of a fetus is determined by the genes inherited from both the mother and the father, but evolution has provided mechanisms through which the genetically determined growth rate can be constrained. Classic experiments using embryo transfers in horses and cattle show that the size of the mother is a primary factor governing fetal growth. Shetland ponies are a small breed of horses, standing at no more than 10 hands (~107 cm), while the Shire horse stands at an impressive 18 hands (180 cm). The foals of these horses are of a size commensurate with their breed. When Shetland mares carry the foals resulting from Shire horse *x* Shetland pony crosses, the genetically large offspring are born at a size similar to the pure Shetland. This form of constraint is in the interest of maternal survival, as carrying a fetus that will become too large to pass through the birth canal is likely to prove fatal to mother and offspring.

Constraint of growth also occurs in response to other characteristics of mothers. A whole range of factors that signal underprivilege or other indicators of a less than optimal environment are associated with lower weights at birth among human babies. One of the strongest predictors of the weight of a baby at birth is the socio-economic class of the mother. In a study of 300 pregnant women from Northampton, United Kingdom (Figure 4.2), average weights at birth were 400 g lower in babies of women from social class V (unemployed) than in babies of women from social class I (professionals; Langley-Evans and Langley-Evans, 2003). Social class is a crude indicator of many different factors that will include family income, nutritional status, access to healthcare services, smoking and other health behaviours. Several of these are known to influence fetal growth in their own right. Maternal smoking during

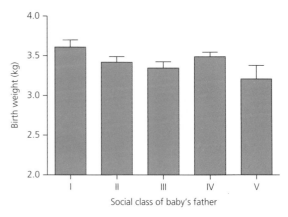

Figure 4.2 Effect of socio-economic status on birth weight. Social class I, professionals; class II, clerical workers; class III, skilled manual or non-manual workers; class IV, unskilled workers; class V, unemployed.

pregnancy, for example, restricts fetal growth and increases risk of low birth weight and premature birth. The same risks are associated with maternal infection and severe maternal distress during pregnancy. Smits and colleagues (2006) studied 1885 Dutch women who were pregnant at the time of the 9/11 terrorist attacks on the World Trade Center. Compared to women giving birth a year later, babies of this cohort were smaller, supporting the hypothesis that psychological stress can impact upon growth and development.

4.2.2.2 Nutrition and the constraint of growth

The ability of maternal nutrition-related factors to constrain fetal growth is an area of some controversy. In populations exposed to famine, it is simple to demonstrate that there is a detrimental impact on fetal growth. The effects are, however, often remarkably small. In the winter of 1944–1945, an area of western Holland was subject to a famine of approximately 6 months' duration as the occupying Nazi forces blocked delivery of rations in reprisal for strike action among Dutch railworkers. At the height of the famine, the adult ration delivered only 500–600 kcal/day. Due to the duration of the famine, some pregnant women were affected over the final stages of pregnancy, while others were undernourished in early pregnancy. Birth weights among babies affected by famine in late gestation were approximately 250 g lower than those of babies born before or conceived after the famine (Roseboom *et al.*, 2001). Surprisingly, the babies caught by famine in the first trimester of gestation were heavier at birth than the Dutch norm for that period.

Women living in rural areas of the Gambia are subject to seasonal variation in nutritional status, which reflects

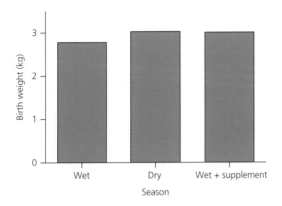

Figure 4.3 Seasonal variation in birth weight among children born in the Gambia. Women are poorly nourished in the wet season and give birth to smaller babies than in the dry season. Supplementation of the diet with energy (431 kcal/day) in the wet season removed the seasonal difference in birth weight, showing that it was related to nutritional status. Reproduced with permission from Prentice *et al.* (1983). © Elsevier.

variation in climate. During the dry season, agriculture is relatively easy as the soil is light and easy to work. Crop growth is good and conditions for food storage are favourable. Thus, at this time, women are relatively well nourished. During the lengthy wet season, however, the women lose 4–5 kg of weight and this is due to a relative scarcity of food, occurring due to inability to keep food stores dry and the difficulty of working the fields and growing viable crops (Moore *et al.*, 1999). The variation in maternal nutritional status between these seasons is reflected in infant birth weights, which are on average 200 g lighter in the wet season than in the dry. Providing women with modest supplements of energy during the wet season has been shown to abolish this difference in birth weight (Figure 4.3).

Among well-nourished populations of women, simple measures of maternal intake tend to be only weakly related to babies' birth weights or other markers of fetal growth. Mathews and colleagues (1999) studied pregnant women living in Portsmouth, United Kingdom, and found that there were no significant associations between babies' weights at birth and maternal intakes of any nutrient. Also, in a UK population, Langley-Evans and Langley-Evans (2003) found that while energy and protein intake in the first trimester of pregnancy were not predictive of later birth weight, the mothers of babies who were born smaller had lower intakes of iron (Figure 4.4). Godfrey and colleagues (1996) reported that birth weights of babies in nearby Southampton were related to maternal intakes of protein in late gestation (low-protein diets were associated with lower birth weights) and maternal sucrose intakes in early gestation

(high sucrose intakes were associated with lower birth weights). Wynn and colleagues (1991) demonstrated that the influence of maternal nutrition may be greater in women of lower socio-economic status, finding that among impoverished women in Hackney, London, intakes of B vitamins were related to birth weight.

The lack of clear and consistent effects of maternal nutrient intakes upon babies' birth weights is unsurprising, as the delivery of nutrients to the fetus in order to drive growth depends upon more than just maternal intakes of those nutrients (Figure 4.5). Well-nourished women will generally have adequate reserves of nutrients and can therefore maintain delivery of most substrates to the fetal tissues even if their intakes are compromised in the short to medium term. Fetal nutrition will also depend upon the ability of the placenta to supply substrates, and this in turn may be influenced by maternal adaptations to pregnancy, nutritional factors and hormonal signals.

4.2.2.3 Fetal growth, health and disease

Constraint of fetal growth, leading to a lower weight at birth, is an indicator that the developing fetus is adapting to aspects of the maternal environment. Given the evidence presented so far, showing that fetal growth can respond to maternal nutritional signals, and that events in early life can programme developing organs and tissues, it is reasonable to assert that maternal nutrition can also affect how mature organs subsequently function and therefore programme aspects of physiology and metabolism, which ultimately determine risk of major disease.

The rate of fetal growth is likely to be set at a very early stage in gestation and could be partly determined by the nutrition of the mother before pregnancy. The availability of plentiful maternal stores may allow the genetically large fetus to get off to a rapid initial growth (Harding, 2004). The rapidly growing fetus may be more vulnerable to undernutrition later on in pregnancy, while a fetus that has been following a slower growth trajectory throughout earlier gestation may be able to maintain this rate of growth even in the face of a nutrient shortage (Figure 4.6).

Some of the first evidence of a possible association between early life nutrition and disease came from simple studies that set out to explore the North–South divide in health noted in England and Wales. In the 1980s, there was a profound difference in risk of coronary heart disease death between the south-eastern corner of England and the industrialized regions of northern England and South Wales. David Barker and colleagues were able to demonstrate that there was a robust association between 1970s coronary mortality rates in the

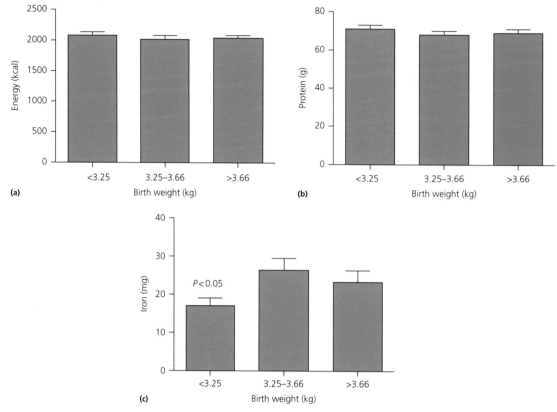

(a)

(b)

(c)

Figure 4.4 The relationship between maternal nutrient intake and birth weight. In a study of 300 pregnant women, the eventual birth weights of their children were not related to energy a), protein b) or other macronutrients in the first trimester of pregnancy. Among the micronutrients, only iron intake c) was associated with weight at birth.

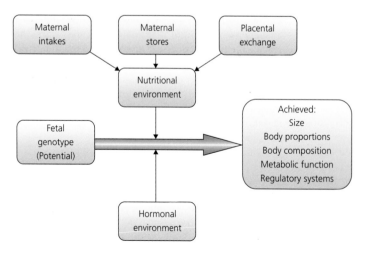

Figure 4.5 Influences upon fetal growth. The growth trajectory of the fetus is determined by the genotype. Genetically determined growth rates may be constrained by influences from the mother or placenta. These can act directly on the fetal tissues, for example, maternal hormones crossing the placenta, or indirectly by modifying the range or concentration of nutrients reaching the fetal tissues.

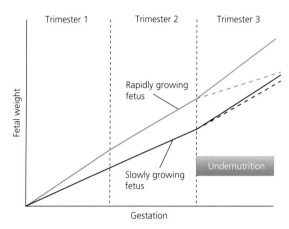

Figure 4.6 Growth is more likely to be constrained in rapidly growing fetuses. Growth of the fetus is primarily set by the genetic potential of the individual. Factors such as maternal undernutrition can constrain this genetic growth rate. The effects of constraint will be greater where growth and the demand for nutrients and oxygen are high. In this example, the slowly growing fetus achieves approximately the same eventual birth weight as the undernourished rapidly growing fetus, irrespective of nutritional status.

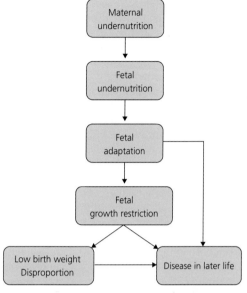

Figure 4.7 The Developmental Origins of Health and Disease hypothesis. Maternal undernutrition promotes fetal undernutrition, which in turn will slow fetal growth rates. The relationship between fetal undernutrition and disease in later life may be directly the result of fetal adaptations to undernutrition or may be related to the restriction of fetal growth and organ development.

different regions and infant death rates some 60 years earlier (Barker and Osmond, 1986). Those parts of the country with high infant mortality early in the twentieth century were the same regions with high coronary death rates. Further investigation of the death certificates of over two million Britons showed that place of birth was a strong predictor of death from coronary heart disease, with greatest risk associated with birth in the industrial north (Bradford, Halifax, Huddersfield, Preston), and lowest risk associated with birth in the south and southeast (East Sussex, West Sussex, Isle of Wight). Most importantly, this risk was independent of subsequent migration, so individuals born in Bradford would retain their greater likelihood of coronary heart disease death later in life, even if they lived out their adult years in Sussex (Osmond *et al.*, 1990). The simplest interpretation of these studies is that adverse factors, such as poor maternal nutrition, during fetal development either led to the death of the infant or prompted physiological adaptations that allowed survival but led to greater risk of cardiovascular disease (CVD) later in life. Such observations were the main spark for Barker's proposal of the Developmental Origins of Adult Disease hypothesis (Barker, 1998).

The Developmental Origins of Adult Disease hypothesis explicitly advances the idea that any form of adverse environment encountered in early life can elicit adaptive responses that modify the future health of the individual. While a range of adverse factors could be responsible

for the developmental programming of health and disease, maternal nutrition was proposed as the main factor that would determine the nature of fetal development (Figure 4.7). The proposal of nutrition as the primary driver of programming stemmed from the fact that the epidemiological evidence suggesting programming of human disease highlighted impaired fetal growth as a predictor of heart disease and diabetes. As will be seen in the following, this evidence mostly came from studies of groups of people born in Britain, early in the twentieth century, a period where undernutrition was rife among young adult women.

4.3 Evidence linking maternal nutrition to disease in later life

4.3.1 Epidemiology

A full exploration of the possible programming relationship between maternal diet and disease in later life would require detailed records of many aspects of maternal diet and lifestyle during pregnancy and long-term follow-up of children into late adulthood. This is not a realistic possibility for most researchers. The alternative approach involves locating adults for whom some indicator of prenatal exposure to putative risk factors is available and then relating these exposure indicators to disease patterns. This is called a retrospective cohort study. Historically, the only data that was reliably recorded about pregnancy outcomes was some simple anthropometric measure of infants, such as birth weight, length at birth and head circumference. These measurements give an imprecise indicator of nutritional influences. As described earlier, undernutrition can constrain growth and reduce birth weight. It is also suggested that the nutritional constraint of birth weight may be greater than that of linear growth, leading to the birth of a baby who is relatively thin (lightweight in relation to body length; Godfrey, 2001).

A unique set of records from the county of Hertfordshire in England provided the basis of the first major epidemiological study to consider relationships between birth anthropometry and disease in later life. Records from 16 000 men and women born in Hertfordshire between 1911 and 1930 were traced. It was found that while mortality rates for all causes were unrelated to size at birth or in infancy, both lower birth weight and lower body weight at 1 year were predictive of increased CVD mortality (Barker *et al.*, 1989). By following up individuals from this cohort who were still living in the county, researchers showed that low weight at birth also predicted risk factors for CVD, including blood pressure, type 2 diabetes and the insulin resistance syndrome (syndrome X) (Hales *et al.*, 1991; Barker *et al.*, 1993a). Infants who weighed less than 5.5 lbs at birth (2.5 kg) were twice as likely to die from coronary heart disease, six and a half times more likely to develop type 2 diabetes and 18 times more likely to develop syndrome X than individuals who weighed greater than 9.5 lbs (4.3 kg). The Hertfordshire study and many similar studies from all over the world showed that low weight at birth was a significant predictor of disease 60–70 years later and supported the concept that maternal undernutrition may programme disease processes (Figure 4.8).

It became clear from a study of a cohort of men and women born in Sheffield, United Kingdom, that body proportions at birth were also significant predictors of CVD risk (Figure 4.9). Among 1586 men born in Sheffield between 1907 and 1923, CVD death rates were not only related to birth weight, but they also rose significantly with decreasing ponderal index (Barker *et al.*, 1993b). The latter (weight/height, kg/m³) is a marker of relative thinness (low ponderal index) or fatness (high ponderal index) at birth. Ponderal index at birth was also a significant predictor of blood pressure. This data therefore showed that babies who were born small and thin were at greater risk of disease in later life. The US

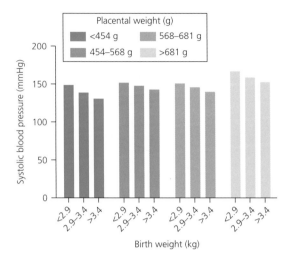

Figure 4.8 Blood pressure in 50-year-old men and women grouped by weight at birth and placental weight. For any birth weight class, blood pressure was higher as placental weight increased. For any placental weight class, a lower weight at birth was associated with higher blood pressure. Reproduced with permission from Barker (1998). © Elsevier.

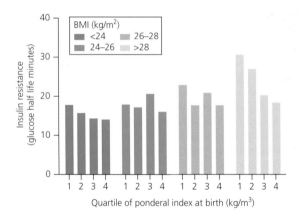

Figure 4.9 Insulin resistance in 50-year-old men and women grouped by ponderal index at birth (PI) and BMI at age 50. For any PI class, insulin resistance was higher as adult BMI increased. For any adult BMI class, a thinness at birth was associated with greater insulin resistance. Quartiles of PI are (1) <20.6 kg/m³, (2) 20.6–22.3 kg/m³, (3) 22.3–25 kg/m³ and (4) >25 kg/m³. Reproduced with permission from Barker (1998). © Elsevier.

Nurses Health Study collected data on birth weight by self-report from 70 297 women and found that among full-term singletons, after adjustment for adult BMI, risk of coronary heart disease and stroke were both related to weight at birth (Curhan *et al.*, 1996). A lower weight at birth increased risk of coronary heart disease (relative risk estimate 0.85 per kg increase in birth weight) and stroke (relative risk estimate 0.85 per kg increase in birth weight) and was associated with higher blood pressure in adult life.

Evidence of associations between characteristics at birth and risk factors for major disease can also be shown in studies of children. Bavdekar *et al.* (1999) studied 8-year-old children in India and found that lower weight at birth was associated with lower sensitivity to insulin and impaired glucose tolerance. In effect, these lower-birth-weight young children were already on the road to type 2 diabetes. This suggests that the programming effects of fetal life impact upon metabolism and physiology immediately after birth and do not depend upon ageing to be expressed.

The most powerful cohort studies to assess possible programming of CVD and diabetes in humans have emerged from investigations of two populations born in Helsinki, Finland (1924–1933 and 1933–1944). Eriksson *et al.* (1999) found that birth weight was inversely associated with risk of both coronary heart disease and stroke-related mortality. Among men, a low ponderal index at birth was also related to risk of coronary heart disease death, if BMI was high in childhood. The most important aspect of the Helsinki 1933–1944 cohort was that the babies had been subject to serial measures of weight and height until age 12. Studies of this cohort showed low birth weight to predict coronary heart disease events, type 2 diabetes and metabolic syndrome and again demonstrated that relative thinness at birth (low ponderal index) and relative fatness in childhood (greater BMI) were associated with risk of these conditions.

An increasing body of evidence from these large cohorts has begun to consider whether there is any interaction between factors that influence fetal growth rates and influences on postnatal growth. For example, it is of interest to know if the fate of the low-birth-weight baby differs depending on how he or she is fed and grows during childhood. Where studies were able to look at postnatal as well as prenatal growth, it is apparent that a rapid gain from birth to adulthood was a risk in addition to prenatal growth restriction. This could be an indicator that the two observations (pre- and postnatal growth) represented independent risk factors, that the most severely constrained babies are subject to postnatal catch-up growth and this is a marker of CVD risk, or that there is a genuine interaction of pre- and early postnatal factors in programming. The Helsinki data suggest the latter, as the fate of individuals with the most rapid rates of infant growth differed depending on their size at birth. Those born small and growing most rapidly in infancy had highest risk of CVD, while those who were larger at birth had lower CVD risk if

weight gain was rapid in infancy. The fact that the small infant at birth who remained small throughout infancy had no increased risk of adult CVD argues that the pre- and postnatal interaction is of prime importance in cardiovascular programming. Figure 4.9 reinforces the importance of the interaction between fetal growth and weight gain in later life. Among 50-year-old men and women, risk of insulin resistance was greatest in those of higher BMI in adulthood. However, at any adult BMI classification, there was also a relationship between insulin resistance and ponderal index at birth. The greatest risk of insulin resistance was observed with relative thinness at birth (low ponderal index) and relative fatness (higher BMI) in adulthood.

The aforementioned studies are limited in that they are only able to report associations between disease states and anthropometric measurements at birth. The latter are only weak markers of the nutritional environment encountered by the fetus during critical periods of development. The Dutch famine, described in Section 4.2.2.2, has been useful in extending the developmental origins hypothesis since it provides an easily accessible population whose mothers were subject to a brief period of food restriction. Follow-up of the Dutch famine babies showed that their health status was poor relative to their contemporaries whose mothers had not been affected by the famine. Exposure to famine in early gestation was associated with greater prevalence of coronary heart disease, with raised circulating lipids, with raised concentrations of blood clotting factors and with more obesity compared to those not exposed to the famine (Roseboom *et al.*, 2001). Exposure to the famine during mid-gestation was associated with microalbuminuria, an indicator of impaired kidney function. Exposure to famine during late gestation was associated with disorders of glucose metabolism that lead to type 2 diabetes.

Similar support for there being an association between maternal nutritional status and disease in later life has been provided by studies of children in Jamaica and the United States. A small-scale study of Jamaican boys aged 10–11 years demonstrated that their blood pressures were related to markers of undernutrition in their mothers during pregnancy (Godfrey *et al.*, 1994). The boys whose mothers had the lowest circulating haemoglobin concentrations (indicating low iron status) and lowest triceps skinfold thicknesses (indicating low body fat reserves) had the highest blood pressures. Blood pressure was also an outcome in Project Viva, a prospective cohort study that aims to follow up the children of women whose nutritional status had been measured in detail in the period prior to and during pregnancy. Gillman and colleagues (2004) reported that maternal calcium supplementation during pregnancy reduced blood pressure in 6-month-old infants. In the same cohort, it was shown that risk of childhood obesity was lower in children of women with the highest intakes of n-3 fatty acids (Donahue *et al.*, 2011). Performance in a test of language skills was better in Project Viva children who were exposed to higher maternal folate intakes during fetal development (Villamor *et al.*, 2012). Together, such studies indicate that higher-quality nutrient intakes in pregnancy are related to better health outcomes in children.

The worldwide increase in the prevalence of overweight and obesity is increasingly impacting across all age groups in the population (Ogden *et al.*, 2013; WHO, 2013). As a result, all developed countries are reporting high levels of obesity among women of childbearing age, and this has important consequences for maternal and fetal health during pregnancy and potentially for the longer-term health of the children of obese women. Pregnancy is recognized as a period during which women are vulnerable to excessive weight gain that they may find difficult to reverse, thereby increasing risk for subsequent pregnancies and their longer-term health.

The effects of maternal obesity and excessive gestational weight gain upon pregnancy outcomes are well documented and described in Section 3.4. The literature that links these factors to programming of disease is less robust but suggestive that overweight may have a long-term effect on offspring health. Several studies point to relationships between maternal weight prior to and during pregnancy and children's weight and adiposity. Oken and colleagues (2007) noted that greater weight gain in pregnancy was associated with higher BMI in 3-year-old children. The risk of overweight in childhood was increased 4.35-fold where maternal weight gain was excessive. Similarly, fat mass in children up to the age of 4 years was greater of women who exceeded the Institute of Medicine (2009) recommendation for gestational weight gain. The Amsterdam Born Children and their Development (ABCD) cohort reported that childhood BMI at age 5–6 years was positively correlated with maternal pre-pregnancy BMI, which was also associated with childhood blood pressure (Gademan *et al.*, 2013). These relationships are often attributed to programming, but this is difficult to separate from possible genetic or other familial influences. A longitudinal study considering the impact of gestational weight gain found that excess maternal weight gain was predictive of more rapid increases in child BMI during adolescence, but the authors concluded that genetic factors may play a role in this (Lawrence *et al.*, 2013).

4.3.2 Criticisms of the programming hypothesis

The compelling epidemiological findings described earlier have major implications for our understanding of how disease processes are initiated and for public health policy across the world. If nutritional programming has a genuine influence on human disease, then interventions designed to prevent disease must be targeted at pregnant women, for the benefit of their children, as well as being aimed at the adults whose lifestyles may increase risk of obesity and related disorders. The developmental origins hypothesis would suggest that altering patterns of disease in populations may be the equivalent of trying to turn around an oil tanker, as effective public health strategies could take decades to come to fruition.

Given the profound implications for public health, it is right that the developmental origins hypothesis should be subjected to close scrutiny and critique. The epidemiology underpinning the hypothesis has been criticized on several different levels. Importantly, most of the epidemiology in this area has focused on measuring disease outcomes in adults aged 50–80 and then attempting to relate these outcomes retrospectively to proxy markers of maternal nutrition from many decades previously. The quality of the data on exposure is therefore very poor and it is relatively easy to invoke the influences of confounding factors that are either not adjusted for (e.g. maternal physical activity, maternal infection, childhood infection, quality of the infant diet in the postnatal period, adult lifestyle factors) or only crudely adjusted for (e.g. social class). Bartley and colleagues (1994) showed how important social class could be in confounding the birth-weight–disease association. Their study showed that individuals born into a poor family tended to be of lower weight at birth. Most individuals born into a family of lower socio-economic class tended to remain in that lower class when they were adults. It is well established that being of lower socio-economic status is a risk factor for CVD, and thus the birth-weight–CVD association could be purely an influence of poverty.

There are also studies that do not fit with the hypothesis. For example, Matthes *et al.* (1994) studied 330 adolescents and found that there was no difference in blood pressure between those who were lighter than 3 kg at birth and those who were 3 kg, or heavier, at birth. Similarly, Falkner *et al.* (1998) found no elevation in blood pressure in young adults who were of low birth weight.

Most epidemiological studies that have examined the maternal diet–later disease association have relied upon birth weight or other proportions at birth as a proxy for maternal nutritional status. This is problematic since, as described earlier, maternal nutrient intakes have only minor influences on fetal growth rates compared to some other factors. Studies of the wartime famines in Holland or the Soviet Union have been widely reported as providing evidence from 'natural experiments' in which we can be sure that the babies born at those times were subject to undernutrition. While they have yielded interesting findings, these studies are subject to important criticisms. During wartime, birth rates can fall dramatically and so it may be that the women having children at these times were in some way not representative of the whole population. Wartime is stressful and maternal stress could programme long-term effects independently of nutrition. It is also apparent that there were ways around rationing and a black market in foodstuffs may have relieved some of the hardships of pregnant women in at least the Dutch famine.

The most potent criticism of the epidemiological studies showing associations between infant birth weights and disease risk indicators in later life has come from the work of Huxley and colleagues (2002). This group performed a meta-analysis of all studies that had considered the association between birth weight and blood pressure in adulthood. Generally, in epidemiology, it is expected that studies with the most subjects give the most reliable and robust findings. Huxley *et al.* (2002) found that the strongest influences of birth weight on blood pressure were reported in small-scale studies, while large cohort studies found the weakest associations. It was concluded that the birth-weight–blood pressure association was partly a product of publication bias (in which small studies showing an effect are prioritized by journal editors over small studies showing no effect) and reflected random error, selective emphasis of particular results, methodological flaws and confounding factors. It is worth noting, however, that other meta-analyses are more supportive of the Developmental Origins hypothesis. Whincup and colleagues found that for every 1 kg higher weight at birth, risk of type 2 diabetes decreased by 23% (Whincup *et al.*, 2008). Low birth weight was shown by White *et al.* (2009) to increase risk of chronic kidney disease (OR 1.73) and end-stage renal disease (OR 1.58). The meta-analysis of Schellong *et al.* (2012) proved counter-intuitive as high birth weight rather than low birth weight was associated with greater risk of adult overweight (OR 1.66).

The criticisms described earlier are inevitable products of the complexity of any likely relationship between nutritional exposures in fetal life and disease outcomes that may not manifest for 60–70 years. It is questionable whether epidemiological approaches have the capacity to investigate these questions at all. Studies such as the Hertfordshire study, which was so influential in promoting interest in developmental programming as a risk factor in human disease, were already no longer representative of influences at work in the modern population, at the time at which they were published. The nutritional and social influences on fetal development operative in the period 1910–1930 were clearly vastly different to those operative in 1990. As alluded to earlier, maternal obesity is now the principal nutritional challenge experienced during fetal life, as opposed to the undernutrition that was prevalent early in the twentieth century. It is possible that the disease consequences that will be observed in 2050 will differ from those noted by Barker and colleagues in the elderly Hertfordshire men and women. It is critical, therefore, that there are studies in this field that can establish the biological plausibility of programming as a risk factor for disease. It is very important to identify the influences of different patterns of diet (e.g. overnutrition as well as undernutrition) upon development and disease and to begin to describe the mechanisms through which programming occurs.

4.3.3 Experimental studies

To perform a study in humans that could adequately test the developmental origins of health and disease hypothesis would require prospective study of women before and during pregnancy, with follow-ups of their children for 50–60 years. Although this is challenging in terms of manpower and cost, several ongoing cohort studies aim to examine the links between early life factors and health. Project Viva (Donahue *et al.*, 2011) recruited 2128 women and their babies between 1999 and 2002 for long-term follow-up. The Millennium cohort in the United Kingdom recruited 19 000 babies born between 2000 and 2001 who are followed up at approximately 2-year intervals. The Southampton Women's Study is the largest European prospective cohort focused upon early life nutrition and later outcomes, with 3156 children born between 1998 and 2007 in the cohort following prospective recruitment of 12 583 women aged 20–34 (Inskip *et al.*, 2006). However, significant insight into the early life antecedents of diseases associated with ageing is not expected from these cohorts for decades. It is not ethically acceptable to manipulate the diets of pregnant women to attempt to influence the future health of their offspring, potentially inducing major disease states. There is, therefore, little alternative to using appropriate animal models to explore the relationship between maternal diet and disease.

Many different animal models have been developed for this purpose, and these will be described later.

Researchers have focused primarily on rodents (rats and mice) for such studies. This is because these species are simple to breed, it is straightforward to modify their diets in pregnancy, gestation is short (rat 22 days, mouse 18 days) and their offspring grow to adulthood very quickly (overall lifespan is around 2 years). There are disadvantages associated with these species, however. The main difference between rodents and humans is that rodents deliver litters of offspring (typically 10–15 pups in the rat) and these offspring are born very immature. Guinea pigs provide an alternative as although these still produce litters of offspring (3–6 pups), gestation is long (68 days), the placenta is more similar to that of the human and the offspring are born at a similar level of maturity to the human infant. The sheep is a broadly favoured species of fetal physiologists, primarily because of the long gestation (147 days) and the fact that the fetus is of similar size to a human (3.5–4 kg). However, as the sheep is a ruminant, the ability to manipulate diet in pregnancy is very limited.

Using these varied species, researchers have attempted to model the developmental origins hypothesis in different ways. Many have sought to simply replicate the relationship between fetal growth retardation and later outcomes. Poore and colleagues (2002) exploited the natural variability in birth weight among litters of piglets and showed that birth weight was inversely associated with blood pressure, just as in humans. This approach is unusual and the relationship is more generally explored by limiting food intake of the pregnant mother and therefore restricting intakes of all macro- and micronutrients (global undernutrition). Some groups take a more drastic approach and retard fetal growth by surgically placing a ligature around the uterine artery to limit the supply of blood and nutrients. Persson and Jansson (1992) showed, using this approach, that growth retardation of the guinea pig fetus resulted in hypertension later in life. Other researchers have chosen to look beyond the birth-weight–disease association and model the effects of specific nutrients in the diet. This allows investigation of the long-term consequences of either nutritional deficit or excess.

4.3.3.1 Global undernutrition

Restriction of overall food intake during pregnancy has a range of different effects that are dependent upon the severity of the restriction imposed and upon the animal species. Woodall and colleagues (1996) reported that feeding pregnant rats only 30% of their normal daily rations led to major retardation of the growth of their fetuses. As adults, these low-birth-weight offspring exhibited high blood pressure and profound obesity. The latter seemed to be caused by an increase in the appetite of the

animals and a reduction in their levels of physical activity. Holemans and colleagues (1999) also worked with pregnant rats and fed 50% of normal rations, but only in the second half of pregnancy. Under these conditions, the offspring did not develop high blood pressure but, as adults, did display abnormalities of cardiovascular function. In the sheep, feeding 50% of nutrient requirements during pregnancy has a number of effects upon the cardiovascular function and metabolic state of the adult lambs. The prenatally nutrient-restricted lamb is generally fatter and has higher blood pressure than a lamb from a well-fed mother, by the age of 3 years (Gardner et al., 2007).

Even mild restriction of maternal food intake in pregnancy can programme the offspring. In the rat, feeding 70% of ad libitum intake produced pups that became hypertensive as adults (Ozaki et al., 2001). Similarly, in guinea pigs, reducing maternal food intake by just 15% was sufficient to programme hypertension and raised blood lipids in the adult offspring (Kind et al., 2002). When pregnant sheep were fed 85% of requirements over the first 70 days of gestation, their fetuses showed altered cardiovascular function at the end of gestation (Hawkins et al., 2000).

4.3.3.2 Micronutrients

Iron deficiency anaemia is the most common nutrient deficiency disorder in the world and particularly impacts upon women during pregnancy. The normal physiological adaptation to pregnancy involves a major expansion of blood volume, and typically, the plasma volume expansion outstrips the production of new red cells and haemoglobin. As a result, blood haemoglobin concentrations fall. Although this sign of iron deficiency may be regarded as a normal part of pregnancy, more severe anaemia is associated with poor pregnancy outcomes. It is estimated that two-thirds of pregnant women will develop some degree of iron deficiency in the course of their pregnancy (see Section 3.3.2). In the pregnant rat, iron deficiency anaemia can be shown to programme fetal development (Gambling et al., 2003). The iron-deficient rat embryo has an abnormally enlarged heart and as an adult will have high blood pressure, suggesting that iron plays a key role in the normal development of the cardiovascular system.

Maternal intakes of calcium are of considerable interest in the programming context. Suboptimal intakes of calcium are relatively common among women of childbearing age, particularly younger women and adolescents. Gillman et al. (2004) showed that increasing intakes of calcium from supplements during pregnancy could lower blood pressure in young children. In rats, the relationship between maternal calcium intake and offspring blood pressure is complex. Rats, whose mothers were fed a calcium-deficient diet, had blood pressures that were 12 mmHg higher than seen in the offspring of rats fed a control diet (Bergel and Belizan, 2002). However, high consumption of calcium in the maternal diet also elevated blood pressures in the offspring, suggesting a U-shaped relationship between calcium intake and later outcomes.

Sodium intake is a major determinant of blood pressure in adults, and there is great concern at the high levels of intake seen within the modern Western diet (see Section "Sodium and blood pressure" in Chapter 8). There have been few studies that have considered the potential for variation in the sodium content of the diet to exert programming effects *in utero*. Battista *et al.* (2002) interestingly showed that a low-sodium diet fed to rats in the last week of their pregnancies induced fetal growth retardation and high blood pressure in their offspring. In stark contrast, Gray *et al.* (2013) reported that loading pregnant rats with a 4% sodium chloride diet (control was 0.26% sodium chloride) resulted in higher arterial blood pressure in their adult offspring.

4.3.3.3 Macronutrients

Protein restriction is one of the mostly widely studied manipulations of the maternal diet in animals. Although protein deficiency per se is relatively rare in most populations of the world, the degree of variation in protein intake both within and between populations is substantial. In the United Kingdom, for example, intakes in pregnancy tend to be lower in women of lower socioeconomic status and in younger mothers. Five to ten per cent of the population may consume protein at less than the 51 g/day RNI for pregnancy (Langley-Evans *et al.*, 2003). On a global scale, access to protein is a significant issue for almost two-thirds of the population, with women in developing countries often subsisting on lower-quality plant protein sources (Figure 4.10).

There is an extensive literature reporting the programming effects of feeding a low-protein diet during rat pregnancy. Relatively mild manipulation of protein intake produces subtle variations in the growth of the offspring, which undergo a late gestation retardation of growth, particularly affecting the development of the truncal organs such as the lungs and kidneys (Langley-Evans *et al.*, 1996a). Although of low to normal birth weight, rats exposed to protein restriction in fetal life develop raised blood pressure by 3–4 weeks of age and this hypertension persists into adult life (Langley-Evans *et al.*, 1994; Langley-Evans and Jackson, 1995). In the postnatal period, these animals have an accelerated progression towards renal failure and their lifespan is significantly shorter than that of rats exposed to a protein-replete diet in fetal life (Aihie Sayer *et al.*, 2001).

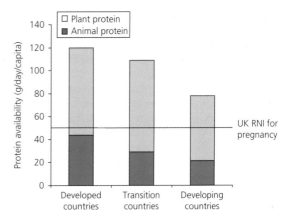

Figure 4.10 Global protein availability statistics. Data extracted from 2004 FAO food balance sheets. Food balance methods only determine the protein available (i.e. produced through agriculture or imported) per head of population. Actual consumption will be below the figures shown and highly variable within each region (e.g. affluent vs poor, urban vs rural). Sixty-five per cent of the world population are likely to consume protein at less than the UK reference nutrient intake and are therefore at risk of low protein intake during pregnancy. Many in developing countries rely on lower-quality plant protein sources.

The offspring of rats fed low-protein diets in pregnancy exhibit a number of age-related disorders that make this an interesting model to study in the context of the metabolic syndrome in humans. Typically, humans become more insulin resistant as they age and develop type 2 diabetes as a consequence. Rats exposed to protein restriction in fetal life are relatively lean in early adult life and show increased sensitivity to insulin. As they age, however, insulin resistance begins to appear and with this the animals develop raised blood lipid profiles and deposit large amounts of fat in their livers (Erhuma *et al.*, 2007).

An excess of protein in the diet is also a major issue in the diets of populations living in the Westernized nations. In parts of Europe and the United States, it is not uncommon for women to consume 120 g protein per day, which is more than double the UK RNI. Daenzer and colleagues (2002) considered the potential programming effects of high-protein diets in pregnant rats. Offspring of rats fed a 40% protein diet were shown to be more prone to obesity, due to reduced total energy expenditure.

In human populations throughout the world, one of the major nutritional concerns is the consumption of diets containing excessive amounts of energy derived from fat and sugar. Rodent studies suggest that such a dietary pattern in pregnancy may programme the later blood pressure and metabolic functions of the resulting offspring. Maternal over-feeding, generally with high-fat diets, has similar programming effects in both rats and mice (Samuelsson *et al.*, 2008; Shankar *et al.*, 2008) with elevated blood pressure, impaired glucose tolerance and dyslipidaemia. Feeding rats a cafeteria diet (a varying menu of highly palatable human foods) prior to pregnancy to induce obesity can impact upon the metabolic function of their later offspring, with changes in glucose homeostasis (Akyol *et al.*, 2012). Using a similar protocol, Bayol *et al.* (2007, 2010) found effects of cafeteria diet upon insulin signalling and glucose metabolism and feeding behaviour in rats.

The most remarkable aspect of all of the animal studies described earlier is the fact that very diverse nutritional manipulations in pregnancy (ranging from severe global undernutrition to an energy-rich, junk-food diet) in a diverse range of species (including rodents and ruminants) can produce very similar effects in the offspring (typically high blood pressure, glucose intolerance and obesity). The commonality of the responses to diverse dietary insults suggests that programming is driven by a small number of common mechanisms, any of which might be initiated by a maternal signal that the nutritional environment is not optimal. Understanding of those mechanisms is of major importance if the Developmental Origins hypothesis is ever to have any significant impact upon the way in which public health problems related to nutrition are treated or prevented.

4.4 Mechanistic basis of fetal programming

4.4.1 Thrifty phenotypes and genotypes
Metabolic 'thrift' is defined as the possession of metabolic and physiological characteristics that ensure the most efficient and effective utilization of substrates. Neel (1962) first proposed this concept, suggesting that in the early evolution of the human species, regular exposure to food shortages would favour the survival of those that carried thrifty genes and that the population would therefore have evolved to store fat during times of plenty and utilize that resource during periods of famine. Clearly, a thrifty genotype would no longer be an advantage in modern society, and the mismatch between our current Westernized lifestyle and the environment that humans have experienced through 99.9% of their history could be invoked as an explanation for modern trends in obesity, CVD and diabetes.

Thrifty genes could influence many aspects of the acquisition and processing of nutrients, and many different candidate genes that confer thrift have been proposed (Breier *et al.*, 2004). These include genes that control

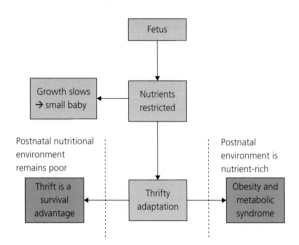

Figure 4.11 The thrifty phenotype hypothesis. Reproduced with permission from Hales and Barker (2001). © Oxford University Press.

feeding behaviour, such as leptin and the melanocortin receptor; genes that are involved in metabolic regulation, such as peroxisome proliferator-activated receptor γ; and genes that play a role in insulin signalling and other signal transduction pathways. Hattersley and Tooke (1999) have proposed that thrifty genotypes could entirely explain the observed association between weight at birth and diabetes in later life. Insulin is an important driver of fetal growth, and so genetic defects of the insulin axis, which would ultimately promote diabetes, might also be associated with fetal growth retardation. Mutations of the glucokinase gene are associated with both maturity onset diabetes and low birth weight in this way. Arguments in favour of a thrifty genotype driving the development of disease are weakened by the fact that while the metabolic diseases (obesity, type 2 diabetes) are very common in Westernized society, mutations of the candidate genes that are proven to be associated with disease are extremely rare.

Thrift, however, remains an important consideration in the diet–disease relationship and comes to the fore in the nutritional programming area. In 1992, Hales and Barker first proposed the thrifty phenotype hypothesis (Figure 4.11). This suggests that the developing fetus, exposed to suboptimal nutrition, undergoes adaptions to key metabolic tissues such as the liver and pancreas. Primarily, these enable the fetus to maximize the resources that are available during that phase of development. However, as programming events are permanent, the thrift that is acquired at the time of undernutrition will remain through to adult life. For our hunter-gatherer ancestors, this would provide the same survival advantage as the thrifty genotype proposed by Neel. In the

Research Highlight 4.1 Thrifty phenotype or thrifty genotype?.

A number of populations around the world are often cited as examples that support the 'Thrifty Phenotype' hypothesis of Hales and Barker (2001). One such population is the group of Ethiopian Jews (Falasha) who migrated from the Gondar region of Ethiopia to Israel in the 1980s. This migration of Falasha was significant in terms of size, as it took the Falasha population of Israel from just 500 in 1980 to over 62 000 by 2001. This large population provides a useful opportunity to examine the changes in health and disease profiles that occurred as a result of moving from rural Africa to the urbanized areas of a Westernized country. The Falasha in Israel tend not to intermarry and so have retained their original genetic background. This makes them an attractive population for the examination of the relative influences of genes and the environment.

On initial inspection, this example appears to support the Hales and Barker hypothesis. However, the Cohen et al. (1988) paper did not define whether the Falasha they studied had developed type 1 or type 2 diabetes. While the thrifty phenotype concept would apply well to type 2 diabetes in which insulin resistance develops alongside obesity and other products of a thrifty metabolism, type 1 diabetes is due to destruction of the pancreatic ß-cells and a failure to produce insulin. Zung et al. (2004) examined Ethiopian Jews in Israel and noted that they exhibited a very high occurrence of a haplotype (DRB1*0301) of the human leukocyte antigen (HLA) genes that is associated with ß-cell destruction and type 1 diabetes. Importantly, the age at which subjects with this haplotype developed their diabetes was dependent on the length of time their families had lived in Israel. This suggested that rather than being programmed for thrift, perhaps the Falasha carry a genotype that promotes diabetes, but only when individuals are exposed to a diabetogenic environment.

The example of the Falasha shows how initial assumptions made about the outcome of epidemiological studies should always be subject to rigorous questioning. While these papers clearly show that the factors in the environment, including diet, can trigger metabolic disease, the question of whether a thrifty phenotype or a thrifty genotype drives the disease process cannot be addressed in this simplistic manner.

modern world, some thrifty individuals would be born into an environment where food shortages still occur and hence would benefit from their fetal experience. However, should the individual programmed to be thrifty be born into an environment where food is plentiful, the thrift would drive excessive fat gain and the development of the associated disease states.

Hales and Barker (1992) proposed several examples of the thrifty phenotype in action. Most of these focused upon populations where it has been shown that rapid changes from a traditional to a Westernized diet have been accompanied by soaring rates of diabetes. The prevalence rate for type 2 diabetes in the population of the Pacific island of Nauru is among the highest in the world. Prior to the Second World War, this population was habitually undernourished, but industrial development since the 1940s sparked an epidemic of diabetes. A further example is provided by the Falasha immigrants in Israel (Research Highlight 4.1).

Observations of twins tend to support the thrifty phenotype hypothesis rather than the concept of a thrifty genotype. Studies of twin pairs (mono- and dizygotic) in which one twin but not the other suffered from diabetes (Poulsen et al., 1997; Bo et al., 2000) showed that insulin

resistance, raised circulating triglycerides and cholesterol were more common in the twin with the lower birth weight. Given that in each case the twins would have very similar or identical genotypes, these findings suggest that fetal growth constraint, perhaps driven by unequal distribution of nutritional resources from the mother, programmed the diabetes.

As many countries around the world acquire greater economic stability and wealth, their populations generally undergo a nutritional transition, moving from a diet rich in complex carbohydrates and low in animal fats and meat to an energy-dense, Westernized diet. The thrifty phenotype hypothesis would predict that in such countries, for example, India, China and Brazil, generations of undernutrition impacting upon pregnant women and their offspring would drive high rates of obesity and diabetes that exceed those seen in the West, where affluent lifestyles have been the norm for several generations. In support of this hypothesis, it is noted that between 1985 and 2010, the prevalence of childhood obesity increased 40-fold in China, with the greatest increase observed in 7–9-year-olds (Song et al., 2013). Among boys, the prevalence of obesity more than doubled between 2000 and 2010.

4.4.2 Mismatched environments

Gluckman and Hanson (2004) have proposed that the thrifty phenotype is just one aspect of a broader phenomenon, which they describe as the 'predictive adaptive response'. This is perhaps better considered as the mismatch between the environments experienced during the developmental period and later life. The concept of 'thrift' is clearly applicable to the handling of energy substrates and metabolic disorders, but does not cover the full gamut of conditions that are programmed by undernutrition. For example, there is a body of evidence that suggests that humans who were of lower weight at birth have a lower complement of nephrons in their kidneys (Hinchliffe *et al.*, 1992). The nephrons are the functional units of the kidney and are responsible for the filtration of the blood and production of urine. Individuals with fewer nephrons are more prone to kidney disease and high blood pressure in later life. If nephron number is programmed in fetal development, this does not indicate a thrifty phenotype. This is more suggestive of an adaptation related to immediate survival of hostile environments that becomes maladaptive if the challenges in the adult environment are grossly different.

When the supply of nutrients to the fetus is restricted or when the passage of hormones from mother to fetus is indicative of stress, the pregnancy may be aborted or the fetus may undergo adaptations to its physiology that ensure immediate survival. Often, these adaptations will relate to a prioritizing of valuable nutrients and resources away from systems that are less critical for fetal survival (e.g. the lungs and kidneys, whose functions are met by the placenta) towards more critical systems such as the brain and circulatory system. This ability to adapt, due to the plasticity of fetal tissues, is clearly advantageous. Disease will only stem from this adaptive response if the new physiological make-up is inappropriate for the environment subsequently encountered by the individual. In the case of the kidney with fewer nephrons, there would be no adverse consequences unless the individual habitually consumed a diet rich in protein or sodium necessitating greater renal function to process the load. On this basis, the responses that we refer to as programming may be considered favourable if the nutritional environment encountered during fetal life is persistent. Like the concept of thrift, a biological response that optimizes development for particular conditions will be advantageous only until those conditions no longer exist.

4.4.3 Tissue remodelling

The thrifty phenotype and mismatch hypotheses are merely conceptual frameworks and do not actually explain the biological processes that link maternal undernutrition, fetal physiology and later disease. One of the simplest mechanisms that can explain these phenomena invokes the process of tissue remodelling. Changes to the numbers of cells or the type of cells present within a tissue would reshape the morphology of that tissue and could have profound effects upon organ function.

The remodelling of organ structure could occur due to disruption of cell proliferation or differentiation at different developmental stages (Figure 4.12). In simple terms, all tissues and organs are derived from small populations of embryonic progenitor cell lines (Figure 4.1). During early embryonic development, these cell lines proliferate, increasing the size of the embryo and early structures. In later fetal periods, they differentiate into specialized cell types, bringing about the maturation of the organs. A lack of nutrients or a disruption of normal endocrine signals during these developmental stages can alter tissue structure, leaving irreversible consequences.

The kidney, as described in Section 4.4.2, provides an example of tissue programming that appears to involve some remodelling of structure. In humans, the number of nephrons is determined before birth. Factors that limit nephron formation will impair renal function, raise local and systemic blood pressure and ultimately promote earlier renal failure. In rats exposed to low-protein diets during fetal development, kidney size is largely unaffected by prenatal nutritional insult, but nephron number is reduced by as much as 30% (Langley-Evans *et al.*, 1999). The decrease in functional units alongside a normal tissue mass indicates that specialized cell types comprising the nephron have been replaced by nonspecialized lineages. This suggests that the vulnerable period for programming of renal development lies in the differentiation phase.

Modifying the numbers and types of cells present within a tissue will have a range of consequences. It is easy to envisage how such changes might impact upon specialized functions that are dependent upon certain structures, as in the case of the kidney. Alterations to the profile of cell types present within a tissue may also modify the capacity of a tissue to produce or respond to hormones, up- or down-regulate essential genes expressed within a tissue or interfere with cell–cell signalling pathways. Some of these changes may have very localized effects, simply impacting upon the function of a particular tissue, but others could disrupt whole-body physiology and metabolic regulation. Studies of rats exposed to maternal low-protein diets during fetal development show that this dietary manipulation results in the offspring developing a pancreas with reduced numbers of islets, which are smaller and less effectively vascularized than in control animals (Snoeck *et al.*, 1990). This has a major impact upon

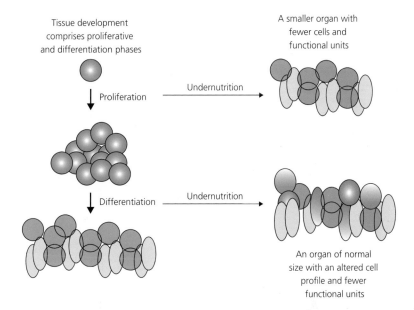

Tissue development
comprises proliferative
and differentiation phases

A smaller organ with
fewer cells and
functional units

Proliferation

Undernutrition

Differentiation

Undernutrition

An organ of normal
size with an altered cell
profile and fewer
functional units

Figure 4.12 The principle of tissue remodelling. During embryonic and fetal life, progenitor cells undergo rounds of proliferative cell division. Following this proliferative phase, the cells undergo differentiation to form diverse cell types that will perform the physiological functions of the mature organ. Adverse environments during either phase will modify the cell numbers or types that appear in the mature organ.

insulin production and hence glucose homeostasis at the whole-body level (Dahri *et al.*, 1991). Similarly, fetal and neonatal undernutrition in the rat alters the size, neuronal density and types of neurone present within the key appetite centres of the hypothalamus (Plagemann *et al.*, 2001).

4.4.4 Endocrine imbalance

The most widely recognized function of the placenta is to permit the exchange of nutrients, gases and waste products between mother and fetus. It should also be appreciated that there are critical endocrine signals that pass between placenta and fetus and between mother and placenta. These regulate aspects of fetal development and also control the partitioning of nutrients to deliver the balance between maternal, placental and fetal requirements (Power and Tardif, 2005). There are hormones of placental origin, which are involved in the maintenance of pregnancy (e.g. progesterone), the preparation of the breasts for lactation (e.g. human chorionic somatomammotropin) and the determination of the timing of labour (e.g. corticotrophin-releasing hormone). Other hormones may move from mother to fetus and these exchanges require tight regulation in order to avoid inappropriate fetal responses.

The glucocorticoids are steroid hormones that have a wide range of different functions. Classically, they act to maintain blood glucose concentrations, generally opposing the effects of insulin (Table 4.1). They are also important stress hormones and have immunosuppressive effects. Most, though not all, of the functions of glucocorticoids are mediated through their binding to

Table 4.1 The classical actions of glucocorticoids.

| **Metabolic** |
| Inhibition of glucose uptake by extra-hepatic tissues |
| Stimulation of hepatic gluconeogenesis |
| Stimulation of lipolysis |
| Mobilization of amino acids from extra-hepatic tissues |
| |
| **Physiological** |
| Suppression of inflammatory responses |
| Inhibition of bone formation |
| Regulation of fluid balance |
| Mediator of stress responses |
| Control of feeding behaviour |

the glucocorticoid receptor (GR). As it is a classical nuclear receptor transcription factor (Figure 4.13), GR is able to bind to glucocorticoid response elements within gene promoters and activate transcription of many different genes. Glucocorticoids are steroid hormones and are therefore able to cross cell membranes through passive diffusion. In the context of maternal–fetal exchange across the placenta, this is potentially problematic as without any barrier mechanism, the hormones should be able to move freely between the mother and the fetus and could therefore up-regulate fetal gene expression at inappropriate stages of development.

There is, however, a protective mechanism that should prevent this from occurring. Placental tissue expresses the enzyme 11ß-hydroxysteroid dehydrogenase-2 (11ßHSD2), which converts active glucocorticoids (e.g. cortisol in humans, corticosterone in rats) to forms that lack physiological activity (e.g. cortisone in humans,

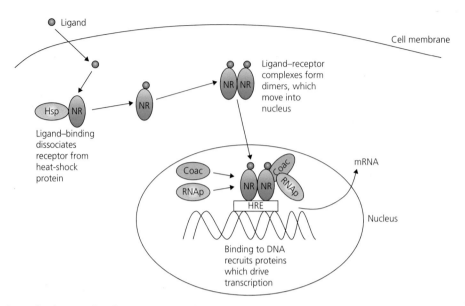

Figure 4.13 The mode of action of nuclear receptors. Nuclear receptors (NR) are typically located in the cytosol associated with heat shock proteins (Hsp). On binding ligand, the ligand–receptor complex forms dimers which bind to hormone response elements (HRE) on DNA, where they promote transcription. Coac, coactivator; RNAp, RNA polymerase.

11-dehydrocorticosterone in rats). 11ßHSD2, therefore, acts as a 'gatekeeper' enzyme that limits the movement of active glucocorticoids into the fetal circulation (Figure 4.14). Indeed, there is a major gradient of glucocorticoids across the placenta, with maternal concentrations maintained at 100–1000-fold greater than in the fetus. This allows the fetal hypothalamic–pituitary–adrenal axis to develop free of maternal influences and also ensures that maternal hormones do not interfere with the normal developmentally regulated patterns of gene expression within fetal tissues.

The consequences of excessive fetal glucocorticoid exposure are well documented. Glucocorticoids have the effect of retarding growth but promoting cellular differentiation, producing a smaller fetus with more mature organs. Synthetic glucocorticoids, which are only weakly metabolized by 11ßHSD2, such as dexamethasone are used clinically to enhance the maturation of the lungs of babies whose mothers are going into premature labour. Benediktsson and colleagues (1993) administered dexamethasone to pregnant rats throughout gestation and then assessed the impact of this treatment on their offspring. The rats exposed to prenatal steroids were smaller at birth, as expected, and as adults had elevated blood pressure. This suggested that glucocorticoids, like maternal undernutrition, could programme long-term health and well-being. The involvement of 11ßHSD2 in this glucocorticoid programming was confirmed by treating pregnant rats with carbenoxolone, which is an inhibitor

of 11ßHSD2 activity. Offspring from such pregnancies also had raised blood pressure as adults (Langley-Evans, 1997). As described in Research Highlight 4.2, inhibitors of 11ßHSD are also seen to have an effect on the children of women who consume them during pregnancy.

While this glucocorticoid-driven mechanism of programming may seem unrelated to nutritional programming, the two processes may be linked. In humans, lower expression or activity of 11ßHSD2 is associated with lower birth weight and greater degrees of illness in premature infants (Kajantie et al., 2006). McTernan and colleagues (2001) reported that 11ßHSD2 mRNA expression in the placenta was lower in pregnancies complicated by intrauterine growth retardation. Most importantly, however, in rats, maternal protein restriction results in a lower activity of placental 11ßHSD2, and this suggests that nutritional factors can alter the capacity of the placenta to protect the fetal tissues from maternal hormone signals (Langley-Evans et al., 1996b). These hormone signals may provide the mechanistic link between undernutrition and long-term ill health. Indeed, treating pregnant rats fed a low-protein diet with a drug that inhibits synthesis of corticosterone prevented their offspring from developing high blood pressure.

There is, therefore, a body of evidence to suggest that undernutrition reduces the capacity of the placenta to maintain the maternal–fetal gradient of glucocorticoid concentrations. Overexposure to steroids of maternal origin will impact on tissue development and programme

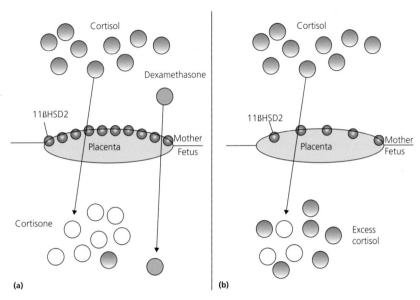

Figure 4.14 Placental 11ß-hydroxysteroid dehydrogenase (11ßHSD2) acts as a barrier to the movement of active glucocorticoids between mother and fetus. a) Normal gatekeeper functions of 11ßHSD2 convert active cortisol to inactive cortisone and hence protect fetal tissues from hormones of maternal origin. Only synthetic glucocorticoids such as dexamethasone may pass across the placenta unchanged. b) In the undernourished mother, expression of 11ßHSD2 in placenta is diminished and hence the fetal tissues are overexposed to active glucocorticoids.

Research Highlight 4.2 Liquorice, glucocorticoids and health.

Liquorice is extracted from the root of *Glycyrrhiza glabra* and is widely used as a flavouring or sweetener in foodstuffs and in tobacco. In addition to the sweet forms of liquorice that are consumed by populations all over the world, people in the countries of Scandinavia, the Baltic states, northern Germany and the Netherlands also enjoy 'salt liquorice' which is made by adding ammonium chloride to the liquorice extract. In Finland, *salmiakki* is a great favourite and is available in super-strength varieties.

The characteristic flavour and sweetness of liquorice is due to glycyrrhizin. This compound is an inhibitor of 11βHSD, and there is a growing literature emerging from Finland that suggests glycyrrhizin has a programming effect if consumed in excess during pregnancy. Strandberg *et al.* (2001, 2002) reported that consuming glycyrrhizin at more than 500 mg/week significantly shortened gestation length and increased the risk of preterm birth by twofold compared to consumption at less than 250 mg/week.

In addition to this effect on gestation length, the children of women who consumed salmiakki while pregnant exhibit signs that cognitive and behavioural functions have been programmed. 8-year-olds with high fetal exposure were 2.6 times more likely to have attention deficit hyperactivity disorder and were more aggressive and more likely to break rules at school (Räikkönen *et al.*, 2009). When exposed to a social stress test, the children of high liquorice consumers had an exaggerated release of cortisol (Räikkönen *et al.*, 2010). This suggests that the liquorice exposure and the resulting greater exposure to maternal glucocorticoid associated with 11βHSD inhibition had a programming effect upon the developing hypothalamic–pituitary–adrenal axis. As this endocrine system plays a major role in homeostasis, effects upon metabolic and physiological function would be expected in these children as they age.

The relationship between high liquorice consumption, pregnancy outcome and the long-term effect of fetal exposure shows that the glucocorticoid programming hypothesis that has extensive support from animal studies also appears to have validity in humans. Factors in the diet that can modify placental 11βHSD activity or expression have the potential to programme long-term disease risk.

disease. It is relatively simple to see how this mechanism could trigger tissue remodelling, as the glucocorticoids would curtail proliferation of cells and promote differentiation. This is just one maternal–fetal hormone exchange that has been examined in the context of fetal programming. There are likely to be other such influences that are, as yet, unidentified.

4.4.5 Nutrient–gene interactions
4.4.5.1 Polymorphisms in humans
It is clear from epidemiological studies that the developmental programming phenomenon involves interactions of early life factors with the genome. Peroxisome proliferator-activated receptor γ2 (PPAR-γ2) is a ligand-dependent transcription factor that is predominantly

expressed in adipose tissue where it regulates fat and energy metabolism. The PPAR-γ2 gene has a polymorphic region within exon B, and individuals may carry either an alanine coding or proline coding allele of the gene depending on their pro12ala genotype. Eriksson and colleagues (2002b) studied the relationship between this polymorphism, birth anthropometry and risk of type 2 diabetes in cohorts of men and women born in Helsinki between 1924 and 1933. The Ala12 allele was shown to be associated with markers of lower diabetes risk in these individuals, but the beneficial effect of the polymorphism was seen only in individuals who had been of lower weight at birth. Low-birth-weight individuals with the Pro12 gene variant were at greater risk of diabetes, hypertension and raised blood lipids, suggesting that a single genotype can give rise to different phenotypes due to variation in early life experience and variation in the quality of early life nutrition.

Osteoporosis is one of the major preventable diseases of adult life that is known to be related to diet and lifestyle factors earlier in the life course. A number of genes that may be involved in determining osteoporosis risk have been mapped, including the vitamin D receptor (VDR) and the type 1 collagen A1 gene (Walker-Bone *et al.*, 2002). For VDR, there are 22 known polymorphisms that in isolation explain only a very small proportion of variation in bone mass. For example, it is estimated that the BB variant of the Bsm I restriction site in VDR can reduce site-specific bone mineral density (a powerful marker of osteoporotic fracture risk) by, at most, 2%. The lack of stronger associations is explained by the fact that the influence of genotype on bone health is modulated by lifestyle and environmental factors. A number of epidemiological studies have suggested that growth *in utero* and in the first year of infancy determine risk of osteoporosis. In a study of the Bsm 1 polymorphism of VDR, Jordan and colleagues (2005) reported that, in men, the B allele increased severity of degenerative bone disease in the lumbar region of the spine and that the impact of the allele was greatest in individuals of lower birth weight. Thus, fetal factors modified the risk associated with this particular VDR genotype.

While these examples generally support the concept that maternal factors operating during development modify the effects of genetically inherited risk factors, not all studies associating single nucleotide polymorphisms with fetal growth favour a programming explanation. Some studies suggest that low birth weight and disease states may share common genetic causes, as proposed by Hattersley and Tooke (1999). A polymorphism of the leptin gene, for example, was related to both birth weight and adult HDL-cholesterol concentrations

(Souren *et al.*, 2008). The Early Growth Genetics Consortium (2013) carried out a meta-analysis that found seven different gene loci where polymorphisms linked birth weight to type 2 diabetes and elevated blood pressure. Some of the genetic associations are relatively weak, however, which very much leaves open the question of fetal gene–environment interactions as drivers of later disease. Winkler and colleagues (2009) found that birth weight was only 81 g lower in individuals carrying the high-risk allele for type 2 diabetes at the HHEX–IDE locus. This is barely outside the limits of reasonable measurement error and does not compare well with the meta-analysis of Whincup *et al.* (2008), reporting a 23% reduction in diabetes risk for every *kilogram* difference in birth weight.

4.4.5.2 Gene expression in animals

The animal studies of programming outlined earlier consistently show that even brief periods of maternal undernutrition have the capacity to impact upon development of major organs (kidney, heart, liver, brain, adipose tissue, skeletal muscle). These changes are associated with disease processes. It is attractive to attempt to explore the mechanistic basis of programming by looking for changes in the expression of genes, proteins and pathways in the affected tissues of adult animals. This would be expected to give insight into the linkage between the fetal nutritional exposure and the physiological or metabolic consequences in the adult.

Many researchers have taken this approach, but the findings of widespread alterations in gene pathways are actually of limited value as the observed changes are likely to be reflecting the programmed disease state or the endocrine, metabolic and physiological elements of the programmed state (Langley-Evans, 2013). For example, in aged rats exposed to low-protein diets during fetal life, the expression of the genes and transcription factors that regulate the synthesis of lipids within the liver are greatly increased. This goes hand-in-hand with the observation that these animals have excess lipid deposits within the tissue. It is likely that the gene expression changes are a result of the non-alcoholic fatty liver disease that the rats have developed, rather than the cause, as the expression of the same genes is suppressed earlier in adulthood (Figure 4.15).

The gene expression changes that occur at the time of the maternal nutritional insult are of much greater interest, as these will show the true primary responses to nutrition that set in train the effects that ultimately lead to disease in later life. Under- or overnutrition during embryonic and fetal development could trigger a series of events, such as tissue remodelling, or less effective regulation of hormone exchange across the placental

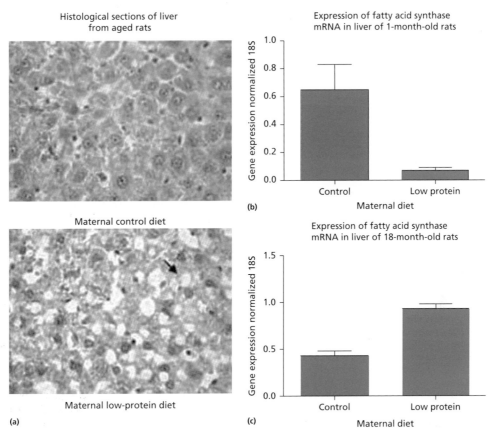

Figure 4.15 Programming of hepatic lipid metabolism by a maternal low-protein diet in the rat. Pregnant rats were fed a low-protein diet throughout pregnancy. a) At 18 months of age, their offspring showed histological evidence of hepatic steatosis (arrow shows white lipid deposits within the liver tissue). b) The mRNA expression of fatty acid synthase, a key enzyme in the synthesis of lipid, was suppressed in the low-protein-exposed offspring at 1 month of age, but c) was elevated in the older animals. Data source: Data from Erhuma *et al.* (2007).

barrier, that in turn have the long-term programming effect on fetal physiology. These primary nutrient–gene interactions may be difficult to observe as they may be transient. During the embryonic stage, even a few hours of up- or down-regulation of key genes could have critical effects on development. Kwong *et al.* (2007) showed that in newly implanted embryos of rats fed low-protein diets, the expression of mRNA for the insulin-like growth factor 2 and the closely related H19 gene were down-regulated. However, in low-protein-exposed fetuses, close to full-term gestation, expression of these genes was similar to levels seen in control pregnancies. Using whole genome microarrays to assess the response of all genes in a tissue to a particular nutritional challenge has enabled the identification of some of the key processes that respond to maternal undernutrition during pregnancy. Mid-gestation rat embryos exposed to either iron deficiency or maternal protein restriction

respond by altering expression of genes that regulate DNA synthesis and cell division and the integrity of the cytoskeleton (Swali *et al.*, 2011, 2012; Altobelli *et al.*, 2013). Most of these gene expression changes are not seen in the same tissues of older animals exposed to the same fetal challenges. Short-term events that impact on cell division can therefore be seen as a means by which the maternal diet irreversibly influences tissue development (remodelling) and hence the way in which the animal will respond physiologically to the conditions it encounters in later life.

4.4.6 Epigenetic regulation

The gene expression patterns described earlier have often been found to represent permanent changes in the level of transcription of specific genes in specific tissues. For such patterns to persist throughout the lifespan of an animal, there must be mechanisms that preserve

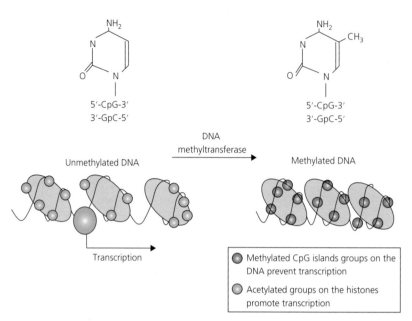

Figure 4.16 DNA methylation and histone acetylation are epigenetic mechanisms that regulate gene transcription. CpG islands in DNA may be methylated or unmethylated. In the unmethylated state, the histone proteins associated with the DNA tend to be acetylated and the DNA is less tightly coiled. Transcription factors and transcription machinery can access gene promoters and hence the unmethylated genes can be expressed. Methylation leads to deacetylation of histones and prevents transcription.

the cellular memory of the events that occurred in early life. Stable changes in the expression of genes can reasonably be attributed to changes in DNA methylation induced by maternal nutritional stimuli. DNA methylation is a potent suppressor of gene expression, either through blocking access of transcriptional machinery to the chromatin structure surrounding specific gene promoters or through interference with the binding of transcription factors to DNA (Figure 4.16). Around the time of embryo implantation, the majority of the genome is unmethylated, and this naïve state is remodelled as a normal element of development. The differentiation of tissues is accompanied by the methylation and silencing of unrequired genes. A series of DNA methyltransferases (DNMT) are responsible for establishing and maintaining the patterns of DNA methylation within cells (Bird, 2002). DNMT1 is important during development, as it maintains the DNA methylation pattern when DNA replicates during cell division. This is essential for normal development and mice deficient for this gene die *in utero*. The other DNMT (DNMT3L, DNMT3a and DNMT3b), which are only expressed in the embryo, are responsible for *de novo* DNA methylation. DNA methylation patterns have been shown to be stably inherited and may therefore allow phenotypic traits, acquired as a result of nutritional programming, to be passed on to subsequent offspring. Thus, a brief period

of undernutrition during embryonic, fetal or even early postnatal development may irreversibly modify DNA methylation in a manner that compromises normal physiology and metabolism.

Epigenetic changes initiated by features of maternal nutritional status are now believed to play an important role in the developmental programming of disease (Burdge *et al.*, 2007). The extensive resetting of DNA methylation marks during the embryonic and fetal period makes this process sensitive to the effects of under- or overnutrition. A wide range of evidence now points to methylation as both a biomarker and mechanism of nutritional programming. For example, differences in methylation were found at the IGF2 locus between individuals exposed to the Dutch famine and their unexposed siblings (Heijmans *et al.*, 2008). There is good evidence from animal models of undernutrition during fetal life that maternal diet can alter the epigenome, particularly DNA methylation, and this may establish changes in gene expression that permanently modify tissue structure or reset the responses to dietary and age-related challenges that occur later in life (Lillycrop *et al.*, 2007; Sinclair *et al.*, 2007; Bogdarina *et al.*, 2010; Altobelli *et al.*, 2013). Exposure to high-fat diets has also been shown to alter DNA methylation and histone marks in rodents, non-human primates and humans, with the brain being particularly sensitive to dietary influences (Jacobsen *et al.*, 2012; Seki *et al.*, 2012; Carlin *et al.*, 2013; Langie *et al.*, 2013).

Changes to the epigenome are likely to have a number of effects upon later health and well-being. Ultimately, the state of the epigenome determines whether genes are to be expressed or silenced. Epigenetic memory of transient nutritional exposures will determine how genes are expressed in response to further environmental challenges. The state of the epigenome is not entirely stable throughout life and so further nutritional or other influences will modify the memory or imprint of early life events. As epigenetic drift occurs, patterns of gene expression within tissues can change and this has been linked to certain cancers and Alzheimer's disease. The nature of age-related drift may be partly mediated by early life events and the state of the epigenome in infancy.

4.5 Implications of the programming hypothesis

4.5.1 Public health interventions

The importance of developmental programming as a risk factor for human disease is currently difficult to estimate. There are, however, some interesting indicators that suggest it may be appropriate to target pregnancy for major health interventions. Depending on age, blood pressure differences between individuals weighing 2.5 kg at birth might be expected to be up to 5 mmHg higher than those who were a kilogram heavier (Barker, 1998). This is a negligible blood pressure difference for an individual, but if blood pressures were to decline by 5 mmHg across the whole population of the United Kingdom, there would be 50 000 fewer deaths from CVD. Developing public health interventions that can prevent adverse nutritional programming, or offset some of the effects of prenatal nutrition, may therefore be worthy of consideration.

For achievement of such goals, there are many possible options that could be considered. The simplest might be to improve the general advice given to pregnant women regarding the quality of their diets. However, more research would be required to determine what might constitute the optimal diet for fetal development. The possibility of using drugs in early life to counteract programming effects of undernutrition was explored by Sherman and Langley-Evans (2000). Pregnant rats were fed control or low-protein diets. Their offspring were then either untreated or administered losartan, an antihypertensive drug, while still being suckled by their mothers. When blood pressure was determined in the adult offspring, while untreated offspring of low-protein fed mothers had raised blood pressure, as expected,

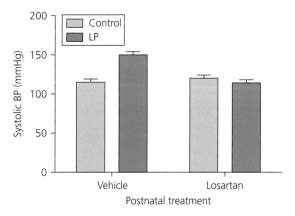

Figure 4.17 Postnatal treatment with antihypertensive drugs reverse programming effects of maternal undernutrition. Pregnant rats were fed control or low-protein (LP) diets in pregnancy. On giving birth, all animals were fed the same diet, but half of the litters from each group were treated with losartan, an antagonist of the angiotensin II AT1 receptor for 2 weeks. Blood pressure was measured 8 weeks later. Blood pressure of offspring from untreated LP-fed rats was elevated compared to controls, but the LP-exposed rats treated with losartan had normal blood pressure. Data source: Data from Sherman and Langley-Evans (2000).

those treated with losartan had normal blood pressure (Figure 4.17). This suggests that postnatal interventions could be designed to overcome the intrauterine effects of nutrition.

Early intervention with drugs to prevent disease would carry many practical and ethical problems. There would be a high risk of adverse effects as well as the intended benefits, and the range of disease states that appear programmed would necessitate a major expansion of the pharmacological arsenal. The development of personalized nutrition advice is a highly desirable alternative. Personalized nutrition is a strategy whereby individuals are given advice about diet, physical activity and lifestyle based upon their genotype for particular traits associated with disease and other characteristics. Our growing knowledge of early life programming mechanisms and the interaction of early life factors and genotype (Research Highlight 4.3) could be used to formulate personalized nutrition approaches based upon the Developmental Origins hypothesis. Personalized nutrition could be used to target pregnant women to optimize the health of their children, or any individual could be given advice based upon a range of factors including genotype and characteristics at birth. Novel approaches to disease prevention will emerge by developing our understanding of how disease is determined through the early life interactions of genotype, epigenetics and the maternal environment (Figure 4.18).

Research Highlight 4.3 Diabetes risk: Genotype, fetal programming or an interaction of the two?.

Type 2 diabetes and birth anthropometry

There are firmly established relationships between characteristics at birth, growth in childhood and risk of diabetes in adulthood (Barker, 1998). Individuals who are born of lower birth weight or who are thin at birth (low ponderal index; Phillips *et al.*, 1994) exhibit significantly greater disease risk, especially if they gain body fat rapidly in adolescence (Eriksson *et al.*, 2002a).

Polymorphisms associated with type 2 diabetes

A number of polymorphisms of genes involved in insulin signalling and metabolic regulation have been identified as playing a causative role in the aetiology of type 2 diabetes. These include the Pro12Ala polymorphism of PPAR-γ2 (Buzzetti *et al.*, 2004), the K121Q polymorphism of glycoprotein 1 (PC1; Pizzuti *et al.*, 1999) and an insertion/deletion (I/D) polymorphism of angiotensin converting enzyme (ACE).

Interaction of programming influences and genotype

The relationship between birth anthropometry and diabetes can be modified by genotype. The Ala12Ala variant of PPAR-γ2 is beneficial to individuals of lower birth weight, and the association of birth weight and diabetes may be confined to individuals with the Pro12Pro genotype (Eriksson *et al.*, 2002b). Some of this interaction may be due to effects on growth. The Ala12 genotype promotes faster growth (Laakso *et al.*, 2010), an effect which is modulated by the method of infant feeding in the first year (Mook-Kanamori *et al.*, 2009). Similarly, the Q variant of the K121Q polymorphism of PC1 is associated with insulin resistance, but only in individuals who were of low weight and shorter stature at birth (Kubaszek *et al.*, 2004).

Genotypes for other genes associated with type 2 diabetes also interact with birth weight, with lower weight associated with a greater influence of the adverse genotype (HHex, Cdkn2A and JAZF1 genotypes; Pulizzi *et al.*, 2009). Single genotypes can therefore give rise to multiple adult phenotypes due to variation in early life experience. Care is needed in interpreting findings relating to both sides of the interaction. The ACE I/D polymorphism exemplifies the fact that genotype may impact upon both disease outcome and birth anthropometry. Individuals with the DD variant are both small at birth and more likely as adults to exhibit a blunted insulin response to glucose (Kajantie *et al.*, 2004).

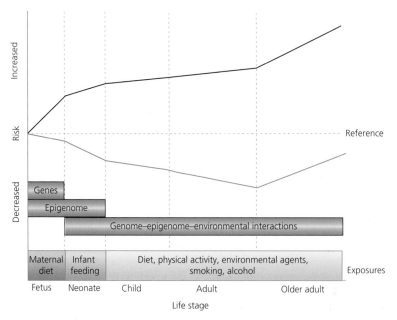

Figure 4.18 Risk of disease is a product of the interaction between the genome, the epigenome and the environment. Risk at any stage of life will be determined by the interaction of multiple genotypes, the epigenetic modification of those genotypes and exposure to the environment, including nutrition. The response to the environment at any stage of life may vary as the epigenetic regulation of genotype will reflect exposures at earlier stages.

4.5.2 Trans-generational transmission of disease risk

It is suggested that the programming influences of the fetal period upon disease in later life become apparent when there is a mismatch between the prenatal and postnatal environment. This is essentially the basis of the thrifty phenotype hypothesis. Babies whose growth was restricted by adverse factors during their fetal growth tend to exhibit catch-up growth in the postnatal period, that is, they grow more rapidly to achieve their genetic potential once the influence of maternal factors is withdrawn. There is good evidence to demonstrate that this rapid catch-up growth following prenatal growth restriction is one of the strongest predictors of the metabolic syndrome (Eriksson *et al.*, 2002a).

In populations that are undergoing economic and nutritional transition from poor to relatively affluent status (e.g. India, China, South Africa), the mismatch of early life influences and the adult diet and lifestyle might therefore be expected to drive an explosion of obesity, type 2 diabetes and CVD. The rapid improvements in maternal nutrition and health that will accompany the nutritional transition in such countries might be expected to lessen the importance of nutritional programming as a contributor to the overall disease burden. However, it is argued that programming could have effects that extend across several generations. The consequences of deficits in maternal nutrition in pregnancy might ultimately be transmitted to grandchildren. This means that across the globe, nutritional/economic transition may represent a sharp decline in malnutrition-related disease to be followed by half a century of unavoidable metabolic disease.

Pembrey (1996) proposed that such an intergenerational feedforward control loop exists, linking the growth and health of an individual with the nutrition of their grandparents. This form of control would be likely to involve some epigenetic marking of genes, with these markers then passed on to subsequent generations. The outcome of such imprinting would be very long-term health consequences for populations that are exposed to either undernutrition or overnutrition at some stage in their history. The complexity of the epidemiological studies that would be necessary to investigate intergenerational programming in human populations largely precludes such work. However, there are some examples that do appear to support the hypothesis advanced by Pembrey. Studies of individuals exposed to the acute but severe famine in wartime Holland indicate that undernutrition of women during pregnancy influenced the nutrition of their daughters, and this subsequently had an impact upon the birth weight of their grandchildren. Intergenerational effects are not necessarily the

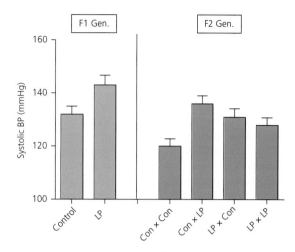

Figure 4.19 Programming of blood pressure across generations. Pregnant rats were fed control or low-protein (LP) diets in pregnancy. On giving birth, all animals were fed the same diet and when adult the offspring were mated to produce four separate crosses (control male × control female, control male × LP female, LP male × control female, LP male × LP female). Blood pressures of first-generation and second-generation offspring were measured at 8 weeks of age. F1, first generation; F2, second generation. Data source: Data from Harrison and Langley-Evans (2009).

product of disturbances in maternal nutrition. Bygren *et al.* (2001) reported that the grandchildren of men who were overfed in the prepubertal growth period had a significantly shorter lifespan.

Intergenerational programming by nutritional insults in fetal life has been noted in studies of animals. Beach *et al.* (1982) assessed immune function in the offspring of mice fed a zinc-deficient diet in pregnancy. This nutritional manipulation in fetal life led to severe immunosuppression in the adult offspring. Surprisingly, even though zinc status was normalized at the end of the original pregnancies, the impact on the immune system persisted into a third generation before resolving. As shown in Figure 4.19, the feeding of a low-protein diet in rat pregnancy produced high blood pressure in the adult offspring. When these adults were mated in all possible combinations of males and females from different dietary backgrounds, the next generation of adults were found to have higher blood pressure if they had at least one parent exposed to undernutrition as a fetus (Harrison and Langley-Evans, 2009). Drake *et al.* (2005) reported that the treatment of pregnant rats with dexamethasone in pregnancy, an intervention known to retard fetal growth and programme hypertension and glucose intolerance in the offspring, produced effects on glucose homeostasis that persisted for two generations.

The main explanation of how programmed traits can be passed on to second or third generation is that the original nutritional insult initiates heritable epigenetic changes to DNA at specific gene loci, as described in Section 4.4.6, and evidence is beginning to emerge to suggest that this is the case. There are, however, other mechanisms that could explain intergenerational programming effects of undernutrition that are specifically transmitted via the maternal line. Rather than genomic imprinting playing a critical role, physiological or endocrine disturbances in mothers, particularly in the response to the challenge of pregnancy, may lead to programming responses in their offspring. For example, undernutrition during fetal life will induce insulin resistance and eventually type 2 diabetes in the resultant adult individual. In women, this will make gestational diabetes more likely to occur, which generally produces an overgrown baby. These babies are more likely to gain excess weight in childhood and adolescence and will themselves be more likely to become diabetic. Studies of rats fed low-protein diets in pregnancy and lactation show that this is in fact the case and that modification of pancreatic function during fetal life has effects that persist for several generations (Reusens and Remacle, 2001).

SUMMARY

- Programming is the process through which exposure of the developing fetus to an insult or stimulus, at a critical stage of development, can permanently alter physiology and metabolism.
- Exposure to undernutrition or overnutrition in early life is a risk factor for major disease states in adulthood.
- Epidemiological studies show that anthropometric measures associated with poor nutrition in fetal life, such as lower birth weight or thinness at birth, predict later risk of coronary heart disease and type 2 diabetes.
- Rapid catch-up growth in infancy, following fetal growth restriction, increases the disease risk associated with a poor maternal diet in pregnancy.
- Animal studies show that restricted intakes or excessive intakes of a variety of macro- and micronutrients in pregnancy programme obesity, glucose intolerance and high blood pressure in the developing fetus.
- Discovery of the mechanisms through which programming occurs will be an important first step in planning future public health interventions that may target pregnancy as a period for preventing major diseases of adulthood.
- Candidate mechanisms that have been proposed to explain the association between maternal nutrition and disease in the offspring include disturbance of maternal–fetal hormone exchange across the placenta, specific nutrient–gene interactions that impact on tissue development and disruption of epigenetic regulation of gene expression.

References

Aihie Sayer, A., Dunn, R., Langley-Evans, S. *et al.* (2001) Prenatal exposure to a maternal low protein diet shortens life span in rats. *Gerontology*, **47**, 9–14.

Akyol, A., McMullen, S. and Langley-Evans, S.C. (2012) Glucose intolerance associated with early-life exposure to maternal cafeteria feeding is dependent upon post-weaning diet. *British Journal of Nutrition*, **107**, 964–978.

Altobelli, G., Bogdarina, I., Stupka, E. *et al.* (2013) Genome-wide methylation and gene expression changes in newborn rats following maternal protein restriction and reversal by folic acid. *PLoS One*, **8**, e82989.

Arai, Y. and Gorski, R.A. (1968) Critical exposure time for androgenization of the developing hypothalamus in the female rat. *Endocrinology*, **82**, 1010–1014.

Barker, D.J. and Osmond, C. (1986) Infant mortality, childhood nutrition, and ischaemic heart disease in England and Wales. *Lancet*, **1**, 1077–1081.

Barker, D.J., Winter, P.D., Osmond, C. *et al.* (1989) Weight in infancy and death from ischaemic heart disease. *Lancet*, **2**, 577–580.

Barker, D.J., Hales, C.N., Fall, C.H. *et al.* (1993a) Type 2 (non-insulin-dependent) diabetes mellitus, hypertension and hyperlipidaemia (syndrome X): relation to reduced fetal growth. *Diabetologia*, **36**, 62–67.

Barker, D.J., Osmond, C., Simmonds, S.J. *et al.* (1993b) The relation of small head circumference and thinness at birth to death from cardiovascular disease in adult life. *British Medical Journal*, **306**, 422–426.

Barker, D.J.P. (1998a) *Mothers, Babies and Health in Later Life*, Churchill Livingstone, Edinburgh.

Bartley, M., Power, C., Blane, D. *et al.* (1994) Birth weight and later socioeconomic disadvantage: evidence from the 1958 British cohort study. *British Medical Journal*, **309**, 1475–1478.

Battista, M.C., Oligny, L.L., St-Louis, J. *et al.* (2002) Intrauterine growth restriction in rats is associated with hypertension and renal dysfunction in adulthood. *American Journal of Physiology*, **283**, E124–E131.

Bavdekar, A., Yajnik, C.S., Fall, C.H. *et al.* (1999) Insulin resistance syndrome in 8-year-old Indian children: small at birth, big at 8 years, or both? *Diabetes*, **48**, 2422–2429.

Bayol, S.A., Farrington, S.J. and Stickland, N.C. (2007) A maternal 'junk food' diet in pregnancy and lactation promotes an exacerbated taste for 'junk food' and a greater propensity for obesity in rat offspring. *British Journal of Nutrition*, **98**, 843–851.

Bayol, S.A., Simbi, B.H., Fowkes, R.C. *et al.* (2010) A maternal 'junk food' diet in pregnancy and lactation promotes nonalcoholic Fatty liver disease in rat offspring. *Endocrinology*, **151**, 1451–1461.

Beach, R.S., Gershwin, M.E. and Hurley, L.S. (1982) Gestational zinc deprivation in mice: persistence of immunodeficiency for three generations. *Science*, **218**, 469–471.

Benediktsson, R., Lindsay, R.S., Noble, J. *et al.* (1993) Glucocorticoid exposure in utero: new model for adult hypertension. *Lancet*, **341**, 339–341.

Bergel, E. and Belizan, J.M. (2002) A deficient maternal calcium intake during pregnancy increases blood pressure of the offspring in adult rats. *British Journal of Obstetrics and Gynaecology*, **109**, 540–545.

Bird, A. (2002) DNA methylation patterns and epigenetic memory. *Genes and Development*, **16**, 6–21.

Bo, S., Cavallo-Perin, P., Scaglione, L. *et al.* (2000) Low birth weight and metabolic abnormalities in twins with increased susceptibility to Type 2 diabetes mellitus. *Diabetic Medicine*, **17**, 365–370.

Bogdarina, I., Haase, A., Langley-Evans, S. *et al.* (2010) Glucocorticoid effects on the programming of AT1b angiotensin receptor gene methylation and expression in the rat. *PLoS One*, **5**, e9237.

Breier, B.H., Krechowec, S.O. and Vickers, M.H. (2004) Maternal nutrition in pregnancy and adiposity in offspring, in *Fetal Nutrition and Adult Disease* (ed S.C. Langley-Evans), CABI Publishing, Wallingford, pp. 211–234.

Burdge, G.C., Hanson, M.A., Slater-Jefferies, J.L. *et al.* (2007) Epigenetic regulation of transcription: a mechanism for inducing variations in phenotype (fetal programming) by differences in nutrition during early life? *The British Journal of Nutrition*, **97** (6), 1036–1046.

Buzzetti, R., Petrone, A., Ribaudo, M.C. *et al.* (2004) The common PPAR-gamma2 Pro12Ala variant is associated with greater insulin sensitivity. *European Journal of Human Genetics*, **12**, 1050–1054.

Bygren, L.O., Kaati, G. and Edvinsson, S. (2001) Longevity determined by paternal ancestors' nutrition during their slow growth period. *Acta Biotheoretica*, **49**, 53–59.

Carlin, J., George, R. and Reyes, T.M. (2013) Methyl donor supplementation blocks the adverse effects of maternal high fat diet on offspring physiology. *PLoS One*, **8**, e63549.

Cohen, M.P., Stern, E., Rusecki, Y. *et al.* (1988) High prevalence of diabetes in young adult Ethiopian immigrants to Israel. *Diabetes*, **37**, 824–828.

Curhan, G.C., Chertow, G.M., Willett, W.C. *et al.* (1996) Birth weight and adult hypertension and obesity in women. *Circulation*, **94**, 1310–1315.

Daenzer, M., Ortmann, S., Klaus, S. *et al.* (2002) Prenatal high protein exposure decreases energy expenditure and increases adiposity in young rats. *Journal of Nutrition*, **132**, 142–144.

Dahri, S., Snoeck, A., Reusens-Billen, B. *et al.* (1991) Islet function in offspring of mothers on low-protein diet during gestation. *Diabetes*, **40** (Suppl 2), 115–120.

Donahue, S.M., Rifas-Shiman, S.L., Gold, D.R. *et al.* (2011) Prenatal fatty acid status and child adiposity at age 3 y: results from a US pregnancy cohort. *American Journal of Clinical Nutrition*, **93**, 780–788.

Drake, A.J., Walker, B.R. and Seckl, J.R. (2005) Intergenerational consequences of fetal programming by in utero exposure to glucocorticoids in rats. *American Journal of Physiology*, **288**, R34–R38.

Early Growth Genetics Consortium (2013) New loci associated with birth weight identify genetic links between intrauterine growth and adult height and metabolism. *Nature Genetics*, **45**, 76–82.

Erhuma, A., Salter, A.M., Sculley, D.V. *et al.* (2007) Prenatal exposure to a low-protein diet programs disordered regulation of lipid metabolism in the aging rat. *American Journal of Physiology*, **292**, E1702–E1714.

Eriksson, J.G., Forsen, T., Tuomilehto, J. *et al.* (1999) Catch-up growth in childhood and death from coronary heart disease: longitudinal study. *British Medical Journal*, **318**, 427–431.

Eriksson, J.G., Forsen, T., Tuomilehto, J. *et al.* (2002a) Effects of size at birth and childhood growth on the insulin resistance syndrome in elderly individuals. *Diabetologia*, **45**, 342–348.

Eriksson, J.G., Lindi, V., Uusitupa, M. *et al.* (2002b) The effects of the Pro12Ala polymorphism of the peroxisome proliferator-activated receptor-gamma2 gene on insulin sensitivity and insulin metabolism interact with size at birth. *Diabetes*, **51**, 2321–2324.

Falkner, B., Hulman, S. and Kushner, H. (1998) Birth weight versus childhood growth as determinants of adult blood pressure. *Hypertension*, **31**, 145–150.

Gademan, M.G., van Eijsden, M., Roseboom, T.J. *et al.* (2013) Maternal prepregnancy body mass index and their children's blood pressure and resting cardiac autonomic balance at age 5 to 6 years. *Hypertension*, **62**, 641–647.

Gambling, L., Dunford, S., Wallace, D.I. *et al.* (2003) Iron deficiency during pregnancy affects postnatal blood pressure in the rat. *Journal of Physiology*, **552**, 603–610.

Gardner, D.S., Bell, R.C. and Symonds, M.E. (2007) Fetal mechanisms that lead to later hypertension. *Current Drug Targets*, **8**, 894–905.

Gillman, M.W., Rifas-Shiman, S.L., Kleinman, K.P. *et al.* (2004) Maternal calcium intake and offspring blood pressure. *Circulation*, **110**, 1990–1995.

Gluckman, P.D. and Hanson, M.A. (2004) Living with the past: evolution, development, and patterns of disease. *Science*, **305**, 1733–1736.

Godfrey, K.M. (2001) The 'gold standard' for optimal fetal growth and development. *Journal of Pediatric Endocrinology and Metabolism*, **14** (Suppl 6), 1507–1513.

Godfrey, K.M., Forrester, T., Barker, D.J. *et al.* (1994) Maternal nutritional status in pregnancy and blood pressure in childhood. *British Journal of Obstetrics and Gynaecology*, **101**, 398–403.

Godfrey, K.M., Robinson, S., Barker, D.J. *et al.* (1996) Maternal nutrition in early and late pregnancy in relation to placental and fetal growth. *British Medical Journal*, **312**, 410–414.

Gray, C., Al-Dujaili, E.A., Sparrow, A.J. *et al.* (2013) Excess maternal salt intake produces sex-specific hypertension in offspring: putative roles for kidney and gastrointestinal sodium handling. *PLoS One*, **8**, e72682.

Hales, C.N. and Barker, D.J. (1992) Type 2 (non-insulin-dependent) diabetes mellitus: the thrifty phenotype hypothesis. *Diabetologia*, **35**, 595–601.

Hales, C.N. and Barker, D.J. (2001) The thrifty phenotype hypothesis. *British Medical Bulletin*, **60**, 5–20.

Hales, C.N., Barker, D.J., Clark, P.M. *et al.* (1991) Fetal and infant growth and impaired glucose tolerance at age 64. *British Medical Journal*, **303**, 1019–1022.

Harding, J. (2004) Nutritional basis for the fetal origins of adult disease, in *Fetal Nutrition and Adult Disease* (ed S.C. Langley-Evans), Cabi, Wallingford, pp. 21–54.

Harrison, M. and Langley-Evans, S.C. (2009) Intergenerational programming of impaired nephrogenesis and hypertension in rats following maternal protein restriction during pregnancy. *British Journal of Nutrition*, **101**, 1020–1030.

Hattersley, A.T. and Tooke, J.E. (1999) The fetal insulin hypothesis: an alternative explanation of the association of low birth weight with diabetes and vascular disease. *Lancet*, **353**, 1789–1792.

Hawkins, P., Steyn, C., Ozaki, T. et al. (2000) Effect of maternal undernutrition in early gestation on ovine fetal blood pressure and cardiovascular reflexes. *American Journal of Physiology*, **279**, R340–R348.

Heijmans, B.T., Tobi, E.W., Stein, A.D. et al. (2008) Persistent epigenetic differences associated with prenatal exposure to famine in humans. *Proceedings of the National Academy of Sciences USA*, **105**, 17046–17049.

Hinchliffe, S.A., Lynch, M.R., Sargent, P.H. et al. (1992) The effect of intrauterine growth retardation on the development of renal nephrons. *British Journal of Obstetrics and Gynaecology*, **99**, 296–301.

Holemans, K., Gerber, R., Meurrens, K. et al. (1999) Maternal food restriction in the second half of pregnancy affects vascular function but not blood pressure of rat female offspring. *British Journal of Nutrition*, **81**, 73–79.

Huxley, R., Neil, A. and Collins, R. (2002) Unravelling the fetal origins hypothesis: is there really an inverse association between birth weight and subsequent blood pressure? *Lancet*, **360**, 659–665.

Inskip, H.M., Godfrey, K.M., Robinson, S.M. et al. (2006) Cohort profile: the Southampton Women's Survey. *International Journal of Epidemiology*, **35** (1), 42–48.

Institute of Medicine (2009) *Weight Gain During Pregnancy: Reexamining the Guidelines*, National Academies Press, Washington, DC.

Jacobsen, S.C., Brøns, C., Bork-Jensen, J. et al. (2012) Effects of short-term high-fat overfeeding on genome-wide DNA methylation in the skeletal muscle of healthy young men. *Diabetologia*, **55** (12), 3341–3349.

Jordan, K.M., Syddall, H., Dennison, E.M. et al. (2005) Birth weight, vitamin D receptor gene polymorphism, and risk of lumbar spine osteoarthritis. *Journal of Rheumatology*, **32**, 678–683.

Kajantie, E., Rautanen, A., Kere, J. et al. (2004) The effects of the ACE gene insertion/deletion polymorphism on glucose tolerance and insulin secretion in elderly people are modified by birth weight. *Journal of Clinical Endocrinology and Metabolism*, **89**, 5738–5741.

Kajantie, E., Dunkel, L., Turpeinen, U. et al. (2006) Placental 11beta-HSD2 activity, early postnatal clinical course, and adrenal function in extremely low birth weight infants. *Pediatric Research*, **59**, 575–578.

Kind, K.L., Simonetta, G., Clifton, P.M. et al. (2002) Effect of maternal feed restriction on blood pressure in the adult guinea pig. *Experimental Physiology*, **87**, 469–477.

Kubaszek, A., Markkanen, A., Eriksson, J.G. et al. (2004) The association of the K121Q polymorphism of the plasma cell glycoprotein-1 gene with type 2 diabetes and hypertension depends on size at birth. *Journal of Clinical Endocrinology and Metabolism*, **89**, 2044–2047.

Kwong, W.Y., Miller, D.J., Wilkins, A.P. et al. (2007) Maternal low protein diet restricted to the preimplantation period induces a gender-specific change on hepatic gene expression in rat fetuses. *Molecular Reproduction and Development*, **74**, 48–56.

Laakso, S., Utriainen, P., Laakso, M. et al. (2010) Polymorphism Pro12Ala of PPARG in prepubertal children with premature adrenarche and its association with growth in healthy children. *Hormone Research Paediatrics*, **74**, 365–371.

Langie, S.A., Achterfeldt, S., Gorniak, J.P. et al. (2013) Maternal folate depletion and high-fat feeding from weaning affects DNA methylation and DNA repair in brain of adult offspring. *FASEB Journal*, **27**, 3323–3334.

Langley-Evans, S.C. (1997) Maternal carbenoxolone treatment lowers birth weight and induces hypertension in the offspring of rats fed a protein-replete diet. *Clinical Science*, **93**, 423–429.

Langley-Evans, S.C. (2013) Fetal programming of CVD and renal disease: animal models and mechanistic considerations. *Proceedings of the Nutrition Society*, **72**, 317–325.

Langley-Evans, S.C. and Jackson, A.A. (1995) Captopril normalises systolic blood pressure in rats with hypertension induced by fetal exposure to maternal low protein diets. *Comparative Biochemistry and Physiology*, **110**, 223–228.

Langley-Evans, A.J. and Langley-Evans, S.C. (2003) Relationship between maternal nutrient intakes in early and late pregnancy and infants weight and proportions at birth: prospective cohort study. *Journal of the Royal Society for the Promotion of Health*, **123**, 210–216.

Langley-Evans, S.C., Phillips, G.J. and Jackson, A.A. (1994) In utero exposure to maternal low protein diets induces hypertension in weanling rats, independently of maternal blood pressure changes. *Clinical Nutrition*, **13**, 319–324.

Langley-Evans, S.C., Gardner, D.S. and Jackson, A.A. (1996a) Association of disproportionate growth of fetal rats in late gestation with raised systolic blood pressure in later life. *Journal of Reproduction and Fertility*, **106**, 307–312.

Langley-Evans, S.C., Phillips, G.J., Benediktsson, R. et al. (1996b) Protein intake in pregnancy, placental glucocorticoid metabolism and the programming of hypertension in the rat. *Placenta*, **17**, 169–172.

Langley-Evans, S.C., Welham, S.J. and Jackson, A.A. (1999) Fetal exposure to a maternal low protein diet impairs nephrogenesis and promotes hypertension in the rat. *Life Science*, **64**, 965–974.

Langley-Evans, S.C., Langley-Evans, A.J. and Marchand, M.C. (2003) Nutritional programming of blood pressure and renal morphology. *Archives of Physiology and Biochemistry*, **111**, 8–16.

Lawrence, G.M., Shulman, S., Friedlander, Y. et al. (2013) Associations of maternal pre-pregnancy and gestational body size with offspring longitudinal change in BMI. *Obesity*, **22**, 1165–1171.

Lillycrop, K.A., Slater-Jefferies, J.L., Hanson, M.A. et al. (2007) Induction of altered epigenetic regulation of the hepatic glucocorticoid receptor in the offspring of rats fed a protein-restricted diet during pregnancy suggests that reduced DNA methyltransferase-1 expression is involved in impaired DNA methylation and changes in histone modifications. *British Journal of Nutrition*, **97**, 1064–1073.

Mathews, F., Yudkin, P. and Neil, A. (1999) Influence of maternal nutrition on outcome of pregnancy: prospective cohort study. *British Medical Journal*, **319**, 339–343.

Matthes, J.W., Lewis, P.A., Davies, D.P. et al. (1994) Relation between birth weight at term and systolic blood pressure in adolescence. *British Medical Journal*, **308**, 1074–1077.

McTernan, C.L., Draper, N., Nicholson, H. et al. (2001) Reduced placental 11beta-hydroxysteroid dehydrogenase type 2 mRNA levels in human pregnancies complicated by intrauterine growth restriction: an analysis of possible mechanisms. *Journal of Clinical Endocrinology and Metabolism*, **86**, 4979–4983.

Mook-Kanamori, D.O., Steegers, E.A., Uitterlinden, A.G. *et al.* (2009) Breast-feeding modifies the association of PPARgamma2 polymorphism Pro12Ala with growth in early life: the Generation R Study. *Diabetes*, **58**, 992–998.

Moore, S.E., Cole, T.J., Collinson, A.C. *et al.* (1999) Prenatal or early postnatal events predict infectious deaths in young adulthood in rural Africa. *International Journal of Epidemiology*, **28**, 1088–1095.

Neel, J.V. (1962) Diabetes mellitus: a 'thrifty' genotype rendered detrimental by 'progress'? *American Journal of Human Genetics*, **14**, 353–362.

Ogden CL, Carroll MD, Kit BK, *et al.*2013). *Prevalence of Obesity Among Adults: United States, 2011–2012*. NCHS Data Brief, No 131. National Center for Health Statistics, Hyattsville, MD.

Oken, E., Taveras, E.M., Kleinman, K.P. *et al.* (2007) Gestational weight gain and child adiposity at age 3 years. *American Journal of Obstetrics and Gynecology*, **196**, 322.

Osmond, C., Barker, D.J. and Slattery, J.M. (1990) Risk of death from cardiovascular disease and chronic bronchitis determined by place of birth in England and Wales. *Journal of Epidemiology and Community Health*, **44**, 139–141.

Ozaki, T., Nishina, H., Hanson, M.A. *et al.* (2001) Dietary restriction in pregnant rats causes gender-related hypertension and vascular dysfunction in offspring. *Journal of Physiology*, **530**, 141–152.

Pembrey, M. (1996) Imprinting and transgenerational modulation of gene expression; human growth as a model. *Acta Geneticae Medicae et Gemellologiae*, **45**, 111–125.

Persson, E. and Jansson, T. (1992) Low birth weight is associated with elevated adult blood pressure in the chronically catheterized guinea-pig. *Acta Physiology Scandinavia*, **145**, 195–196.

Phillips, D.I., Barker, D.J., Hales, C.N. *et al.* (1994) Thinness at birth and insulin resistance in adult life. *Diabetologia*, **37**, 150–154.

Pizzuti, A., Frittitta, L., Argiolas, A. *et al.* (1999) A polymorphism (K121Q) of the human glycoprotein PC-1 gene coding region is strongly associated with insulin resistance. *Diabetes*, **48**, 1881–1884.

Plagemann, A., Harder, T., Rake, A. *et al.* (2001) Hypothalamic nuclei are malformed in weanling offspring of low protein malnourished rat dams. *Journal of Nutrition*, **130**, 2582–2589.

Poore, K.R., Forhead, A.J., Gardner, D.S. *et al.* (2002) The effects of birth weight on basal cardiovascular function in pigs at 3 months of age. *Journal of Physiology*, **539**, 969–978.

Poulsen, P., Vaag, A.A., Kyvik, K.O. *et al.* (1997) Low birth weight is associated with NIDDM in discordant monozygotic and dizygotic twin pairs. *Diabetologia*, **40**, 439–446.

Power, M.L. and Tardif, S.D. (2005) Maternal nutrition and metabolic control of pregnancy, in *Birth, Distress and Disease* (eds M.L. Power and J. Schulkin), Cambridge University Press, New York, pp. 88–113.

Prentice, A.M., Whitehead, R.G., Watkinson, M. *et al.* (1983) Prenatal dietary supplementation of African women and birth-weight. *Lancet*, **321**, 489–492.

Pulizzi, N., Lyssenko, V., Jonsson, A. *et al.* (2009) Interaction between prenatal growth and high-risk genotypes in the development of type 2 diabetes. *Diabetologia*, **52**, 825–829.

Räikkönen, K., Pesonen, A.K., Heinonen, K. *et al.* (2009) Maternal licorice consumption and detrimental cognitive and psychiatric outcomes in children. *American Journal of Epidemiology*, **170**, 1137–1146.

Räikkönen, K., Seckl, J.R., Heinonen, K. *et al.* (2010) Maternal prenatal licorice consumption alters hypothalamic-pituitary-adrenocortical axis function in children. *Psychoneuroendocrinology*, **35**, 1587–1593.

Reusens, B. and Remacle, C. (2001) Intergenerational effect of an adverse intrauterine environment on perturbation of glucose metabolism. *Twin Research*, **4**, 406–11.

Roseboom, T.J., Van Der Meulen, J.H., Ravelli, A.C. *et al.* (2001) Effects of prenatal exposure to the Dutch famine on adult disease in later life: an overview. *Molecular and Cellular Endocrinology*, **185**, 93–98.

Samuelsson, A.M., Matthews, P.A., Argenton, M. *et al.* (2008) Diet-induced obesity in female mice leads to offspring hyperphagia, adiposity, hypertension, and insulin resistance: a novel murine model of developmental programming. *Hypertension*, **51**, 383–392.

Schellong, K., Schulz, S., Harder, T. *et al.* (2012) Birth weight and long-term overweight risk: systematic review and a meta-analysis including 643,902 persons from 66 studies and 26 countries globally. *PLoS One*, **7**, e47776.

Seki, Y., Williams, L., Vuguin, P.M. *et al.* (2012) Minireview: Epigenetic programming of diabetes and obesity: animal models. *Endocrinology*, **153**, 1031–1038.

Shankar, K., Harrell, A., Liu, X. *et al.* (2008) Maternal obesity at conception programs obesity in the offspring. *American Journal of Physiology*, **294**, R528–R538.

Sherman, R.C. and Langley-Evans, S.C. (2000) Antihypertensive treatment in early postnatal life modulates prenatal dietary influences upon blood pressure in the rat. *Clinical Science*, **98**, 269–275.

Sinclair, K.D., Allegrucci, C., Singh, R. *et al.* (2007) DNA methylation, insulin resistance, and blood pressure in offspring determined by maternal periconceptional B vitamin and methionine status. *Proceedings of the National Academy of Sciences*, **104**, 19351–19356.

Smits, L., Krabbendam, L., de Bie, R. *et al.* (2006) Lower birth weight of Dutch neonates who were in utero at the time of the 9/11 attacks. *Journal of Psychosomatic Research*, **61**, 715–717.

Snoeck, A., Remacle, C., Reusens, B. *et al.* (1990) Effect of a low protein diet during pregnancy on the fetal rat endocrine pancreas. *Biology of the Neonate*, **57**, 107–118.

Song, Y., Wang, H.J., Ma, J. *et al.* (2013) Secular trends of obesity prevalence in urban Chinese children from 1985 to 2010: gender disparity. *PLoS One*, **8**, e53069.

Souren, N.Y., Paulussen, A.D., Steyls, A. *et al.* (2008) Common SNPs in LEP and LEPR associated with birth weight and type 2 diabetes-related metabolic risk factors in twins. *International Journal of Obesity*, **32** (8), 1233–1239.

Strandberg, T.E., Järvenpää, A.L., Vanhanen, H. *et al.* (2001) Birth outcome in relation to licorice consumption during pregnancy. *American Journal of Epidemiology*, **153**, 1085–1088.

Strandberg, T.E., Andersson, S., Järvenpää, A.L. *et al.* (2002) Preterm birth and licorice consumption during pregnancy. *American Journal of Epidemiology*, **156**, 803–805.

Swali, A., McMullen, S., Hayes, H. *et al.* (2011) Cell cycle regulation and cytoskeletal remodelling are critical processes in the nutritional programming of embryonic development. *PLoS One*, **6**, e23189.

Swali, A., McMullen, S., Hayes, H. *et al.* (2012) Processes underlying the nutritional programming of embryonic development by iron deficiency in the rat. *PLoS One*, **7**, e48133.

Villamor, E., Rifas-Shiman, S.L., Gillman, M.W. *et al.* (2012) Maternal intake of methyl-donor nutrients and child cognition at 3 years of age. *Paediatric and Perinatal Epidemiology*, **26**, 328–335.

Walker-Bone, K., Walter, G. and Cooper, C. (2002) Recent developments in the epidemiology of osteoporosis. *Current Opinions in Rheumatology*, **14**, 411–415.

Whincup, P.H., Kaye, S.J., Owen, C.G. *et al.* (2008) Birth weight and risk of type 2 diabetes: a systematic review. *Journal of the American Medical Association*, **300**, 2886–2897.

White, S.L., Perkovic, V., Cass, A. *et al.* (2009) Is low birth weight an antecedent of CKD in later life? A systematic review of observational studies. *American Journal of Kidney Disease*, **54**, 248–261.

Winkler, C., Illig, T., Koczwara, K. *et al.* (2009) HHEX-IDE polymorphism is associated with low birth weight in offspring with a family history of type 1 diabetes. *Journal of Clinical Endocrinology and Metabolism*, **94**, 4113–4115.

Woodall, S.M., Johnston, B.M., Breier, B.H. *et al.* (1996) Chronic maternal undernutrition in the rat leads to delayed postnatal growth and elevated blood pressure of offspring. *Pediatric Research*, **40**, 438–443.

World Health Organization (WHO) (2013) *Obesity and Overweight*. WHO Factsheet 311, http://www.who.int/media centre/factsheets/fs311/en/ (accessed 28 January 2014).

Wynn, A.H., Crawford, M.A., Doyle, W. *et al.* (1991) Nutrition of women in anticipation of pregnancy. *Nutrition and Health*, **7**, 69–88.

Zung, A., Elizur, M., Weintrob, N. *et al.* (2004) Type 1 diabetes in Jewish Ethiopian immigrants in Israel: HLA class II immunogenetics and contribution of new environment. *Human Immunology*, **65**, 1463–1468.

Additional reading

If you would like to find out more about the material discussed in this chapter, the following sources may be of interest.

Barker, D.J.P. (1998b) *Mothers, Babies and Health in Later Life*, Churchill Livingstone, Edinburgh.

Gluckman, P.D. and Hanson, M.A. (2008) *Mismatch: The Lifestyle Diseases Timebomb*, Oxford University Press, Oxford.

Kok, F., Bouwman, L. and Desiere, F. (eds) (2008) *Personalized Nutrition. Principles and Applications*, Taylor and Francis, Boca Raton, FL.

CHAPTER 5

Lactation and infant feeding

LEARNING OBJECTIVES

This chapter will enable the reader to:
- Describe the anatomy of the human breast and the synthesis of milk within mammary alveolar tissue
- Demonstrate an understanding of the endocrine control of lactation
- Discuss the extra nutrient demands that are imposed by lactation and the maternal dietary changes that may be required to meet those demands

- Critically review the evidence that breastfeeding is beneficial for the health and well-being of mothers and their infants
- Describe trends in infant feeding behaviours seen in developed countries and discuss the global strategies that have been developed to promote breastfeeding
- Discuss the composition of infant formula milks and describe the need for specialized formulas for premature babies and infants with food allergies and intolerances

5.1 Introduction

The period of early infancy and the provision of nutrients in an optimal balance are critical for the immediate health and well-being of the child. It is also becoming clear that events that occur during this phase of development can also have a major impact upon the long-term physiology, metabolism and disease risk of the individual (Chapter 4). There are different strategies available for feeding infants in the first 4–6 months of life, and these include breastfeeding, bottle-feeding a formula and a mixed approach utilizing both breast and formula milks. The health of both the infant and the mother is best served by exclusive breastfeeding. This chapter will review the processes through which human milk is produced and why breastfeeding is optimal for health and development. The chapter will also describe the composition of formula milks and how these can be shaped to meet the varying demands of life stage and special clinical circumstances.

5.2 The physiology of lactation

5.2.1 Anatomy of the breast

The anatomy of the human mammary gland is shown in Figure 5.1. The breast is a major site of fat deposition, particularly during pregnancy when high levels of oestrogen promote storage in preparation for later lactation. This fat underlies the skin of the breast and provides protection for the ducts and alveolar structures that are required for milk production. There are four key structures within the breast to be aware of in the context of lactation.

5.2.1.1 The nipple and areola

The nipples are surrounded by a dark pigmented region termed the areola. Both structures contain smooth muscle cells that will contract when mechanically stimulated, allowing the nipple to stiffen. This is essential to allow the suckling baby to grip the nipple and to take the whole of the area into its mouth (see 'The rooting reflex'). The nipple and areola also have structures

Nutrition, Health and Disease: A Lifespan Approach, Second Edition. Simon Langley-Evans.
© 2015 John Wiley & Sons, Ltd. Published 2015 by John Wiley & Sons, Ltd.
Companion website: www.wiley.com/go/langleyevans/lifespan

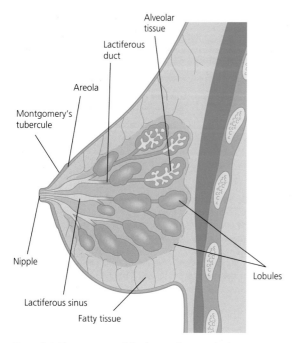

Figure 5.1 The anatomy of the human breast. The breast comprises 10–12 lobules, each containing mammary alveolar tissue with associated lactiferous ducts. The ducts terminate at the lactiferous sinuses that discharge via the nipple.

Table 5.1 The composition of human milk.

	Units per 100 g milk		
	Colostrum	Transitional milk	Mature milk
Energy (kcal)	56.0	67.0	69.0
Protein (g)	2.0	1.5	1.3
Protein (% energy)	14.0	9.0	8.0
Fat (total, g)	2.6	3.7	4.1
Fat (% energy)	42.0	51.0	53.0
Carbohydrate (g)	6.6	6.9	7.2
Carbohydrate (% energy)	44.0	40.0	39.0
Calcium (mg)	28.0	25.0	34.0
Phosphorus (mg)	14.0	16.0	15.0
Sodium (mg)	47.0	30.0	15.0
Zinc (mg)	0.6	0.3	0.3
Riboflavin (mg)	0.03	0.03	0.03
Nicotinic acid (mg)	0.8	0.6	0.7
Vitamin B6 (µg)	Trace	Trace	0.01
Folate (µg)	2.0	3.0	5.0
Vitamin C (mg)	7.0	6.0	4.0
Vitamin A (µg)	177.5	91.2	62.0

Source: Data from Holland *et al.* (1991).
Selected nutrients.

called Montgomery's tubercles, which are sebaceous glands that produce lubricants during suckling.

5.2.1.2 The lactiferous ducts
Each breast has 15–20 lobes in which the machinery for production of milk develops. Within each lobe lies a lactiferous duct that links the milk-producing tissues to the nipple where milk is released.

5.2.1.3 The lactiferous sinuses
The lactiferous sinuses lie at the nipple end of each duct. These sinuses provide some limited capacity for storage of milk between feeds but more importantly are lined with contractile myoepithelial cells that have the role of ejecting milk from the nipple when the baby suckles.

5.2.1.4 The alveolar cells
The mammary alveoli are the site of milk synthesis. The key cells in these structures are the epithelial cells, which form a single layer around the alveolar lumen that drains into the lactiferous duct. Alveolar epithelial cells are polar in nature, meaning that there are specialized organelles on the basal side (the side of the cell in contact with the vascular system) and on the apical side (the side of the cell in contact with the alveolar lumen). This reflects the

function of these cells, which requires uptake of nutrients from the blood and secretion of milk. The apical side of the cells is therefore packed with secretory structures (Golgi apparatus, secretory vesicles and fat droplets).

5.2.1.5 The rooting reflex
Successful suckling requires that the baby correctly takes the nipple into the mouth and stimulates the nerve endings that lie beneath the areola. To achieve this, correct 'latching-on', the human infant is born with an innate response called the rooting reflex. All newborn babies will turn their heads towards anything that strokes their cheek or mouth and open the mouth. Thus, brushing the cheek with the nipple will cause the baby to take it into the mouth and initiate suckling. The nipple is drawn up to the palate, and the tongue and palate then squeeze together to draw milk from the sinuses. The baby then starts the actual milking action, which involves a tongue movement from areola to nipple. These movements are instinctively coordinated with breathing and swallowing.

5.2.2 Synthesis of milk
The average composition of mature human milk is shown in Table 5.1. Generally speaking, women will produce 750–800 ml of milk per day at the peak of lactation, and

within this milk, approximately 50% of the energy will be delivered as fat and 40% as carbohydrate. Carbohydrate is primarily delivered in the form of lactose and fats as triacylglycerols. Protein comprises casein and the whey proteins (α-lactalbumin, lactoferrin).

The true composition of human milk is highly complex as there are a number of non-nutritional components in addition to the basic nutritional requirements of the infant. There is also a wide variation in composition between women and between breasts within the same woman. Some of this variation may be explained by the differences in quality of maternal diet and maternal body composition and stores. Human milk also changes in composition at different stages across the full lactation period, with time of day and within the course of a feed.

5.2.2.1 Foremilk and hindmilk

The first milk to be released during a feed is called the foremilk. Once the full letdown of milk occurs (see the following text), hindmilk is released. Foremilk tends to be more watery than hindmilk and may serve primarily to meet the thirst of the infant and provide some instant satisfaction of the desire to feed. The foremilk is lower in fat content and richer in lactose than the hindmilk and is therefore less energy and nutrient dense. As the hindmilk provides more of the energy requirements of the infant, it is important for the breast to be fully drained at each feed, rather than adopt the strategy of allowing the infant to suckle for a few minutes on each breast at each feed.

5.2.2.2 Time of day

Several studies have documented that the composition of human milk varies during the course of the day. Lubetzky *et al.* (2006) reported that in mothers of premature infants who were expressing milk for their babies, the fat content of the milk was greater in the evening than in the morning. Similarly, Mitoulas and colleagues (2003) found that the fatty acid composition of milk from mothers of full-term infants varied over the day, with generally more fat produced in the evenings. The dynamic quality of milk composition may be explained by the diurnal variation in nutrient reserves of the mother or possibly by endocrine factors.

5.2.2.3 Course of lactation

The greatest variation in milk composition is associated with the developmental stage of the infant (Table 5.1). Mothers of premature babies produce milk that differs in composition to mothers of full-term babies. Preterm milk contains greater concentrations of protein, non-protein nitrogen, arachidonic acid and docosahexaenoic acid (DHA) (Kovacs *et al.*, 2005).

The first secretions of the mammary gland following the birth of the baby are called colostrum. Colostrum is a thick, sticky, yellowish fluid produced in small quantities (around 100 ml/day). Due to the low quantity produced, it has long been believed that colostrum has little nutritive function and that it is instead a protective secretion that minimizes the infants' risk of infection and promotes maturation of the gut. Colostrum has a low content of lactose and fat and has a protein concentration that is considerably greater than in mature milk (Table 5.1). Most of the proteins in colostrum are protective factors, the principal elements being the secretory immunoglobulin IgA and lactoferrin. Colostrum is also rich in vitamin A.

Between 3 and 7 days post-partum, the mammary gland switches from the production of colostrum to the synthesis of *transitional milk*. This milk is produced in a larger volume and has a lower protein and sodium content than colostrum. Lactose and fat concentrations are more similar to mature milk. Mature milk will be secreted from around 14 days post-partum.

5.2.2.4 Synthesis of carbohydrates

The primary carbohydrate within milk is lactose, which comprises approximately 80% of the total carbohydrate load. The remaining carbohydrate is in the form of oligosaccharides that are believed to have an immunoprotective role. Oligosaccharides escape digestion within the small intestine and pass to the colon where they act as prebiotics. Prebiotic compounds provide substrates for the growth of bacteria within the colon. Maintaining a healthy population of *Lactobacillus* and *Bifidobacterium* species appears to reduce the risk of infection with diarrhoea-causing species.

Lactose is synthesized from glucose in the polar alveolar epithelial cells (Figure 5.2). Galactose is primarily synthesized de novo from glucose, although some galactose will be taken up from the maternal diet. Lactose is synthesized from glucose and galactose through the action of lactose synthetase, which is a multi-enzyme complex comprising galactosyltransferase and α-lactalbumin. Galactosyltransferase is expressed in the mammary glands during pregnancy, but as there is little α-lactalbumin, the mature complex cannot be formed.

Lactose synthesis occurs within the Golgi apparatus on the apical side of the alveolar epithelial cell. Lactose is packaged into secretory vesicles, and due to the high osmolality of the disaccharide, the vesicles take up water and electrolytes such as potassium and sodium. Lactose synthesis is therefore responsible for generating the fluid portion of the milk. Secretory vesicles and their contents are discharged into the alveolar lumen by exocytosis.

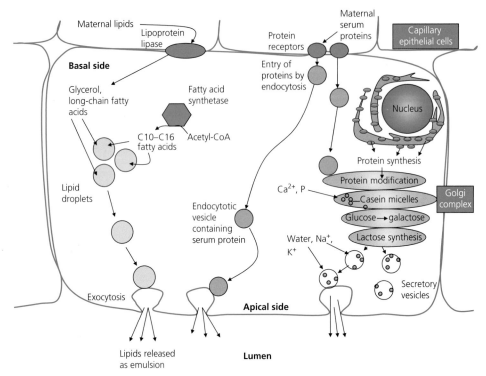

Figure 5.2 Synthesis of human milk. Milk synthesis occurs in the polar alveolar cells of the mammary tissue. Substrates for milk production are either synthesized de novo within the cytoplasm and Golgi complexes of the alveolar cell or are imported from the maternal circulation through endocytotic uptake on the basal side of the cell. Lipid droplets and maternal circulation-derived proteins are discharged to the alveolar lumen by exocytosis. Lactose, casein micelles, water and micronutrients are secreted to the lumen from the Golgi apparatus.

5.2.2.5 Origins of milk fats

Milk contains fat in the form of emulsified droplets that consist of a mixture of triacylglycerides, diacylglycerides, monoacylglycerides, free fatty acids, cholesterol and phospholipids. Ninety-eight percent of the fat is in the form of triacylglycerides. Lipid droplets are formed within the alveolar epithelial cells as lipids that are derived from maternal circulation or from de novo synthesis coalesce and migrate towards the apical side of the cell. The droplets are eliminated from the cells by exocytosis, and in this process, a small portion of the apical cell membrane is lost. This will therefore deliver some maternal phospholipids and cell membrane proteins into the milk (Figure 5.2).

Glycerol for the synthesis of triacylglycerides is derived from the maternal circulation. This along with the longer-chain fatty acids (16 or more carbon chain) is cleaved from triacylglycerides by the action of lipoprotein lipase in the mammary capillaries. As these fatty acids are derived from the maternal diet, the composition of breast milk will therefore reflect the composition of the fats consumed by the mother. Shorter-chain fatty acids are synthesized within the cytosol of the alveolar cells. Acetyl-CoA, which

is generated from the citric acid cycle in the mitochondria, is transported to the cytosol via the acetyl-group shuttle. Carboxylation generates malonyl-CoA, which is the substrate for the fatty acid synthetase complex, which progressively conjugates two carbon units up to C16 palmitic acid. Fatty acids of C10–C16 length synthesized in this manner will be incorporated into milk fat.

5.2.2.6 Milk proteins

Human milk contains a broad array of proteins, many of which have non-nutritive functions. In addition to the major milk proteins, casein, α-lactalbumin and β-lactoglobulin, which are synthesized de novo within the mammary epithelial cells, there are proteins that are derived from the maternal circulation. These include secretory IgA, lactoferrin, antiviral agents, enzymes and growth factors (insulin-like growth factor 1, mammary-derived growth factor, insulin and nerve growth factor). Immunoglobulin A that is secreted into milk will reflect the antigen exposures of the mother and serves to protect the infant from gastrointestinal infection and to prime the neonatal immune system. Lactoferrin is an

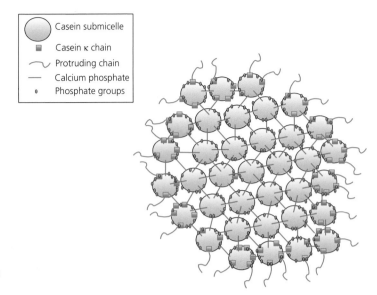

Casein submicelle
Casein κ chain
Protruding chain
Calcium phosphate
Phosphate groups

Figure 5.3 The structure of a casein micelle. Micelles bind and transport calcium and phosphate in milk. The internal sub-micelles comprise hydrophobic α and β caseins, while those on the external surface of the structures incorporate hydrophilic κ casein chains.

iron-binding protein that minimizes risk of infection of the infant gut by removing iron that could be used as a bacterial substrate.

Blood-borne proteins, including IgA, generally enter the alveolar cells from the basal side through passive mechanisms (Figure 5.2). Endocytotic vesicles will either deliver the proteins to the Golgi complex for packaging into the same secretory vesicles that deliver lactose and water to the lumen or will move across to the apical side of the cell and discharge the proteins through exocytosis. Proteins that are synthesized de novo within the alveolar cells are transported to the Golgi complex for post-translational modification and secretion. Casein (of which there are α_{s1}, α_{s2}, β and κ forms), for example, is combined with calcium and phosphate to form a complex micelle structure (Figure 5.3). Hydrophobic α and β caseins form the core of these spherical structures with hydrophilic κ casein on the external surface (Phadungath, 2005). These casein micelles not only give milk many of its physical characteristics, for example, the white colour, but also have an important biological function. Micelles carry large amounts of highly insoluble calcium phosphate in a liquid form. They then form a clot in the neonatal stomach, which increases the efficiency of absorption of these minerals. Micelles also deliver citrate, electrolytes and digestive enzymes such as lipase.

5.2.3 Endocrine control of lactation

Once established, lactation is under the control of a cascade of hormones of hypothalamic and pituitary origin. However, the actions of sex steroids produced during pregnancy and endocrine factors produced from the

placenta are also critical in stimulating the maturation of the breast tissue and ensuring that milk production does not occur until after the birth of the infant.

5.2.3.1 The breast during pregnancy

The mammary glands are extremely sensitive to the actions of the sex steroids, oestrogen and progesterone. The development of the breast is primarily driven by these hormones and occurs in a number of distinct stages. The early stages occur during puberty in direct response to the rising concentrations of oestrogen and progesterone that occur at this time. The actions of these hormones produce the structures shown in Figure 5.1. However, the full functional differentiation of the breast tissue does not occur until pregnancy. With the establishment of pregnancy, the breast undergoes extensive changes that are an essential preparation for feeding the baby after delivery. Oestrogen acts, along with growth hormone, to stimulate elongation of the lactiferous ducts. Progesterone and prolactin trigger alveologenesis where, essentially, new ducts are formed branching off from the ducts formed during pubertal breast development and a new alveolar tissue is laid down around these ducts. While oestrogen and progesterone will be produced from the placenta, prolactin is a product of the anterior pituitary.

The main function of prolactin is to stimulate secretion of milk, but during pregnancy, the high circulating concentrations of progesterone and oestrogen inhibit this process. However, prolactin and the placentally derived human chorionic somatomammotropin are still able to act on alveolar cells to stimulate the maturation of the enzyme systems that will be required for milk production. Genes that encode human milk proteins have been shown to be expressed from mid-gestation, and this expression is under the control of prolactin.

5.2.3.2 Established lactation

After delivery of the baby, concentrations of progesterone and oestrogen fall rapidly, and inhibition of the effect of prolactin on alveolar cells is lifted. Lactation is now principally governed by prolactin and the posterior pituitary hormone oxytocin. These are produced in a coordinated manner that ensures that milk synthesis and release are coupled together (Figure 5.4).

The suckling of the baby provides stimulation to the mechanoreceptors that are located in the nipple. This sends nerve signals to the hypothalamus, which then coordinates the response. The hypothalamus releases prolactin-releasing hormone (PRH), which stimulates secretion of prolactin. Prolactin acts on the alveolar epithelial cells of the breast, and milk is released into the alveolar lumen. Simultaneously, the synthesis of more milk is activated. Secretion of oxytocin by the posterior pituitary is stimulated by nerve impulses from the hypothalamus. Oxytocin acts on the myoepithelial cells surrounding the alveolar lumen, and contractions move milk into the ducts, where further contractions forcibly eject the milk from the nipple (Figure 5.4). The ejection of milk should, in a correctly latched on baby, lead to the transfer of milk directly to the throat of the baby. As a result, the baby does not need to suck, but simply stimulate the nipple through action of its gums. This suckling 'technique' is markedly different from that required by a bottle-fed baby, which has to suck the teat to access the milk.

The coordinated secretion of prolactin and oxytocin is called the letdown reflex. In new mothers, letdown will be triggered solely by the mechanical stimulation of the nipples, but in women who have a well-established lactation or who have previously breastfed a baby, letdown can be triggered by other cues such as the sound of their baby crying. The coupling of milk synthesis and release means that lactation is a demand-led process. Essentially, the more a baby suckles at the breast, the greater the stimulation of prolactin secretion and the more milk will be produced. This important principle lies at the heart of the advice to breastfeeding women to do so on demand. While bottle-fed babies are usually fed to a strict (usually four hourly) schedule, breastfed babies need to control the feeding schedule to ensure that the supply is sufficient to meet their requirements.

In the very early stages of lactation, the baby will receive only small amounts of colostrum, which will not satisfy hunger. As a result, the baby may suckle 12–18 times in a 24-h period. This gruelling period for the new mother serves to establish a good supply of milk once inhibition of prolactin effects is lifted. Within a few weeks, a more predictable pattern of feeding (6–10 feeds per day) will develop, and the breasts will produce sufficient milk to satiate the baby, which in the process develops the capacity to regulate its own food intake. During phases of more rapid growth, the baby will suckle more to obtain the extra energy and nutrients required, and the stimulus to the breasts will increase milk production accordingly.

5.2.3.3 The breast after weaning

Once lactation is ended, the stimulation of mammary tissue by prolactin comes to an end. Remarkably, the remodelling of the breast tissue that occurred during

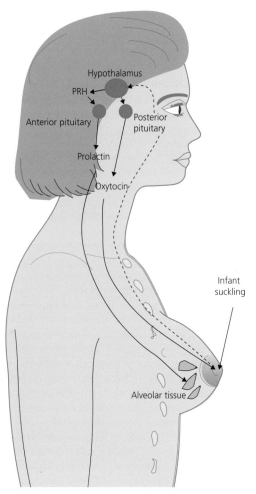

Figure 5.4 The neuroendocrine control of lactation. Milk letdown is stimulated by activation of mechanoreceptors in the nipple. The hypothalamus coordinates the response to stimulation, involving oxytocin and prolactin, thereby ensuring that milk synthesis and release occur simultaneously.

pregnancy is then largely reversed, as the milk production apparatus is essentially dismantled and reconstructed for any subsequent pregnancies. This process, termed involution, involves apoptosis of the epithelial cells of the mammary alveoli and recruitment of inflammatory cells to the breast tissue. Most of the new ducts and alveolar tissue are removed in this process, and the breasts enter a resting phase. Only the myoepithelial cells of the ducts and some secretory cells are retained, with the bulk of the alveolar tissue laid down in pregnancy replaced by fibrous tissue. At the end of reproductive life, complete involution occurs and the breast structure returns to the virgin-like state.

During involution, the composition of human milk undergoes a change (Table 5.1). If weaning is gradual rather than abrupt, then this will impact upon the delivery of nutrients to the infant. Involutional milk is lower in lactose content but is richer in protein, fat and sodium. The composition changes occur because retention of unused milk in the breast forces apart tight cell junctions, allowing flow of extracellular fluids containing non-milk proteins and electrolytes into the ducts.

5.2.4 Maintenance of lactation

The demand-led nature of lactation means that it can be maintained for as long as the baby is suckled. In most Westernized countries, breastfeeding beyond 9–12 months is an unusual behaviour, but in many other societies, prolonged breastfeeding (sometimes up to 3 years) is relatively commonplace. In such circumstances, the demand-led nature of the process means that women can maintain production of around 500 ml milk per day. Similarly, women who are feeding twins will produce twice as much milk as women feeding a singleton baby, as milk production matches demand. Lactation will come to an end only when the stimulus of suckling is withdrawn for 7–14 days. This results in a cessation of prolactin secretion and subsequently the cessation of milk production and breast involution.

Lactation is remarkably robust and even malnourished women appear able to maintain successful breastfeeding. Prentice *et al.* (1994) noted that extreme malnutrition (famine or near-famine conditions) is the only state in which milk production will be significantly impaired. There is no detectable relationship between the body mass index (BMI) of the mother and the volume or composition of the milk she produces. Very thin women (BMI< 18.5) appear capable of maintaining normal lactational performance.

There are circumstances where it may be necessary to temporarily avoid suckling the baby but maintain the lactation. Such a situation may arise if the woman requires a short period of medical treatment with drugs

that are excreted into breast milk. This can be achieved through artificial withdrawal of milk from the breast using a breast pump. This process is termed expressing. In circumstances where the milk may be a hazard to the infant, an artificial formula can be used and the expressed breast milk discarded until safe to resume feeding. In circumstances where the baby is unable to feed, for example, due to prematurity, ill health or surgery, expressed milk can be safely stored and given from a bottle or mixed with solids at a later date.

5.2.5 Nutritional demands of lactation

Lactation is a highly demanding state for the mother, and there are undoubted increases in requirements for a broad range of nutrients while breastfeeding continues. However, with the exception of protein and energy, the exact nature of the altered requirements is generally poorly understood, and it is difficult to conclude whether lactating women need to make significant changes to the quality of their diet. Table 5.2 shows the increments for lactation that are added to UK reference nutrient intakes. For many nutrients, these levels of intake are likely to be met within the normal diets of women in Westernized countries.

The micronutrient composition of human milk is relatively constant. Studies of women in developing countries where micronutrient deficiencies are relatively common show that milk composition is most affected by maternal deficiencies of the water-soluble vitamins, thiamin, riboflavin, vitamin C, vitamin B6 and vitamin B12. Marginal maternal deficiency of these factors will limit milk concentrations, and supplementation restores milk vitamin

Table 5.2 UK reference nutrient intakes (RNI) for lactating women.

Nutrient	UK RNI for lactation*	Estimated intake for UK women[†]
	(Lactation increment)	Mean (standard deviation)
Protein (g/day)	45.0 (+11)	63.7 (16.6)
Riboflavin (mg/day)	1.11 (+0.5)	1.6 (0.6)
Vitamin B12 (µg/day)	1.5 (+0.5)	4.8 (2.7)
Folate	200 (+60)	251 (90)
Vitamin C (mg/day)	40 (+30)	109 (63–160)
Vitamin A (µg/day)	600 (+350)	671 (633)
Calcium (mg/day)	800 (+550)	777 (268)
Magnesium (mg/day)	270 (+50)	229 (70)
Zinc (mg/day)	7.0 (+6.0)	7.4 (2.1)
Copper (mg/day)	1.2 (+0.3)	1.03 (0.38)

Sources: Department of Health (1991), Henderson *et al.* (2002).
*For the first 4–6 months of lactation.
[†]Non-pregnant, non-lactating women.

content. The fat-soluble vitamins are less influential on milk composition, although maternal vitamin A status is to some extent reflected in milk. With respect to folic acid and all of the minerals, very severe maternal deficiency has to occur before any appreciable decline in milk concentrations is observed. This protection of milk composition against variation in maternal intake is achieved through mobilization of maternal reserves. For example, if intakes are less than optimal, calcium will be released from the skeleton in order to maintain milk calcium concentrations. Dijkhuizen and colleagues (2001) studied mother–infant pairs in Java and found that the micronutrient deficiencies (vitamin A deficiency, iron deficiency anaemia) observed in the mothers tended also to occur in their children. However, this was not well explained by the micronutrient composition of breast milk. Only 13% of variation in milk retinol and 24% of variation in milk β-carotene were explained by variation in maternal plasma concentrations. Compromised accumulation of infant reserves during fetal development or use of weaning diets low in these nutrients would be a greater risk factor for infant deficiency.

The energy requirements for lactation are extremely high, and over the first 6 months of lactation, a woman will need to mobilize approximately 115 000 kcal (481 MJ) for milk production. These figures are calculated on the basis that human milk has an energy content of around 0.67 kcal/g, that the conversion of maternal energy to milk energy is around 80% and that women will secrete around 750 ml milk per day. Thus, the energy cost of lactation is around 640 kcal (2.7 MJ) per day in the first 6 months of lactation, declining to around 510 kcal (2.1 MJ) per day beyond 6 months.

Most of the extra energy requirement will need to be derived from increasing energy intake within the maternal diet. Although some studies have suggested that there are metabolic adaptations to conserve energy, the balance of opinion is that resting metabolic rate and thermogenesis do not change in lactation. Physical activity levels tend to be lower in women in the first 4–6 weeks after childbirth, but energy savings achieved through a sedentary lifestyle are unlikely to have much impact on availability of energy for lactation. Most women will lose around 2 kg body weight per month during lactation, and this provides around 150 kcal/day for milk production. It is suggested therefore that women require approximately 500 kcal (2.1 MJ) per day extra within the diet to meet requirements during lactation.

The protein content of milk varies with the stage of lactation (colostrum contains 30 g protein/l, while mature milk is 8–9 g/l). It is estimated that women require an extra 11 g protein/day over the first 6-month lactation, falling to 8 g/day for more prolonged breastfeeding in order to meet this demand. In developed countries, most women consume protein well in excess of this requirement and would not need to alter diet during lactation (Table 5.2). Studies of animals suggest that the protein content of the maternal diet has an influence upon the quantity and quality of milk produced, but it is not clear whether this is also true of humans. Generally, a higher protein intake is believed to increase milk volume, but variation in protein intake within normal ranges does not appear to alter milk composition. Some studies have shown that short-term reductions in maternal protein intake decrease milk protein and non-protein nitrogen content, but it is unclear whether longer-term reductions in protein intake have the same effect.

5.3 The advantages of breastfeeding

5.3.1 Advantages for the mother

Breastfeeding an infant carries a number of advantages for the mother, which encompass both the ease of child-rearing and her short- and long-term health (Table 5.3). The most obvious advantage is the convenience of being able to feed the baby on demand, at any time and in any place without the need for special preparation. Moreover, breastfeeding costs nothing, in contrast to bottle-feeding that carries the cost of bottles, teats, sterilizing equipment and of course the infant formula itself. A typical infant milk formula in the United Kingdom is likely to cost a family £6 (US$10) per week, which for a lower-income family is a significant investment. Milk voucher schemes

Table 5.3 The health benefits of breastfeeding for women and their babies.

Women
Promotes uterine recovery
Reduced risk of post-partum haemorrhage
Delayed menstruation promotes recovery of iron stores
Delayed menstruation may be contraceptive
Reduced anxiety and better emotional bond with baby
Lower risk of breast cancer
Lower risk of endometrial and ovarian cancer
Improved bone mass and reduced risk of osteoporosis
Babies
Priming of the immune system and reduced infection risk
Lower risk of sudden infant death syndrome
Less constipation and improved gastrointestinal function
Reduced risk of childhood leukaemia
Lower risk of type 1 diabetes
Better IQ, developmental scores and behavioural traits in childhood
Lower risk of childhood obesity
Reduced atopy in children with a family history of allergy

exist to assist with this cost in some countries but are often unclaimed by parents.

Breastfeeding helps to develop the emotional bond between the mother and baby. The act of feeding involves close physical contact and eye contact (termed mutual gazing), which is suggested to increase the quality of the mother–child relationship. Oxytocin secretion associated with the letdown reflex has the effect of reducing anxiety through increasing activity of the parasympathetic nervous system. This helps the mother to develop the emotional bond with her child and promotes her sensitivity to the needs of the infant.

Breastfeeding aids the maternal recovery from pregnancy in a number of ways. Primarily, the early initiation of feeding promotes the involution of the uterus and reduces the risk that the mother will suffer a post-partum haemorrhage, as the uterus is a target for actions of oxytocin. Endocrine factors that control lactation also delay the onset of reproductive cycling, and this means that women who breastfeed will have a longer delay before resumption of their normal periods. Suckling inhibits the production of follicle-stimulating hormone and luteinizing hormone from the anterior pituitary. This lactational amenorrhoea confers two benefits. Firstly, reduced blood losses help to preserve iron stores and hence lead to a more rapid recovery of normal iron status after pregnancy. Secondly, lactational amenorrhoea acts as a natural form of contraception. In populations where other forms of contraception are not readily available, this approach (which is estimated to be 90% effective in women fully breastfeeding for 6 months) helps to space out pregnancies. This has a number of benefits for maternal health, allowing full recovery between successive pregnancies, and in turn reduces the likelihood of children being of low birth weight and hence at greater risk of neonatal mortality.

Pregnancy is associated with extensive deposition of fat reserves that are primarily intended for mobilization during lactation to meet the energy requirements of milk production. It has been widely assumed therefore that breastfeeding will promote a more rapid loss of weight gained during pregnancy because of the high energy expenditure associated with lactation. The evidence suggests that the influence of breastfeeding is actually very slight. Martin and colleagues (2012) found that maternal weight at 12 months post-partum was not related to infant feeding methods with slightly more weight retention among women who had exclusively breastfed for 3 months. In contrast, Janney *et al.* (1997) found that breastfeeding women achieved their pre-pregnancy weight on average 6 months faster than women who had not breastfed. Where greater weight loss is noted in breastfeeding women compared to formula-feeding women, the effect is generally confined to those with a healthy BMI (Lovelady, 2011). The interpretation of data around breastfeeding and maternal weight retention is complicated by the fact that obese women are a population subgroup who either choose not to breastfeed or have difficulties with establishing and maintaining lactation (Lepe *et al.*, 2011). The findings of an extensive systematic review of the literature (Ip *et al.*, 2007) indicated that breastfeeding had negligible impact on return to pre-pregnancy weight and no clear benefits for post-partum weight loss.

Evidence is emerging to suggest that risk of cancer is lower in women who breastfeed their infants. Danforth and colleagues (2007) carried out an analysis of the two US Nurses' Health Studies, which included approximately 150 000 women who had children. Risk of ovarian cancer in these women was reduced by 14% (not statistically significant) when comparing 'ever breastfed' with 'never breastfed' groups. However, risk of ovarian cancer was shown to decrease by 2% for every month of breastfeeding and was 34% lower in women who had breastfed their children for more than 18 months. A meta-analysis of studies considering the relationship between breastfeeding and epithelial ovarian cancer reported a 24% reduction in risk when comparing women who had at least initiated breastfeeding with those who had not. Longer-duration breastfeeding carried additional benefits, with an 8% reduction in cancer risk with every 5 months of lactation (Ip *et al.*, 2007).

Risk of breast cancer is significantly reduced simply by having a child. As childbearing and breastfeeding are closely related activities, it can be difficult to independently evaluate the extent to which breastfeeding impacts upon cancer risk. The Collaborative Group on Hormonal Factors in Breast Cancer (2002) examined data from 47 epidemiological studies encompassing 50 302 women with breast cancer and 96 973 controls across 30 different countries. The data confirmed the protective effect of childbearing and showed that having a larger family (three or more children) was most protective. Risk of breast cancer was reduced by 7% for every birth. On top of this, each year of breastfeeding reduced risk by 4.3%. The systematic review of Anothaisintawee and colleagues (2013) found that breastfeeding for any period of time was associated with a 30% reduction of breast cancer risk. The mechanisms by which this reduction in risk occurs are yet to be identified, but it is likely that the major contributors are a reduced number of menstrual cycles and the differentiation of breast tissue that occurs with pregnancy and lactation. It has also been suggested that alpha-lactalbumin in milk may have local anti-tumour effects.

The benefits of breastfeeding for breast cancer appear small, but applying these data to breastfeeding prevalence and duration rates in developed countries suggests that a high proportion of the difference in breast cancer prevalence between developed and developing countries might be explained by infant feeding practices. For example, in Germany where only 10% of women breastfeed their infants to 6 months of age, breast cancer prevalence rates are 1030 cases per 100000 population compared to around 75 per 100000 population in most African countries, where long-duration breastfeeding is commonplace. The Collaborative Group on Hormonal Factors in Breast Cancer study (2002) suggested that if children in developed countries were breastfed for 6 months longer than at present, 5% of breast cancers (25000 cases) would be prevented.

A number of studies have evaluated the impact of lactation upon maternal bone health. Milk production places heavy demands for calcium, and it is estimated that 200–225 mg calcium/day is transferred from mother to infant via breast milk. Over a period of 6-month lactation, this equates to an additional calcium requirement of between 35 and 40 g. Bone is a dynamic tissue and acts as a reserve for calcium that can be readily released in order to support the lactation. This results in changes in the level of bone mineral present within the maternal skeleton. This can be measured using the technique of dual x-ray absorptiometry, which determines the amount of bone mineral present per unit area of skeleton (bone mineral density, BMD). Typically, lactation for a period of 6 months results in loss of around 4–6% of BMD, with most losses coming from the spine and hip (Karlsson *et al.*, 2005). This loss of bone mineral occurs despite the fact that most lactating women reduce their intakes of alcohol and caffeine, which are known to exert negative influences on BMD. It is probably driven by low levels of oestrogen, resulting from suppression of the hypothalamic–pituitary–ovarian axis.

With these negative influences of lactation upon the skeleton, it is clearly important to evaluate whether breastfeeding is associated with long-term risk of osteoporosis, a disease associated with increased risk of bone fracture in the elderly. As with cancer, it is difficult to dissociate the influences of breastfeeding and childbearing upon osteoporosis risk. It is clear though that in women who have had children, BMD is typically 3–5% *higher* than in women who have never had children. Ip and colleagues, however, concluded from a review of six case–control and four long-term prospective cohort studies that breastfeeding was not associated with osteoporosis. Unlike cancer, prolonged (more than 12 months) lactation, particularly in younger women, may be associated with lower BMD post-menopause and greater risk of osteoporosis (Okyay *et al.*, 2013).

The lack of evidence of increased osteoporosis risk associated with lactation in most women is explained by the fact that BMD is fully recovered once the infant is weaned

and lactation ends. Most studies show that all bone mineral lost during lactation is replaced within 12–18 months of giving birth. A number of adaptive mechanisms appear to conserve calcium and promote remineralization, of which the most important is an increase in the capacity to absorb calcium from the diet. Bioavailability of calcium, that is, the proportion of dietary intake that is taken up across the gut, in non-lactating women is approximately 25–30%. This increases with lactation to between 32 and 52% but to an extent that reflects habitual intake. In a study of well-nourished US women, using radioisotope tracers, Ritchie and colleagues (1998) showed that early lactation was not associated with a significant increase in calcium absorption, but that renal losses of calcium were reduced to around half of pre-pregnancy levels. This renal conservation was maintained at 5 months past the resumption of reproductive cycling.

5.3.2 Advantages for the infant

As described earlier in this chapter, the composition of human milk changes with the stage of infant development, across the day and across the course of a feed. These compositional changes and the robust nature of milk production, which ensures nutrient content is maintained even by relatively poorly nourished mothers, guarantee that the nutrient availability for the infant is optimal. This aspect of breastfeeding can clearly be viewed from a teleological perspective, as ensuring that there are health advantages for the infant in the short term. Similarly, from what is known about early life influences on long-term health and well-being (Chapter 4), it is reasonable to propose that breastfeeding will confer lifelong benefits.

In the short term, one of the most important advantages for the infant is derived from the immunoprotective factors that are present in milk and that are indirectly associated with the process of breastfeeding (Table 5.3). Among the developing countries in particular where hygiene and sanitation standards may be poor, the major hazards to infants are diarrhoeal infections and infections of the respiratory tract. Breastfeeding provides clear protection against both. Arifeen and colleagues (2001) reported on the prevalence of infection-related deaths in the slums of Dhaka, Bangladesh. In this population, 11% of infants died within the first 12 months of life, and 45% of these deaths were attributable to either acute respiratory infection or diarrhoea. Infants who were not breastfed or who were partially breastfed were 2.40 times more likely to die of respiratory infection than those breastfed and were 3.94 times more likely to die from diarrhoeal infections.

A large proportion of this protective effect can be attributed to the presence of immunoglobulins, lactoferrin, B lymphocytes, complement proteins and macrophages in human milk. These factors provide the capacity to actively combat infection and also bind out substrates that may be beneficial for bacterial growth. Breastfeeding is also protective against gastrointestinal infection as provision of human milk ensures that fluids consumed by the infant are clean and free of contaminating factors. Poor sterilization of bottle-feeding equipment, or the use of infected water supplies for formula preparation, is an avoidable cause of infection.

The term sudden infant death syndrome (SIDS) describes the sudden unexplained death of an infant under 1 year of age. Risk of SIDS is increased by parental smoking and alcohol use and by placing infants to sleep on their stomachs. Some studies have suggested that SIDS is more prevalent in formula-fed infants than breastfed infants. Alm and colleagues (2002) examined 244 cases of SIDS from Scandinavia. After careful adjustment for potential confounding factors, it was found that short-duration breastfeeding (<4 weeks) increased risk of SIDS by 5.1-fold, compared to breastfeeding for longer than 15 weeks. Similarly, Ford et al. (1993) reported that risk of SIDS was almost doubled in non-breastfed infants compared to those breastfed. A meta-analysis by Ip et al. (2007) concluded that breastfeeding reduced SIDS risk by 36%. Hauck and colleagues later confirmed the benefits of breastfeeding, with their analysis showing that any breastfeeding and exclusive breastfeeding for up to 2 months reduced SIDS risk by 62 and 73%, respectively. The possible explanation for the reduction in risk associated with breastfeeding could be a reduction in the occurrence of respiratory infections.

Advocacy of breastfeeding to reduce risk of SIDS creates an ethical dilemma. Risk of SIDS is increased by the practice of bed sharing (in which the baby sleeps with the parents). As bed sharing facilitates the establishment of breastfeeding, parents are faced with potentially contradictory advice about infant feeding and sleeping arrangements. There is some concern that parents may receive mixed messages relating to SIDS that will ultimately discourage breastfeeding.

The last trimester of pregnancy and the first 2 years of life are the most rapid stage of brain development in humans. The brain increases in size from around 350g at birth to 1100g at 12 months of age. This rapid growth makes the brain vulnerable to adverse environments during this time, including undernutrition. Grantham-McGregor and colleagues (1991) showed in a group of stunted Jamaican infants that a combination of nutritional supplements and stimulation through play increased developmental scores. This, like most other studies of this kind, indicated that the main effects of nutrition upon brain development were on the development of locomotor abilities. This is in keeping with the idea that rather than overall brain growth being

vulnerable to undernutrition, it is specific brain functions that may suffer if nutrition is less than optimal.

There are a number of studies that have demonstrated that the manner of infant feeding can impact upon the cognitive development of infants. Some of the best documented are those of Lucas and Morley who have considered several cohorts of preterm or low-birth-weight infants. These have shown that in low-birth-weight infants, feeding of the mothers own milk via an enteral tube produced an eight-point difference in the Bayley score compared to feeding of an infant formula. The Bayley score measures the mental and motor development of infants, and the observed differences persisted until at least 7.5–8 years of age (Morley et al., 1988).

Several studies have suggested that breastfeeding has a positive effect on the development of intelligence. However, the literature in this area is very variable in terms of the conclusions that can be drawn and is invariably confounded by the fact that it is generally considered neither ethical nor feasible to perform a randomized controlled trial of breastfeeding compared to formula feeding (although Kramer and colleagues performed this intervention in Belarus). As a result, maternal characteristics and environment will have a strong bearing on any studies that attempt to relate measures of childhood intelligence (intelligence quotient (IQ)) to infant feeding methods. Jain and colleagues (2002) performed a systematic review of the literature and found that most studies conclude that breastfeeding does improve later IQ scores. Few studies have specifically studied full-term rather than preterm infants, and higher-quality studies suggest no clear effect. Smithers et al.'s (2012) study of the Avon Longitudinal Study of Parents and Children (ALSPAC) cohort reported that there was a two-point higher IQ in 8-year-olds who had still been breastfed at 6 months of age and who were weaned onto home-made rather than ready-prepared foods. This finding of a very minor influence of breastfeeding bears out the conclusions of Eriksen and colleagues (2013) who reported that in the Danish Birth Cohort, the IQ of 5-year-olds were largely explained by maternal IQ and parental education, with breastfeeding having an effect of limited magnitude. A systematic review of 84 studies found that most of the reported relationship between breastfeeding and IQ is explained by confounding factors (Walfisch et al., 2013). Only a study designed to compare siblings who differ in their infant feeding experience would be able to resolve whether breastfeeding really improves cognitive development.

It is argued that many of the observed differences in behavioural and developmental outcomes noted between infants fed human milk and formula milk are explained by the provision of particular fatty acids. In terms of composition, the brain is around 60% lipid, and in particular, it is rich in long-chain polyunsaturated fatty acids (PUFA), arachidonic acid and DHA. Both become concentrated in the cell membranes of non-myelinated cells of the brain and in the retina and accumulate during the rapid phase of brain growth. DHA has been shown to be critical for the normal development of a number of visual and mental functions (Carlson *et al.*, 1994). Extrapolation from animal studies suggests that over the first 6 months of life, infants accumulate high quantities of DHA of which approximately 50% will be incorporated into the brain (Cunnane *et al.*, 2000).

DHA is not widely found in the diet and is chiefly derived from fish oils. It can be synthesized from α-linolenic acid via a series of desaturase- and elongase-catalysed reactions, but it is generally considered that this pathway cannot support the high demand of the infant brain for this fatty acid. Thus, the delivery of DHA in a pre-synthesized form in breast milk may represent a significant advantage during the brain growth spurt. The DHA content of human milk varies considerably and generally reflects the maternal diet. Studies have shown that supplementation of women with fish oils can boost DHA excretion in their milk. Typically, DHA constitutes between 0.3 and 0.4% of the fatty acids present in human milk. In the past, infant formula used in bottle-feeding contained negligible amounts of DHA, but many formula manufacturers now include long-chain fatty acids derived from egg, and these milks contain DHA at a level around 0.2% of total fatty acids. A number of international expert groups have published recommendations for optimal levels of DHA and arachidonic acid supplementation in term infant formula. Recommendations of 0.2–0.4% fatty acids for DHA and between 0.35 and 0.7% fatty acids for arachidonic acid are based on the median worldwide range of concentrations of these fatty acids in breast milk. A randomized controlled trial of long-chain PUFA-enriched formulas (0.64% fatty acids as arachidonic acid and up to 0.96% fatty acids as DHA) against standard formula found that at age 5–6 years children performed better in tests of intelligence, vocabulary and rule learning, but not advanced problem-solving or spatial memory (Colombo *et al.*, 2013).

Research Highlight 5.1 Breastfeeding and the risk of childhood obesity.

It was first suggested that breastfeeding might provide protection against the development of later obesity in the early 1980s. However, definitive exploration of this hypothesis was problematic due to inconsistencies in the methods used for breastfeeding data collection, definitions of breastfeeding and confounding factors that inevitably arise in such research. For example, women who are better educated and wealthier are more likely to breastfeed their infants and are more likely to have children that consume a healthy diet and exercise, hence avoiding obesity.

Systematic reviews and meta-analysis

Arenz and colleagues (2004) performed a systematic review of the literature published between 1966 and 2003 to address the possible association between breastfeeding and childhood obesity. The meta-analysis associated with this review incorporated data from 9 studies including 69 000 participants, aged from 3 to 26 years. Breastfeeding was found to significantly reduce the risk of childhood obesity with an adjusted odds ratio (OR) of 0.78 (95% confidence intervals 0.71–0.85). In four of the nine studies, duration of breastfeeding was shown to be an important factor. Von Kries *et al.* (1999) reported that while 4.5% of 6-year-olds who were never breastfed were obese, only 3.8% of those breastfed for 3–5 months and 0.8% of those breastfed for 12 months were obese. Similar findings emerged from the systematic review of Weng *et al.* (2012), who found that the risk of childhood overweight was lower in breastfed compared to non-breastfed individuals (OR 0.85 (0.75–0.99)). A systematic review, which included unpublished 'grey literature', by Owen and colleagues (2005) found that although being breastfed was associated with lower BMI in childhood, adolescence and adult life, the effect was marginal and likely to be a result of inadequate adjustment for confounding factors and publication bias. There is clearly a need for well-designed, robust studies to firmly resolve this issue.

Protective mechanism

A number of putative mechanisms have been suggested to explain a potential protective effect of breastfeeding:

- Bottle-feeding leads to an earlier adiposity rebound (see Chapter 6). BMI in children normally increases rapidly in the first year of life and then declines reaching a minimum point around age 5–6, before rising again. The point of minimum BMI (maximum leanness) is termed the adiposity rebound point. Early adiposity rebound is predictive of obesity later in life.
- Breastfeeding is demand led and the infant controls energy intake. With bottle-feeding, loss of infant control over intake causes the normal hypothalamic regulators of appetite to develop in a way that favours excess intake in the longer term.
- Bottle-fed infants have higher plasma insulin concentrations than breastfed infants. This favours early deposition of fat and an increase in fat cell number.
- Human milk contains bioactive factors that maintain a pattern of growth that favours a leaner body mass.
- The lower ratio of n-3 to n-6 fatty acids in formula milk compared to human milk promotes adipose tissue development.

Some controversy surrounds claims that breastfeeding is protective against the development of obesity in childhood (Research Highlight 5.1). The rising prevalence of overweight and obesity among children across the globe has prompted interest in the possible contribution of early life nutrition to this problem. In many developed countries, the beginning of an upward trend in childhood overweight coincided with widespread rejection of breastfeeding. Although difficult to demonstrate in single studies, large-scale analyses of available data sets indicate that the risk of obesity in childhood is reduced by around 22% by breastfeeding compared to bottle-feeding with an infant formula. This area of research highlights the need for collection of robust exposure data (breastfeeding is socially desirable and so may be inaccurately reported by mothers) and adjustment for all possible confounding factors in epidemiological studies.

It has been suggested that breastfeeding may have an influence on the development of allergies in children, which will most commonly manifest as either atopic dermatitis (allergic eczema) or asthma. The main reasoning here is that formula feeding generally involves exposure of the infant to cow's milk proteins at an early stage of development. Allergies to cow's milk proteins are among the most common food allergies noted in children, but while using modified hydrolysed formulas (Section 5.6.4) reduces risk of allergy to cow's milk protein compared to standard formulas in high-risk infants, there is no robust evidence that breastfeeding is protective (de Silva *et al.*, 2014). Clearly, breastfeeding prevents this early exposure and sensitization but could also be beneficial since human milk provides passive immunity and promotes the development of the infant immune system. However, it is also clear that proteins and peptides can cross from the maternal circulation into milk, and so some argue that breastfeeding could increase risk of allergic sensitization by exposing the infant to allergens consumed by the mother. Some groups have argued that women who show allergic tendencies themselves should restrict intakes of dairy products, nuts and other common food allergens while breastfeeding to lower risk in their children, but the evidence base suggests that this is not necessary or effective (de Silva *et al.*, 2014). A growing literature is also suggesting that early and frequent exposure to small amounts of antigens may be beneficial in preventing food allergies.

Atopy, a tendency to develop allergies, is strongly associated with genetic components, and the impact of breastfeeding on risk of atopic dermatitis varies between children that have a family history of atopy and those that do not. In children with no atopic heredity, there is no clear evidence that breastfeeding has either a beneficial or detrimental effect on risk of atopic dermatitis. However, Kramer and colleagues (2001), who are to date the only group to carry out a randomized controlled trial of breastfeeding versus formula feeding, reported a 46% decrease in risk of atopic dermatitis when children were exclusively breastfed for 3 months. In children with a family history of atopy, the benefits of breastfeeding are clear, with significant reductions in childhood eczema associated with breastfeeding for up to 4 months. Kerkhof *et al.* (2003) reported that in the children of women with a history of allergic asthma, breastfeeding for 13 weeks or more reduced prevalence of atopic dermatitis by 40%. However, the current balance of opinion is that most reported benefits of breastfeeding in atopy are explained by confounding factors (Matheson *et al.*, 2012). The development of allergies is, for example, strongly related to respiratory infections in infancy. It is well established that breastfeeding reduces the prevalence of such infections.

5.3.3 Recommendation to feed to 6 months

In 1990, participants at a World Health Organization (WHO)/UNICEF policymakers' meeting on breastfeeding produced the Innocenti Declaration. This was in recognition of the fact that breastfeeding provides optimal infant nutrition and carries significant benefits for the health of infants and their mothers. The declaration set out a number of global goals and operational targets. The central aims were as follows:

- To ensure optimal maternal and child health, all women should be enabled to practise exclusive breastfeeding for 4–6 months.
- To reinforce a breastfeeding culture and defend this against development of a bottle-feeding culture.
- To increase confidence of women in their ability to breastfeed.
- To ensure that women are adequately nourished.

The declaration called upon all governments to take effective steps to centrally coordinate breastfeeding promotion and enact legislation to protect the rights of women to breastfeed. International organizations were called upon to develop action plans to promote and support breastfeeding and to support national governments in delivering breastfeeding policies.

The main outcome of the Innocenti Declaration was the establishment of a global policy for the promotion of breastfeeding. At the heart of this is the WHO/UNICEF recommendation that infants should be exclusively breastfed for the first 6 months of life. The benefits of such a policy for infant and maternal health are clear, particularly in the developing countries. The most important advantage is the reduction in the risk of gastrointestinal infection, which is a major killer of infants. Globally, diarrhoeal disease is a cause of up to 2 million deaths among under-5s each year.

Research Highlight 5.2 Is 6-month exclusive breastfeeding appropriate for all infants?.

In 2001, the World Health Organization (WHO) issued the global recommendation that all infants should be exclusively breastfed for 6 months. Not all countries adopted this advice, and while the United Kingdom and Australia are among the developed countries recommending the WHO guidance to mothers, the majority of European countries and the United States have alternative guidance. The WHO recommendations were largely based upon the systematic review of Kramer and Kakuma (2002) which had evaluated the impact of exclusive breastfeeding upon maternal and infant health. This showed clear benefits in terms of infant growth, maternal recovery of iron stores post-partum and most importantly a reduction in infection among infants.

The relevance of the WHO recommendations for developing countries where infectious disease is the driver of high infant mortality is not disputed. For developed countries, however, where the morbidity and mortality associated with infection are controlled through other means, there are important concerns about the appropriateness of the guidance to exclusively breastfeed for 6 months (Fewtrell, 2011). The concerns are:

- The nutritional adequacy of exclusive breastfeeding. Iron deficiency is the major concern as human milk is a poor source of iron, and infants must rely on stores accrued before birth. Chantry *et al.* (2007) reported that among US infants exclusively breastfed for more than 6 months, there was a 10% prevalence of iron deficiency anaemia compared to 2.3% among children exclusively breastfed for 4 months up to 6 months. Iron deficiency anaemia in infants is associated with irreversible deficits in motor, cognitive and social development (Lozoff and Georgieff, 2006; Algarín *et al.*, 2013), and the risk of deficiency must be carefully weighted against the immune benefits of breastfeeding.
- Coeliac disease: There is some evidence that there is an optimal time frame for exposure of the gastrointestinal tract to allergens such as gluten. Olsson *et al.* (2008) reported that in Sweden a change of advice to introduce gluten to infants at 6 months rather than 4 months resulted in an increase in incidence of early-onset coeliac disease.

An update of the Kramer and Kakuma review (2012) concluded that there were no deficits in infant growth associated with 6-month exclusive breastfeeding in either developed or developing countries. Risk of iron deficiency was confined to developing countries where the iron stores accrued by the infant *in utero* may be compromised by poor maternal iron status. Breastfeeding with iron supplementation may be an effective strategy for preventing iron deficiency in infants who are exclusively breastfed. Wells and colleagues (2012) conducted a randomized controlled trial in Iceland where infants were randomized to either 4- or 6-month exclusive breastfeeding. In keeping with the Kramer and Kakuma evidence, the study found no deficits in infant growth, body composition or energy intake associated with longer-duration exclusive breastfeeding.

While any public health nutrition policy will clearly focus on the potential benefits to the population, it is important to also consider potential hazards. Some studies have suggested that exclusive breastfeeding can lead to poor iron status in infants if maternal iron status is suboptimal (a commonplace scenario throughout the developing countries). It is unclear whether the same risk applies to other micronutrients. While the overwhelming benefits of exclusive breastfeeding for 6 months outweigh potential hazards in most developing countries, there are some suggestions that 4–6 months might be a more appropriate guideline in developed countries (Research Highlight 5.2).

5.4 Trends in breastfeeding behaviour

Despite the clear evidence that breastfeeding is the best infant feeding option for the health of both the mother and her infant, the majority of babies in Westernized countries are bottle-fed with artificial formula preparations. The WHO recommends that all babies are *exclusively* breastfed until 6 months of age in order to maximize the benefits for the infant. However, in the United States and most European countries, exclusive breastfeeding is an activity pursued by a very small minority of women, and bottle-feeding or a mixed feeding regime is the norm.

Understanding the literature on breastfeeding trends and breastfeeding in relation to health can often be confusing due to the different terms used to describe and define approaches to infant feeding. Table 5.4 provides an overview of some of these terms. Looking at trends over time or making comparisons between countries is particularly difficult due to variation in these definitions. In general, the rates of breastfeeding have been increasing across the Western world over the last two to three decades, as increasingly women become aware of the positive impact this has on the development of their babies. However, in some countries, the significant increase has come from a very low base, and so breastfeeding rates remain low. In the United States, for example, a mere 25% of babies born in 1970 were *ever breastfed*. By 1994, this had risen to 57.4%, and in 2009, the figure was around 77% with considerable variation related to ethnicity and social class.

In the United Kingdom, increases in the rates of breastfeeding were noted from a low base in the mid-1970s through to the 1980s, taking the overall numbers of babies who were *ever* breastfed to around 65% of the population. Since then, considerable progress has been made in the promotion of breastfeeding, and

Table 5.4 Definitions of breastfeeding behaviour.

Breastfeeding*	Process of feeding baby human milk either directly from the breast or in expressed[†] form
Ever breastfed	Infant has been breastfed on at least one occasion
Exclusive breastfeeding	Infant has only ever been fed with breast milk. No other liquids or solids have been introduced, with the exception of vitamin and mineral supplements
Predominant breastfeeding	Infant has mainly been breastfed but may have consumed water, fruit juices, teas or oral rehydration fluids
Full breastfeeding	Includes both exclusive and predominant breastfeeding behaviour
Bottle-feeding[‡]	Process of feeding baby liquid or semi-solid foods via a bottle with a teat. Generally, this refers to feeding a cow's milk-derived substitute to human milk
Mixed feeding	Process through which an infant is nourished through a combination of breastfeeding and bottle-feeding
Complementary feeding	The infant is nourished through a combination of breastfeeding and solid or semi-solid foods

*Successful breastfeeding is generally baby led. Baby is fed on demand rather than to a timed schedule.

[†]Expressing refers to the technique of manually drawing milk off the breast for administration via a bottle or through mixing with solid foods.

[‡]Bottle-fed babies are generally fed to a timed schedule, for example, a bottle every 4 h.

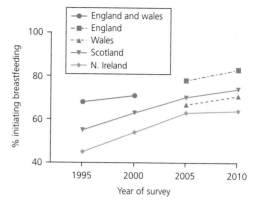

Figure 5.5 Breastfeeding trends in the United Kingdom from 1995 to 2010.

the 2010 Office for National Statistics Infant Feeding Survey (McAndrew *et al.*, 2012) found 81% of British babies were *ever* breastfed (Figure 5.5). Like the United States, Britain sees variation related to ethnicity (over 95% of non-white Caucasian women initiate breastfeeding) and social class (90% of women in managerial and professional occupations breastfeed). As can be seen in Figure 5.5, there is also a tremendous regional variation, and despite large increases in breastfeeding rates in Wales, Scotland and Northern Ireland in recent years, these countries within the United Kingdom lag behind England in terms of uptake of breastfeeding. The relatively low rates of breastfeeding seen in the United Kingdom (bearing in mind that the 81% figure reported previously really only represents the percentage of women who initiate breastfeeding) are atypical of much of Europe, and only France, Belgium, Malta and Ireland have lower initiation of breastfeeding than the United Kingdom. The Scandinavian countries (Denmark, Norway and Sweden), Slovenia and Turkey have the highest rates

of breastfeeding of any of the Westernized countries, achieving close to 100% initiation of breastfeeding (Yngve and Sjöström, 2001).

While trends in the initiation of breastfeeding are encouraging, exclusive breastfeeding for 6 months as recommended by the WHO is considerably less commonplace (Figure 5.6). Exclusive breastfeeding rates are highest in the least developed countries, but even in those regions, around 50% of women opt for other feeding strategies. Exclusive breastfeeding to 6 months is not widely seen in developed countries with 25% of Canadian mothers, 16% of US mothers and just 1% of UK mothers adhering to the WHO recommendation. Even in Scandinavia where initiation is almost universal, exclusive breastfeeding to 6 months is provided to less than 10% of infants.

While across Europe breastfeeding is initiated by between 70 and 98% of women, the dropout rate is very high, and as noted previously, the numbers of infants who are exclusively breastfed to 6 months of age are typically low. Figure 5.7 shows the fall-off in the number of breastfed infants in the United Kingdom (McAndrew *et al.*, 2012). It can be clearly seen that of the women who initiate breastfeeding at birth of their babies, a more than a quarter will give up within the first 4 weeks, with especially high attrition in the first 2 weeks. Two-thirds of mothers will switch to bottle-feeding or mixed feeding within 10 weeks, and only 20% will maintain breastfeeding out to 4–6 months. These trends apply across all European states, and the dropout rate is similar even in Sweden, where breastfeeding is most actively promoted and supported (Yngve and Sjöström, 2001). The observation that large numbers of women initiate breastfeeding but soon switch to bottle-feeding or mixed feeding approaches provides a major clue to the fact that breastfeeding can be very difficult for many women to sustain.

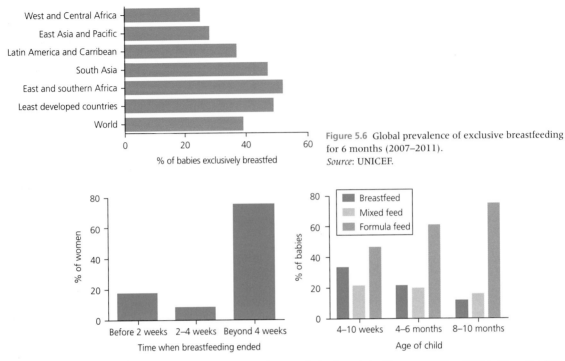

Figure 5.6 Global prevalence of exclusive breastfeeding for 6 months (2007–2011). *Source*: UNICEF.

Figure 5.7 Attrition among breastfeeding women is high in the United Kingdom. A significant proportion (25%) of breastfeeding women give up within the first 4 weeks. By 4–10 weeks after birth, only 33% of babies are solely breastfed. *Source*: McAndrew *et al.* (2012).

5.4.1 Reasons why women do not breastfeed

In considering why bottle-feeding is the preferred infant feeding method for most women in Western countries, we need to consider two sets of factors. The first are the factors that prevent women from initiating breastfeeding in the first place, and the second group of factors are those that lead women to give up breastfeeding at some stage in the first 6 months.

Most of the factors that women cite as important in leading them to choose bottle-feeding in preference to breastfeeding are socially and culturally related. For example, in the United States, the 2005 Women's Health Survey found that Hispanic women were most likely to breastfeed, while non-Hispanic blacks were least likely. In European studies, the women who are least likely to breastfeed are younger mothers, women with low educational attainment and women from a lower-income family. Figure 5.8 shows data from a survey of 300 women from Northampton, United Kingdom, who were surveyed in the final trimester of pregnancy. The data show that among higher social classes, the intention to breastfeed was indicated by a number of women that were well above the national average, while only 50–60% of single

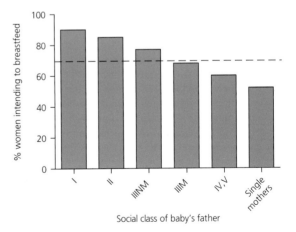

Figure 5.8 Socio-economic factors are a strong determinant of breastfeeding behaviour. Three hundred pregnant women from Northampton, United Kingdom, were interviewed regarding their breastfeeding intentions in the 32nd week of pregnancy (Langley-Evans and Langley-Evans, 2003). The dotted line shows the proportion of women in the United Kingdom who would be expected to breastfeed (Hamlyn *et al.*, 2002). Social class I, professionals; II, clerical workers; IIINM, skilled non-manual workers; IIIM, skilled manual workers; IV, partly skilled workers; V, unskilled workers.

mothers and women of lower socio-economic class indicated that they would breastfeed their babies.

These behaviours almost certainly arise from women's perception of the social acceptability of breastfeeding. Women who choose not to breastfeed may do so because of embarrassment at breastfeeding in public, as in the Western world the breast is perceived as a sexual object. The attitudes of their partners may also shape this viewpoint. Women may also need to return to work early after delivery, and patterns of breastfeeding can easily be seen to reflect the financial support offered by governments to support parents. Countries such as Slovenia and Denmark where up to 1 year of maternal leave at full pay can be taken see initiation of breastfeeding in approximately 97% of mothers. Similarly, in Slovakia and Austria where up to 3-year fully paid leave is available, around 90% of women will breastfeed. Lower uptake of breastfeeding is noted where there are less liberal arrangements. In the United Kingdom, for example, statutory maternity leave is less generous (6 weeks at 90% of full pay, 33 weeks at a lower rate and 13 weeks unpaid), and women of lower socio-economic class, for example, may not be able to afford an extended period of leave after having their babies.

Women who have previously breastfed and had a negative experience are also disinclined to repeat the process. Some women also report that they would like to share feeding of their baby with other family members and thereby spread the burden of childcare. The experience of members of the extended family is of major importance, and women will often take advice from and mirror the behaviours of their mothers. In some cultures, this influence can produce quite extreme feeding practices. In some parts of Canada, including Newfoundland, breastfeeding rates are very low (around 40% initiate breastfeeding), and there is a tradition of feeding babies evaporated or condensed cow's milk, which is passed on from mothers to daughters and through social networks (Matthews *et al.*, 1998). Although this practice, based on saving money, has been suggested to cause harm to infants due to the high associated protein and solute loads, it remains prevalent among aboriginal groups and low-income families.

It has also been suggested that the media contributes to the negative stereotypes that women may develop in relation to breastfeeding. A US study showed that exposure to print media relating to formula feeding significantly impacted on choice of infant feeding method, with lower likelihood of initiating breastfeeding and breastfeeding for shorter periods (Zhang *et al.*, 2013). Henderson and colleagues (2000) studied UK newspaper, television and radio coverage of infant feeding during the month of March 1999. It was apparent from this study that not only was bottle-feeding more commonly portrayed (82% of all

references to feeding), but it was also presented as simpler and more socially integrated. Breastfeeding tended to be presented as 'problematic, funny, embarrassing, and actively associated with women who were middle class or celebrities'. In contrast, women seeing other women breastfeeding are more likely to initiate breastfeeding themselves, emphasizing the importance of the perception of social acceptability in shaping decision making about infant feeding.

Successful breastfeeding requires a good technique, and problems with establishing this technique and in overcoming the difficulties of the first few days of lactation account for the very high dropout in the first weeks after birth. Latching the baby on to the nipple correctly is something that has to be learned by all women. Incorrect latching-on such that the baby grips solely the nipple, rather than taking the whole of the areola into the mouth, will lead to soreness and in the worst cases blistering and bleeding of the nipple tissue. Even with correct technique and with experience of previous breastfeeding, the early days of feeding are likely to be uncomfortable, and hence, some women will look for alternatives. Breast engorgement may also lead women to give up breastfeeding. After 2–3 days beyond birth, the decline in production of the sex steroids lifts the inhibitory effect upon prolactin stimulus of milk synthesis. The breasts begin to produce mature milk in large quantities due to the high level of stimulation from the baby over the preceding days. The breasts become large, hard and painful, and it can be difficult to continue feeding. As this engorgement generally coincides with an emotional low that is also associated with falling progesterone and oestrogen concentrations, women are liable to give up feeding at this point.

Breast engorgement and sore or bleeding nipples do not preclude maintaining breastfeeding for women who are prepared to work through the difficult early days. With an engorged breast, the solution is to manually express milk to soften the breast tissue sufficiently for the baby to be able to suckle and drain off the engorgement, which will pass within a few days. Sore nipples can be treated with ointments and by exposing to the air between feeds to promote healing.

Other problems that can arise with breastfeeding, at any time, can also be debilitating and discourage further maintenance of feeding. These include infection of the nipple with *Candida albicans* and mastitis. The latter arises either through infection of damaged nipples or due to breast engorgement or blockage of ducts. Mastitis due to infection can produce severe flu-like symptoms and requires treatment with a suitable antibiotic to resolve it. Mastitis due to non-infective causes is generally a consequence of the breast not being fully drained at each feed.

Table 5.5 Ten steps to successful breastfeeding.

Facilities providing maternity services and care for newborn infants should:

1 Have a written breastfeeding policy that is routinely communicated to all healthcare staff
2 Train all healthcare staff in skills necessary to implement this policy
3 Inform all pregnant women about the benefits and management of breastfeeding
4 Help mothers in initiating breastfeeding within half an hour of birth
5 Show mothers how to breastfeed and how to maintain lactation if separated from their infants
6 Give newborn infants no food or drink other than breast milk, unless medically indicated
7 Practise rooming-in. Mothers and infants to remain together at all times
8 Encourage breastfeeding on demand
9 Give no artificial teats or pacifiers to breastfeeding infants
10 Foster the establishment of breastfeeding support groups and refer mothers to them on discharge from the hospital

WHO/UNICEF (1989).

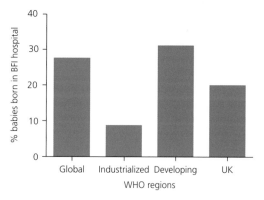

Figure 5.9 Globally, a minority of babies are born in baby-friendly hospitals. Most industrialized nations lag behind developing countries in ensuring the BFI standards.
Source: UNICEF.

This can promote localized infections, and so the breast needs to be manually drained through massage, and relief from symptoms can be gained through cooling with wet towels, ice packs or even cabbage leaves.

While these physical problems account for much of the early drop-off in breastfeeding rates, the decision to stop feeding after the first few weeks is generally because women perceive that they are producing insufficient milk (Colin and Scott, 2002). Due to lactation being a demand-led process, it is highly unlikely that the capacity to produce milk will be genuinely outstripped by infant requirements in the first 4–6 months of life. Agostoni *et al.* (1999) clearly showed that in fact over the first 6 months of life, exclusively breastfed babies grew faster than formula-fed babies. However, many women perceive unsettled behaviour in their children as a sign of hunger and may start to introduce solid foods or formula top-up feeds in addition to breastfeeding or cease breastfeeding completely in response. Stress related to feeding the infant, or the inevitable fatigue associated with a 24-h demand-feeding schedule, can inhibit the letdown reflex and hence interfere with successful lactation.

5.4.2 Promoting breastfeeding

Across Europe, Australasia and North America, there is an active support for the aims of the Innocenti Declaration, and there are a number of organizations and initiatives that aim to promote breastfeeding and provide support for breastfeeding mothers. The most important development on a global scale is the UNICEF Baby-Friendly Hospital Initiative (BFHI). This worldwide programme of the WHO and UNICEF was launched in 1992 to encourage maternity hospitals to implement the 10 steps to successful breastfeeding (Table 5.5) and to practise in accordance with the International Code of Marketing of Breastmilk Substitutes, which seeks to limit the promotion of formula milks to mothers.

The BFHI is coordinated in individual countries by local organizations. The attainment of sufficiently high standards to gain baby-friendly status and the implementation of the BFHI seven-point plan are relatively low across the world and are variable both within and between countries (Figure 5.9). Sweden was an early adopter, and by 1998, all 65 maternity hospitals in the country had full accreditation. In the United Kingdom, 20 years on from the launch of BFHI, accreditation has been given to less than 20% of maternity units, and these are spread unevenly around the country. For example, in Scotland, 81% of babies are born in baby-friendly hospitals, while in other areas in such as southeast England, no hospitals have accredited status. Barriers to uptake of BFHI by hospitals include a lack of willingness and awareness among national and local health authorities and a low perceived value among parents and legislators.

BFHI standards do provide a clear benefit in terms of increasing uptake of advice to breastfeed. Broadfoot and colleagues (2005) considered the impact of BFHI in Scotland, where breastfeeding rates are below the UK average. Babies born in BFHI-accredited hospitals were 28% more likely to be still breastfed at 7 days of age than those born elsewhere, and the rates of breastfeeding initiation had increased more rapidly in BFHI-accredited hospitals than in non-accredited hospitals. A study from Switzerland (Merten *et al.*, 2005) showed that babies born in baby-friendly hospitals were more likely to be breastfed for longer duration. This is not a universal benefit however. A UK study found that babies born in baby-friendly hospitals were no more likely to be still breastfed at 4 weeks than those who were not (Bartington *et al.*, 2006). In the United States, a survey of women who gave birth in hospitals that had BFHI accreditation showed that only 35% had experienced all seven of the standards associated with accreditation and that 25% had even been provided with gift packs of formula milk (Hawkins *et al.*, 2014). In this study, BFHI accreditation had no effect on duration of breastfeeding and only increased initiation of breastfeeding among women with low educational attainment.

BFHI promotes and supports breastfeeding through national health services and may therefore be effective only in the first few days of breastfeeding when women are in close contact with midwives. Other organizations exist to provide support and encouragement outside the healthcare setting. The United Kingdom has a national breastfeeding helpline operated by the Breastfeeding Network, enabling women experiencing difficulties to seek telephone support from experienced breastfeeders. The La Leche League (international) and the National Childbirth Trust (United Kingdom) are charitable organizations that can be easily accessed by women requiring support. La Leche League, in particular, is involved in training of health professionals and providing peer counsellors who can give practical advice and moral support to breastfeeding mothers in difficulty.

Just as social networks can strongly influence the initial decision on whether to breastfeed or bottle-feed, peer support groups can be very important in helping women to continue breastfeeding and overcome the challenges faced in the early weeks. For example, Vari and colleagues (2000) reported that women were more able to maintain exclusive breastfeeding for longer if they were given professional advice about breastfeeding as a group during pregnancy, with follow-up sessions from women who were currently breastfeeding to demonstrate the technique and provide later breastfeeding support. One-to-one informal peer support in addition to more formal antenatal education is an effective way of promoting breastfeeding initiation among low-income women (Dyson *et al.*, 2014). Continuing that support into the postnatal period also reduces the risk that breastfeeding will be discontinued by approximately 30% (Kaunonen *et al.*, 2012; Sudfeld *et al.*, 2012). Postnatal support from trained peer supporters is however only effective in low- and middle-income countries, with much less effect seen in high-income countries such as the United Kingdom. Ingram (2013) reported an evaluation of a peer support programme in deprived areas of Bristol (United

Kingdom) where women had access to peer support antenatally and in the first two weeks after delivery. This had negligible benefits for breastfeeding maintenance to 8 weeks.

5.5 Situations in which breastfeeding is not advised

There may be circumstances in which breastfeeding is not advised, as to do so would put the infant at risk. This may occur due to maternal exposure to toxic agents that are excreted in the milk, for example, heavy metals, or through maternal usage of prescription or non-prescription drugs that might have a negative impact on the infant. Drugs and other exogenous organic chemicals, perhaps encountered in the workplace, undergo a two-phase metabolism in the liver. Phase I metabolism comprises oxidation, reduction or hydrolytic reactions catalysed by the cytochrome P450s, yielding stable products that are targets for phase II metabolism. This consists of conjugation with either glucuronide, sulphonate or amino acids. The conjugated products are then excreted, and in lactating women, excretion into breast milk is one route of disposal. The pharmacokinetics of all prescription drugs are well characterized, and women will be advised accordingly if it is necessary to administer a drug likely to appear in the milk in this way.

There are also a number of inborn errors of metabolism that may make breastfeeding inadvisable or difficult to pursue (Figure 5.10). Galactosaemia is an inherited disorder in which individuals lack the enzyme galactose-1-phosphate uridyl transferase. This occurs in approximately 1 in 45 000 live births in the United Kingdom. In the absence of this enzyme, galactose will accumulate, and this leads to extensive damage in the liver and kidney. Individuals with galactosaemia therefore have to restrict galactose consumption throughout life, but even with restrictive diets, there are many long-term complications that cannot be avoided. Clearly, as lactose is metabolized to glucose and galactose, consumption of human or normal formula milk is impossible, and infants with galactosaemia cannot be breastfed. There are galactose-free formulas available for use in this situation.

It has been widely supposed that most inborn errors of metabolism may preclude breastfeeding, but this need not be the case if mothers want to confer some of the health benefits of human milk upon their children. There are two approaches that can be taken to achieve this. Firstly, expressed milk mixed with other required ingredients can be fed via a bottle. Secondly, infants can be breastfed on demand but pre-fed with

Galactosaemia

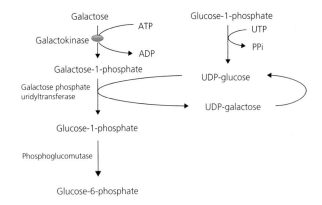

Phenylketonuria

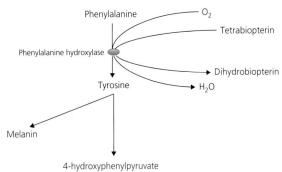

Figure 5.10 Inborn errors of metabolism can make breastfeeding hazardous to child health. Galactosaemia and phenylketonuria necessitate the feeding of special infant formulas.

specialized formula to limit intake. Phenylketonuria (PKU) provides a good example of the possibilities of the latter approach.

Infants with PKU lack the enzyme phenylalanine hydroxylase and as a result have to restrict intake of phenylalanine (Figure 5.10). Human milk has a relatively low content of phenylalanine. Some mothers feed their infants weighed quantities of expressed milk in order to regulate phenylalanine intake. More commonly, women will breastfeed but begin each feed by giving a measured amount of a phenylalanine formula, following up with breastfeeding until the infant is satiated. Another possible approach is to adopt a mixed feeding schedule in which infants are alternately breastfed and bottle-fed with low-phenylalanine formula.

There are situations where breastfeeding can increase the risk of transmission of disease from mother to infant, either through direct passage of infective organisms via the milk (e.g. HIV) or through the close contact between baby and infected mother (e.g. tuberculosis). The ideal protocols for dealing with these situations will depend upon other factors in the maternal–infant environment but could involve the use of an alternative to breastfeeding.

HIV infection of the infant during breastfeeding is believed to occur due to movement of virus in maternal milk into the infant circulation through uptake at points in the mouth, throat or intestine where the integrity of the mucosal cells lining the digestive tract is compromised (e.g. due to ulcers or inflammation). The most likely cause of a breakdown in the mucosal integrity is the introduction of solid foods. Given this significant risk of direct transmission of HIV from mother to infant during breastfeeding, in developed countries, maternal HIV infection would normally be regarded as a contraindication for breastfeeding.

The WHO updated their guidance for women who are HIV positive in developing countries in 2010 (WHO, 2010). The WHO recommends that women should either exclusively formula feed or breastfeed for a minimum of 12 months alongside the use of antiretroviral (AVT) drugs. AVT can be provided either to the infant (option A) or to the mother (option B+). Breastfeeding and AVT should be used only in situations where diarrhoeal disease and malnutrition are a major cause of infant mortality, with formula preferred if it is safe, feasible and affordable to do so. The clear concern about formula feeding is that children are vulnerable to malnutrition if families cannot afford or access formula and to infection if clean water supplies to make up formula are not secured. Some women also feel that formula feeding will identify them as being HIV positive, and thus, their feeding behaviour effectively stigmatizes them. Breastfeeding with option B+ AVT avoids this stigma and the concern that antiretrovirals might have adverse effects if given prophylactically to infants. This concern and uncertain access to formula milk lead some women to take a mixed feeding approach (Coutsoudis *et al.*, 2008).

The implementation of the WHO policy on infant feeding with HIV is down to national governments, and in many countries, this is proving successful. The Prevention of Mother-to-Child Transmission programme in Botswana, for example, encourages HIV-positive women to exclusively formula feed for 6 months and provides all formula requirements for 12 months (NACA, 2012). However, this approach also results in a high prevalence of diarrhoeal disease and malnutrition once complementary feeding begins (McGrath *et al.*, 2012).

Where HIV-positive women are breastfeeding, keeping the transition from breastfeeding only to a diet comprising solids and formula milk as short as possible may minimize the risk of mother-to-child transmission of HIV. Taha *et al.* (2007) studied Malawian mother–infant pairs in which the women were HIV positive, but infants were uninfected at 6 weeks of age. Mother-to-child transmission of HIV during infancy occurred in 9.7% of the mother–infant pairs over the ensuing 2 years, with most infections occurring after the critical 6-month point. Although this supports the proposal for abrupt cessation of breastfeeding at 6 months, there is concern that this will increase vulnerability to diarrhoeal infections.

Tuberculosis is becoming increasingly common on a global scale and in many areas occurs alongside HIV infection. In the past, it was common practice to separate women with tuberculosis from their infants in order to prevent cross infection, but in developing countries, this would tend to increase infant death rates due to loss of the immunoprotective effects of breast milk. It is now recognized that the best way to prevent tuberculosis infection of infants is to immunize the infant, treat the disease in the mother and maintain exclusive breastfeeding for 6 months, if compatible with management of HIV. In the absence of HIV, women with tuberculosis should continue breastfeeding with complementary foods for up to 2 years.

5.6 Alternatives to breastfeeding

The evidence that breastfeeding carries both short- and long-term health benefits for both mother and infant is overwhelming. However, for the vast majority of infants born in Westernized countries, feeding will be largely based upon the use of artificial milk formulas fed via a bottle. The main benefit of this approach to feeding is that it reduces the dependency of the infant upon the mother as the main carer and allows closer bonding with other family members. Bottle-feeding is also clearly advantageous to women who need to return to work early after the delivery of their baby.

As described previously, there are some hazards and drawbacks associated with formula feeding that may make it an inappropriate choice for families on low incomes and for women in developing countries where a clean water supply cannot be guaranteed. It should also be appreciated that formula feeding can increase the risk of allergic sensitization to cow's milk protein and can be hazardous if feeds are not prepared according to manufacturers' instructions. Under-concentrating milk formula, that is, adding less milk powder per unit volume, is a strategy that may be adopted by families on low incomes to make the formula last longer and can lead to infant malnutrition. Over-concentration of the formula, that is, adding too much milk powder per unit volume, can lead to dehydration of the infant, as more water will have to be excreted to deal with the ingested protein and electrolytes.

There is a huge array of different milk formulas available to consumers. These vary little in their composition as there are strict regulations that limit the capacity of manufacturers to alter formula constituents. As will be described in the following text, however, there are formulas designed for specific situations, and formulas may vary in composition in order to deliver an optimal balance of nutrients according to the developmental stage of the infant.

5.6.1 Cow's milk formulas
Most infant formulas are based upon cow's milk, modified to produce a composition that is more similar to the average composition of human milk. Unmodified cow's milk should not be given to infants below the age of 12 months, although it can be mixed with solids as part of complementary feeding before this time. Unmodified cow's milk would promote the development of nutrient deficiencies in infants as it is low in vitamin C, vitamin

E, essential fatty acids and iron. Iron deficiency would also be promoted as adverse reactions to components of cow's milk would promote blood loss in the digestive tract. Importantly, the high nitrogen, calcium, phosphorus, sodium, potassium and chloride content of cow's milk would promote dehydration as water would be required to excrete the excess solute load.

Figure 5.11 shows a comparison of the macronutrient and micronutrient composition of human, cow and a typical formula milk. Cow's milk contains almost three-fold more protein than human milk and has a lower sugar content, and so the main modifications made during formula production include processing to remove protein and the addition of lactose. Many of the raw materials used in the production of infant formulas are actually waste products from other areas of the dairy industry, and generally, the starting material for formula production is not whole, unmodified milk. The processing to remove protein may involve a variety of steps including evaporation, condensation and hydrolysis, and other components of the cow's milk will be lost along the way. Much of the whey protein that is included in formula milks is discarded during cheese manufacture and when added to formula mixes will consist of demineralized, fat-free whey protein (Jost *et al.*, 1999). All infant formulas will contain vegetable oils added to attain the required total fat content. Between 25 and 75% of fats in formulas may be of vegetable origin, and this will clearly impact upon the overall fatty acid composition of the formula.

It is a relatively simple process for manufacturers to add vitamins and minerals to achieve optimal concentrations, and indeed, this is necessary if processing demineralizes the raw materials that comprise the basis of the formula. For many micronutrients, this addition will need to take into account the bioavailability of the nutrient from the formula milk matrix. This is exemplified by iron, which in human milk is present in the highly absorbed haem form, but in formula milk, it is in the non-haem form. It is therefore necessary to add iron to cow's milk formula at a concentration 10-fold greater than seen in either human milk or the cow's milk from which the formula is derived (Figure 5.11).

5.6.1.1 Milk stages and follow-on milk

In the processing of cow's milk to produce formula, it becomes possible to manipulate the casein/whey ratio of the proteins in the milk. Unmodified cow's milk has a casein/whey ratio of 80:20, which is markedly different to human milk where the ratio is 40:60. Most manufacturers take advantage of the ability to alter this ratio to market separate *first-stage* and *second-stage* milks. First-stage milks are whey-rich products and have a casein/whey ratio that mimics mature human milk. Second-stage milks provide the 80:20 ratio seen in cow's milk and are proposed to be more difficult to digest within the infant gut but to have a more satiating effect on infant appetite.

It is suggested that feeding a whey-rich formula may have a number of benefits for the infant. The predominant whey proteins in infant formulas derived from cow's milk are β-lactoglobulin and α-lactalbumin. β-Lactoglobulin is not found in human milk, but α-lactalbumin is the dominant whey protein consumed by breastfed infants. Some formulas are manufactured to contain a level of α-lactalbumin that is similar to human

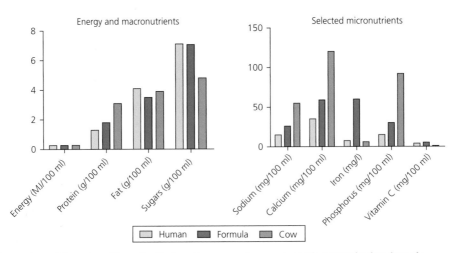

Figure 5.11 Comparison of the compositions of milks from humans and cows, alongside a typical infant formula. *Source*: Data from Holland *et al.* (1991).

milk. It is suggested that these enriched formulas may aid in the neurodevelopment of infants as they increase circulating concentrations of tryptophan, an amino acid that plays an important role in brain development (Lien, 2003). Other whey proteins that are present in whey-rich formulas may provide some antimicrobial protection for infants. Lactoferrin, for example, has been shown in animal studies to have immune system priming actions and may therefore help the maturation of the cellular immunity of infants. The lactoferricin B fragment of bovine lactoferrin, which is generated during digestion within the stomach (Kuwata *et al.*, 1998), has been shown to have the capacity to damage cell membranes and inhibit growth of a number of food-borne pathogens, including *Salmonella, Listeria* and *Campylobacter* species.

The progression from whey-rich to casein-rich formulas is not an absolute necessity. Feeding casein-rich formula at an earlier age would do no harm, and the whey-rich formulation can sustain the nutritional requirements of an infant up to 6 months of age. At 6 months, however, it is advisable for parents to switch formula and introduce a follow-on (stage 3) milk to their infant. Follow-on milks derived from cow's milk are less modified than the milks produced for younger infants and therefore contain more protein and minerals to meet the increasing demands of the infant past 6 months. Follow-on milks are used as a mixer during weaning or as a drink during complementary feeding.

5.6.2 Preterm formulas

Approximately 6% of all infants born in the United Kingdom are born prematurely (<38-week gestation). The infants at greatest risk of significant morbidity are those born before 32-week gestation, which make up around one-third of all preterm deliveries. This latter group of preterm infants poses a number of problems from a nutritional point of view, as they have high demands for nutrients and yet cannot be fed by conventional means.

As seen in earlier chapters of this book, the organs develop and mature at differing rates. Organs and systems that mature relatively late in gestation are those which will be least mature in a preterm infant. Lung immaturity leads to life-threatening complications that significantly raise nutrient demands due to the need for mechanical ventilation. Immaturity of the digestive system poses considerable problems in terms of feeding strategies. Before 32-week gestation, the infant lacks the rooting reflex and so is unable to breastfeed. The digestive system is so underdeveloped that the stomach capacity is only around 3 ml for a 1.5 kg infant, and this clearly limits the quantity of food that can be taken via the enteral route. The gut is also functionally immature and lacks effective peristalsis and the key enzymes and other factors required for digestion.

The last stages of gestation are normally a time when the fetus acquires nutrients for storage from the mother. In terms of energy, for example, the full-term 40-week-gestation infant has fat reserves of approximately 450 g (4530 kcal, 18.98 MJ), whereas a 26-week-gestation infant has a meagre 20 g fat (320 kcal, 1.34 MJ). The nutritional status of preterm infants is therefore often poor at earlier stages of their clinical management, as they have low intakes of nutrients, low reserves and high demands associated with trauma and their high growth rate (human body weight normally doubles between 28- and 40-week gestation).

Strategies for feeding preterm infants will depend upon their size and their gestational age. For infants born prior to 34 weeks, normal bottle-feeding or breast-feeding is not possible, and the infant will need artificial feeding using a tube via the enteral route (a nasogastric tube carries milk directly to the stomach) or using a parenteral feeding (intravenous feeding of nutrients in the simplest form, e.g. free fatty acids, glucose and amino acids) protocol. Human milk may be fed to older preterm babies via a tube. Ideally, this is milk expressed by the babies' own mother, which will have a composition suited to the stage of development. Mothers of preterm infants are reported to produce a more energy-dense milk with a greater protein, fat and sodium content than mothers of full-term infants. Feeding human milk conveys the immunological benefits to the infant, but does carry some risk. Osteopenia of prematurity is a condition of bone in which bone mineralization is compromised. This can arise due to the low calcium and phosphate content of human milk. Thus, when human milk is used as the basis of enteral feeding for premature babies, it is mixed with fortifiers to increase the vitamin and mineral content (Schanler, 1995).

Where preterm infants are fed with formula milk, it is inappropriate to use a normal full-term formula as the nutrient density is insufficient to meet demands. Given the lower capacity of the premature gut and raised nutrient demands, most constituents are needed at greater concentrations than in term formula. Preterm formulas are based upon β-lactoglobulin as the protein source and are hence whey rich. Due to the functional immaturity of the gut, the fat and sugar components are delivered as mixtures that are more easily digested and which do not overwhelm the existing enzyme systems. Sugars are provided as a mixture of lactose and glucose polymers, while fats are provided as a mixture of long-chain and medium-chain

Table 5.6 Comparison of full-term and preterm infant formula composition (selected nutrients).

Nutrient	Formula content/100 ml reconstituted milk	
	Term formula	Preterm formula
Energy (kcal)	70.0	70.0
Protein (g)	1.5	1.9
Calcium (mg)	48.0	120.0
Phosphate (mg)	35.0	59.0
Iron (mg)	1.2	1.2
Sodium (mg)	20.0	30.0
Vitamin A (µg retinol equivalents)	100.0	350.0
Vitamin D (µg)	1.0	3.0
Vitamin C (mg)	5.8	24.0

triglycerides. Table 5.6 shows a comparison of the nutrient composition of preterm and full-term formulas, highlighting their differing nutrient density.

5.6.3 Soy formulas

Some infants are intolerant of cow's milk-derived formulas, which is usually because of lactose intolerance, and may therefore require a lactose-free alternative. Soy formulas are produced from isolated soy protein and provide sugar as glucose rather than lactose. Originally, soy-based formulas were developed for infants with cow's milk protein allergy, but as the proteins in these formulas cross-react with cow's milk protein to a large extent, infants allergic to cow's milk are highly likely to respond to soy formulas in the same way. Soy formulas should not be confused with standard soy milk. They should only be used on medical advice, and there are some concerns that there are implications for the development of the reproductive tract and fertility in male babies exposed to phytoestrogens in soy formulas.

5.6.4 Hydrolysed protein and amino acid-based formulas

Cow's milk protein allergy is the most common food allergy seen in children. The only effective treatment is the exclusion of all dairy produce from the diet, and this means that for formula-fed infants, specialized products have to be introduced. Soy formula is generally inappropriate as described previously, and approximately 50% of all children who are allergic to cow's milk will be allergic to soy formula. Osborn and Sinn (2004) performed a systematic review of the literature and found that in children with a family history of atopy, feeding a soy formula also increased risk of soy

protein allergy by twofold compared to feeding standard formula. This suggests that soy formulas would not be the ideal choice of feed for infants at risk of allergies.

The alternative is to feed infants with either extensively hydrolysed protein or amino acid-based formulas. Hydrolysed protein formulas are generally based upon the whey fraction of cow's milk, with the major proteins hydrolysed to smaller peptides that are less allergenic than the native proteins. Extensively hydrolysed protein formulas do not prevent the development of allergies, but are an effective treatment for managing children with established cow's milk protein allergy. Amino acid-based formulas play the same role and are formulations that are free of intact proteins and peptides, instead providing all nitrogen in the form of isolated amino acids. Not all infants are able to tolerate hydrolysed protein formulas, and the study of Niggemann et al. (2001) suggested that children with intolerance or allergy to cow's milk had better growth rates when fed amino acid-based formula compared to hydrolysed proteins. An Australian consensus panel (Kemp et al., 2008) recommended that on diagnosis of cow's milk protein allergy, children under the age of 6 months should be fed extensively hydrolysed formula with amino acid formula reserved for infants with more severe allergy or other complications. Taylor et al. (2012) found that there were no major differences in clinical outcomes between amino acid formulas and extensively hydrolysed formulas and that the hydrolysed formula was the more cost-effective option.

5.6.5 Other formulas

Formula milks based upon sheep or goat's milk may be promoted as an alternative to cow's milk formula, the argument being that consumption of such milks would reduce risk of allergy to cow's milk protein. The milk proteins of sheep and goats are very similar to those of cows and so this argument is fatuous. Milk from sheep or goats provides an inadequate supply of folic acid, iron and vitamins A, D and C, and so formulas from these sources should not be given to infants. Infant formulas and follow-on formulas based on sheep or goat milk have not been approved for use in Europe, but full-fat sheep or goat's milks can be used for preparing sauces that are used in complementary feeds from 6 months of age. Zhou et al. (2014) however carried out a double-blind randomized controlled trial of a goat formula compared to standard formula in term infants. There were no differences in infant growth, occurrence of allergy or dermatitis or serious adverse health outcomes. This suggests that concerns about safety may be unfounded, but further trials would be required.

SUMMARY

- Mammary alveoli are the sites of milk synthesis. This process involves de novo synthesis of lactose, fatty acids and proteins.
- Human milk production is under endocrine control through actions of prolactin and oxytocin. Hypothalamic integration of the secretion of these hormones ensures that milk supply meets infant demand.
- Lactation increases maternal demand for energy, protein and micronutrients.
- Breastfeeding confers health benefits upon lactating women, including a more rapid recovery from childbirth, suppression of reproductive cycling and protection against breast and ovarian cancers.
- Breastfeeding delivers immunoprotective factors to the infant, in addition to nutrients in an optimal formulation. Immunoprotective cells and proteins reduce the risk of gastrointestinal and respiratory tract infections.
- Breastfeeding is associated with lower risk of sudden infant death syndrome, childhood obesity and allergies in susceptible infants. The delivery of docosahexaenoic acid in human milk is believed to enhance infant brain development.
- The World Health Organization recommends that infants are exclusively breastfed for the first 6 months of life. The only exceptions to this are where children have inborn errors of metabolism or where mothers are HIV positive.
- Despite the advantages of breastfeeding for mothers and infants, the majority of infants in developed countries do not experience the recommended 6 months of exclusive breastfeeding. The decision to use alternative feeding methods is largely shaped by social and cultural factors.
- Promotion of breastfeeding through initiatives such as the Baby-Friendly Hospital Initiative contributes to greater initial rates of breastfeeding. Peer support interventions may help women maintain breastfeeding beyond the early weeks.
- Formulas designed for bottle-fed babies are generally manufactured using modified by-products of the dairy industry. Their composition mimics average human milk and must comply with strict legislation.
- Specialized infant formulas are used for the feeding of preterm infants and infants with confirmed allergies or intolerance to cow's milk.

References

Agostoni, C., Grandi, F., Gianni, M.L. *et al.* (1999) Growth patterns of breast fed and formula fed infants in the first 12 months of life: an Italian study. *Archives of Disease in Childhood*, **81**, 395–399.

Algarín, C., Nelson, C.A., Peirano, P. *et al.* (2013) Iron-deficiency anemia in infancy and poorer cognitive inhibitory control at age 10 years. *Developmental Medicine and Child Neurology*, **55**, 453–458.

Alm, B., Wennergren, G., Norvenius, S.G. *et al.* (2002) Breast feeding and the sudden infant death syndrome in Scandinavia 1992–1995. *Archives Disease in Childhood*, **86**, 400–402.

Anothaisintawee, T., Wiratkapun, C., Lerdsitthichai, P. *et al.* (2013) Risk factors of breast cancer: a systematic review and meta-analysis. *Asia-Pacific Journal of Public Health*, **25**, 368–387.

Arenz, S., Ruckerl, R., Koletzko, B. *et al.* (2004) Breast-feeding and childhood obesity – a systematic review. *International Journal of Obesity*, **28**, 1247–1256.

Arifeen, S., Black, R.E., Antelman, G. *et al.* (2001) Exclusive breast-feeding reduces acute respiratory infection and diarrhea deaths among infants in Dhaka slums. *Pediatrics*, **108**, E67.

Bartington, S., Griffiths, L.J., Tate, A.R. *et al.* and Millennium Cohort Study Health Group (2006) Are breastfeeding rates higher among mothers delivering in Baby Friendly accredited maternity units in the UK? *International Journal of Epidemiology*, **35**, 1178–1186.

Broadfoot, M., Britten, J., Tappin, D. *et al.* (2005) The Baby Friendly Hospital initiative and breast-feeding rates in Scotland. *Archives of Disease in Childhood*, **90**, F114–F116.

Carlson, S.E., Werkman, S.H., Peeples, J.M. *et al.* (1994) Long-chain fatty acids and early visual and cognitive development of preterm infants. *European Journal of Clinical Nutrition*, **48** (Suppl 2), S27–S30.

Chantry, C.J., Howard, C.R. and Auinger, P. (2007) Full breast-feeding duration and risk for iron deficiency in U.S. infants. *Breastfeeding Medicine*, **2**, 63–73.

Colin, W.B. and Scott, J.A. (2002) Breast-feeding: reasons for starting, reasons for stopping and problems along the way. *Breastfeeding Reviews*, **10**, 13–19.

Collaborative Group on Hormonal Factors in Breast Cancer (2002) Breast cancer and breast-feeding: collaborative reanalysis of individual data from 47 epidemiological studies in 30 countries, including 50 302 women with breast cancer and 96 973 women without the disease. *Lancet*, **360**, 187–195.

Colombo, J., Carlson, S.E., Cheatham, C.L. *et al.* (2013) Long-term effects of LCPUFA supplementation on childhood cognitive outcomes. *American Journal of Clinical Nutrition*, **98**, 403–412.

Coutsoudis, A., Coovadia, H.M. and Wilfert, C.M. (2008) HIV, Infant feeding and more perils for poor people: new WHO guidelines encourage review of formula milk practices. *Bulletin of the World Health Organization*, **86**, 210–214.

Cunnane, S.C., Francescutti, V., Brenna, J.T. *et al.* (2000) Breast-fed infants achieve a higher rate of brain and whole body docosahexaenoate accumulation than formula-fed infants not consuming dietary docosahexaenoate. *Lipids*, **35**, 105–111.

Danforth, K.N., Tworoger, S.S., Hecht, J.L. *et al.* (2007) Breast-feeding and risk of ovarian cancer in two prospective cohorts. *Cancer Causes and Control*, **18**, 517–523.

Department of Health (1991) *Dietary Reference Values for Food Energy and Nutrients for the United Kingdom*, The Stationery Office, Norwich.

de Silva, D., Geromi, M., Halken, S. *et al.* (2014) Primary prevention of food allergy in children and adults: systematic review. *Allergy*, **69**, 581–589.

Dijkhuizen, M.A., Wieringa, F.T., West, C.E. *et al.* (2001) Concurrent micronutrient deficiencies in lactating mothers and their infants in Indonesia. *American Journal of Clinical Nutrition*, **73**, 786–791.

Dyson, L., McCormick, F.M. and Renfrew, M.J. (2014) Interventions for promoting the initiation of breastfeeding. *São Paulo Medical Journal*, **132**, 68.

Eriksen, H.L., Kesmodel, U.S., Underbjerg, M. *et al.* (2013) Predictors of intelligence at the age of 5: family, pregnancy and birth characteristics, postnatal influences, and postnatal growth. *PLoS One*, **8**, e79200.

Fewtrell, M.S. (2011) The evidence for public health recommendations on infant feeding. *Early Human Development*, **87**, 715–721.

Ford, R.P., Taylor, B.J., Mitchell, E.A. *et al.* (1993) Breastfeeding and the risk of sudden infant death syndrome. *International Journal of Epidemiology*, **22**, 885–890.

Grantham-McGregor, S.M., Powell, C.A., Walker, S.P. *et al.* (1991) Nutritional supplementation, psychosocial stimulation, and mental development of stunted children: the Jamaican Study. *Lancet*, **338**, 1–5.

Hamlyn, B., Brooker, S., Oleinikova, K. *et al.* (2002) *Infant Feeding 2000*, Department of Health, London.

Hawkins, S.S., Stern, A.D., Baum, C.F. *et al.* (2014) Compliance with the Baby-Friendly Hospital Initiative and impact on breastfeeding rates. *Archives of Disease in Childhood*, **99**, F138–F143.

Henderson, L., Kitzinger, J. and Green, J. (2000) Representing infant feeding: content analysis of British media portrayals of bottle feeding and breast feeding. *British Medical Journal*, **321**, 1196–1198.

Henderson, L., Gregory, J. and Swan, G. (2002) *National Diet and Nutrition Survey: Adults Aged 19–64 Years*, Office of National Statistics, London.

Holland, B., Welch, A.A., Unwin, I.D. *et al.* (1991) *McCance and Widdowson's The Composition of Foods*, 5th edn, Royal Society of Chemistry, Cambridge.

Ingram, J. (2013) A mixed methods evaluation of peer support in Bristol, UK: mothers', midwives' and peer supporters' views and the effects on breastfeeding. *BMC Pregnancy and Childbirth*, **13**, 192.

Ip, S., Chung, M., Raman, G. *et al.* (2007) Breastfeeding and maternal and infant health outcomes in developed countries. *Evidence Report/Technology Assessment*, **153**, 1–186.

Jain, A., Concato, J. and Leventhal, J.M. (2002) How good is the evidence linking breast-feeding and intelligence. *Pediatrics*, **109**, 1044–1053.

Janney, C.A., Zhang, D. and Sowers, M. (1997) Lactation and weight retention. *American Journal of Clinical Nutrition*, **66**, 1116–1124.

Jost, R., Maire, J.-C., Maynard, F. *et al.* (1999) Aspects of whey protein usage in infant nutrition, a brief review. *International Journal of Food Science and Technology*, **34**, 533–542.

Karlsson, M.K., Ahlborg, H.G. and Karlsson, C. (2005) Maternity and bone density. *Acta Orthopaedica*, **76**, 2–13.

Kaunonen, M., Hannula, L. and Tarkka, M.T. (2012) A systematic review of peer support interventions for breastfeeding. *Journal of Clinical Nursing*, **21**, 1943–1954.

Kemp, A.S., Hill, D.J., Allen, K.J. *et al.* (2008) Guidelines for the use of infant formulas to treat cows milk protein allergy: an Australian consensus panel opinion. *Medical Journal of Australia*, **188**, 109–112.

Kerkhof, M., Koopman, L.P., van Strien, R.T. *et al.* (2003) Risk factors for atopic dermatitis in infants at high risk of allergy: the PIAMA study. *Clinical and Experimental Allergy*, **33**, 1336–1341.

Kovacs, A., Funke, S., Marosvolgyi, T. *et al.* (2005) Fatty acids in early human milk after preterm and full-term delivery. *Journal of Pediatric Gastroenterology and Nutrition*, **41**, 454–459.

Kramer, M.S. and Kakuma, R. (2002) Optimal duration of exclusive breastfeeding. *Cochrane Database of Systematic Reviews*, **1**, CD003517.

Kramer, M.S. and Kakuma, R. (2012) Optimal duration of exclusive breastfeeding. *Cochrane Database of Systematic Reviews*, **8**, CD003517.

Kramer, M.S., Chalmers, B., Hodnett, E.D. *et al.* (2001) Promotion of breast-feeding intervention trial (PROBIT): a randomized trial in the Republic of Belarus. *Journal of the American Medical Association*, **285**, 413–420.

Kuwata, H., Yip, T.T., Yamauchi, K. *et al.* (1998) The survival of ingested lactoferrin in the gastrointestinal tract of adult mice. *Biochemical Journal*, **334**, 321–323.

Langley-Evans, A.J. and Langley-Evans, S.C. (2003) Relationship between maternal nutrient intakes in early and late pregnancy and infants weight and proportions at birth: prospective cohort study. *Journal of the Royal Society for the Promotion of Health*, **123**, 210–216.

Lepe, M., Bacardí Gascón, M., Castañeda-González, L.M. *et al.* (2011) Effect of maternal obesity on lactation: systematic review. *Nutrición Hospitalaria*, **26**, 1266–1269.

Lien, E.L. (2003) Infant formulas with increased concentrations of α-lactalbumin. *American Journal of Clinical Nutrition*, **77** (suppl), 1555S–1558S.

Lovelady, C. (2011) Balancing exercise and food intake with lactation to promote post-partum weight loss. *Proceedings of the Nutrition Society*, **70**, 181–184.

Lozoff, B. and Georgieff, M.K. (2006) Iron deficiency and brain development. *Seminars in Paediatric Neurology*, **13**, 158–165.

Lubetzky, R., Littner, Y., Mimouni, F.B. *et al.* (2006) Circadian variations in fat content of expressed breast milk from mothers of preterm infants. *Journal of the American College of Nutrition*, **25**, 151–154.

Martin, J.E., Hure, A.J., Macdonald-Wicks, L., *et al.* (2012) *Predictors of post-partum weight retention in a prospective longitudinal study. Maternal & Child Nutrition*. DOI:10.1111.

Matheson, M.C., Allen, K.J. and Tang, M.L. (2012) Understanding the evidence for and against the role of breastfeeding in allergy prevention. *Clinical and Experimental Allergy*, **42**, 827–851.

Matthews, K., Webber, K., McKim, E. *et al.* (1998) Maternal infant-feeding decisions: reasons and influences. *Canadian Journal of Nursing Research*, **30**, 177–198.

McAndrew, F., Thompson, J., Fellows, L. *et al.* (2012) *Infant Feeding Survey 2010*, Health and Social Care Information Centre, Leeds.

Mcgrath, C.J., Nduati, R., Richardson, B.A. *et al.* (2012) The prevalence of stunting is high in HIV-1-exposed uninfected infants in Kenya. *Journal of Nutrition*, **142**, 757–763.

Merten, S., Dratva, J. and Ackermann-Liebrich, U. (2005) Do baby-friendly hospitals influence breast-feeding duration on a national level? *Pediatrics*, **116**, E702–E708.

Mitoulas, L.R., Gurrin, L.C., Doherty, D.A. *et al.* (2003) Infant intake of fatty acids from human milk over the first year of lactation. *British Journal of Nutrition*, **90**, 979–986.

Morley, R., Cole, T.J., Powell, R. *et al.* (1988) Mothers choice to provide breast milk and developmental outcome. *Archives of Disease in Childhood*, **63**, 1382–1385.

NACA (National Aids Coordinating Agency). (2012) *Botswana National Policy on HIV/AIDS 2012*, http://www.naca.gov.bw/node/2054 (accessed 28 December 2014).

Niggemann, B., Binder, C., Dupont, C. *et al.* (2001) Prospective, controlled, multi-center study on the effect of an amino-acid-based formula in infants with cow's milk allergy/intolerance and atopic dermatitis. *Pediatric Allergy and Immunology*, **12**, 78–82.

Okyay, D.O., Okyay, E., Dogan, E. *et al.* (2013) Prolonged breast-feeding is an independent risk factor for postmenopausal osteoporosis. *Maturitas*, **74**, 270–275.

Olsson, C., Hernell, O., Hörnell, A. *et al.* (2008) Difference in celiac disease risk between Swedish birth cohorts suggests an opportunity for primary prevention. *Pediatrics*, **122**, 528–534.

Osborn, D.A. and Sinn, J. (2004) *Soy formula for prevention of allergy and food intolerance in infants. Cochrane Database of Systematic Reviews*, CD003741.

Owen, C.G., Martin, R.M., Whincup, P.H. *et al.* (2005) The effect of breastfeeding on mean body mass index throughout life: a quantitative review of published and unpublished observational evidence. *American Journal of Clinical Nutrition*, **82**, 1298–1307.

Phadungath, C. (2005) Casein micelle structure: a concise review. *Songklanakarin Journal of Science and Technology*, **27**, 201–212.

Prentice, A.M., Goldberg, G.R. and Prentice, A. (1994) Body mass index and lactation performance. *European Journal of Clinical Nutrition*, **48** (Suppl 3), S78–S86.

Ritchie, L.D., Fung, E.B., Halloran, B.P. *et al.* (1998) A longitudinal study of calcium homeostasis during human pregnancy and lactation and after resumption of menses. *American Journal of Clinical Nutrition*, **67**, 693–701.

Schanler, R.J. (1995) Suitability of human milk for the low-birthweight infant. *Clinics in Perinatology*, **22**, 207–222.

Smithers, L.G., Golley, R.K., Mittinty, M.N. *et al.* (2012) Dietary patterns at 6, 15 and 24 months of age are associated with IQ at 8 years of age. *European Journal of Epidemiology*, **27**, 525–535.

Sudfeld, C.R., Fawzi, W.W. and Lahariya, C. (2012) Peer support and exclusive breastfeeding duration in low and middle-income countries: a systematic review and meta-analysis. *PLoS One*, **7**, e45143.

Taha, T.E., Hoover, D.R. and Kumwenda, N.I. (2007) Late postnatal transmission of HIV-1 and associated factors. *Journal of Infectious Disease*, **196**, 10–14.

Taylor, R.R., Sladkevicius, E., Panca, M. *et al.* (2012) Cost-effectiveness of using an extensively hydrolysed formula compared to an amino acid formula as first-line treatment for cow milk allergy in the UK. *Pediatric Allergy and Immunology*, **23**, 240–249.

Vari, P.M., Camburn, J. and Henly, S.J. (2000) Professionally mediated peer support and early breast-feeding success. *Journal of Perinatal Education*, **9**, 22–30.

von Kries, R., Koletzko, B., Sauerwald, T. *et al.* (1999) Breast feeding and obesity: cross sectional study. *British Medical Journal*, **319**, 147–150.

Walfisch, A., Sermer, C., Cressman, A. *et al.* (2013) Breast milk and cognitive development – the role of confounders: a systematic review. *British Medical Journal Open*, **3**, e003259.

Wells, J.C., Jonsdottir, O.H., Hibberd, P.L. *et al.* (2012) Randomized controlled trial of 4 compared with 6 mo of exclusive breastfeeding in Iceland: differences in breast-milk intake by stable-isotope probe. *American Journal of Clinical Nutrition*, **96**, 73–79.

Weng, S.F., Redsell, S.A., Swift, J.A. *et al.* (2012) Systematic review and meta-analyses of risk factors for childhood overweight identifiable during infancy. *Archives of Disease in Childhood*, **97**, 1019–1026.

WHO (2010) *Guidelines on HIV and Infant Feeding 2010: Principles and Recommendations for Infant Feeding in the Context of HIV and a Summary of Evidence*, WHO, Geneva.

WHO/UNICEF (1989) *Protecting, Promoting and Supporting Breast-feeding: The Special Role of Maternity Services*, WHO, Geneva.

Yngve, A. and Sjöström, M. (2001) Breast-feeding in countries of the European Union and EFTA: current and proposed recommendations, rationale, prevalence, duration and trends. *Public Health Nutrition*, **4**, 631–645.

Zhang, Y., Carlton, E. and Fein, S.B. (2013) The association of prenatal media marketing exposure recall with breastfeeding intentions, initiation, and duration. *Journal of Human Lactation*, **29**, 500–509.

Zhou, S.J., Sullivan, T., Gibson, R.A. *et al.* (2014) Nutritional adequacy of goat milk infant formulas for term infants: a double-blind randomised controlled trial. *British Journal of Nutrition*, **111**, 1641–1651.

Additional reading

If you would like to find out more about the material discussed in this chapter, the following sources may be of interest:

Dobbing, J. (ed) (2013) *Brain, Behavior and Iron in the Infant Diet*, Springer Verlag, London.

Morgan, J.B. and Dickerson, J.W.T. (eds) (2002) *Nutrition in Early Life*, John Wiley & Sons, Ltd, Chichester.

Riordan, J. and Wambach, K. (eds) (2008) *Breastfeeding and Human Lactation*, James and Bartlett Publishers, Burlington, MA.

CHAPTER 6
Nutrition and childhood

LEARNING OBJECTIVES

This chapter will enable the reader to:
- Explain that growth is the most important physiological process determining the nutrient and energy requirements of children
- Show an appreciation of why the requirements of children must be delivered through a nutrient-dense dietary pattern
- Describe how infectious disease and catch-up growth can promote micronutrient deficiencies among children in developing countries
- Discuss the importance of nutrition during infancy in establishing lifelong food preferences and the opportunities for health promotion that arise during this life stage
- Demonstrate understanding of the key issues surrounding the weaning process, with particular emphasis on the timing of the introduction of complementary foods
- Discuss the contribution of child poverty to both malnutrition and occurrence of overweight in the population
- Describe the susceptibility of children to advertising of energy-dense, nutrient-poor foods and beverages and highlight the importance of regulation of such marketing to ongoing health promotion strategies
- Show an awareness of how schools contribute to health promotion among school-age children
- Describe global trends in childhood obesity prevalence
- Discuss the significant contribution that genetic factors make to early-onset obesity
- Demonstrate understanding of the contribution that the modern environment makes to obesity and overweight among children
- Critically evaluate the evidence that suggests that childhood obesity is predictive of obesity and related disorders in adult life
- Describe optimal strategies for the prevention and treatment of obesity in children

6.1 Introduction

Humans are almost unique among mammalian species in that there is an extended period of growth and development between birth and adulthood. Even among our closest relatives, the great apes, where lifespan is typically 30–50 years, full maturity is achieved after just 7–13 years. Human childhood represents an important physiological and psychosocial stage of the lifespan. During this time, the individual attains full adult stature and full functional capacity of organs and systems, achieves a mature view of the world and develops independence from parents. Childhood is the phase of maximum growth, enlargement of the skeleton and remodelling of body composition. These changes are driven by surges in, and maturation of, the activities of key endocrine systems, including the somatotropic, hypothalamic–pituitary–gonadal and hypothalamic–pituitary–adrenal axes. Nutrition plays a paramount role during this time as the provision of an adequate and balanced supply of energy and nutrients is essential to maintain a normal developmental profile, to provide resistance against infectious disease and to ensure good health at later stages of life. Within this book, the childhood years have been divided into three stages: infancy, childhood and adolescence. The latter will be discussed in Chapter 7.

6.2 Infancy (birth to five)

6.2.1 The key developmental milestones
Nutritional demands over the first 5 years of life are very much shaped by the physiological and developmental processes associated with this life stage. Achieving the physical milestones sets a relatively high demand for energy and nutrients, but the psychosocial

Nutrition, Health and Disease: A Lifespan Approach, Second Edition. Simon Langley-Evans.
© 2015 John Wiley & Sons, Ltd. Published 2015 by John Wiley & Sons, Ltd.
Companion website: www.wiley.com/go/langleyevans/lifespan

and behavioural milestones should not be ignored, as these impact upon how nutrient demands are delivered and upon the development of attitudes and behaviours that help to shape long-term health and well-being. Alongside the development of the physical systems of the body and the ability to communicate and learn about the world around them, children at this preschool stage are undergoing a radical reshaping of their dietary pattern. The infant must make the transition from the milk-only diet of the first 4–6 months of life to a diet that comprises solids, but which remains energy dense, and then to a pattern of food intake that more resembles that which they will follow in their adult years.

Growth is the most important physiological process for the preschool child and largely explains the high nutrient requirements of infancy. The first year of life has the most rapid growth rate of any life stage, and during this period, the infant will triple body weight and increase height by approximately 75%. Growth rates slow thereafter, but growth continues to be a major demand process (Figure 6.1). Growth rates for boys and girls are similar over the first 5 years.

In addition to growth, the body is undergoing a series of changes in terms of composition and proportions, along with maturation of organ systems. For example, the lungs continue to undergo the process of branching off new alveoli until the age of 7–8 years. At birth, the human head is disproportionately large in relation to the trunk and the limbs are relatively short. Over the first 5 years, truncal and limb growth is prioritized. Between birth and 1 year of age, there is considerable deposition of fat reserves, taking the proportion of the body that is fat from 14% to around 25%. Over years 1–4, the absolute fat mass in the body stays relatively stable, but increasing lean body mass (increases from

14% of body mass at birth to 20% by age 5 years) results in fat proportions declining to around 20%. Body water is repartitioned in infancy. Initially, a greater proportion of water is held in the extracellular compartment making the infant more vulnerable to dehydration. Shifting of fluid to the intracellular compartment reduces this risk in the older child.

While growth of the trunk and limbs is greatest during infancy, the brain still grows at a rapid rate at this time. Brain size doubles over the first year of life, which can be observed as an increase in head circumference. Average head circumference at birth is around 34 cm, and the first year sees an increase of 12 cm. Over the next year (1–2), this slows to a gain of just 2 cm, but despite this, the brain increases in size by around 50% between the ages of 1 and 5 years and by the end of this period is around 90% of adult size.

Changes in brain size are accompanied by profound changes in the abilities of the child. At birth, the infant is relatively helpless, and while it has well-developed sensory neurones, the motor neurones are extremely immature. Over the early years, rapid development is seen in terms of these motor systems and their integration with sensory inputs. As a result, the infant years see the acquisition of key skills such as speech, walking and the ability to interact with family members and other children. Table 6.1 summarizes some of the key developmental milestones achieved by infants. The acquisition of these new physical and social skills impacts upon the nutrition of the child, who is effectively developing a physical and psychosocial independence from his/her mother. Considering the supply and demand model outlined in Chapter 1, on the demand side, growth and maturation increase requirements for nutrients in relation to body size. On the supply side, there are factors such as attaining the ability to self-feed or snack, the development of preferences and attitudes about food and the interaction with adults and peers, which will all determine the quality and possibly quantity of nutrient inputs.

6.2.2 Nutrient requirements

Over the first 5 years of life, there is a need for a pattern of dietary intake that is both energy and nutrient dense in order to meet high metabolic demands. With their short stature, preschool children are unable to consume and process sufficient bulk of food to meet their needs. While in absolute terms the nutrient requirements of young children are well below those of older children and adults, on a per-body-weight basis, they can be many times higher than at the later life stages. Table 6.2 shows how energy requirements are threefold higher in infancy than in adulthood and requirements for many micronutrients are elevated to a similar extent.

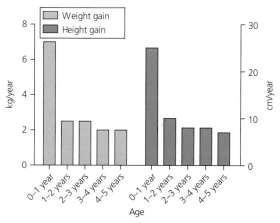

Figure 6.1 Rates of growth in preschool children. *Source*: Data compiled from Freeman *et al.* (1995).

Table 6.1 Developmental milestones for infants.

Age (years)	Physical changes and abilities	Psychosocial changes and food-related behaviour
0–1	Rapid growth	Dependent on parent
	Hand–eye coordination	Good appetite
	Sitting	Enjoys food
	Crawling	
	Convey food to mouth	
	Eruption of teeth	
1–2	Walking	Good appetite
	Chewing	Enjoys food but less experimental
	Use of baby cup	Developing verbal communication skills
	Manipulation of food items	
2–3	Running and jumping	Appetite slows
	Fine motor skills	Fluent speech
	Use of cup	Uses tantrums to influence the behaviour of others
	Use of cutlery	
3–4	Hopping	Picky/faddy eating
	Balancing	Develops independent food preferences
	Self-feeding	
4–5	Adult range of dexterity	Receptive to attitudes of others
		Develops a circle of peers

Table 6.2 A comparison of nutrient requirements* between adults and children under the age of 5 years.

Nutrient[†]	Age			
	1–3	4–6	19–50 (male)	19–50 (female)
Energy (kcal/kg/day)	95.8	91.6	34.5	32.3
Protein (g/kg/day)	0.94	0.83	0.60	0.62
Folate (µg/kg/day)	4.0	4.21	2.02	2.50
Ascorbate (mg/kg/day)	1.6	1.12	0.29	0.36
Cobalamin (µg/kg/day)	0.032	0.039	0.017	0.021
Iron (mg/kg/day)	0.42	0.26	0.09	0.19
Zinc (mg/kg/day)	0.30	0.28	0.10	0.09
Calcium (mg/kg/day)	22.0	19.7	7.1	8.8

Data derived from UK estimated average requirements (Department of Health, 1998) and assuming body weights of 12.5 (1–3 years), 17.8 (4–6 years), 74 (adult male) and 60 kg (adult female).
*Selected nutrients.
[†]All figures are shown adjusted for body weight.

One of the major challenges for delivery of nutrient requirements to this age group is to provide an appropriate balance of all nutrients, within the restrictions placed by the fact that children often have a limited range of preferred foods. Snacks are extremely important for the nutrition of younger children as they allow the supply of nutrients to be maintained throughout the day and compensate for the limited quantity of food that can be consumed at mealtimes. Selection of snacks needs to remain focused upon nutrient rather than energy density.

During this period of life, children move through the major transitions of weaning and from a childhood dietary pattern to an adult diet. This latter transition is substantial as the infant diet essentially delivers around 50% of energy as fat and 40% as simple sugars, with very little dietary fibre. In contrast, the adult diet should deliver no more than 35% of energy of fat and is mostly based upon bulky complex carbohydrates. Throughout this period, children need to be encouraged to experiment with a wide range of different foods, flavours and textures in order to establish healthy food preferences later in life.

6.2.2.1 Macronutrients and energy

As in adults, total energy expenditure (TEE) in childhood is defined in terms of the resting energy expenditure (REE) plus energy expended in diet-induced thermogenesis and physical activity. For children, however, overall energy requirement is not solely defined by TEE, as there are also considerations in relation to growth and losses through urine and faeces. The latter are minor components, but compared to adults, in children constitute a significant element of energy expenditure. Growth impacts upon energy requirements as the fat and protein deposited in growing tissue has an energy value and because energy must be expended in order to carry out the synthetic processes that yield new tissues (Torun, 2005).

Over the first year of life, energy requirements are exceptionally high and can be between three and four times greater (on a per-body-weight basis) than in adulthood. This high demand is only partly explained by the energy requirements of growth. Torun (2005) estimated the energy cost of growth for infants at around 4 kcal (17 kJ) per gram of weight gain. In a 2-year-old, this would equate to around 26.4 kcal (112.2 kJ) per day, which is clearly a very minor component (around 2%) of estimated average requirement

(EAR). In the neonate, the energy demand for growth is much greater but at most amounts to a third of overall energy requirement. TEE in infants is in fact mostly related to REE, which increases steadily over the first 5 years in proportion to body weight. The smaller bodies of children compared to adults have a greater surface area to volume ratio, and as a result, more energy must be expended to maintain normal body temperature.

Children in developing countries are subject to a number of specific factors that may elevate their dietary energy requirements to a greater extent than those seen in more affluent settings. Micronutrient deficiencies are commonplace in developing countries, particularly in rural populations. If any micronutrient is limiting within the diet, then this will impact upon the efficiency of utilization of energy substrates and hence the capacity to meet demands for energy (Prentice and Paul, 2000). Moreover, infectious diseases are common in these communities, and this promotes negative energy balance by increasing demand and reducing intakes. Fever has an anorectic influence and gastrointestinal infection, or the presence of gastrointestinal parasites, increases losses of energy and nutrients. Periods of acute infection are often followed by catch-up growth, effectively maintaining energy requirements at a higher level over a longer period of time (Prentice and Paul, 2000). Such requirements are likely to outstrip the supply of energy from the diet, and as a result, growth will falter. Lost growth will result in either stunting (failure of linear growth) or wasting (failure to gain weight; Figure 6.2). Children in this age group are the most vulnerable to protein–energy malnutrition and associated morbidities, mortality and long-term deficits of stature, cognitive function and health.

The requirements of preschool children for protein that are shown in Table 6.2 and considered in more detail in the various dietary reference value systems produced by the World Health Organization and national governments are estimates that are contested by some researchers in the field. Protein requirements for children have been estimated using nitrogen balance studies, usually performed on older individuals, integrated with estimates of the nitrogen content of tissues and rates of tissue accretion. It has been noted that the actual protein intakes of breastfed infants are below these estimates and yet growth and development are maintained. It may therefore be inferred that the estimated requirements are in excess of true values. As amino acids regulate growth and development, it is possible that consumption in excess could have negative consequences. Garlick (2006) reported the findings of potassium balance studies in young children. Potassium balance is closely correlated with nitrogen balance, and using relevant regression models, it was suggested that the average protein requirement of a 6-month-old would be 1.12 g/kg body weight/day, declining to 0.74 g/kg/day by 10 years.

Provision of fat is an important consideration in the diets of preschool children as fat plays an important role in the provision of energy, maturation of organ systems and maintenance of immune function (Butte, 2005). There are no recommendations regarding the fat intakes of children before the age of 2, but it is estimated that, at this stage, fat should be providing around 50% of total energy. It is suggested that between 2 and 5 years of age, fat should provide a minimum of 15% of dietary energy and ideally between 30 and 40%. Including fat in the

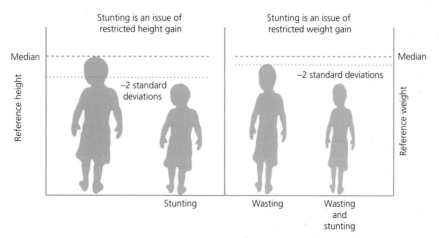

Figure 6.2 Stunting and wasting. Stunting is defined as height which is two standard deviations or more below the median height for age for an appropriate reference population. Wasting is defined as weight which is two standard deviations or more below the weight for age for an appropriate reference population.

diet is important as it is the most effective means of delivering the required energy density of the infant diet. There is good evidence that restricting fat intake can impact adversely upon rates of growth. Fat may be of greater importance in some populations than in others. Children in developing countries generally expend more energy through physical activity and therefore become dependent on fat oxidation as glycogen reserves are rapidly depleted (Prentice and Paul, 2000). Immune cells preferentially use fat oxidation to provide energy for their function; so again, children in developing countries may require more lipid for this purpose, in the face of regular infection. Essential fatty acids give rise to inflammatory mediators and therefore also make a contribution to this role. Long-chain fatty acids such as arachidonic acid and docosahexaenoic acid are required for the growth and maturation of the brain and visual apparatus. Given the rapid growth of the infant brain over the first 5 years, provision of sufficient essential fatty acids of the n-3 and n-6 series is a critical element of a healthy diet for infants.

6.2.2.2 Micronutrients

All of the vitamins and minerals are essential for the growth and well-being of children at this age. Infants are especially vulnerable to the development of deficiency diseases and subclinical deficiencies as they have high nutrient demands and generally low stores of micronutrients. Micronutrients can be limiting factors in the diet, causing growth faltering. Classical studies of children being treated for malnutrition in the Caribbean showed that growth of infants receiving supplemental protein and energy was heavily dependent upon adequate provision of zinc, for example.

Given the high demand for all micronutrients, this text will not focus upon specific requirements in any detail and the reader is advised to consult relevant texts listing dietary reference values for more detailed information (e.g. Department of Health, 1998). However, some nutrients are noteworthy as there are either special guidelines in place or major concerns about the adequacy of their provision to infants. Calcium and vitamin D, for example, are considered important at this time as early growth and mineralization of the skeleton may boost the peak bone mass attained in early adulthood and reduce risk of osteoporosis in later life. Infants should therefore consume good sources of calcium, such as milk, and fortified sources of vitamin D.

Fluoride is important for the formation of the teeth and as a defence against dental caries. Caries are caused by demineralization of apatite in tooth enamel, an effect of organic acid production by bacterial species such as *Streptococcus mutans*. Fluoride supplementation (0.25 mg/ day for under 1-year-olds, 0.5 mg/day for older infants) is recommended where fluoride is not available through other means (see Research Highlight 6.1).

Sodium should be restricted in the diet of infants and young children need to be taught the importance of selecting low-salt foods and not adding salt to meals, either during cooking or at the table. The Scientific Advisory Committee on Nutrition (SACN, 2003) in the United Kingdom issued guidelines for salt intake in the under-fives. Their recommendation was for children under 1 year to consume no more than 1 g salt (400 mg sodium) per day, with this rising to 2 g salt (800 mg sodium) between 2 and 6 years.

6.2.3 Nutrient intakes and infants

The diets of young children are often quite limited in their range and can exclude foods that would actually be ideal for the delivery of the required nutrient and energy density. This limitation may be a product of children's responses to newly introduced foods, a lack of parental knowledge or the use of a limited variety of food items during weaning. The rolling programme of the National Diet and Nutrition Surveys in the United Kingdom has included two large studies of the diets of children (1995 and 2002). The findings of the 2008/2009 and 2009/2010 survey (Bates *et al.*, 2011) showed that among under 11-year-olds, there was high consumption of rice, pasta and cereals, cheese, white bread, biscuits, confectionery, snack foods, fruit juices and soft drinks. Consumption of non-milk extrinsic sugars (free sugar) was above the <11% of energy guidance (14.4% in boys and 14.3% in girls), and more children than expected were consuming vitamin A and zinc at below the LRNI (10% of 4–10-year-old girls had low zinc intakes). Similar trends were also apparent in the subsequent 2011/2012 survey (Bates *et al.*, 2014) which also reported higher than recommended intakes of salt in 4–6-year-olds (mean intake 3.7 g/day). The previous National Diet and Nutrition Surveys have highlighted that young children have low intakes of green leafy vegetables, citrus fruits and eggs (Gregory *et al.*, 2000).

Studies of toddlers (0–2-year-olds) in the United States have also indicated a relatively narrow range of foods as the main staples. Fox *et al.* (2006) found that cereals and milk were the major sources of micronutrients in the diet and that for 1–2-year-olds milk, cheese, bread, chicken and turkey, eggs and fruit juices were the major sources of energy and protein. In developing countries, the range of foods available to infants is generally considerably lower than noted for the developed countries, particularly in impoverished communities and rural areas. Even where choice is limited by overall availability, food-related behaviours of children may limit their

Research Highlight 6.1 Fluoride and dental caries.

Caries

Dental caries, or tooth decay, is the consequence of bacterial infection of the tooth surface. Bacteria are present in the plaque that coats the teeth after ingestion of food and utilize food material for fermentation processes that generate lactic acid, which then demineralizes enamel surface of the teeth. This can produce cavities that will accumulate increasing numbers of bacteria leading to extensive acid erosion. If untreated, the infection will destroy the pulp, leading to loss of the tooth or infection of the tissue of the gum and underlying bone. Caries are highly prevalent in children, with 28% of English 5-year-olds (Public Health England, 2012) and 42% of US 2–11-year-olds (NIDCR, 2014) reported to have experienced caries in their milk teeth. Other countries have much greater problems (e.g. China 55%, Philippines 92%, Peru 79%; Bagramian *et al.*, 2009). Five key factors are associated with risk of caries: *S. mutans* infection, high dietary sucrose intake, frequent consumption of food, low saliva production and low fluoride status.

Effect of fluoride

Enamel is the hard material that makes up the external surface of the tooth. Enamel comprises crystals of hydroxyapatite, which is a mineral with the formula $Ca_5(PO_4)_3(OH)$. Within hydroxyapatite, the hydroxyl groups can be replaced with carbonate, chloride (chloroapatite) or fluoride (fluoroapatite). The formation of fluoroapatite increases resistance to acid erosion and is therefore beneficial in prevention of caries. For this reason, strategies to limit caries in children and adults focus on increasing fluoride intake or topical application of fluoride in toothpastes and dental coatings. Water fluoridation has been one of the most important public health measures designed to combat caries.

Water fluoridation and fluorosis

The addition of fluoride in the form of calcium fluoride to water has been common practice since the 1960s in many countries, including New Zealand, Australia, the United States, Canada and much of South America. In the United States, around 62% of the population consume water containing fluoride at between 0.7 and 1.2 ppm (Truman *et al.*, 2002), but in Europe, the approach is less common. In the United Kingdom, only 10% of the population receive fluoridated water, but local health authorities can implement fluoridation in response to monitoring of dental health among children. In Germany and the Netherlands, fluoridation has been discontinued, and many European nations use fluoridated salt as an alternative route of fortification (Schulte, 2005). Where water fluoridation was introduced in the United States, it is estimated that there were decreases in prevalence of caries of up to 40% over follow-up periods of 3–12 years (Truman *et al.*, 2002). The systematic review of McDonagh *et al.* (2000) suggests that water fluoridation has significant benefits in terms of the numbers of children with caries and the number of decayed, filled and missing teeth among children in fluoridated areas versus non-fluoridated areas. Fluoridation is opposed by many, on the grounds of effectiveness, personal autonomy and safety concerns. The effectiveness of water fluoridation has undoubtedly been lowered by the introduction of fluoridated toothpastes, but in areas where water fluoridation has been withdrawn, the prevalence of caries is noted to increase by around 18% over the subsequent 6–10 years (Truman *et al.*, 2002). Safety concerns have included greater risk of cancer, Alzheimer's disease, Down's syndrome and goitre, but there is no strong evidence to justify these fears (McDonagh *et al.*, 2000). High consumption of fluoride due to the combination of water fluoridation and use of fluoride toothpastes do however result in dental fluorosis which will be present in 48% of the population exposed to fluoridated water. In most cases, fluorosis goes unnoticed beyond white specks in the tooth enamel, but 12% of the population may develop mottling of the tooth enamel, with a rough pitted tooth surface that is difficult to clean.

preferences even further. Lutter and Rivera (2003) noted that among children who were undernourished and growth retarded, up to 25% of food offered was not consumed. Often, foods in these situations are low in fat and lack nutrient density. Fat is important in stimulating the appetite by virtue of its contribution to aroma, flavour and texture of food. Palatability is a particularly important determinant of food intake and choice in children.

Observations that milk is a major source of nutrients in these studies are encouraging. It is generally considered that milk should be a major staple in the diets of infants by virtue of its capacity to deliver a high proportion of required nutrients and energy, either as a drink, as a component of sauces used in cooking or added to breakfast cereals. Consuming 440 ml/day of whole milk will deliver 25–32% of daily energy requirements for a 1–4-year-old and up to 60% of protein requirement and all of the requirements for vitamin A, calcium and several B vitamins (e.g. riboflavin). To maintain energy density and intakes of fat-soluble vitamins, it is suggested that under-fives should consume whole milk but that semi-skimmed milk is acceptable for children over the age of 2 years. The UK National Diet and Nutrition Survey (Bates *et al.*, 2011) showed that milk provided up to 15% of energy and 22% of protein intake of 4–10-year-olds, with the majority consuming semi-skimmed milk.

Vitamin and mineral supplements are often provided to infants by their parents and in the past have been recommended for infants who were breastfed. In a study from the United States, Briefel and colleagues (2006) noted that 16% of children aged 4 months to 2 years were given supplements, with a much greater proportion (31%) between the ages of 1 and 2. Leaf (2007) highlights UK recommendations that younger children should be supplemented with vitamin D, unless consuming fortified sources. The Healthy Start Service operated in this country ensures that supplements are freely available, along with milk, for under-4s from poor families. However, uptake of the scheme has been shown to be low due to lack of awareness among families and poor access to the service (Jessiman *et al.*, 2013). There are some concerns that supplements may be more likely to be provided by better educated and more affluent parents to children who do not really need them. A study from Belgium found high use of supplements among preschool children of highly educated, non-smoking parents. Although for some of this group supplements helped in achieving recommended intakes of vitamin D, intakes of other nutrients such as zinc were excessive (Huybrechts *et al.*, 2010). Briefel *et al.* (2006) found that nutrient intakes were not compromised in infants who did not receive supplements and found excessive intakes of folate, zinc and vitamin A in supplemented children due to the additive effects of supplements on top of fortified food sources.

6.2.4 Transition to an adult pattern of food intake

The infant years are a time of major physical and psychological development and represent an intense period of change to the diet. There are two key changes that occur between 6 months and the age of 5. The first is the process of weaning, which generally results in the child moving from a complete dependence upon milk for all nutrition to a diet that provides most nutrients from non-milk sources by the age of 1 year. The second is a decrease in the energy and nutrient density of the diet as the pattern of intake shifts to include foods that are lower in fat content and richer in complex carbohydrates. Accomplishing the dietary transitions of infancy should be done in such a way that the child learns dietary behaviours that will reduce risk of obesity and related disorders later in his/her life.

6.2.4.1 Complementary feeding

The introduction of complementary feeding (weaning) is the process through which the infant makes the transition from a milk-only diet, whether breast- or formula-fed, to a diet that contains solid foods and non-milk drinks (complementary foods). This is a key developmental milestone that exerts powerful changes in terms of functional changes to the gastrointestinal tract, the immune system and metabolic processes. From a nutritional perspective, the diversification of the diet that accompanies the introduction of complementary foods has profound effects. The weaned infant becomes exposed to a greater range of fatty acids and proteins, and these, and associated micronutrients, must be absorbed from a more varied food matrix. While in early infancy feeding occurs throughout the day and night, with no meal-based pattern, with the introduction of complementary foods, the infant moves to having two to three set meals per day, with snacks in between, and often ceases night feeding. This changes metabolic parameters markedly, producing bigger fluctuations in glucose and insulin concentrations between the fasted and fed states.

Complementary feeding is critical for a number of reasons. First of all, it is essential to ensure that the requirements of the infant for nutrients are met by the dietary supply. Milk is a poor source of certain nutrients, particularly iron, zinc, vitamin D and vitamin A, all of which are essential for the maintenance of normal growth and function. Prior to weaning, the infant, particularly if breastfed, is reliant upon stores of these nutrients that were accrued in the last trimester of pregnancy. These stores are largely depleted by the age of 6 months. The introduction of solid foods also serves to stimulate the development of the reflexes that coordinate biting and chewing with swallowing of food. Weaning is also the transition to a dietary pattern that includes most of the normal range of foods consumed by the mature individual. This process provides a useful opportunity to promote development of food preferences and feeding behaviours that will be associated with good health later in life.

The initiation of complementary feeding can be seen as a hazardous process. In developing countries, the transition from sterile breast milk greatly increases vulnerability of infants to food- and waterborne infection. It can also promote malnutrition, as children from poor communities may be weaned onto low-quality foods that lack essential nutrients, or which cannot provide the necessary energy and nutrient densities. It is this latter point that has prompted the World Health Organization to issue advice relating to weaning, which should ideally be adopted on a global scale. Essentially, parents are advised that all babies should be exclusively breastfed for the first 6 months of life, with no introduction of complementary foods prior to this time. At 6 months, nutritionally adequate complementary foods should be introduced, with continuation of breastfeeding to 2 years of age. This policy is likely to be highly effective in rural populations in developing countries, where access to clean water and uncontaminated foods is difficult. Later weaning reduces the likelihood of diarrhoeal disease and associated mortality and has been shown to have no detriment in terms of the growth of children. In developed countries, however, many have questioned the appropriateness of this advice, which represents a significant shift away from the long-held view that weaning after 4 months but no later than 6 months should be normal practice (Fewtrell, 2011). The current view is that the timing of weaning should ideally correspond with the World Health Organization advice but that health professionals should give flexible advice to parents, on a case-by-case basis (Foote and Marriott, 2003). This affirms the view of Lanigan *et al.* (2001) who suggested that delaying weaning until 6 months had no clear detrimental effect on infant growth but that there were subgroups in the population that would benefit from earlier introduction of complementary foods. Essentially, larger, more rapidly growing babies are likely to need weaning at an earlier stage than their smaller counterparts. It has also been argued that babies who may be at risk of allergy due to an atopic family history should be weaned between 4 and 6 months (Anderson and Dinulos, 2009). Guidelines on the approach to weaning are presented in Table 6.3, and Research Highlight 6.2 discusses the relationship between weaning and childhood obesity.

In most developed countries, weaning earlier than 6 months of age is the norm. The UK Infant Feeding Survey 2010 (Health and Social Care Information Centre, 2012) found that although fewer babies were introduced to solids before 4 months of age (30%) than in 2005 (51%), 75% of babies had been fed solids by the age of 5 months. Introduction of solids before 6 months was more common where mothers were of low income and was less prevalent among ethnic minority groups than in white Caucasian families. Older mothers were more likely to delay introduction of solids beyond 4 months. Confusion created by two changes in guidance over a 10-year period has been an issue for parents, and many reject the advice of health professionals (Moore *et al.*, 2012) and make use of possibly unreliable Internet-based sources to inform judgements about timing and pattern of introduction of complementary foods (Figure 6.3).

Complementary feeding with solids prior to 4 months of age is not advisable and may be detrimental to the health of the child. Prior to this age, most babies are unable to masticate and swallow solids safely and are therefore at risk of choking. Moreover, the immaturity of the kidneys and gastrointestinal tract presents a significant hazard. The introduction of solid foods increases the quantity of nitrogen and solutes delivered to the body. This can overwhelm the excretory capacity of the

Table 6.3 Complementary feeding stages.

	First introduction 17–26 weeks	26–30 weeks	30–39 weeks	40–52 weeks
Foods to introduce*	Baby rice, ground oat porridge, cooked starchy vegetables, banana, cooked fruit	Meat, fish, poultry Noodles, pasta Full fat yoghurt, custard, fromage frais, cheese, well-cooked eggs	Well-cooked shellfish Raw soft vegetables Raw soft fruit, citrus fruit	
Food preparation	Pureed with milk	Finely mashed and mixed with milk	Mashed with small lumps. Provide finger foods	Chopped, minced family foods, with finger foods
Frequency	A few teaspoons once per day	Two solid feeds per day	Three solid feeds per day	Aim for three to four servings of starchy foods and three to four servings of fruits and vegetables, with two servings of protein-rich foods per day
Foods to avoid	Foods with high salt, added salt in cooking and serving, foods with high sugar content, low-fat foods, honey, whole nuts, unpasteurized dairy products			

In the early stages of weaning, foods should be pureed or mashed mixed with either breast milk or an appropriate formula to give an easily swallowed texture and consistency. Finger foods are easily handled food items that babies can pick up and convey to the mouth, for example, bite-sized pieces of fruit. This encourages biting, chewing and swallowing, along with independent feeding and developing coordination skills.
*Foods which are highly allergenic (wheat products, eggs, fish, shellfish, foods containing nuts) may be introduced at any time but should be given one at a time with a gap of 2–3 days in between to monitor for a reaction.

Research Highlight 6.2 Weaning and the risk of childhood obesity.

With rising prevalence of childhood obesity, there has been considerable interest in the possibility that elements of the early diet may be risk factors for adiposity in childhood. Early complementary feeding may be one such risk factor for childhood obesity. Brophy et al. (2009) reported that in the UK Millennium Cohort, children who had been weaned before 3 months of age were more likely to be obese at age 5 years (OR for obesity 1.2 [1.02–1.5]). A US study found that delaying weaning reduced the risk of childhood obesity by 0.1% for every month delay beyond 4 months (Hediger et al., 2001). In contrast, studies of the ALSPAC and Southampton Women's study cohorts in the United Kingdom reported no association between age at introduction of complementary feeding and childhood obesity (Reilly et al., 2005; Robinson et al., 2009). Most of the literature showing effects of timing of weaning upon subsequent obesity, however, comprises small studies with poor adjustment for confounding effects of breastfeeding exposure, maternal education, socio-economic status and birth weight, all of which are also related to obesity. The systematic review of Pearce et al. (2013) concluded that the timing of the introduction of complementary foods has no clear association with childhood obesity, although very early introduction of solid foods (≤4 months of age) may result in higher childhood BMI.

The types of food used in weaning may also influence infant weight gain and hence the development of adiposity and obesity. Several studies have considered the impact of protein intake during infancy but appear to show that it is the level of protein in the diet in the second year of life rather than the weaning diet which is important. Günther et al. (2007a, b) reported that infants with high intakes of protein, and in particular meat and dairy protein at 12 months, had higher BMI at age 7, but these studies are contradicted by others (Hoppe et al., 2004). One study found that a high energy intake at 4 months was associated with higher BMI and body fatness at age 5, but only in formula-fed infants (Ong et al., 2006). The risk of overweight (BMI over the 85th centile) was 25% greater for every 100 kcal/day increase in energy intake. The systematic review of Pearce and Langley-Evans (2013) found limited but suggestive evidence that complementary feeding may be related to childhood adiposity but that specific foods were less important than adherence to current guidelines on making the transition from milk to consumption of healthy family meals.

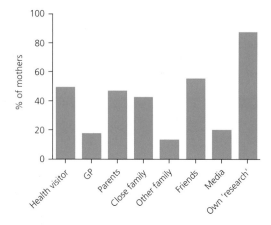

Figure 6.3 A UK survey of 474 mothers of young infants showed that the most trusted source of advice on when and how to introduced complementary foods was their 'own research', which included accessing Internet articles and reading books. General practitioners were the least trusted source of information (Spray and Langley-Evans, unpublished data).

kidneys, promoting dehydration. The immature gut does not produce the full range of pancreatic and intestinal secretions, so solid food may remain undigested in the gut for longer periods. This can promote gastroenteritis and damage to the lining of the tract. Moreover, the immature gut is more permeable and will allow larger proteins to cross into systemic circulation. This can promote allergic sensitization.

Late weaning (i.e. beyond 6 months of age) may also be a cause for concern. This is more likely to be associated with certain ethnic subgroups in the population. In the UK Infant Feeding Survey 2000 (Hamlyn et al., 2002), it was noted that mothers from Asian backgrounds were most likely to delay weaning and in some Muslim communities the first stage of weaning involved a switch to whole cow's milk, accompanied by lengthy use of convenience weaning foods. In developing countries, later weaning reduces morbidity and mortality among infants, but where infectious disease is not a major issue, it is of greater concern that late-weaned infants may become malnourished due to depletion of nutrient stores.

The introduction of complementary foods should be accomplished gradually and the full process of weaning will typically take 6 months. Throughout that time, milk should remain a key part of the diet. Feeds of breast milk or appropriate follow-on formula should continue, with both later being used for drinks and mixing with solid foods. Weaning foods must be prepared to a consistency that is appropriate to the neuromuscular development of the child (Table 6.3). This means that initially foods need to be pureed and should contain no lumps that may cause choking. Over time, this should give way to mashed and finely chopped food and eventually to normal family foods. To help children become familiar with biting and chewing and the conveyance of food from hand to mouth, it is suggested that children of around 6 months of age should be given 'finger foods', which might be pieces of bread, rusks, biscuits, fruit or raw vegetables. The first foods during weaning have more to do with giving the baby the experience of food and portion sizes and meal frequency are not a consideration. To aid acceptance of food and to avoid these early experiences displacing nutrients from milk, solids should be offered to the child immediately after a milk feed.

The foods that should be used in weaning can generally be normal family foods that have been prepared to suit the stage of the child, as described earlier. A key part of the process is providing the child with a varied range of flavours, textures and aromas as this should help with acceptance of a broad range of foods later in life. Most parents introduce new foods one at a time in order to check whether any might produce an adverse reaction. The energy density of the food needs to be high (more than 4.2 kJ/g food) and the salt content should be low. If the diet does not include meat, then an alternative source of iron (generally fortified cereals) should be included. Infants require a diet that is low in phytate to maximize the absorption of micronutrients. Foods that are at risk of being infected with pathogens, for example, unpasteurized soft cheeses, raw or only lightly cooked eggs and pate, should be avoided. The introduction of foods that are commonly associated with food allergy in children (eggs, milk, soya, wheat, peanuts) can proceed at any stage of weaning but with close and careful monitoring for reactions following first use.

There are a vast range of commercially available weaning foods. These certainly do not disadvantage infant growth and development and their major downside is their expense. As these foods are formulated in a way that ensures they meet with regulations on salt and provision of a balanced nutrient content, they may to some extent be superior to home-made foods used in early weaning. For example, many babies' first experience of food may be pureed fruit. This has inadequate energy and nutrient density and a better choice would be a milk-based nonwheat porridge or baby cereal. In many developing countries, the move of populations from rural to urban areas is increasing the proportion of food that is purchased rather than grown, particularly in Latin America and the Caribbean. This provides an opportunity to address some of the problems of malnutrition that are associated with weaning onto inadequate diets. Lutter and Dewey (2003) proposed the development of a low-cost fortified processed complementary food that could be introduced into such areas and ensure an adequate energy and nutrient intake.

In the United Kingdom, the practice of baby-led weaning has become popular among middle–high-income families. Baby-led weaning involves allowing the child to self-feed from the first introduction of solids. There is no use of spoons and no requirement to puree or mash foods. Providing finger foods is supposed to encourage babies to experiment with textures and flavours and to develop skills required for self-feeding. Although popular, there is a very limited evidence base on which to judge the potential benefits and safety of baby-led weaning. Townsend and Pitchford (2012) reported that baby-led weaning reduced the prevalence of obesity among children aged 20–78 months. However, this study controlled poorly for social confounders and breastfeeding exposure. Mothers who adopt baby-led weaning are also more likely to breastfeed and to follow the 6-month guidance on introduction of solids (Brown and Lee, 2011). Cameron and colleagues (2013) reported that the majority of parents reporting to be following a baby-led approach were not actually doing so in a strict manner. This would make interpretation of any published studies problematic.

6.2.4.2 Nutrition-related problems

Infants are vulnerable to micronutrient deficiencies, which are often not detected until at an advanced stage. This vulnerability arises in part due to a lack of extensive reserves of nutrients but also due to factors that impact upon nutrient intakes, nutrient losses and the bioavailability of nutrients. Nutrient intake is most often compromised due to poverty but may also arise because children are provided with an insufficiently varied diet. For example, in many parts of the world, children will live on rice as a staple food, which is often not adequately complemented by other nutrient sources. Rice is a poor source of vitamin A, and as a consequence, vitamin A deficiency becomes rife among children in these regions. Cooking methods or food processing that leaches nutrients from raw food ingredients may also limit the nutrient supply to children. Losses of nutrients via the kidneys or digestive tract may be a consequence of infectious disease. Infection and chronic disease processes can lead to malabsorption of micronutrients. For example, children with cystic fibrosis are vulnerable to deficiencies of fat-soluble vitamins due to the accumulation of mucous in the digestive tract. Foods that are rich in phytates, as are commonly used in weaning in some cultures, limit the bioavailability of micronutrients. In addition, short-term periods of malnutrition, for example, following repeated episodes of infection, will stimulate catch-up growth. This rapid growth may increase demands for micronutrients beyond the capacity of the diet to supply them.

6.2.4.2.1 Zinc deficiency

Zinc deficiency is difficult to detect as it has few clinical signs and biochemical assessment of zinc status is far from straightforward. It is estimated that zinc deficiency may occur in one-third of the world population (Shamah and Villalpando, 2006) and in children it will impair growth, immune function and brain development. Zinc deficiency is most commonly seen in children who do not eat meat, either by virtue of cultural background or due to poverty, and where the diet is rich in cereal fibre (containing phytic acid; Figure 6.4). Zinc deficiency can also arise as a consequence of diarrhoeal disease, which increases losses. Zinc is a major component of digestive enzymes secreted into the small intestine, and so maintaining zinc status is dependent upon reuptake from the gut. Reuptake of zinc is impaired by gastrointestinal infection. Although clinically relevant zinc deficiency is mostly seen in developing countries, low intakes of zinc during childhood are also a cause for concern in more affluent populations (Cowin and Emmett, 2007; Bates *et al.*, 2011).

Zinc is a prerequisite for growth as it is required for the synthesis of DNA during cell replication. Growth faltering is therefore the main clinical indicator of deficiency. Zinc is also essential for brain development during infancy, partly due to the need for cell division during brain growth but also because zinc is required for neurotransmitter release. There are reports that zinc deficiency may be associated with poor cognitive development, but the balance of evidence suggests that it mostly limits the motor skills of infants. Supplementation of children with zinc deficiency increases their activity and ability to explore the world, possibly increasing their ability to exploit learning opportunities in their environment (Black, 2003). Animal studies indicate that zinc deficiency impairs development of the frontal lobes of the brain and the cerebellum. These are important areas in determining memory (Georgieff, 2007).

The immune function of zinc-deficient children is impaired, increasing their vulnerability to infectious diseases. In some parts of the world, diarrhoeal infection is considered to be a symptom of deficiency (Calder and Jackson, 2000). Osendarp *et al.* (2002) reported that supplementation of Bangladeshi infants with 5 mg/day zinc between 4 and 24 weeks of age produced better weight gains and reduced the risk of respiratory infection by 70%. These benefits were confined to the children who were zinc deficient at baseline. Ten milligram per day zinc supplements given to Indian under-5s over a 4-month period were shown by Bhandari and colleagues (2002) to reduce the occurrence of diarrhoea, the duration of episodes of diarrhoea and the recurrence of diarrhoea. As diarrhoeal infection is a major cause of infant death in such populations, this has important public health implications.

6.2.4.2.2 Vitamin D deficiency

Poor vitamin D status is commonplace among children, with deficiency defined as a circulating concentration of 25-hydroxy-vitamin D below 50 nmol/l and insufficiency as a concentration between 50 and 100 nmol/l. Clinically, vitamin D deficiency manifests as rickets in children who are undergoing rapid growth. Rickets is characterized by soft, malleable bones that in weight-bearing locations become deformed. This gives deficient children a characteristic bow-leggedness. Rickets also causes swelling of joints and of the skull. Although easily avoided through supplementation, or consumption of fortified sources, rickets and vitamin D insufficiency continues to occur in children in Northern latitudes with low levels of sunlight during the winter months. Gordon and colleagues (2008) reported vitamin D deficiency in 12% of a population of American toddlers, and Absoud *et al.* (2011) found that 35.1% of a population of UK 4–17-year-olds were deficient. The National Diet and Nutrition Survey in the United Kingdom reported that 7.5% of 1.5–3-year-olds had 25-hydroxy-vitamin D concentrations below 25 nmol/l (Bates *et al.*, 2014). High prevalence of deficiency and insufficiency are also noted in sunnier climates, with 22% deficiency

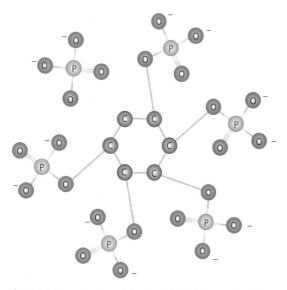

Figure 6.4 The structure of phytic acid. Phytates are found in many cereals and legumes, where they occur bound to proteins and starches. The phosphate groups of phytic acid are able to chelate cations, and as a result, phytate in the gut will reduce bioavailability of minerals such as zinc, calcium and magnesium.

reported in the Northern Territory of Australia (Dyson *et al.*, 2014) and 58.8% deficiency in the winter months in Algeria (Djennane *et al.*, 2014). In the United Kingdom and northern Europe, deficiency is most common in the Asian population (Shaw and Pal, 2002) where it is a product of low synthesis within the skin due to dark pigmentation, low skin exposure to sunlight due to wearing of traditional clothing and the consumption of foods rich in phytate. This limits calcium absorption and hence the response to vitamin D. Infants may also be prone to vitamin D deficiency due to limited transfer from their mothers. Poor vitamin D status is near universal among Asian adults in northern countries during the winter months, and for many women, this is not fully redressed in the summer. During pregnancy, competition for vitamin D between mother and fetus may limit transfer to fetal tissues, and this may be exacerbated postnatally through low vitamin D concentrations in breast milk.

6.2.4.2.3 Iron deficiency

Iron deficiency is the most common micronutrient deficiency in children. It is rarely seen in infants under the age of 4 months due to accrual of iron of maternal origin in the fetal period. Beyond 4 months, the rapid growth of infants means that requirements for iron can often outstrip supply from breast milk and foods used in weaning. The introduction of unmodified cow's milk to the diet between 6 and 12 months of age increases the risk of iron deficiency in infants, and this may stem from gastrointestinal blood losses triggered by the presence of cow's milk proteins (Booth and Aukett, 1997).

Iron deficiency anaemia in young children has a number of adverse consequences. It is more common in children from poor families and in the developed countries is most often seen in children from ethnic minorities. In the United Kingdom, for example, Asian children are most at risk as they are more likely to be weaned onto vegetarian diets (providing iron in the less well-absorbed nonheme form) or to be breastfed for an extended period. Iron deficiency slows the growth of children and increases their susceptibility to infectious disease. The mechanisms through which iron deficiency suppresses immune function are unclear and may involve effects on the metabolism of other nutrients such as vitamin A (Muñoz *et al.*, 2000). Iron-deficient children have impaired capacity to produce T cells and their phagocytes are less active. Although iron supplements can reverse these impairments of immunity, care needs to be taken in any intervention programme to support populations where deficiency is common. Iron is utilized by pathogens as well as host tissues. Although some studies show that treating iron deficiency can reduce infant morbidity and mortality, others show increased infection following supplementation of children (Calder and Jackson, 2000). The parasite responsible for malaria, for example, depends on erythrocytes to complete its life cycle. In malarial areas, iron deficiency anaemia has a protective effect and supplementation of children has to be targeted outside the malarial season. Sazawal *et al.* (2006) showed that in a high malaria risk population in East Africa, supplements of iron (12.5 mg/day), folate (50 µg/day) and zinc (10 mg/day) increased prevalence of malaria infection, hospitalization and malarial death.

Iron deficiency anaemia is associated with developmental delay in preschool children, as it interferes with growth of the brain. In contrast to zinc deficiency, which impacts mainly upon motor development, iron deficiency has a detrimental effect upon the capacity to learn (Booth and Aukett, 1997). Children with iron deficiency have low developmental scores and poor ability to process information and are less happy, more wary and more dependent upon their mothers for social support (Lozoff *et al.*, 2006). While long-term iron supplementation can overcome many of the developmental problems associated with deficiency, some consequences may be longer lasting. Animal studies suggest that during periods of brain development and maturation, iron deficiency impacts upon expression of tyrosine hydroxylase and tryptophan hydroxylase. These are enzymes involved in the synthesis of the neurotransmitters dopamine and serotonin, respectively (Lozoff *et al.*, 2006). Reduced expression during critical developmental stages appears to change densities of dopaminergic and serotonergic neurones in brain regions such as the substantia nigra. Congdon *et al.* (2012) reported that brain activity in 10-year-old children who had suffered from iron deficiency anaemia was different to that of children who had not, even after anaemia had been successfully treated. Changes during development may not be corrected later in life so any functional deficits may be irreversible. A range of studies suggest that low haemoglobin concentrations between 6 and 9 months of age may be predictive of lower IQ at ages up to 9 years. Lozoff *et al.* (2013) reported that the educational achievement and some emotional and social indices remained lower in young adults who had suffered chronic iron deficiency anaemia as infants (Figure 6.5).

6.2.4.2.4 Food additives and hyperactivity

While micronutrient deficiencies present a significant threat to the health and development of very young children, there is also concern that the use of food colourings, preservatives and flavourings may also impact

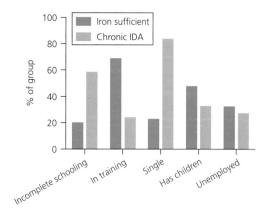

Figure 6.5 Iron deficiency anaemia has long-term effects on cognitive development and life opportunities. Costa Rican 25-year-olds who had either been chronically iron deficient (IDA) or iron sufficient in infancy were more likely to have failed to complete secondary school, were less likely to be in training during early adulthood and were more likely to be unmarried. *Source*: Lozoff *et al.* (2013).

upon well-being. These agents are commonly used in processed foods and especially those that are marketed at children, for example, fizzy drinks, sweets and frozen ready meals. There has been concern since the 1970s that artificial colourings, in particular, may be associated with hyperactive behaviour (i.e. impulsiveness, overactivity, poor attention span).

There is now little doubt that in some children who have a confirmed diagnosis of attention deficit hyperactivity disorder (ADHD), restriction of the diet to exclude artificial colourings and other additives can improve behaviour (Kemp, 2008). A meta-analysis by Nigg *et al.* (2012) suggested that 8% of children with ADHD may benefit from a restricted diet with no artificial colourings. Whether the additives have a causal role in the development of hyperactive disorders in otherwise normally behaved children is unclear. Meta-analyses show that almost all effects of additives on behaviour are restricted to children with ADHD and there is little robust evidence to suggest any impact upon the broader population (Schab and Trinh, 2004). However, debate in this area was fuelled by the findings of a double-blind randomized placebo trial in two groups of children aged 3 and 9 years (McCann *et al.*, 2007). When 3-year-olds were given either a placebo or one of two mixtures of additives, it was shown that children receiving a mixture of sodium benzoate, sunset yellow, carmoisine, tartrazine and Ponceau 4R exhibited more hyperactive behaviours over the subsequent week. In contrast, a randomized controlled trial of artificial colourings and sodium benzoate concluded

that these agents had no impact upon behaviour in a group of 8–9-year-olds (Lok *et al.*, 2013).

6.2.4.3 Barriers to healthy nutrition

As described earlier, infants are vulnerable to a number of nutrition-related problems. These often arise due to a lack of parental knowledge and understanding of what constitutes a balanced diet or due to disease and other organic causes. While these nutrition-related problems are relatively uncommon in developed countries, the majority of parents express the concern that the diets their very young children consume are not healthy. This may be a misperception arising because parents do not understand that the diet that is optimal for an infant is very different to that which would be recommended for an adult. The snacks that infants depend upon are perceived as a negative element of the diet and fussy eating behaviours, which are common in infants, also cause parents a lot of concern. Although many parental worries are unfounded, modern society does impose genuine barriers to developing healthy nutrition and food-related behaviours in young children.

6.2.4.3.1 Faddy eating

In developed countries, most parents of children below the age of 5 will readily voice concerns about the quality and quantity of nutrients in their children's diets. These are often only perceived problems and are generally not backed up by hard evidence of growth faltering or other manifestations of undernutrition. The negative perceptions of parents are explained by two common food-related behaviours in young children: food neophobia and faddy (picky) eating.

Food neophobia is an inherent trait seen in most children that may well have evolved in order to prevent poisoning. Essentially, it involves the rejection of foods that have not been previously encountered (Dovey *et al.*, 2008). Neophobic behaviour is at a low level around the time of weaning, when children are very open to experimentation with flavours and textures, but steadily increases thereafter, reaching a peak between the ages of 2 and 6 years. It has been suggested that neophobia occurs, as children are especially averse to bitter tastes. Most of the foods rejected by neophobic children are fruits and vegetables, and these often contain chemicals that have a bitter tang that is no longer perceived by the more mature adult palate. However, much of the food neophobia response appears to be based in the visual domain. In other words, children appear to reject foods that do not look right and cannot be persuaded to taste the items and confirm their negative assessment. It may well be that this rejection is based upon previous taste experience. For example, a green food (e.g. Brussels sprouts) might be tasted in early infancy and found unpleasant, and thereafter all green foods are rejected on the basis that they will be similarly unpalatable.

Most food neophobia disappears by the time the child reaches early adolescence, and repeated exposures to food items will generally result in their acceptance. Social influences are important. Acceptance of novel food items is more likely to occur if the child is in the company of a group of other people who are also consuming that foodstuff (Dovey *et al.*, 2008). At this age, this is most likely to be other family members, but as the circle of friends of the same age begins to grow, 'peer pressure' may help to bring an end to neophobic behaviours.

Food neophobia, when combined with the growing independence of the preschool child, can be a trigger for faddy eating behaviours and make mealtimes an area of tension within families. Faddy or picky eating is best defined as a behaviour pattern in which a child either refuses to eat or will only eat a limited range of foods. It is perhaps best regarded as a flexing of muscle and a testing of developing powers of communication and control of the behaviour of other family members. Young children crave attention of any sort from their parents and other caregivers, and mealtimes provide an ideal opportunity to gain that attention. By refusing to eat, children can gain a response from an adult and become the centre of attention.

Faddy eating behaviours are highly unpredictable and variable. Some children demonstrate a good appetite but only for a limited range of foods, while others may consume a broad range of foods but only intermittently. A food that appears to be the favourite of a child on 1 day may be rejected out of hand the next. Even within a mealtime, a display of temper and refusal to eat may give way to normal eating of a full portion if the child is somehow distracted. Wright and colleagues (2007) found that 8% of parents of 30-month-old children reported faddy eating behaviours. The responses of the parents were often to try and mollify children by providing rewards for eating their meals and offering alternatives to the rejected food items or distract the children by providing television during mealtimes. These are generally considered inappropriate responses to faddy eating, as in effect they reward and reinforce the behaviour. An angry response accompanied by punishment is also inappropriate. The best response to faddy eating is to ignore the behaviour and to try and encourage eating by making mealtimes into pleasant, social occasions in which normal eating is praised.

It has generally been assumed that faddy eating, except in extreme forms, has little impact upon the nutritional status of infants. Children will often put on a

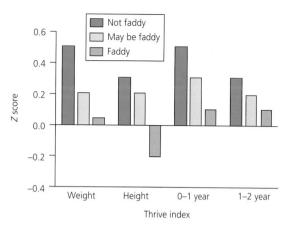

Figure 6.6 Faddy eating has no major effect on the growth of infants. No statistically significant differences in weight or height among 455 British infants aged 30 months were noted when they were classified by parental report of faddy eating. Thrive Index is a measure of growth over a year.
Source: Wright *et al.* (2007).

'performance' to gain attention at one meal per day and then compensate for any lost intake through other meals and snacks throughout the rest of the day. Indeed, there is little evidence that faddy eaters are more prone to growth faltering despite their apparently limited range of preferred foods (Figure 6.6; Wright *et al.*, 2007). Galloway and colleagues (2003), however, reported that the altered patterns of food intake that are associated with faddy eating can impact upon nutrient intakes. Girls who were faddy eaters tended to consume less fruits and vegetables and hence have lower intakes of fibre, folate, ascorbate and vitamin E and compensated for lower food intakes by consuming more fat.

The role of parents in managing both food neophobia and faddy eating is critical and, as in many aspects of promoting healthy eating to children, the simplest approach is to lead through positive examples. The study of Galloway *et al.* (2003) noted that girls were more likely to consume fruits and vegetables if they observed their mothers doing so. This agrees with the findings of Cooke *et al.* (2004) who reported that among nursery school children, parental consumption of fruits and vegetables was the major predictor of fruit and vegetable intakes.

6.2.4.3.2 Poverty

Child poverty is the major cause of malnutrition and associated disease and death among the under-5s. It is rife on a global scale and UNICEF estimates that more than a billion children live in conditions that are unacceptable, with poor housing, limited sanitation and chronic food insecurity. The alleviation of child poverty is one of the key Millennium Development Goals set out by the United Nations in 2005. Poverty is not limited to the developing countries of the world. High rates are noted in developed regions and in some of the most affluent countries of the world (Figure 6.7), and this poverty has a significant impact upon the nutrition of infants and older children.

Poverty is defined using a variety of different measures. The UN Millennium project uses an income of less than US$1/day to define unacceptable poverty. Although more than half of children living in developing countries live in such conditions, there are estimated to be in excess of 50 million European children living in poverty by this measure, mostly centred in Russia, the former republics of the Soviet Union and the Balkan states (Bulgaria, Romania). The less than US$1/day definition is unrealistic as a tool for measuring poverty in richer countries, and instead poverty tends to be defined as living on an income that is less than half of the median income for the national population. As can be seen in Figure 6.7, using this definition, poverty rates among families are very high and more than 1 in 10 children is likely to be affected in the developed nations. There are major variations in poverty levels depending on ethnicity and regions within countries. In the United States, for example, 22% of children live below the Federal Poverty Level (US$23550/year for a family of four). The highest rates of US child poverty are seen in rural counties of the southern states (28% of children, compared to 17% in urban areas), with some communities in South Dakota and Mississippi having child poverty rates between 60 and 70%. US children are more likely to live in poverty if they are black American or native American. Similarly, poverty rates are highest in immigrant populations and among indigenous peoples of Canada. In the United Kingdom, it is estimated that 3.5 million children (27% of children) are raised in poverty, with much higher rates (40–50%) seen in parts of London, the North West region, Midlands and Northern Ireland. Again, ethnic minorities, particularly Asians, are most affected (Child Poverty Action Group, 2014). For many of these affected families, poverty may be borderline or short term, but significant numbers of children live in households where substantial meals may not be provided on at least 1 day each fortnight and where meat or suitable vegetarian alternatives are available only on every other day (EU-SILC, 2007).

The impact of poverty on the nutrition and health and young children is well documented. Nelson (2000) reported important differences in the pattern of diet consumed by 1–5-year-olds from socially deprived families compared to other children. The children from poor backgrounds consumed more white bread and sugar-coated cereals, more fatty food (pies, pastries, fried food, chips) and less fruit, vegetables, meat and poultry. Their diets contained more salt, more fat and less iron, calcium, iodine, β-carotene and vitamin C. Food insecurity associated with poverty impacted upon diets of 3-year-olds in Southampton, United Kingdom (Pilgrim *et al.*, 2012). Infants from poor families consumed less vegetables, more chips, more white bread and more processed meats than those from food-secure homes. Sausenthaler *et al.* (2007) reported that 2-year-olds whose parents were on low incomes and who had lower educational achievement consumed more hydrogenated vegetable fats and less milk, less fresh fruit and cooked vegetables. Food insecurity is greater where children do no have access to safety nets such as the US School Breakfast Program (Bartfeld and Ahn, 2011). Children from poor backgrounds suffer from a greater number of dental caries and have slower rates of recovery from infection (Nelson, 2000). They are more likely to be obese (Freedman *et al.*, 2007) and to suffer from specific nutrient deficiencies, such as iron deficiency anaemia (Booth and Aukett, 1997).

Attempts to combat child poverty on a global scale have had limited success. The Millennium Development Goal to halve world hunger by 2015 is doomed to failure. Although child hunger has been reduced in Latin America, South and Southeast Asia and North Africa, there has been insufficient progress or increase in hunger in sub-Saharan Africa, the west of Asia and Oceania (UN, 2013). Achieving improvements in developing

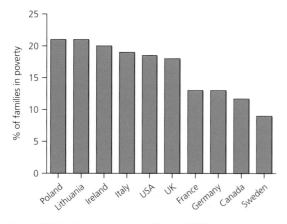

Figure 6.7 Social deprivation in children. Within developed countries, poverty is defined as a family income below 50% of the population median wage. Levels of poverty experienced by children are variable throughout the developed countries, generally being highest in eastern and southern Europe. Data shown represents figures for the period 2002–2007.

countries depends upon cooperation between national governments, non-governmental organizations and aid agencies. In the developed countries, tackling child poverty and the impact this has on nutrition in the short and long term is a matter for national governments. A number of strategies can be considered as a means to ensure that all children are adequately fed. One approach would be to provide more food directly to children. The US School Breakfast Program (see Section 6.3.3) does this, through provision of free or low-cost breakfasts and lunches to children from low-income families. In the United Kingdom, the government introduced a scheme to provide free school meals to all children aged 4–7 in 2014, which supplements the existing provision of free school meals to children whose families claim certain state benefits. While this is feasible with school-age children (e.g. by providing free school milk and meals), it is more problematic for the preschool infant. Establishing breakfast clubs and the provision of milk and healthy snacks in nurseries and playgroups are approaches that can provide poor children with at least one nutritious meal per day. Providing food through state-sponsored interventions can be very effective. Schemes such as the School Breakfast Program help to reduce family concerns about food and remove some households from marginal food insecurity (Bartfeld and Ahn, 2011). Alternatively, governments can increase the money available to poor families by increasing benefits and reducing taxation. Kukrety (2007) advocates direct transfers of cash from governments to families as a means of helping households cope with either short-term financial crises or chronic poverty. This is an approach often used in humanitarian aid, and experience in Asia and Africa shows that families spend a high proportion of such money on food. In some states, this approach is done in a way that ensures money can only be spent on food, for example, by issuing food vouchers (Nelson, 2000). Implicit in this are a lack of trust in families and the view that they will waste the money on non-essential items. All the evidence suggests that making provision of money conditional is unnecessary and that most poor families are very efficient in budgeting and targeting funds at essential items such as food (Kukrety, 2007). In the United Kingdom, low-income families with children under 4 are eligible for Healthy Start vouchers, which can be spent on milk, fruits and vegetables. Healthy Start vouchers improve the quantity and range of fruit and vegetable consumption by families but can be challenging to apply for and are only usable in registered retailers and their value does not keep up with rising food prices (McFadden et al., 2014). Similar schemes exist elsewhere and are shown to be effective in improving food purchases. A New Zealand study by Smith et al. (2013) found that families provided with vouchers increased their total spend on food but that vouchers did not influence the types of foods purchased.

6.2.4.3.3 The impact of advertising

The advertisement of unhealthy foods and beverages to children is a significant negative influence that works against the efforts of parents, health professionals and educators to promote the establishment of healthy eating and behaviours in children. Preschool children are avid watchers of television and are increasingly exposed to movies in cinemas and unregulated media such as the Internet. For children under the age of 5, there is little perception of the difference between advertisements and the actual programme content they are watching. This makes them an ideal and particularly receptive audience for the advertising of a range of items, including food and drink. Although these infants are not in direct control of food purchasing in a household, they can very effectively influence parental choices through demanding behaviour.

The budgets available to spend on advertising of food and drink are staggering and make the sums allocated for health education and health promotion pale into insignificance. In the United States alone, food and drink companies spend $10 billion/year on advertising of products aimed specifically at children (Robinson et al., 2007). In contrast, the annual budget of the World Health Organization for all of its varied activities is $4.5 billion. Neville and colleagues (2005) monitored Australian television networks and found that there were 8.2 advertisements for food and drink per hour of broadcasting, of which 55% were for foods that were high in fat and sugar. Half of these advertisements were placed during programming aimed at children. In contrast, only 0.1% of food advertising was for fruits and vegetables. Food and beverage advertising is also appearing on the Internet and sites that allow children access to free games and cartoons generally advertise confectionary and fast-food restaurants such as McDonald's (Alvy and Calvert, 2008). Much of the literature that evaluates the impact this has on children's food choices and health is focused upon older children and generally shows a detrimental influence. Dixon et al. (2007) found that among children aged between 10 and 12, television advertising produced more positive attitudes towards junk foods and was associated with greater consumption of such items. Kopelman et al. (2007) noted very high recognition of brands in 9–11-year-olds. Overweight children have been shown to have better brand recognition than appropriate weight children (Keller et al., 2012).

It is becoming clear that the preschool child is also susceptible to advertising messages and this may be more insidious due to the critical impact that this stage of life has upon future health behaviours. Goris and colleagues (2010) estimated that in the United States, as much as 40% of childhood obesity risk may be explained by exposure to food advertising. Advertisers use branding of products to increase recognition. Associating positive messages with a brand is designed to gain lifelong customers (Connor, 2006). By the age of 2, children are already able to recognize well-advertised food brands and have certain value beliefs attached to those brands (Robinson *et al.*, 2007). Two- to six-year-olds are aware of brand names and have strong recognition of logos and packaging. Advertisement of brands and logos is a widely used tactic in the battle to gain very young children as customers. Connor (2006) found that on commercial children's channels in the United States, 96 half-hour blocks of programming contained 130 advertisements for food and drink, of which half were for fast-food outlets and sugar-coated cereals and aimed directly at the children. Advertisers frequently associate cartoon characters, sports personalities and superheroes with brands and children in this age group are adept at linking the characters to the brands. In an experiment with children aged between 2 and 6 years, Borzekowski and Robinson (2001) showed that when exposed to just 30 s of brand advertising within a 30 min session of watching cartoons, children were up to three times more likely to choose a branded item when it was offered alongside an identical product presented in similar but unbranded packaging. Similarly, when 3–5-year-olds were offered a choice of identical foods but with one item packaged plainly and the other in McDonald's branded materials, they were up to six times more likely to choose the branded item (Robinson *et al.*, 2007). When offered branded or equivalent unbranded meals, 4–6-year-old girls consumed significantly more energy with the branded meal (732 ± 199 kcal vs 632 ± 197 kcal; Keller *et al.*, 2012). Exposure to snack food advertising can impact upon the quantity and type of foods consumed by children during television viewing, showing an immediate effect in addition to the brand-loyalty effect (Figure 6.8; Halford *et al.*, 2007).

Finding solutions to this problem will not be easy, particularly with the growth of the Internet, which crosses national borders and therefore largely escapes robust legislation. Ustjanauskas *et al.* (2014) reported that Internet sites specifically aimed at children hosted 3.4 billion food advertisements, of which 84% were for foods high in fat, sugar and sodium. Given the ready acceptance of branding and logos by very young children, it may be opportune to use this high exposure to

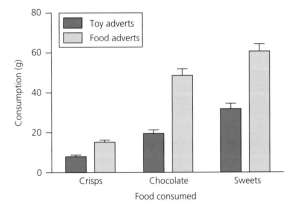

Figure 6.8 Advertising impacts upon the snacking habits of children. Infants were exposed to 30 min of cartoons with advertisements for either toys or snack foods. With free access to a range of snacks, the exposure to food adverts increased consumption. *Source*: Halford *et al.* (2007).

advertising messages in a positive manner, for example, branding fruits and vegetables or healthier cereals. There are some examples of this, but generally food producers and supermarkets are reluctant to interfere with their very successful marketing of less healthy foods. Several studies have shown that advertising of healthy foods can increase nutritional knowledge in children but has little impact upon food choice.

The World Health Organization (2011) published 12 recommendations on the advertising of food and non-alcoholic beverages, which overall put the onus upon governments to reduce the exposure of children to marketing of foods that are high in sugar, fat and salt. Very few countries have such policies. In the United Kingdom, legislation introduced in 2007 effectively banned the advertising of foods high in sugar and fat during television programmes aimed at the under-9s, and this policy was extended to programming for under-16s in 2009. Although initial analysis suggested that this had markedly reduced exposure to advertising of unhealthy foods, Adams and colleagues (2012) reported that post-ban the exposure of children to unhealthy foods through television advertising had actually increased. Total food advertising had almost twice as many exposures to high sugar, fat and salt products, and overall advertising across all categories showed a 1.5–fold increase in junk-food adverts. The key problem with the UK ban is that it only affected specific children's programming and fails to cover all programmes that may be watched by a household (including children). Other countries (Norway, Sweden, Canada) have adopted restrictions or total bans on any advertising that may be viewed by children. Quebec is the only province of Canada to have such a ban, and it is estimated that this has reduced sales of fast food by US$88 million per annum (Dhar and Bayliss, 2011).

6.2.4.3.4 Restrictive dietary practices

Some infants may be fed diets that restrict specific foods or food groups. This is often due to religious, ethical or health-related beliefs held by parents, which are imposed upon the children. In most cases, these practices do not have any detrimental impact upon nutritional status or health, but careful management may be necessary to avoid problems. Hindu and Buddhist families, for example, may follow vegetarian diets, and although there are reports that infants weaned onto such diets suffer a greater incidence of iron deficiency anaemia, growth is generally maintained at a rate equivalent to omnivores. Children following vegetarian diets have been shown to maintain normal prepubertal growth patterns but only if the diet is managed to include an appropriate diversity of nutrient sources (Hackett *et al.*, 1998). Vegan diets provide a greater challenge as they are of low energy density. To maintain growth, careful planning of diets for vegan children to include varied sources of protein (tofu, beans and meat analogues) and more energy-dense items such as avocados and vegetable oils is essential (Mangels and Messina, 2001). There are many reports of vitamin B12 deficiency in vegan children, so supplements should be provided to such infants.

There are other circumstances in which parents may restrict the foods that are provided for young children, with negative outcomes for growth. There are reported cases of failure to thrive in children whose parents have, in good faith, introduced a low-fat, high-fibre diet that accords with guidelines for healthy eating in adults. This is inappropriate for young children as the bulk of food required to deliver nutrient requirements is not feasible. The introduction of adult healthy eating recommendations should be delayed until the end of the infant stage but applied flexibly. While, on average, the age of 5 years would be appropriate to adopt a high-fibre, low-fat diet, for slow-growing children, this may be too soon and for children on a more rapid trajectory it should come earlier, but certainly not before the age of 2 years.

Fear of food allergies and intolerances may also prompt restrictions in children's diets. The prevalence of adverse reactions to food is estimated at between 4 and 8% of the childhood populations. Parents often mistakenly believe that their child has an allergy to food, and the parental report of adverse reactions is at a level three to four times above the true prevalence (Noimark and Cox, 2008). Where adverse reactions are suspected, parents may act unilaterally to remove the suspect food

from the diet and in so doing exclude important sources of nutrients. Even where expert advice is given and allergy confirmed, parents may be overzealous in the interpretation of that advice and take actions to restrict the diet without providing suitable alternative sources of nutrients and energy. This can contribute to growth faltering.

6.3 Childhood (5–13)

6.3.1 Nutrient requirements of the older child

In contrast to the earlier stages of childhood, the period between the age of 5 and puberty is characterized by a relative absence of nutritional problems and rapidly declining nutrient demands. Growth continues to keep nutrient requirements above those of adults, but it is striking that despite demands of growth and their larger body size, children of this age have requirements for energy and nutrients that are not grossly dissimilar to those of under-5s. As shown in Table 6.4, energy requirements on a per-kilogram-body-weight basis fall sharply throughout this period.

While still a problem in many regions, the impact of micronutrient deficiencies upon older children is less severe. Although stunting of growth remains a significant issue, the high rates of morbidity and mortality associated with undernutrition in younger children are not seen in the older age groups. This stems from more robust immune function, less vulnerability to dehydration associated with diarrhoeal disease and a longer period of time in which to accrue viable nutrient reserves. In the developed countries, the major nutritional concerns at this stage of life are overweight and obesity, which will be discussed in greater detail later in this chapter.

Children at this stage are increasing their independence from their parents and begin to hold their own

Table 6.4 Energy requirements of children.

Age (years)	UK estimated average requirement (kcal/day)		Energy requirement (kcal/kg body weight/day)	
	Boys	**Girls**	**Boys**	**Girls**
3	1490	1370	97	92
5	1720	1550	88	82
7	1890	1680	78	71
9	2040	1790	69	61

Data from Department of Health (1998).

strong views about food, physical activity and health. They take a greater role in the acquisition of the food that they will consume and, as they begin to experience more life outside the home through going to school, become more likely to purchase meals and snacks for their own consumption. Education about food, nutrition and health, therefore, becomes an important priority in the development of these children. By this stage of life, it is important for them to begin to follow a model along the lines of the Eatwell plate or similar schemes such as the US Food Pyramid in order to develop eating habits that lower fat intake and promote consumption of starchy foods and fruits and vegetables.

6.3.2 School meals and the promotion of healthy eating

All over the world, schools provide meals for children. These are generally optional, giving children the opportunity to either bring in their own lunches from home or to purchase a cooked meal in school. While lunches brought in from home are the responsibility of parents, it is now common for schools and government agencies to provide information and advice to ensure that these meals are based upon basic principles of healthy eating. Schools, and the meals that they provide, are well placed to influence the dietary choices of children who are easily influenced, receptive to health education messages and interested in cooking and helping with food-related activities.

The meals that are provided within schools are increasingly subject to formal regulation to ensure their quality, particularly in the light of concern about rising levels of childhood obesity. These meals may be provided free of charge to children from poor backgrounds as a means of combating undernutrition. The United Kingdom provides a useful example of how legislation can be introduced to ensure that school meals fulfil nutritional standards. In 2006, in response to public concerns at the levels of fat in school meals and the widespread use of low grade, mechanically reclaimed meat and fish, new regulations were introduced to ensure that caterers were properly trained and used higher-quality ingredients, included at least two portions of fruits or vegetables and provided sources of complex carbohydrate (bread, cereals or potatoes) in every meal. The provision of fried foods was limited to no more than once per week, and fizzy drinks, crisps and confectionary were banned from school vending machines and meal provision. Under these guidelines, school lunches must provide 30% of the EAR for energy, at least 30% of the RNI for protein and at least 40% of the RNI for iron, zinc, calcium, vitamin A, vitamin C and folate. Meals should contain no more than 30% of

the SACN guidelines for salt (no more than 1.8 g salt for this age group). New regulations introduced in 2015 set limitations on provision of fruit juices to limit sugar intakes, with an emphasis on drinking water instead. The new regulations also limit fried foods and pastries and require at least three different fruits and three different vegetables to be offered during the school week. School meal provision is now an element of the inspection programme that ensures overall quality standards of UK education. This emphasizes the growing importance of food, nutrition and health in the overall curriculum, which encourages children to engage more with food production and increase their knowledge of how diet impacts upon health and well-being. School caterers are expected to modify recipes, portion sizes and food selection protocols to ensure that meals fit the standards. Unfortunately, these regulations apply only to government-run schools, so private schools and the rapidly growing self-governing academy sector in the United Kingdom are exempt, meaning that coverage is not universal. However, where implemented, it is reported that children increase intakes of water, vegetables and salad, fruit and starchy foods while decreasing intakes of fried starchy foods and non-fruit desserts. Overall intakes of protein, fibre and most micronutrients are increased, while energy, fat, sodium and non-milk extrinsic sugars are lower (School Food Trust, 2012). In 2010, the United States passed the Healthy, Hunger-Free Kids act, which introduced new nutritional standards. This policy informs programmes such as the School Breakfast Program and the National School Lunch Program, setting standards on intakes of grains, fruits, vegetables, sodium, milk and trans-fatty acids.

School meals are often just one element of a wider range of health interventions in schools, which also target physical activity and health education. Again, in the United Kingdom, the government introduced the National School Fruit and Vegetable Scheme in 2004 with the aim of providing one portion of fruit per day to school children aged between 4 and 6 years. The aim was to improve nutrient intakes and promote the five-a-day message to children. Evaluations of this programme have shown that while the scheme improved intakes of fruit while children were in the age group covered by the scheme, once they moved out of the targeted provision, their intakes declined to where they were at baseline (Fogarty et al., 2007; Ransley et al., 2007). This is unsurprising as the scheme merely adds to what children may consume at home and does not change family behaviours outside school. Longer and more sustained interventions would be required to obtain any lasting benefits. The evaluation of the scheme by Hughes et al. (2012) showed that the scheme increased both fruit and vegetable intakes in all areas where it was implemented, but could not override the effect of social deprivation upon children's access to fruits and vegetables. A similar scheme in Norway increased children's intake of fruits, but not vegetables (Bere *et al.*, 2010).

6.3.3 The importance of breakfast

Breakfast is an important contributor to the overall dietary quality of children. It has been estimated that it provides between 275 and 670 kcal energy, which is delivered mostly from carbohydrate (50–72% of energy) and fat (14–40% of energy). The major breakfast foods consumed by children in developed countries are milk, fruit juices, breads and fortified cereals (Rampersaud *et al.*, 2005). Generally, breakfast will be delivering approximately 20% of daily energy intake and a greater proportion of micronutrients if based upon fortified cereals. It has an important metabolic role in that it ends the overnight period of fasting during which glycogen stores become depleted. Breakfast induces a rise in blood glucose concentrations, which will be sustained over a longer period if the meal contains a high proportion of complex carbohydrates.

Despite its importance, breakfast is the most likely meal of the day to be missed by children. Utter *et al.* (2007) found that 3.7% of New Zealand children missed breakfast on most days and that 12.8% failed to eat it every day. These figures are similar to reports from other countries, with a prevalence of breakfast skipping of 8% in Australia and 18% in England reported by Mullan *et al.* (2014). Breakfast consumption is not universal even among very young children, with up to 5% of a sample of Dutch 2–5-year-olds missing breakfast regularly (Küpers *et al.*, 2014). Children who skip breakfast have been shown to have greater intakes of less healthy snack foods at other points in the day and to often have irregular meal patterns. Typically, their intakes of fruits and vegetables tend to be lower than seen in regular breakfast consumers. Breakfast skipping is therefore a good indicator of unhealthy food choices in children. In the study of Utter and colleagues, skipping breakfast was also associated with greater body mass index (BMI), consistent with other reports that although they consume less energy during the day, children who skip breakfast are more likely to be overweight (Rampersaud *et al.*, 2005). Although replicated in many studies (Figure 6.9), the relationship is not consistent across all age groups (Küpers *et al.*, 2014), and it is likely that breakfast skipping is an indicator of an unhealthy pattern of eating which promotes obesity rather than a causal factor in the development of obesity.

There are many reports that breakfast benefits cognitive processes and boosts performance in school. Observational

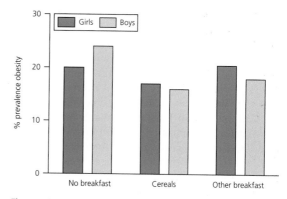

Figure 6.9 Boys who miss breakfast are more likely to be obese than those who consume a breakfast cereal or other breakfast foods on a regular basis.
Source: Deshmukh-Taskar *et al.* (2010), 9–13-year-olds in the 1999–2006 US NHANES survey.

studies based in school and home settings and experimental studies generally show that consumption of a breakfast that is rich in complex carbohydrate improves school attendance rates, boosts academic attainment and improves both short- and long-term memories. Liu *et al.* (2013) reported that among 6-year-olds, IQ was higher in children who regularly consumed breakfast. Higher scores in cognitive tests were observed among 14–15-year-olds who had consumed breakfast compared to those who had not (Wesnes *et al.*, 2012). It has been argued that this stems from the effect of breakfast upon blood glucose concentrations or possibly through modulation of neurotransmitter functions. A study by Brindal *et al.* (2012) could find no evidence of an effect of blood glucose, with no difference in cognitive function in 12-year-olds who were fed breakfasts where protein was replaced by carbohydrate sources with differing glycemic index. Ells *et al.* (2008) suggest that reports of improved cognitive performance should be treated with caution as experiments are mostly performed in small cohorts of children and over short periods of time. Studies that are based in school breakfast clubs may be confounded by the social benefits of eating breakfast with peers and in younger children by poverty and family lifestyle.

The provision of breakfast in schools is seen as an important tool for dietary intervention to improve the quality of children's diets. As missing breakfast is a behaviour that is more common in socially deprived children from low-income families, this may be a useful approach to target this population group (Moore *et al.*, 2007). In the United States, the Department of Agriculture (USDA) oversees the School Breakfast Program, which is a major initiative to assist children from poor social backgrounds across the nation. The programme provides breakfast to children of all backgrounds but is subsidized so that the price paid depends upon family income. Children from the poorest families receive breakfast free of charge. In 2012, 89 000 schools and institutions were involved with the programme and 12.9 million children were given breakfast every day. New nutritional standards were introduced in 2010. The implementation of the School Breakfast Program standards in schools in Los Angeles and Illinois resulted in provision of meals with lower energy, salt and sugar content (Cummings *et al.*, 2014). The programme provides a breakfast based upon 240 ml milk, 120 ml fruit or vegetable juice, one slice of bread or an alternative and 28 g of meat or an alternative (Kennedy and Davis, 1998). This provides one-quarter of the RDA for energy and a significant proportion of requirements for other nutrients. Evaluations of this scheme have shown that it improves the nutrient intakes of participants and has benefits for school attendance and performance.

In schools where breakfast clubs and other schemes along the lines of the USDA School Breakfast Program are operating, there is a major opportunity for health promotion and to make improvements to the quality of diets consumed by children. The USDA scheme, for example, engages schools with resources on healthy snacks and school wellness policies. Children participating in breakfast schemes may also consume lunch within school. A high proportion of daily food intake can therefore be managed and planned to fit well with health priorities. The importance of effective school-based interventions will be further explored in Section 6.4.5.

6.4 Obesity in children

6.4.1 The rising prevalence of obesity

Obesity and overweight are a major health concern at all points across the lifespan. Chapter 8 will set out in detail the evidence that the prevalence of overweight and obesity in adults increased by twofold between 1990 and 2000 in the developed countries and is increasing at an alarming rate all across the world. The prevalence of obesity in childhood is also increasing rapidly in all parts of the world, and this may be of greater significance in terms of the future public health burden.

One of the challenges in following trends in childhood obesity over time is the often very different definitions that have been used in surveys and research papers over recent decades. In adults, BMI cut-off values can be simply applied (25 kg/m² for overweight, 30 kg/m² for obesity), and although there are many concerns about the accuracy of BMI in predicting body fatness and the suitability of these standard cut-offs for

all ethnic groups, this gives a reasonable estimate of population-wide overweight and obesity rates. In children, as shown in Figure 6.10, BMI varies with age and in a nonlinear manner, so simple cut-off values are inappropriate. Instead, clinicians and researchers make reference to centile charts for BMI to define obesity. Typically, clinical reports are more stringent and define obesity as having BMI above the 98th centile (i.e. the BMI of the child is in the top 2% for the population at that age). Research reports using data collected prior to 2002 tended to define overweight as BMI above the 90th centile and obesity above the 95th centile. In an attempt to provide a standard classification to be applied globally, the International Obesity Taskforce (IOTF; now the World Obesity Federation) suggested that the centile value at any given age should be projected forward to age 18 and then the cut-offs of 25 kg/m² for overweight and 30 kg/m² for obesity applied. On this basis, obese children lie just above the 98th centile for BMI, and overweight is defined as just above the 90th centile.

There is a wealth of evidence to suggest that the prevalence of obesity has increased at a similar rate to that seen in adults over recent decades. Global estimates suggest that 170 million children are overweight or obese and the prevalence more than doubled between 1974 and 2004 (Swinburn *et al.*, 2011). Of particular concern is the high prevalence of overweight and obesity in the under-5s.

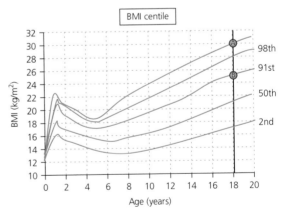

Figure 6.10 Body mass index centiles. The most robust definitions of overweight and obesity are based upon tracking the current BMI centile of any child under the age of 18 through to the BMI value for that centile at age 18. Standard BMI cut-offs of 25 and 30 kg/m² for overweight and obesity, respectively, can then be applied. On this basis, a child following the centile marked A on the chart would be defined as obese, while a child following the centile marked B would be defined as overweight.
Source: Data compiled from Cole *et al.* (1995). This chart is shown for illustrative purposes only and is not for clinical use.

There are 42 million overweight children in this age group, of which 35 million live in developing countries.

Evidence from the United Kingdom suggests that a rapid rate of increase in prevalence of obesity increased over the 1990s, with a near doubling, reported in the under-5s and a two- to threefold increase reported in 4–11-year-olds (Bundred *et al.*, 2001; Chinn and Rona, 2001). Rudolf and colleagues (2001) showed that in 9–11-year-olds, obesity prevalence had increased by four-fold over the period 1975–2000. The annual UK National Child Measurement Programme for 2012–2013 reported that 18.9% of 10–11-year-olds were obese and 14% were overweight. This represented a year-on-year increase over the 7 years of the survey. In contrast, prevalence in 4–5-year-olds appeared to have fallen slightly over the same period. However, such measurements focus on BMI rather than other measures of obesity. Griffiths *et al.* (2013) followed a cohort of nearly 700 British children from ages 11 to 12 for 5 years. Over this period, the prevalence of obesity as assessed by BMI decreased, but measures of weight circumference suggest that the children, and in particular the girls, increased central adiposity dramatically across the study. This implies that estimates of obesity that suggest a levelling off of prevalence may be missing changes in the prevalence of central obesity.

The trends for increasing prevalence of obesity that have been noted in the United Kingdom are typical of all of the developed countries. Analysis of the 1976–1980, 2003–2004 and 2009–2010 NHANES studies from the United States indicates that among 6–11-year-olds, obesity prevalence increased from 7 to 18%, while for 12–19-year-olds, the increase was from 5 to 21% over the same period. In the European region, the prevalence of obesity among 7–11-year-olds ranged from 3% in the Netherlands to 12% in Malta in 2005. It was estimated that in the early part of this century, the number of overweight and obese children in the European Union increased by 500 000–700 000 every year (out of a total population of 75 million). This is an incidence rate of close to 1%/year. Figure 6.11 shows the prevalence of obesity in children in selected countries. Highest prevalence is noted in the United States, the United Kingdom, Mediterranean countries and Australasia.

6.4.2 The causes of obesity in childhood

On a simplistic level, the causes of obesity at any age are obvious. Obesity represents the excess accumulation of body fat as a consequence of positive energy balance. In other words, the amount of energy consumed is in excess of requirement for metabolic and physiological processes. To put this another way, childhood obesity is the product of excess food intake and insufficient energy expenditure through physical activity. This explanation is, however, a superficial viewpoint and is unhelpful as it serves to perpetuate the false idea that all obese children are greedy and lazy.

Obesity is multifactorial in origin and represents an interaction between a genetic predisposition and the environment. Obesity can be generated without gross imbalances of energy supply and demand. A habitual positive energy balance of just 10–20 kcal/day can result in a significant accumulation of excess body fat over a period of a few years. It is generally argued that the modern obesity 'epidemic' that afflicts children is a consequence of the mismatch between the biological evolution of humans and the technological revolution of recent times. This 'discordance hypothesis' suggests that early humans evolved for subsistence on a food supply

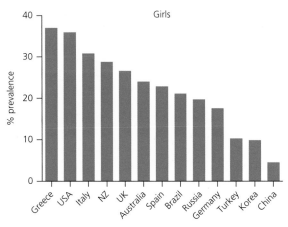
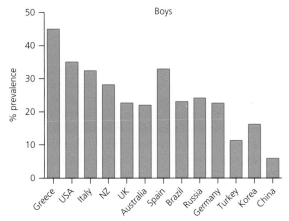

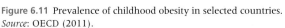

Figure 6.11 Prevalence of childhood obesity in selected countries. *Source*: OECD (2011).

that was insecure and where considerable amounts of energy had to be expended in order to gain access to food, either through hunting or foraging. As a result, the human genome evolved to favour efficient energy storage. The modern environment is at odds with this biological background and daily consumption of energy-rich foods, with low energy expenditure through activity (Eaton *et al.*, 1988; Hill and Peters, 1998). It is proposed that obesity genes carried by many humans achieve their expression in the 'obesogenic' environment that has been constructed through social and technological changes.

Obesity-promoting genes may play an important role in determining risk of childhood obesity. It is estimated that between 33 and 50% of the risk to any individual is derived from genetic inheritance. In a powerful analysis, Wardle and colleagues (2008) studied twins aged between 8 and 11, a study therefore free of many confounding influences seen in earlier studies of adult twins, and noted that 77% of the variation in BMI and waist circumference could be explained by genetic factors. Given that many monogenic causes of obesity are likely to be of early onset, they may contribute significantly to observed levels of childhood obesity. Despite the major influence of genetic factors, it has to be recognized that the modern obesity crisis has developed over the last 20–30 years and that the human gene pool will have been relatively stable for tens of thousands of years. The overwhelming view of researchers in the field is that environmental factors explain current trends.

6.4.2.1 Physical activity

Physical activity is seen as an important element of normal healthy development and provides protection against weight gain and related disorders later in life while promoting bone mineralization and optimal growth. Some points in childhood appear to be more important than others in terms of the health gain associated with activity, for example, the preschool years and the later stages of adolescence. This may be because these are stages at which attitudes to exercise are shaped, therefore influencing activity levels at future life stages. Physical activity levels often decline with age, reflecting patterns of play in children, which often change from free, unstructured and active games (e.g. spontaneous games of chase and tag) to a more regimented sports-based pattern in early adolescence (Must and Tybor, 2005).

Declining levels of physical activity are seen as a major contributor to obesity in children. The modern environment encourages low levels of physical activity in children for a number of reasons. Firstly, modern

transport networks discourage walking or cycling, and many parents will choose to drive their children to school and other activities by car even over relatively short distances. This may be due to concerns about children's safety when out and about but may also be a product of the fact that driving is easier and faster and a simpler way to integrate children's activities into busy family life. Within schools, the prioritization of academic subjects and testing over time spent in physical education, sport, dance and other more active subjects has led to a progressive fall in levels of physical activity within the working week. Alternative activities outside school can be difficult for some children to access due to cost, location or a general lack of availability.

The flip side of the coin in consideration of declining physical activity is the increase in the amount of time spent on sedentary activities. These are generally leisure activities that involve little more than the resting level of energy expenditure. In developed countries, children spend 4–6 h/day either watching television or using computers and games consoles. Exceeding a recommended 2 h/day sedentary screen time is the norm for children in most developed countries (Figure 6.12). These are now the preferred leisure activities of most children and are favoured by many parents as they keep the child in a safe and controlled environment.

Although physical activity is seen as a key contributor to obesity risk in children, it is difficult to quantify the extent of that risk with any certainty. Within populations, levels of physical activity are extremely variable and it is highly problematic to quantify actual energy expenditure through activity, using validated methods (Rennie *et al.*, 2006). Most of the literature is therefore based upon indirect and subjective measurements (e.g. self-report of the hours spent watching television). Moreover, cross-sectional

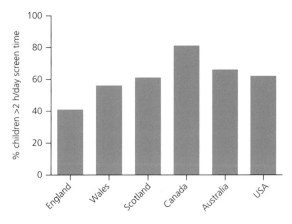

Figure 6.12 Children's daily exposure to television or other screen-based activities.

studies that attempt to examine relationships between activity and obesity are confounded by the fact that causality cannot be shown. In general, overweight and obese children *will* be less active than their lean counterparts as they find physical activity and sport more difficult and less enjoyable (Must and Tybor, 2005).

Despite these methodological issues, from the available information, it seems likely that leisure inactivity is a critical component of the modern obesogenic environment that is driving childhood obesity. Prospective studies that have considered how childhood BMI changes over time are related to activity levels consistently show strong negative associations between the two variables. Sedentary behaviours are strongly predictive of greater BMI (Must and Tybor, 2005). A systematic review found that 94/119 cross-sectional studies reported that longer periods of time engaged in sedentary activities were associated with greater BMI, fat mass and risk of overweight in children. Similarly, 19/28 longitudinal studies found that greater sedentary time was associated with faster rates of increase in BMI and fat mass (Tremblay *et al.*, 2011). More than 2 h/day of watching television was associated with greater risk of obesity, with a dose-dependent effect of every additional hour over 2 h. A key step in the reduction of obesity risk may therefore be to promote the avoidance of sedentary behaviour rather than participation in high-impact physical activities. Interventions which target sedentary activities such as screen watching significantly impact on BMI in children and are more effective than interventions that target sedentary behaviour alongside dietary change and increasing physical activity (Liao *et al.*, 2014). Television watching may be doubly insidious in that not only is it a sedentary activity, but it also changes dietary behaviours, promoting consumption of soft drinks, snack foods and convenience foods. This may be a response to advertising of such items. Lobstein and Dibb (2005) found that in the United States, Australia and a number of European countries, there was a positive association between children's exposure to advertisements for energy-dense, micronutrient poor foods and levels of overweight and obesity in the population.

6.4.2.2 Food intake

From the aforementioned discussion, it should be clear that energy expenditure through physical activity among children has declined markedly over recent decades. James (2008a) highlighted the fact that this has impacted particularly heavily on the rapidly developing countries such as China and India. In China, changes in technology and increasing use of motorized transport mean that energy requirements for children are markedly lower than they were 40 years ago. Whereas, in the past, children were engaged in work-related activities for much of their time, modernization and urbanization may have reduced energy requirements by 200 kcal/day. Alongside these shifts in activity levels, the nature of the diet has undergone a revolution in almost all parts of the world, producing an increase in energy intakes and energy density of foodstuffs. Interestingly, among Chinese children, significant decreases in energy intake between 1991 and 2009 were reported by Cui and Dibley (2012), but against that backdrop, the proportion of energy from fat was seen to have increased from 26.3 to 34.6% among urban children. Low dietary diversity has been reported in overweight Chinese children (Li *et al.*, 2011). It can therefore be strongly asserted that the modern environment simultaneously promotes reduced energy expenditure and increased consumption.

Studies that have sought to establish the links between dietary intakes and obesity in children have generally produced inconclusive results and at best indicate weak relationships between specific dietary factors and obesity in childhood. For example, Guillaume *et al.* (1998) found no association between energy intake from fat and body fatness in 6–12-year-olds. Similarly, Maffeis *et al.* (1998) could find no association between body fatness and intakes of macronutrients in children. Robertson and colleagues (1999) considered fatness using a comprehensive series of skinfold measurements and showed that children with more body fat had higher intakes of energy, but not of any specific macronutrient. Reilly *et al.* (2005) found no contribution of dietary factors to difference in risk of overweight among 7-year-old children, even when comparing children with an established preference for a diet rich in chocolate, crisps and sugar-sweetened beverages to those with diets rich in complex carbohydrates and protein.

There are major challenges in attempting such studies, and this may be responsible for the lack of consistency in the literature. Firstly, confounding factors need to be taken into account, including body weight at birth and parental BMI. Moreover, as individuals of greater weight require more energy to maintain that weight, studies are best performed using a longitudinal design to monitor the associations between dietary factors and weight or fat gain over a period of time. Obtaining accurate measurements of dietary intake is difficult at any stage of life but is particularly difficult in children and their parents, who may fail to recall and fully record their intakes. As described in Section 6.4.1, even the anthropometric classification of overweight and obesity is far from straightforward.

Magarey *et al.* (2001) used robust methods in order to avoid the pitfalls identified earlier, in a study of 2–15-year-old Australian children. However, no clear influence of macronutrient intake upon BMI or body fatness measured using skinfolds could be identified. In contrast, Skinner and colleagues (2004) found associations between macronutrient intakes and change in BMI between 2 months and 8 years of age. Regular assessment of dietary intake using weighed records and 24-h maternal recall allowed determination of longitudinal patterns of protein, carbohydrate and fat consumption, alongside changes in BMI. Protein and fat intakes were positively associated with BMI, while carbohydrate intake was negatively associated. Surprisingly, total energy intake was not predictive of BMI. BMI at 8 years was most strongly related to BMI at age 2 and the timing of the adiposity rebound (Figure 6.13), indicating that factors in early infancy may be critical in setting the risk of overweight and obesity and reinforcing the importance of infant feeding methods in this context (see Research Highlight 6.2).

While the macronutrient composition of the diet cannot be strongly related to body fatness in children, there is clear evidence that meal patterns, portion sizes and the energy density of foods consumed play an important role in determining risk of overweight and obesity. Dubois and colleagues (2008), for example, considered energy and macronutrient intakes in a cohort of Canadian children. These children were divided into a group who consumed breakfast on a daily basis (90% of the study population) and those who missed breakfast

on at least 1 day each week (10% of population). Those who skipped breakfast had different overall dietary patterns to the breakfast consumers. They consumed more energy in total, consumed less protein and energy from protein and ate a greater number of carbohydrate-rich snacks. Risk of overweight among the breakfast-skipping children was increased by 2.27-fold (95% CI 1.33–3.88). The study could not discount the fact that breakfast skipping could be a marker for other confounding factors, such as sedentary behaviour, but nonetheless showed how patterns of intake within the day could influence body fatness. While in the reference group BMI was unrelated to intakes at specific points in the day, in children who skipped breakfast, consumption of over 700 kcal at lunchtime was a predictor of overweight. This suggests that meal frequency could impact on energy balance or appetite regulation.

Increased energy density of foodstuffs has also been proposed as a factor driving the increase in childhood obesity. Changes in family lifestyle, where the need for both parents to be out of the house in paid employment, have increased the consumption of preprepared convenience foods. These are generally rich in fats and sugars and have a higher energy density than meals prepared at home, from fresh ingredients. Moreover, children are consuming increasing amounts of snack foods, in addition to meals, and these also increase the energy density of the overall diet. It is logical to assume that this change in food consumption has an impact upon overall energy intake in children, but once again methodological issues have made it difficult to demonstrate a relationship between energy density and obesity risk. McCaffrey *et al.* (2008) investigated this potential association using a 7-year follow-up to a study initially conducted in primary school children (aged 6–8). No relationship was noted between energy density of the children's diets and the gain in fat mass over this period. In contrast, Johnson and colleagues (2008) found that fat mass in 9-year-old children was related to energy density of the diet and dietary fat intake and inversely related to intakes of dietary fibre.

Regular consumption of 'fast food' is recognized as a behaviour that increases energy density of the diet and hence overall energy intake. Fast food can be defined as foodstuffs that are mass-produced convenience foods, generally purchased from self-service or takeaway outlets. There is a huge market for these foods, and in the United States, this represents the most rapidly expanding sector of the food industry. Fifty per cent of food expenditure in the United States is on fast food (Rosenheck, 2008). Analysis of the 2009–2010 US NHANES data set showed that 21% of 2–5-year-olds and 46% of 12–18-year-olds were fast-food consumers and that 35% of added sugar and solid fat consumption came from fast-food outlets (Poti *et al.*, 2013). Bowman *et al.* (2004) explored the

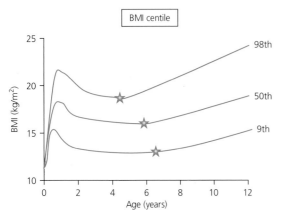

Figure 6.13 The adiposity rebound. In early childhood, the weight gain of children outstrips their height gain, and as a result, BMI rises rapidly. Beyond the first year of life, height gain tends to exceed weight gain and so BMI declines. Between the ages of 4 and 8, the BMI begins to increase again and this point is termed the adiposity rebound. Having an earlier adiposity rebound appears to be predictive of obesity in childhood, and it can be clearly seen on the graph that for children on a higher BMI centile, the rebound (marked by the stars) occurs at an earlier age. Earlier adiposity rebound is noted in formula-fed compared to breastfed infants.

dietary patterns of US children and found that 30% consumed fast food on a typical day. Among these children, this increased energy density by 0.29 kcal/g food, increased intakes of fat, carbohydrate and sugar-sweetened beverages and was associated with lower intakes of milk, fruits and vegetables. Fast-food consumers on average consumed an extra 187 kcal/day. A review of experimental and cohort studies of fast-food consumption and obesity risk (Rosenheck, 2008) concluded that, in children, although fast-food consumption increases energy intake, there is no clear effect upon BMI and weight gain. However, Thompson and colleagues (2006) found that after 4–10 years of follow-up, girls who consumed fast food twice or more per week at a baseline survey exhibited a greater increase in BMI than those who did not. Studies from the United States and the United Kingdom suggest that ready accessibility to fast-food outlets is associated with greater body fatness and risk of obesity (Fraser *et al.*, 2012). Although the evidence is equivocal, it is suggested that fast-food consumption in childhood helps to establish a pattern of behaviour and food preferences that may increase risk later in life.

Sugar-sweetened beverages are an important element of the energy-dense diet that is associated with fast-food consumption. These drinks can contribute significantly to energy intake in children. Pure fruit juices are also considered in this category, even though parents widely perceive these to be a healthy alternative to other drinks, including water. A 100 ml serving of apple juice, for example, can deliver 11.8 g of sugar (a nearly identical quantity to a similar serving of cola), and consumption may displace less energy-dense, more nutrient-dense drinks such as milk (Table 6.5). Wang *et al.* (2008) reported that in the United States, energy intakes in children from sugar-sweetened beverages and fruit juices accounted for 10–15% of total energy intakes. The consumption of sugar-sweetened beverages appears to be a

major culprit in weight gain associated with dietary patterns that include fast food. Although there was initial caution as to whether sugar-sweetened beverages caused weight gain (Ludwig *et al.*, 2001), there is now clear evidence that they play a role in determining childhood body weight. Lim *et al.* (2009) followed a population of African-American preschool children over 2 years and found that there was a significant risk of obesity associated with high consumption of sugar-sweetened beverages. Odds of overweight increased by 4% for every 28 ml consumed per day. Similarly, a case–control study of Spanish 5–18-year-olds noted a 3.46-fold (95% CI 1.24–9.62) increase in risk of obesity with greater than 4 servings per week (Martin-Calvo *et al.*, 2015). The meta-analysis of Te Morenga *et al.* (2012) suggested that odds of overweight were higher (OR 1.55, 95% CI 1.32–1.82) in groups with the highest compared to the lowest intakes. These drinks may be particularly important in promoting weight gain, as the hypothalamic systems that regulate appetite and energy balance do not compensate for liquid food sources as efficiently as they do for solids.

6.4.2.3 Genetic disorders

There are a number of single-gene mutations that are known to promote early-onset obesity (Table 6.6). Until recently, it has always been assumed that these are extremely rare and account for only a small proportion of childhood and adult obesity cases. The use of modern

Table 6.5 Energy and sugar content of beverages commonly consumed by children.

Beverage	Per 100 ml serving		
	Energy (kcal)	Energy (KJ)	Sugars (g)
Cow's milk (whole)	66	277	5.6
Apple juice (unsweetened)	49	205	11.8
Orange juice (unsweetened)	49	205	11.1
Fruit squash	55	230	12.8
Lemonade	63	264	15.9
Cola	43	180	11.9

Table 6.6 Genetic disorders associated with early-onset obesity.

Condition	Gene defect(s)	Contribution to obesity
Melanocortin receptor defects	MC1R, MC2R, MC3R, MC4R, MC5R	MC4R defects may explain 5% of all childhood obesity cases
FTO polymorphisms	FTO	Explains 1% of variation in population BMI. Sixteen per cent of population homozygous for obesity-related allele
Prader–Willi syndrome	Abnormalities of chromosome 15	One in 12 000–15 000 births
Leptin receptor defects	LepR	Up to 3% of cases of childhood obesity
Bardet–Biedl syndrome	Abnormalities of chromosomes 11 and 16	One in 125 000 births
MOMO	Unknown	Only five confirmed cases
Congenital leptin deficiency	Leptin	Only 12 confirmed cases

MOMO, macrosomia, obesity, macrocephaly and ocular abnormalities.

molecular techniques for population screening and the discovery of new gene targets are starting to change this perception, and it appears that up to 10% of all obese children may have an underlying genetic disorder. For example, confirmed deficiency of the leptin receptor had only been observed in a single family, but a screen of 300 individuals with early-onset obesity revealed LepR defects in 3% of cases (Farooqi *et al.*, 2007). The *FTO* gene has been highlighted as a novel gene target for obesity research. Single nucleotide polymorphisms in *FTO* are common in the population (between 14 and 52%) and are associated with greater BMI. Individuals who are homozygous for the at-risk form of the *FTO* allele have 1.67-fold greater risk of obesity (Loos and Bouchard, 2008).

Many of the genetic disorders linked to obesity are associated with other abnormalities. In Bardet–Biedl syndrome, for example, obesity is just one outcome amidst a myriad of abnormalities of growth and development, affecting the eyes, the gastrointestinal tract and the cardiovascular system. Other disorders induce obesity through effects upon the neuroendocrine control of appetite. Defects of MC4R (the melanocortin 4 receptor, Research Highlight 6.3) are associated with binge eating disorders (Loos *et al.*, 2008). In Prader–Willi syndrome (PWS), there are defects of the chromosome 15q11–13 region that stem from either deletion of paternally derived alleles or epigenetic silencing (DNA methylation) of paternal alleles (Goldstone, 2004). PWS-affected children have a number of neurological defects and generally have learning difficulties. In infancy, they often fail-to-thrive as they are unable to feed normally but between 1 and 6 years gain weight at a prodigious rate due to extreme hyperphagia. Some adolescents with PWS will consume in excess of 5000 kcal/day if given free access to food. Management of the condition therefore requires strict control over portion sizes and the availability of food. This can involve extreme measures such as locking fridges and larders.

6.4.3 The consequences of childhood obesity

Soaring rates of childhood overweight and obesity have prompted fears about the impact of these trends upon the health of populations. Clearly, these concerns must focus upon the immediate health of the affected children, but it is also of importance to consider whether obesity in childhood increases risk of obesity and related disorders later in life.

6.4.3.1 Immediate health consequences

Obesity and overweight have important physical and psychological effects upon children and adolescents. Overweight children tend to grow and mature more rapidly and so attain a greater height than their leaner peers. In girls, the greater level of body fat drives earlier menarche (see Chapter 2). Overweight has important metabolic consequences and, as a result, disease states that were once extremely rare among children are increasing in prevalence. The metabolic syndrome, also referred to as the insulin resistance syndrome, is defined as the combined presence of hyperinsulinaemia, hypertriglyceridaemia and cardiovascular disorders (hypertension). It is primarily a condition of adulthood, with a prevalence of just 4% in children. There are reports that in overweight children and adolescents, this may increase to 30–50% (Daniels *et al.*, 2005). Individual components of the syndrome are also noted in a high proportion of overweight children, who are more likely to have a profile of circulating lipids that is associated with greater risk of cardiovascular disease (elevated low-density lipoprotein (LDL)-cholesterol and triglycerides, lower concentrations of high-density lipoprotein-cholesterol). Glucose intolerance is also more likely, leading to a marked increase in the prevalence of non-insulin-dependent diabetes in children (Dietz, 1998). Pinhas-Hamiel and colleagues (1996) reported a tenfold increase in the number of US adolescents diagnosed with diabetes between 1982 and 1995. Although type 1 diabetes is generally regarded as the early-onset form of diabetes, among US children, the prevalence of type 1 diabetes is now markedly lower (1.7 cases/1000 children) than that of type 2 diabetes (4.1 cases/1000 children) (Daniels *et al.*, 2005).

Overweight impacts upon liver function and obese children are more prone to hepatic steatosis and gallstones. High blood pressure is reported to be on the increase among obese children (Dietz, 1998). Cerebral hypertension can manifest as pseudotumour cerebri. Carrying excess weight puts strain upon the growing skeleton. Two-thirds of patients diagnosed with Blount's disease, a bone-deformation condition of childhood, are obese. Thirty to fifty per cent of children with slipped capital femoral epiphysis, a defect of the growth plate in the thigh bone, are overweight or obese.

From a psychological perspective, overweight in the childhood years can be extremely destructive, lowering self-esteem, promoting depression and preventing happy social interactions. Children who are overweight are more likely to be bullied at school and are often discriminated against by their peers. Even very young children show a preference for thinner children as playmates and will equate obesity with laziness and other undesirable descriptions (Dietz, 1998).

6.4.3.2 Tracking of obesity: Consequences for the future

In the context of obesity, 'tracking' is the term used to describe the situation where body fatness at one stage of life correlates strongly with a later stage. For example,

Research highlight 6.3

Melanocortin

The human hypothalamus, anterior pituitary and brainstem express the 241-amino-acid peptide pro-opiomelanocortin. This peptide is relatively inert but is cleaved to produce a series of biologically active peptide hormones including β-endorphin, adrenocorticotrophin and the melanocortins α-MSH, β-MSH and γ-MSH. Melanocortins have varied functions. In the periphery, α-MSH (12-amino-acid residues) is an inflammatory mediator and promotes skin pigmentation but within the central nervous system is an important regulator of energy balance and food intake. β-MSH (22-amino-acid residues) has similar functions. The functions of γ-MSH are poorly defined.

The melanocortin receptors

There are five melanocortin receptors (MC1R, MC2R, MC3R, MC4R and MC5R), which are expressed in many tissues. MC3R and MC4R are expressed in the regions of the hypothalamus that are involved in the regulation of appetite and energy balance (Coll, 2007). Both may contribute to this process, but MC4R is known to play the more important role. MC4R is a G-protein-coupled receptor and binds both α- and β-MSH. Following consumption of food, or in an energy-rich situation, production of leptin from adipose tissue simultaneously stimulates synthesis of melanocortins and suppresses production of agouti-related protein (AgRP). Binding of α-MSH to MC4R suppresses food intake. As AgRP is an antagonist of the receptor, this aspect of leptin signalling optimizes melanocortin binding (Coll, 2007).

Melanocortin and control of appetite

Studies of rodents have shown that MC4R plays a critical role in controlling food intake and weight gain. Animals with MC4R deficiency become hyperphagic, obese and insulin resistant. Selective knockout of MC4R in the paraventricular nucleus duplicates this effect (Garza et al., 2008). In humans, mutations of MC4R are relatively common and are noted in 0.1% of the UK population (O'Rahilly, 2007). Although there may be marked differences in prevalence in different ethnic groups (Lee et al., 2008), MC4R mutations represent the major monogenic forms of obesity. In some populations, 5% of early-onset obesity appears related to MC4R defects. The interaction of leptin receptor and MC4R mutations may also be important in determining risk of obesity (Hart Sailors et al., 2007). Interestingly, MC4R mutations also promote increases in lean mass, so affected children are often taller as well as fatter (Coll, 2007).

Future therapeutics

MC4R may be an important target for the development of future therapies for obesity. Possibilities include transgenic approaches to increase expression of melanocortins. In obese rodents, overproduction of α- and β-MSH reduces weight gain and body fatness. Melanocortin agonists have been developed for use as anti-obesity drugs but to date have proved unsuitable as they impact upon skin pigmentation and sexual function as well as food intake and energy homeostasis (Coll, 2007).

if underweight children grow up to become underweight adults, their body fatness will be said to have tracked from one stage to another (Figure 6.14). Similarly, if overweight infants remain overweight in adolescence, their body fatness will be described as having tracked throughout childhood. Identification of tracking of overweight and obesity from childhood to adulthood and of risk factors for such tracking is important for two reasons. Firstly, strong evidence of tracking would indicate that high levels of childhood obesity will exert effects upon adult body fatness and related health problems for many decades to come. In other words, if obese children grow up to be obese adults, then the current generation of children may grow up with a major burden of type 2 diabetes and cardiovascular disease. Secondly, if overweight and obesity really do track to adulthood, then it may be possible to identify individuals at greatest risk of obesity and related disorders at an early phase of life and intervene at that stage.

In general, the literature in relation to obesity tracking shows only a moderate, weak association between BMI in childhood and adulthood but stronger associations between BMI in adolescence and later life. Studies that consider tracking are often limited by the span of time that can be reasonably covered by a follow-up study and by the confounding influences of parental BMI and genetic factors.

The Thousand Families cohort, a study of children born in the city of Newcastle between May and June 1947, provided a useful opportunity to consider tracking of body fatness from childhood to middle age. BMI at age 9 was weakly correlated with adult BMI, but this relationship was explained by lean, rather than fat, mass (Wright et al., 2001). There was evidence of tracking from ages 13 to 50 and children whose BMI was in the top quartile for the population were twice as likely to be in the top quartile for body fatness at age 50. However, as obesity was relatively uncommon in the

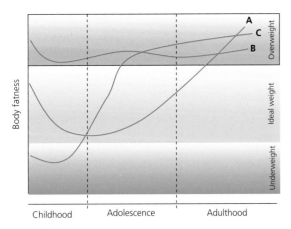

Figure 6.14 Tracking of overweight. An individual whose weight (body fatness) classification changes from childhood to adulthood is not said to be tracking (e.g. line A shows an adult onset of overweight). Where weight classification remains the same from childhood to adulthood (line B) or from adolescence to adulthood (line C), weight is tracking. The evidence of tracking of overweight is strongest from adolescence to adulthood.

1950s and as the drivers of childhood obesity at that time may well be different to contemporary populations, the generalizability of these data may be questioned. Moreover, this study reported that most obese 50-year-olds had not been overweight as children. In contrast, Johannsson *et al.* (2006) suggested that tracking from infancy to adolescence meant that BMI in childhood was a strong predictor of overweight or obesity at age 15. Being overweight at age 6 or 9 was found to increase risk of overweight at 15 by 10.4- and 18.6-fold, respectively. Fifty-one per cent of overweight 6-year-olds remained overweight after puberty. The Bogalusa Heart Study was a prospective cohort study from the United States, with adults who were initially studied at ages 9–11 followed up to 19–35 years of age. Within this more contemporary study, overall tracking of overweight from childhood to adulthood was found to be around 22.5%, compared to 40% tracking of normal weight (Deshmukh-Taskar *et al.*, 2006).

The evidence to support the view that overweight in childhood predisposes the individual to overweight and obesity in adulthood is, therefore, rather modest. While it is clear that there is some influence of childhood body fatness on later weight classification, this is just one component of a more complex aetiology for adult obesity. However, it is important to also consider whether childhood overweight and obesity might be an independent risk factor for adult disease states. Few studies have the power to consider this question in detail. The Thousand Families study surprisingly found that after adjusting for adult body fat, there was an inverse

relationship between BMI at 9 years and adult total cholesterol and triglyceride concentrations, but only for women. Other cardiovascular risk factors were unrelated to childhood BMI, and BMI at age 13 was completely unrelated to adult risk profile (Wright *et al.*, 2001). The greatest risk for adult disease appeared to be predicted by the combination of underweight during childhood and obesity in adulthood.

Juonala *et al.* (2005) found strong evidence of tracking of overweight from early childhood to adulthood. Individuals with BMI over the 80th centile between 3 and 9 years had triple the risk of obesity between 24 and 39 years, and this risk increased to fourfold in those who were overweight in adolescence. Measurements of carotid intima-media thickness as a proxy for early stages of atherosclerosis, however, showed no risk of cardiovascular disease associated with childhood or adolescent obesity. All disease risk was related to adult obesity. Freedman and colleagues (2001) examined relationships between risk factors for cardiovascular disease and BMI in childhood. Although individuals who had been obese in childhood tended to have high circulating total cholesterol, LDL-cholesterol, insulin and triglyceride concentrations and higher blood pressure, these effects were all explained by their greater body fatness in adulthood (Figure 6.15). Systematic reviews of the relationship between childhood obesity and adult cardiovascular (Lloyd *et al.*, 2010) and metabolic (Lloyd *et al.*, 2012) disease found little evidence to suggest that childhood obesity is an independent risk factor. Risk appears entirely related to adult fatness and so tracking of obesity, particularly from adolescence, needs to be prevented.

Although there is a lack of strong evidence to suggest that the obese child is at greater risk of disease in adulthood by virtue of his/her childhood adiposity, the balance of opinion appears to be that the obese child is more likely to be an obese adult and hence develop a high-risk metabolic profile. The treatment and prevention of paediatric obesity is therefore considered to be a very high priority for public health and clinical practice.

6.4.4 Treatment of childhood obesity

Once identified as being overweight or obese, children require rapid and well-thought-out intervention to limit the risk of health problems and of becoming an obese adult with related metabolic and cardiovascular disorders. However, the treatment of obese children poses special problems, as there is a need to maintain normal rates of growth, while simultaneously promoting loss of excess weight and reduction of fat mass. The strategy to be employed will depend upon the age of the child, partly because his/her capacity for

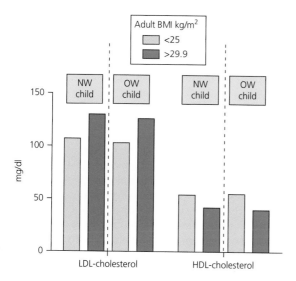

Figure 6.15 Risk factors for coronary heart disease in relation to childhood or adult overweight. Adult obesity is associated with raised circulating LDL-cholesterol and lower HDL-cholesterol concentrations. These are established risk factors for coronary heart disease. In adult individuals who were overweight during childhood, the risk profile associated with obesity is no different to that seen in adults who were of normal weight in childhood. These data suggest that adult risk of coronary heart disease is not directly influenced by childhood weight status. NW, normal weight; OW, overweight. *Source*: Data drawn from Freedman *et al.* (2001).

autonomous decision making will change markedly between childhood and later adolescence but also because of the influence of normal growth. For very young children, for example, reducing rates of weight gain may be sufficient to correct overweight and obesity as the child will normalize body weight and fat mass through the growth process.

The overriding aim in treating childhood obesity is to promote only slow and gradual reductions in fat mass and loss of excess weight. Slower rates of fat loss are easier to sustain and the gradual approach can be advantageous as children and their parents can be set simply achieved goals. With achievement of those goals comes the self-esteem and confidence that is necessary to achieve longer-term aims. However, the absence of an obvious and rapid change can also be disheartening. In some cases, fat loss may occur without any change or even an increase in body weight due to growth. Obese children and their parents therefore require close supervision and encouragement in order to sustain successful treatment.

Treating paediatric obesity requires a close integration of multiple approaches that include changes in nutrition, physical activity levels, sedentary time and wholesale lifestyle modifications that ideally impact upon whole families. The physical activity component can be particularly difficult to introduce as many overweight and obese children find exercise difficult and embarrassing. To promote fat loss, children need to engage in around 60 min/day of aerobic exercise, such as cycling, swimming, dancing or walking. To ensure compliance with any exercise programme, it is essential that the activities increase in intensity at a gradual rate and that the activities are tailored to the individual children. If the exercise is enjoyable, then the children will maintain their involvement, whereas humiliating boot camp experiences will achieve no more than a short-term gain in energy expenditure. When children can be encouraged to take part in activities where they can succeed and show some mastery, self-esteem is increased, boosting motivation and the desire to stay active even at the end of treatment (Craig *et al.*, 1996). Alongside increased levels of exercise, parents should remove or limit access to elements of the environment that promote sedentary activity, for example, televisions and computer games. Many of these changes are perhaps most effective if they are incorporated into whole lifestyle changes in which activity becomes a part of everyday life, for example, walking or cycling to school and other activities.

Dietary modifications to treat obesity must be introduced as long-term changes. It is obvious that any short-term dietary change that ceases as soon as an acceptable BMI is achieved will fail, as the individual will simply revert to his/her old eating habits and regain weight at the end of the treatment. With children, dietary changes should not be referred to as dieting and must be treated as a wholly positive experience. Rather than labelling certain foods as forbidden and to be wholly excluded, children should be encouraged to consume a pattern of diet that is healthier overall but which still includes their preferred options such as sweets and chocolate (Grace, 2001). The overweight child requires a diet that delivers sufficient energy and nutrients to support growth that is based upon foods that are acceptable to children and that are easy to acquire and prepare. Epstein and colleagues (2008) compared the approaches of promoting healthy eating against restricting energy-dense foods in a group of children aged between 8 and 12. All children and their parents were given the goal of keeping energy intake to between 1000 and 1500 kcal/day and taught a traffic light classification of foodstuffs. One group was instructed to limit intakes of red light foods (high in sugar and fat), while the other was instructed to consume greater amounts of green light foods (mostly fruits and vegetables). At follow-ups 12–24 months after the intervention, both groups of children had improved their BMI, but the healthy

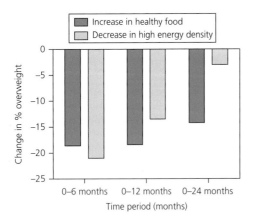

Figure 6.16 Managing obesity in children is more effective where a healthy rather than a restrictive diet is promoted. Weight loss was sustained for a longer period by children who were advised to increase their intakes of 'healthy' foods than among children advised to reduce intake of foods with high energy density.
Source: Epstein *et al.* (2008).

eating group had fared significantly better (Figure 6.16). This study highlights the importance of promoting a healthy lifestyle rather than simply dictating a restrictive diet. When given greater access to healthier foods, children find it easier to consume these as alternatives for energy-dense choices.

For most overweight and obese children, small gradual changes are sufficient to manage weight gain. For those with more severe or morbid obesity, the strategy is different as more rapid weight loss is necessary to avoid ill health. In these cases, low-calorie or very-low-calorie diets (800 kcal/day or less) may be merited but only under strict medical supervision (Caroli and Burniat, 2002).

Parents play a central role in the treatment of obese children. With younger children (under 11), at least, parents will generally have full control over food purchase and preparation, access to exercise opportunities and leisure activities and as such need to be the main targets for education and advice during periods of treatment (Golan *et al.*, 1998). Where at least one parent is actively participating in a weight loss programme alongside their children, the chances of success are increased (McLean *et al.*, 2003). Children enjoy monitoring the progress of their parents and setting their goals and rewards. This stimulates active engagement with treatment programmes. The influence of parents should ideally be applied to all children in a family. It is clearly unreasonable to expect an obese child to change his/her diet and increase activity levels, if other family members do not.

With parents at the heart of treatment strategies, it is of concern to note that many parents of obese children do not recognize that their children have a problem. Carnell *et al.* (2005) surveyed parents of 3–5-year-old children through nursery and primary schools in London and found that only 1.9% of parents with overweight children and 17.1% of parents with obese children described their children as overweight. None of the parents described their children as 'very overweight', even though the prevalence of obesity among the children was actually 7.3%. However, although they were unable to correctly classify their children's body weights, the parents of overweight and obese infants were more than twice as likely than other parents to express concerns that their children may become obese later in life. Successful treatment of paediatric obesity can only begin once parents are ready to recognize the issue and engage with the relevant professionals. Parents are more likely to do this if their overweight child is older, if the parents are themselves overweight or obese and if there is a belief that the health of the child may be at risk (Rhee *et al.*, 2005).

6.4.5 Prevention of childhood obesity

In the United Kingdom, the government's chief scientist published the Foresight Report in 2007. This report highlighted obesity as a major public health problem, which by 2050 would be expected to cost the country £45 billion/year. Within this report, obesity was regarded as the normal passive physiological response to the modern obesogenic environment. To tackle the problem, there has to be massive societal change that changes the environment, as the epidemic cannot be prevented through individual action alone. These conclusions echo the statement made by the World Health Organization in 1997, 'Obesity cannot be prevented or managed solely at the individual level. Committees, governments, the media and the food industry need to work together to modify the environment so that it is less conducive to weight gain'.

Prevention of obesity is a far more effective public health strategy than treatment at any stage of life. Targeting prevention strategies at children is considered to be of primary importance, partly due to the evidence that suggests that obesity may track from childhood to adulthood, but primarily because sweeping lifestyle changes at this stage of life are more likely to be sustained by individuals over the longer term. While prevention strategies require a multi-agency approach that involves families, schools, the food industry and governments (Figure 6.17), they may be more effective if tailored to suit the specific targets in the population. For

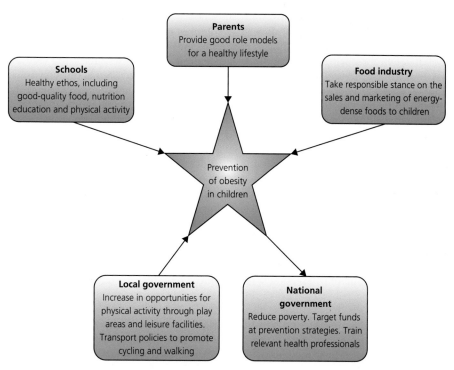

Figure 6.17 The prevention of childhood obesity depends upon the involvement of parents and families, food producers, schools and government agencies. None of these stakeholders have sufficient influence to be able to tackle the obesity problem in isolation.

example, interventions that promote breastfeeding may be an effective way of prevention obesity in infants, while targeting schools to increase physical activity, include more health-related subjects in the curriculum and limit access to energy-dense snacks would be an effective strategy for older school-age children (Daniels *et al.*, 2005).

The influence of parents and family upon the food choices and lifestyle behaviours of children is immense. Implementation of population-wide strategies for prevention of childhood obesity requires all members of the community to recognize the benefits of a healthy diet and greater level of physical activity. The food choices, attitudes and levels of activity adopted by parents will tend to be copied by their children. Parents undoubtedly shape the food choices of young children and even their ability to regulate their own intake and appetite (Birch and Davison, 2001; Cooke *et al.*, 2004). Campaigns to promote awareness of key issues are essential, and the constant coverage of the obesity epidemic and its causes through the printed and broadcast media should play a positive role.

Aside from parents and siblings, schools are the most important influence upon the health behaviours and knowledge of children. Schools are therefore seen as an ideal environment to set obesity prevention strategies and interventions. Schools can change behaviour in a number of different ways:

- Inclusion of healthy eating messages in the curriculum
- Promotion of healthy living to both children and their parents
- Inclusion of physical activity sessions across the whole curriculum on all days of the school week
- Provision of open spaces and active play equipment
- Limiting access to energy-dense snack foods through appropriate policies and removal of vending machines
- Provision of healthy school meals

There have been many published reports of school-based interventions, and these have yielded rather patchy results. These generally show that interventions can be effective in promoting physical activity and/or dietary choices, but often without long-term effects, or observable impact upon risk of overweight. The SMART lunchbox intervention in the United Kingdom (Evans *et al.*, 2010) showed that materials targeting 8–9-year-olds and their parents could improve the quality of packed lunches taken into school, with greater adherence to government standards on school meals. Ribeiro and Alves (2014) showed the efficacy of two school-based programmes in increasing physical activity, reducing sedentary time, improving intakes of fruits and vegetables and reducing fat consumption. The Eat Well and Keep Moving intervention in the United States (Gortmaker *et al.*, 1999) was based upon taught sessions from teachers in all curriculum areas. It achieved improvements in physical activity and dietary quality over a period of 2 years. Kipping *et al.* (2008, 2010) showed that the same programme could be imported into the United Kingdom, again with improvements in activity and intakes of fruits and vegetables over unhealthy snacks. None of these studies, however, reported any benefits in terms of obesity.

Sahota and colleagues (2001) attempted a very broad school-based intervention in primary schools in Leeds, United Kingdom. A group of five schools serving 5–11-year-olds were subjected to a 1-year multidisciplinary programme designed to influence diet, physical activity and knowledge. Teachers underwent relevant training, school meals quality was reviewed and improved, dietitians went into schools to teach sessions to children, physical education classes were altered to emphasize physical fitness, school health resources were improved, playground equipment renewed, and parents encouraged to provide healthier packed lunches. At the end of the intervention period, the schools were compared to five similar schools where no intervention had taken place. Within the intervention schools, the overall ethos had changed considerably and children showed much greater knowledge and understanding of how to change their own behaviour in relation to health. However, despite this, there was no difference in levels of obesity and overweight. In the intervention schools, while consumption of vegetables increased, fruit consumption decreased. Physical activity patterns were unchanged by the intervention. This study highlights the need for engagement with obesity prevention from more than just one agency. Schools alone cannot succeed in reversing obesity trends, if influences and opportunities outside school hours are operating in the opposite direction. The systematic review of Nixon *et al.* (2012) found that randomized controlled trials of school-based interventions were effective in improving dietary choices, physical activity and measures of obesity only if there was high engagement of parents within the intervention. A meta-analysis of 37 randomized controlled trials (Waters *et al.*, 2011) showed that despite great heterogeneity between the effects of individual programmes,

school-based interventions among 6–11-year-olds reduced age-adjusted BMI by $0.15\,kg/m^2$. The review concluded that although the observed benefit was small, it was sufficient to justify continued efforts to target children in schools through approaches based upon education, improving school meals and physical activities and engaging with parents.

The food industry, supermarkets and all elements of the food distribution network have a powerful influence upon the eating habits of the population and must therefore play a critical role in any obesity prevention strategy. To achieve societal change, the industry needs to be persuaded or forced by government to make changes to pricing, availability and marketing of energy-dense, high-fat and high-sugar foodstuffs in order to discourage their consumption (Dehghan *et al.*, 2005; James, 2008b). In some parts of the United States and Canada, taxes have been introduced in order to increase the price of unhealthy foods and snacks, but this might be seen by consumers as heavy-handed and an infringement of their right to choice. It might be more appropriate to lead consumers to make healthier choices through other means, such as improved labelling of foods. James (2008b) points out that the food industry has responded well to other health concerns and should be in a position to do so again. Effective marketing, pricing and control of availability have manipulated population-wide consumption of saturated fats such that intakes have declined and intakes of polyunsaturated fats have increased, with clear benefits in cardiovascular health across northern Europe and America. The UK Department of Health has established the Public Health Responsibility Deal to encourage organizations to commit to taking action by changing commercial activity. The major food companies are signatories to the Responsibility Deal and have initiated action on reducing portion sizes, sugar content of drinks and launches of lower-energy products.

Governments at national and local levels can have a major impact upon the fight against childhood obesity through the influence that they have upon all of the other agencies and individuals described earlier. Introducing policies, taxes or incentives that can influence food purchasing and consumer choices is one tool that could be applied. Similarly, governments can shape education policy and the priorities within school curricula. Changes to the built environment to encourage more leisure facilities, safe open spaces and the introduction of walking and cycling networks can help to promote physical activity.

SUMMARY

- Compared to adults, the energy and nutrient requirements of children are high. Increased demands are a product of growth and maturation. A nutrient- and energy-dense diet is essential to meet these demands as the small size of children means that they are unable to process a bulky diet.

- Children are vulnerable to micronutrient deficiencies and protein–energy malnutrition. Growth faltering is a common sign of these problems. Poverty, infectious disease or restrictive dietary practices are the major factors that drive undernutrition.

- Weaning is the introduction of complementary foods to the infant diet. The overall transition from a milk-based diet to a diet comprising an adult pattern of eating is an opportunity to teach children to follow a healthy lifestyle and comply with guidelines for healthy eating. The range of preferred foods that is actually consumed by children is rather narrow but strongly influenced by parental choices.

- Schools provide suitable environments for the promotion of health in children. This can be achieved through placing health and nutrition in a prominent position in the curriculum, by encouraging daily physical activity and through introduction of high-quality school meals, breakfast clubs and other food-based initiatives.

- The prevalence of overweight and obesity in children has more than doubled in the first decade of the twenty-first century. This increase is primarily driven by increased consumption of energy-dense foodstuffs and declining energy expenditure associated with sedentary leisure activities.

- Successful strategies for the prevention of childhood obesity at the population level are dependent upon integrated activities of all stakeholders, including parents and children, schools, the food industry and local and national governments.

References

Absoud, M., Cummins, C., Lim, M.J. *et al.* (2011) Prevalence and predictors of vitamin D insufficiency in children: a Great Britain population based study. *PLoS One*, **6**, e22179.

Adams, J., Tyrrell, R., Adamson, A.J. *et al.* (2012) Effect of restrictions on television food advertising to children on exposure to advertisements for 'less healthy' foods: repeat cross-sectional study. *PLoS One*, **7**, e31578.

Alvy, L.M. and Calvert, S.L. (2008) Food marketing on popular children's web sites: a content analysis. *Journal of the American Dietetic Association*, **108**, 710–713.

Anderson, P.C. and Dinulos, J.G. (2009) Atopic dermatitis and alternative management strategies. *Current Opinion in Pediatrics*, **21**, 131–138.

Bagramian, R.A., Garcia-Godoy, F. and Volpe, A.R. (2009) The global increase in dental caries. A pending public health crisis. *American Journal of Dentistry*, **22**, 3–8.

Bartfeld, J.S. and Ahn, H.M. (2011) The School Breakfast Program strengthens household food security among low-income households with elementary school children. *Journal of Nutrition*, **141**, 470–475.

Bates, B., Lennox, A., Prentice, A. *et al.* (2011) *National Diet and Nutrition Survey Headline Results from Years 1, 2 and 3 (Combined) of the Rolling Programme (2008/2009–2010/11)*, Public Health England, London.

Bates, B., Lennox, A., Prentice, A. *et al.* (2014) *National Diet and Nutrition Survey: Results from Years 1-4 (combined) of the Rolling Programme (2008/2009 – 2011/12)*, Public Health England, London.

Bere, E., Hilsen, M. and Klepp, K.I. (2010) Effect of the nationwide free school fruit scheme in Norway. *British Journal of Nutrition*, **104**, 589–594.

Bhandari, N., Bahl, R., Taneja, S. *et al.* (2002) Substantial reduction in severe diarrheal morbidity by daily zinc supplementation in young north Indian children. *Pediatrics*, **109**, e86.

Birch, L.L. and Davison, K.K. (2001) Family environmental factors influencing the developing behavioral controls of food intake and childhood overweight. *Pediatric Clinics of North America*, **48**, 893–907.

Black, M.M. (2003) The evidence linking zinc deficiency with children's cognitive and motor functioning. *Journal of Nutrition*, **133**, 1473S–1476S.

Booth, I.W. and Aukett, M.A. (1997) Iron deficiency anaemia in infancy and early childhood. *Archives of Disease in Childhood*, **76**, 549–553.

Borzekowski, D.L. and Robinson, T.N. (2001) The 30-second effect: an experiment revealing the impact of television commercials on food preferences of preschoolers. *Journal of the American Dietetic Association*, **101**, 42–46.

Bowman, S.A., Gortmaker, S.L., Ebbeling, C.B. *et al.* (2004) Effects of fast-food consumption on energy intake and diet quality among children in a national household survey. *Pediatrics*, **113**, 112–118.

Briefel, R., Hanson, C., Fox, M.K. *et al.* (2006) Feeding Infants and Toddlers Study: do vitamin and mineral supplements contribute to nutrient adequacy or excess among US infants and toddlers? *Journal of the American Dietetic Association*, **106**, S52–S65.

Brindal, E., Baird, D., Danthiir, V. *et al.* (2012) Ingesting breakfast meals of different glycaemic load does not alter cognition and satiety in children. *European Journal of Clinical Nutrition*, **66**, 1166–1171.

Brophy, S., Cooksey, R., Gravenor, M.B. *et al.* (2009) Risk factors for childhood obesity at age 5: analysis of the millennium cohort study. *BMC Public Health*, **9**, 467.

Brown, A. and Lee, M. (2011) A descriptive study investigating the use and nature of baby-led weaning in a UK sample of mothers. *Maternal & Child Nutrition*, **7**, 34–47.

Bundred, P., Kitchiner, D. and Buchan, I. (2001) Prevalence of overweight and obese children between 1989 and 1998: population based series of cross sectional studies. *British Medical Journal*, **322**, 326–328.

Butte, N.F. (2005) Energy requirements of infants and children. *Nestle Nutrition Workshop Series: Pediatric Programme*, **58**, 19–32.

Calder, P.C. and Jackson, A.A. (2000) Undernutrition, infection and immune function. *Nutrition Research Reviews*, **13**, 3–29.

Cameron, S.L., Taylor, R.W. and Heath, A.L. (2013) Parent-led or baby-led? Associations between complementary feeding practices and health-related behaviours in a survey of New Zealand families. *BMJ Open*, **3**, e003946.

Carnell, S., Edwards, C., Croker, H. *et al.* (2005) Parental perceptions of overweight in 3–5 y olds. *International Journal of Obesity*, **29**, 353–355.

Caroli, M. and Burniat, W. (2002) Dietary management, in *Child and Adolescent Obesity. Causes, Consequences and Management* (eds W. Burniat, T. Cole, I. Lissau and E. Poskitt), Cambridge University Press, New York, pp. 282–306.

Child Poverty Action Group. (2014) *Child poverty facts and figures*, http://www.cpag.org.uk/child-poverty-facts-and-figures (accessed 20 May 2014).

Chinn, S. and Rona, R.J. (2001) Prevalence and trends in overweight and obesity in three cross sectional studies of British children, 1974–94. *British Medical Journal*, **322**, 24–26.

Cole, T.J., Freeman, J.V. and Preece, M.A. (1995) Body mass index reference curves for the UK, 1990. *Archives of Disease in Childhood*, **73**, 25–29.

Coll, A.P. (2007) Effects of pro-opiomelanocortin (POMC) on food intake and body weight: mechanisms and therapeutic potential? *Clinical Science*, **113**, 171–182.

Congdon, E.L., Westerlund, A., Algarin, C.R. *et al.* (2012) Iron deficiency in infancy is associated with altered neural correlates of recognition memory at 10 years. *Journal of Pediatrics*, **160**, 1027–1033.

Connor, S.M. (2006) Food-related advertising on preschool television: building brand recognition in young viewers. *Pediatrics*, **118**, 1478–1485.

Cooke, L.J., Wardle, J., Gibson, E.L. *et al.* (2004) Demographic, familial and trait predictors of fruit and vegetable consumption by pre-school children. *Public Health Nutrition*, **7**, 295–302.

Cowin, I. and Emmett, P. (2007) ALSPAC Study Team. Diet in a group of 18-month-old children in South West England, and comparison with the results of a national survey. *Journal of Human Nutrition and Dietetics*, **20**, 254–267.

Craig, S., Goldberg, J. and Dietz, W.H. (1996) Psychosocial correlates of physical activity among fifth and eighth graders. *Preventive Medicine*, **25**, 506–513.

Cui, Z. and Dibley, M.J. (2012) Trends in dietary energy, fat, carbohydrate and protein intake in Chinese children and adolescents from 1991 to 2009. *The British Journal of Nutrition*, **108** (7), 1292–1299.

Cummings, P.L., Welch, S.B., Mason, M. *et al.* (2014) Nutrient content of school meals before and after implementation of nutrition recommendations in five school districts across two U.S. counties. *Preventive Medicine*, **67** Suppl 1, S21–S27.

Daniels, S.R., Arnett, D.K., Eckel, R.H. *et al.* (2005) Overweight in children and adolescents: pathophysiology, consequences, prevention, and treatment. *Circulation*, **111**, 1999–2012.

Dehghan, M., Akhtar-Danesh, N. and Merchant, A.T. (2005) Childhood obesity, prevalence and prevention. *Nutrition Journal*, **2**, 4–24.

Department of Health (1998) *Dietary Reference Values for Energy and Nutrients for the United Kingdom*, Stationary Office, London.

Deshmukh-Taskar, P., Nicklas, T.A., Morales, M. *et al.* (2006) Tracking of overweight status from childhood to young adulthood: the Bogalusa Heart Study. *European Journal of Clinical Nutrition*, **60**, 48–57.

Deshmukh-Taskar, P.R., Nicklas, T.A., O'Neil, C.E. *et al.* (2010) The relationship of breakfast skipping and type of breakfast consumption with nutrient intake and weight status in children and adolescents: the National Health and Nutrition Examination Survey 1999-2006. *Journal of the American Dietetic Association*, **110**, 869–878.

Dhar, T. and Baylis, K. (2011) Fast-food consumption and the ban on advertising targeting children: the Quebec experience. *Journal of Marketing Research*, **48**, 799–813.

Dietz, W.H. (1998) Childhood weight affects adult morbidity and mortality. *Journal of Nutrition*, **128**, 411S–414S.

Dixon, H.G., Scully, M.L., Wakefield, M.A. *et al.* (2007) The effects of television advertisements for junk food versus nutritious food on children's food attitudes and preferences. *Social Science and Medicine*, **65**, 1311–1323.

Djennane, M., Lebbah, S., Roux, C. *et al.* (2014) Vitamin D status of schoolchildren in Northern Algeria, seasonal variations and determinants of vitamin D deficiency. *Osteoporosis International*, **25**, 1493–1502.

Dovey, T.M., Staples, P.A., Gibson, E.L. *et al.* (2008) Food neophobia and 'picky/fussy' eating in children: a review. *Appetite*, **50**, 181–193.

Dubois, L., Farmer, A., Girard, M. *et al.* (2008) Social factors and television use during meals and snacks is associated with higher BMI among pre-school children. *Public Health Nutrition*, **12**, 1–13.

Dyson, A., Pizzutto, S.J., MacLennan, C. *et al.* (2014) The prevalence of vitamin D deficiency in children in the Northern Territory. *Journal of Paediatrics and Child Health*, **50**, 47–50.

Eaton, S.B., Konner, M. and Shostak, M. (1988) Stone agers in the fast lane: chronic degenerative diseases in evolutionary perspective. *American Journal of Medicine*, **84**, 739–749.

Ells, L.J., Hillier, F.C., Shucksmith, J. *et al.* (2008) A systematic review of the effect of dietary exposure that could be achieved through normal dietary intake on learning and performance of school-aged children of relevance to UK schools. *British Journal of Nutrition*, **100**, 927–936.

Epstein, L.H., Paluch, R.A., Beecher, M.D. *et al.* (2008) Increasing healthy eating vs. reducing high energy-dense foods to treat pediatric obesity. *Obesity*, **16**, 318–326.

EU-SILC (2007) *EU Survey on Income and Living Conditions*, The Stationery Office, Dublin.

Evans, C.E., Greenwood, D.C., Thomas, J.D. *et al.* (2010) SMART lunch box intervention to improve the food and nutrient content of children's packed lunches: UK wide cluster randomised controlled trial. *Journal of Epidemiology and Community Health*, **64**, 970–976.

Farooqi, I.S., Wangensteen, T., Collins, S. *et al.* (2007) Clinical and molecular genetic spectrum of congenital deficiency of the leptin receptor. *New England Journal of Medicine*, **356**, 237–247.

Fewtrell, M.S. (2011) The evidence for public health recommendations on infant feeding. *Early Human Development*, **87**, 715–721.

Fogarty, A.W., Antoniak, M., Venn, A.J. *et al.* (2007) Does participation in a population-based dietary intervention scheme have a lasting impact on fruit intake in young children? *International Journal of Epidemiology*, **36**, 1080–1085.

Foote, K.D. and Marriott, L.D. (2003) Weaning of infants. *Archives of Disease in Childhood*, **88**, 488–492.

Fox, M.K., Reidy, K., Novak, T. *et al.* (2006) Sources of energy and nutrients in the diets of infants and toddlers. *Journal of the American Dietetic Association*, **106**, S28–S42.

Fraser, L.K., Clarke, G.P., Cade, J.E. *et al.* (2012) Fast food and obesity: a spatial analysis in a large United Kingdom population of children aged 13-15. *American Journal of Preventive Medicine*, **42**, e77–e85.

Freedman, D.S., Khan, L.K., Dietz, W.H. *et al.* (2001) Relationship of childhood obesity to coronary heart disease risk factors in adulthood: the Bogalusa Heart Study. *Pediatrics*, **108**, 712–718.

Freedman, D.S., Ogden, C.L., Flegal, K.M. *et al.* (2007) Childhood overweight and family income. *Medscape General Medicine*, **9**, 26.

Freeman, J.V., Cole, T.J., Chinn, S. *et al.* (1995) Cross sectional stature and weight reference curves for the UK, 1990. *Archives of Disease in Childhood*, **73** (1), 17–24.

Galloway, A.T., Lee, Y. and Birch, L.L. (2003) Predictors and consequences of food neophobia and pickiness in young girls. *Journal of the American Dietetic Association*, **103**, 692–698.

Garlick, P.J. (2006) Protein requirements of infants and children. *Nestle Nutrition Workshop Series: Pediatric Programme*, **58**, 39–47.

Garza, J.C., Kim, C.S., Liu, J. *et al.* (2008) Adeno-associated virus-mediated knockdown of melanocortin-4 receptor in the paraventricular nucleus of the hypothalamus promotes high-fat diet-induced hyperphagia and obesity. *Journal of Endocrinology*, **197**, 471–482.

Georgieff, M.K. (2007) Nutrition and the developing brain: nutrient priorities and measurement. *American Journal of Clinical Nutrition*, **85**, 614S–620S.

Golan, M., Weizman, A., Apter, A. *et al.* (1998) Parents as the exclusive agents of change in the treatment of childhood obesity. *American Journal of Clinical Nutrition*, **67**, 1130–1135.

Goldstone, A.P. (2004) Prader-Willi syndrome: advances in genetics, pathophysiology and treatment. *Trends in Endocrinology and Metabolism*, **15**, 12–20.

Gordon, C.M., Feldman, H.A., Sinclair, L. *et al.* (2008) Prevalence of vitamin D deficiency among healthy infants and toddlers. *Archives of Pediatrics and Adolescent Medicine*, **162**, 505–512.

Goris, J.M., Petersen, S., Stamatakis, E. *et al.* (2010) Television food advertising and the prevalence of childhood overweight and obesity: a multicountry comparison. *Public Health Nutrition*, **13**, 1003–1012.

Gortmaker, S.L., Cheung, L.W., Peterson, K.E. *et al.* (1999) Impact of a school-based interdisciplinary intervention on diet and physical activity among urban primary school children: eat well and keep moving. *Archives of Pediatrics and Adolescent Medicine*, **153**, 975–983.

Grace, C.M. (2001) Dietary management of obesity, in *Management of Obesity and Related Disorders* (ed P.G. Kopelman), Martin Dunitz, London, pp. 129–164.

Gregory, J., Lowe, S., Bates, C.J. *et al.* (2000) *National diet and nutrition survey: young people aged 4 to 18 years, volume 1: report of the diet and nutrition survey*, The Stationery Office, London.

Griffiths, C., Gately, P., Marchant, P.R. *et al.* (2013) A five year longitudinal study investigating the prevalence of childhood obesity: comparison of BMI and waist circumference. *Public Health*, **127**, 1090–1096.

Guillaume, M., Lapidus, L. and Lambert, A. (1998) Obesity and nutrition in children. The Belgian Luxembourg Child Study IV. *European Journal of Clinical Nutrition*, **52**, 323–328.

Günther, A.L., Buyken, A.E. and Kroke, A. (2007a) Protein intake during the period of complementary feeding and early childhood and the association with body mass index and percentage body fat at 7 y of age. *American Journal of Clinical Nutrition*, **85**, 1626–1633.

Günther, A.L., Remer, T., Kroke, A. *et al.* (2007b) Early protein intake and later obesity risk: which protein sources at which time points throughout infancy and childhood are important for body mass index and body fat percentage at 7 y of age? *American Journal of Clinical Nutrition*, **86**, 1765–1772.

Hackett, A., Nathan, I. and Burgess, L. (1998) Is a vegetarian diet adequate for children. *Nutrition and Health*, **12**, 189–195.

Halford, J.C., Boyland, E.J., Hughes, G. *et al.* (2007) Beyond-brand effect of television (TV) food advertisements/commercials on caloric intake and food choice of 5-7-year-old children. *Appetite*, **49**, 263–267.

Hamlyn, B., Brooker, S., Oleinikova, K. *et al.* (2002) *Infant Feeding 2000*, The Stationery Office, London.

Hart Sailors, M.L., Folsom, A.R., Ballantyne, C.M. *et al.* (2007) Genetic variation and decreased risk for obesity in the Atherosclerosis Risk in Communities Study. *Diabetes Obesity and Metabolism*, **9**, 548–557.

Health and Social Care Information Centre (2012) *National Statistics Infant Feeding Survey - UK, 2010*, Health and Social Care Information Centre, Leeds.

Hediger, M.L., Overpeck, M.D., Kuczmarski, R.J. *et al.* (2001) Association between infant breastfeeding and overweight in young children. *Journal of the American Medical Association*, **285**, 2453–2460.

Hill, J.O. and Peters, J.C. (1998) Environmental contributions to the obesity epidemic. *Science*, **280**, 1371–1374.

Hoppe, C., Mølgaard, C., Thomsen, B.L. *et al.* (2004) Protein intake at 9 mo of age is associated with body size but not with body fat in 10-y-old Danish children. *American Journal of Clinical Nutrition*, **79**, 494–501.

Hughes, R.J., Edwards, K.L., Clarke, G.P. *et al.* (2012) Childhood consumption of fruit and vegetables across England: a study of 2306 6-7-year-olds in 2007. *British Journal of Nutrition*, **108**, 733–742.

Huybrechts, I., Maes, L., Vereecken, C. *et al.* (2010) High dietary supplement intakes among Flemish preschoolers. *Appetite*, **54**, 340–345.

James, W.P. (2008a) The fundamental drivers of the obesity epidemic. *Obesity Reviews*, **9**, 6–13.

James, W.P. (2008b) The epidemiology of obesity: the size of the problem. *Journal of Internal Medicine*, **263**, 336–352.

Jessiman, T., Cameron, A., Wiggins, M. *et al.* (2013) A qualitative study of uptake of free vitamins in England. *Archives of Disease in Childhood*, **98**, 587–591.

Johannsson, E., Arngrimsson, S.A., Thorsdottir, I. *et al.* (2006) Tracking of overweight from early childhood to adolescence in cohorts born 1988 and 1994: overweight in a high birth weight population. *International Journal of Obesity*, **30**, 1265–1271.

Johnson, L., Mander, A.P., Jones, L.R. *et al.* (2008) Energy-dense, low-fiber, high-fat dietary pattern is associated with increased fatness in childhood. *American Journal of Clinical Nutrition*, **87**, 846–854.

Juonala, M., Raitakari, M.S.A., Viikari, J. *et al.* (2005) Obesity in youth is not an independent predictor of carotid IMT in adulthood. The cardiovascular risk in Young Finns Study. *Atherosclerosis*, **185**, 388–393.

Keller, K.L., Kuilema, L.G., Lee, N. *et al.* (2012) The impact of food branding on children's eating behavior and obesity. *Physiology & Behaviour*, **106**, 379–386.

Kemp, A. (2008) Food additives and hyperactivity. *British Medical Journal*, **336**, 1144.

Kennedy, E. and Davis, C. (1998) US department of agriculture school breakfast program. *American Journal of Clinical Nutrition*, **67**, 798S–803S.

Kipping, R.R., Payne, C. and Lawlor, D.A. (2008) Randomised controlled trial adapting US school obesity prevention to England. *Archives of Disease in Childhood*, **93**, 469–473.

Kipping, R.R., Jago, R. and Lawlor, D.A. (2010) Diet outcomes of a pilot school-based randomised controlled obesity prevention study with 9-10 year olds in England. *Preventive Medicine*, **51**, 56–62.

Kopelman, C.A., Roberts, L.M. and Adab, P. (2007) Advertising of food to children: is brand logo recognition related to their food knowledge, eating behaviours and food preferences? *Journal of Public Health*, **29**, 358–367.

Kukrety, N. (2007) *Investing in the Future*, Save the Children, London.

Küpers, L.K., de Pijper, J.J., Sauer, P.J. *et al.* (2014) Skipping breakfast and overweight in 2- and 5-year-old Dutch children-the GECKO Drenthe cohort. *International Journal of Obesity*, **38**, 569–571.

Lanigan, J.A., Bishop, J., Kimber, A.C. *et al.* (2001) Systematic review concerning the age of introduction of complementary foods to the healthy full-term infant. *European Journal of Clinical Nutrition*, **55**, 309–320.

Leaf, A.A. (2007) RCPCH standing committee on nutrition. Vitamins for babies and young children. *Archives of Disease in Childhood*, **92**, 160–164.

Lee, Y.S., Poh, L.K., Kek, B.L. *et al.* (2008) Novel melanocortin 4 receptor gene mutations in severely obese children. *Clinical Endocrinology*, **68**, 529–535.

Li, Y., Wedick, N.M., Lai, J. *et al.* (2011) Lack of dietary diversity and dyslipidaemia among stunted overweight children: the 2002 China National Nutrition and Health Survey. *Public Health Nutrition*, **14**, 896–903.

Liao, Y., Liao, J., Durand, C.P. *et al.* (2014) Which type of sedentary behaviour intervention is more effective at reducing body mass index in children? A meta-analytic review. *Obesity Reviews*, **15**, 159–168.

Lim, S., Zoellner, J.M., Lee, J.M. *et al.* (2009) Obesity and sugar-sweetened beverages in African-American preschool children: a longitudinal study. *Obesity*, **17**, 1262–1268.

Liu, J., Hwang, W.T., Dickerman, B. *et al.* (2013) Regular breakfast consumption is associated with increased IQ in kindergarten children. *Early Human Development*, **89**, 257–262.

Lloyd, L.J., Langley-Evans, S.C. and McMullen, S. (2010) Childhood obesity and adult cardiovascular disease risk: a systematic review. *International Journal of Obesity*, **34**, 18–28.

Lloyd, L.J., Langley-Evans, S.C. and McMullen, S. (2012) Childhood obesity and risk of the adult metabolic syndrome: a systematic review. *International Journal of Obesity*, **36**, 1–11.

Lobstein, T. and Dibb, S. (2005) Evidence of a possible link between obesogenic food advertising and child overweight. *Obesity Reviews*, **6**, 203–208.

Lok, K.Y., Chan, R.S., Lee, V.W. *et al.* (2013) Food additives and behavior in 8- to 9-year-old children in Hong Kong: a randomized, double-blind, placebo-controlled trial. *Journal of Developmental and Behavioral Pediatrics*, **34**, 642–650.

Loos, R.J. and Bouchard, C. (2008) FTO: the first gene contributing to common forms of human obesity. *Obesity Reviews*, **9**, 246–250.

Loos, R.J., Lindgren, C.M., Li, S. *et al.* (2008) Common variants near MC4R are associated with fat mass, weight and risk of obesity. *Nature Genetics*, **40**, 768–775.

Lozoff, B., Beard, J., Connor, J. *et al.* (2006) Long-lasting neural and behavioral effects of iron deficiency in infancy. *Nutrition Reviews*, **64**, S34–S43.

Lozoff, B., Smith, J.B., Kaciroti, N. *et al.* (2013) Functional significance of early-life iron deficiency: outcomes at 25 years. *Journal of Pediatrics*, **163**, 1260–1266.

Ludwig, D.S., Peterson, K.E. and Gortmaker, S.L. (2001) Relation between consumption of sugar-sweetened drinks and childhood obesity: a prospective, observational analysis. *Lancet*, **357**, 505–508.

Lutter, C.K. and Dewey, K.G. (2003) Proposed nutrient composition for fortified complementary foods. *Journal of Nutrition*, **133**, 3011S–3020S.

Lutter, C.K. and Rivera, J.A. (2003) Nutritional status of infants and young children and characteristics of their diets. *Journal of Nutrition*, **133**, 2941S–2949S.

Maffeis, C., Talamini, G. and Tatò, L. (1998) Influence of diet, physical activity and parents' obesity on children's adiposity: a four-year longitudinal study. *International Journal of Obesity*, **22**, 758–764.

Magarey, A.M., Daniels, L.A., Boulton, T.J. *et al.* (2001) Does fat intake predict adiposity in healthy children and adolescents aged 2–15 y? A longitudinal analysis. *European Journal of Clinical Nutrition*, **55**, 471–481.

Mangels, A.R. and Messina, V. (2001) Considerations in planning vegan diets: infants. *Journal of the American Dietetic Association*, **101**, 670–677.

Martin-Calvo, N., Martínez-González, M.A., Bes-Rastrollo, M. *et al.* (2015) *Sugar-sweetened carbonated beverage consumption and childhood/adolescent obesity: a case-control study*. Public Health Nutrition In Press.

McCaffrey, T.A., Rennie, K.L., Kerr, M.A. *et al.* (2008) Energy density of the diet and change in body fatness from childhood to adolescence; is there a relation? *American Journal of Clinical Nutrition*, **87**, 1230–1237.

McCann, D., Barrett, A., Cooper, A. *et al.* (2007) Food additives and hyperactive behaviour in 3-year-old and 8/9-year-old children in the community: a randomised, double-blinded, placebo controlled trial. *Lancet*, **370**, 1560–1567.

McDonagh, M.S., Whiting, P.F., Wilson, P.M. *et al.* (2000) Systematic review of water fluoridation. *British Medical Journal*, **321**, 855–859.

McFadden, A., Green, J.M., Williams, V. *et al.* (2014) Can food vouchers improve nutrition and reduce health inequalities in low-income mothers and young children: a multi-method evaluation of the experiences of beneficiaries and practitioners of the Healthy Start programme in England. *BMC Public Health*, **14**, 148.

McLean, N., Griffin, S., Toney, K. *et al.* (2003) Family involvement in weight control, weight maintenance and weight-loss interventions: a systematic review of randomised trials. *International Journal of Obesity*, **27**, 987–1005.

Moore, G.F., Tapper, K., Murphy, S. *et al.* (2007) Associations between deprivation, attitudes towards eating breakfast and breakfast eating behaviours in 9–11-year-olds. *Public Health Nutrition*, **10**, 582–589.

Moore, A.P., Milligan, P., Rivas, C. *et al.* (2012) Sources of weaning advice, comparisons between formal and informal advice, and associations with weaning timing in a survey of UK first-time mothers. *Public Health Nutrition*, **15**, 1661–1669.

Mullan, B., Wong, C., Kothe, E. *et al.* (2014) An examination of the demographic predictors of adolescent breakfast consumption, content, and context. *BMC Public Health*, **14**, 264.

Muñoz, E.C., Rosado, J.L., López, P. *et al.* (2000) Iron and zinc supplementation improves indicators of vitamin A status of Mexican preschoolers. *American Journal of Clinical Nutrition*, **71**, 789–794.

Must, A. and Tybor, D.J. (2005) Physical activity and sedentary behavior: a review of longitudinal studies of weight and adiposity in youth. *International Journal of Obesity*, **29**, S84–S96.

National Institute of Dental and Craniofacial Research. (2014) *Dental caries in children (aged 2-11)*, http://www.nidcr.nih.gov/DataStatistics/FindDataByTopic/DentalCaries/DentalCariesChildren2to11 (accessed 20 May 2014).

Nelson, M. (2000) Childhood nutrition and poverty. *Proceedings of the Nutrition Society*, **59**, 307–315.

Neville, L., Thomas, M. and Bauman, A. (2005) Food advertising on Australian television: the extent of children's exposure. *Health Promotion International*, **20**, 105–112.

Nigg, J.T., Lewis, K., Edinger, T. *et al.* (2012) Meta-analysis of attention-deficit/hyperactivity disorder or attention-deficit/hyperactivity disorder symptoms, restriction diet, and synthetic food color additives. *Journal of the American Academy of Child and Adolescent Psychiatry*, **51**, 86–97.

Nixon, C.A., Moore, H.J., Douthwaite, W. *et al.* (2012) Identifying effective behavioural models and behaviour change strategies underpinning preschool- and school-based obesity prevention interventions aimed at 4-6-year-olds: a systematic review. *Obesity Reviews*, **13** (Suppl 1), 106–117.

Noimark, L. and Cox, H.E. (2008) Nutritional problems related to food allergy in childhood. *Pediatric Allergy and Immunology*, **19**, 188–195.

O'Rahilly, S. (2007) Human obesity and insulin resistance: lessons from experiments of nature. *Biochemical Society Transactions*, **35**, 33–36.

OECD. (2011) *Overweight and obesity among children*, http://www.oecd-ilibrary.org/sites/health_glance-2011-en/02/04/index.html;jsessionid=cglsg3b4phjf.x-oecd-live-01?contentType=&itemId=%2Fcontent%2Fchapter%2Fhealth_glance-2011-19-en&mimeType=text%2Fhtml&containerItemId=%2Fcontent%2Fserial%2F19991312&accessItemIds=%2Fcontent%2Fbook%2Fhealth_glance-2011-en (accessed 20 May 2014).

Ong, K.K., Emmett, P.M., Noble, S. *et al.* (2006) Dietary energy intake at the age of 4 months predicts postnatal weight gain and childhood body mass index. *Pediatrics*, **117**, e503–508.

Osendarp, S.J., Santosham, M., Black, R.E. *et al.* (2002) Effect of zinc supplementation between 1 and 6 mo of life on growth and morbidity of Bangladeshi infants in urban slums. *American Journal of Clinical Nutrition*, **76**, 1401–1408.

Pearce, J. and Langley-Evans, S.C. (2013) The types of food introduced during complementary feeding and risk of childhood obesity: a systematic review. *International Journal of Obesity*, **37**, 477–485.

Pearce, J., Taylor, M.A. and Langley-Evans, S.C. (2013) Timing of the introduction of complementary feeding and risk of childhood obesity: a systematic review. *International Journal of Obesity*, **37**, 1295–1306.

Pilgrim, A., Barker, M., Jackson, A. *et al.* (2012) Does living in a food insecure household impact on the diets and body composition of young children? Findings from the Southampton Women's Survey. *Journal of Epidemiology and Community Health*, **66**, e6.

Pinhas-Hamiel, O., Dolan, L.M., Daniels, S.R. *et al.* (1996) Increased incidence of non-insulin-dependent diabetes mellitus among adolescents. *Journal of Pediatrics*, **128**, 608–615.

Poti, J.M., Slining, M.M. and Popkin, B.M. (2013) Where are kids getting their empty calories? Stores, schools, and fast-food restaurants each played an important role in empty calorie intake among US children during 2009-2010. *Journal of the Academy of Food and Dietetics*, **114**, 908–917.

Prentice, A.M. and Paul, A.A. (2000) Fat and energy needs of children in developing countries. *American Journal of Clinical Nutrition*, **72**, 1253S–1265S.

Public Health England (2012) *National Dental Epidemiology Programme for England: Oral Health Survey of Five-Year-Old Children 2012*, Public Health England, London.

Rampersaud, G.C., Pereira, M.A., Girard, B.L. *et al.* (2005) Breakfast habits, nutritional status, body weight, and academic performance in children and adolescents. *Journal of the American Dietetic Association*, **105**, 743–760.

Ransley, J.K., Greenwood, D.C., Cade, J.E. *et al.* (2007) Does the school fruit and vegetable scheme improve children's diet? A non-randomised controlled trial. *Journal of Epidemiology and Community Health*, **61**, 699–703.

Reilly, J.J., Armstrong, J., Dorosty, A.R. *et al.* (2005) Avon longitudinal study of parents and children study team. Early life risk factors for obesity in childhood: cohort study. *British Medical Journal*, **330**, 1357.

Rennie, K.L., Wells, J.C., McCaffrey, T.A. *et al.* (2006) The effect of physical activity on body fatness in children and adolescents. *Proceedings of the Nutrition Society*, **65**, 393–402.

Rhee, K.E., De Lago, C.W., Arscott-Mills, T. *et al.* (2005) Factors associated with parental readiness to make changes for overweight children. *Pediatrics*, **116**, e94–e101.

Ribeiro, R.Q. and Alves, L. (2014) Comparison of two school-based programmes for health behaviour change: the Belo Horizonte Heart Study randomized trial. *Public Health Nutrition*, **17**, 1195–1204.

Robertson, S.M., Cullen, K.W., Baranowski, J. *et al.* (1999) Factors related to adiposity among children aged 3 to 7 years. *Journal of the American Dietetic Association*, **99**, 938–943.

Robinson, T.N., Borzekowski, D.L., Matheson, D.M. *et al.* (2007) Effects of fast food branding on young children's taste preferences. *Archives of Pediatrics and Adolescent Medicine*, **161**, 792–797.

Robinson, S.M., Marriott, L.D., Crozier, S.R. *et al.* (2009) Variations in infant feeding practice are associated with body composition in childhood: a prospective cohort study. *Journal of Clinical Endocrinology and Metabolism*, **94**, 2799–2805.

Rosenheck, R. (2008) Fast food consumption and increased caloric intake: a systematic review of a trajectory towards weight gain and obesity risk. *Obesity Reviews*, **9**, 518–521.

Rudolf, M.C., Sahota, P., Barth, J.H. *et al.* (2001) Increasing prevalence of obesity in primary school children: cohort study. *British Medical Journal*, **322**, 1094–1095.

SACN (2003) *Salt and Health*, The Stationery Office, London.

Sahota, P., Rudolf, M.C., Dixey, R. *et al.* (2001) Randomised controlled trial of primary school based intervention to reduce risk factors for obesity. *British Medical Journal*, **323**, 1029–1032.

Sausenthaler, S., Kompauer, I., Mielck, A. *et al.* (2007) Impact of parental education and income inequality on children's food intake. *Public Health Nutrition*, **10**, 24–33.

Sazawal, S., Black, R.E., Ramsan, M. *et al.* (2006) Effects of routine prophylactic supplementation with iron and folic acid on admission to hospital and mortality in preschool children in a high malaria transmission setting: community-based, randomised, placebo-controlled trial. *Lancet*, **367**, 133–143.

Schab, D.W. and Trinh, N.H. (2004) Do artificial food colors promote hyperactivity in children with hyperactive syndromes? A meta-analysis of double-blind placebo-controlled trials. *Journal of Developmental and Behavioral Pediatrics*, **25**, 423–434.

School Food Trust. (2012) *Final food-based standards for school lunches*, http://www.childrensfoodtrust.org.uk/the-standards/the-food-based-standards/final-food-based-standards (accessed 20 May 2014).

Schulte, A.G. (2005) Salt fluoridation in Germany since 1991. *Schweizerische Monatsschrift für Zahnmedizin*, **115**, 659–662.

Shamah, T. and Villalpando, S. (2006) The role of enriched foods in infant and child nutrition. *British Journal of Nutrition*, **96**, S73–S77.

Shaw, N.J. and Pal, B.R. (2002) Vitamin D deficiency in UK Asian families: activating a new concern. *Archives of Disease in Childhood*, **86**, 147–149.

Skinner, J.D., Bounds, W., Carruth, B.R. *et al.* (2004) Predictors of children's body mass index: a longitudinal study of diet and growth in children aged 2–8 y. *International Journal of Obesity*, **28**, 476–482.

Smith, C., Parnell, W.R., Brown, R.C. *et al.* (2013) Providing additional money to food-insecure households and its effect on food expenditure: a randomized controlled trial. *Public Health Nutrition*, **16**, 1507–1515.

Swinburn, B.A., Sacks, G., Hall, K.D. *et al.* (2011) The global obesity pandemic: shaped by global drivers and local environments. *Lancet*, **378**, 804–814.

Te Morenga, L., Mallard, S. and Mann, J. (2012) Dietary sugars and body weight: systematic review and meta-analyses of randomised controlled trials and cohort studies. *British Medical Journal*, **346**, e7492.

Thompson, O.M., Ballew, C., Resnicow, K. *et al.* (2006) Dietary pattern as a predictor of change in BMI z-score among girls. *International Journal of Obesity*, **30**, 176–182.

Torun, B. (2005) Energy requirements of children and adolescents. *Public Health Nutrition*, **8**, 968–993.

Townsend, E. and Pitchford, N.J. (2012) Baby knows best? The impact of weaning style on food preferences and body mass index in early childhood in a case-controlled sample. *BMJ Open*, **2**, e000298.

Tremblay, M.S., LeBlanc, A.G., Kho, M.E. *et al.* (2011) Systematic review of sedentary behaviour and health indicators in school-aged children and youth. *International Journal of Behavioral Nutrition and Physical Activity*, **8**, 98.

Truman, B.I., Gooch, B.F., Sulemana, I. *et al.* (2002) Reviews of evidence on interventions to prevent dental caries, oral and pharyngeal cancers, and sports-related craniofacial injuries. *American Journal of Preventive Medicine*, **23** (1 Suppl), 21–54.

United Nations. (2013) *The Millennium Development Goals Report 2013*, http://www.un.org/millenniumgoals/pdf/report-2013/mdg-report-2013-english.pdf (accessed 8 January 2015).

Ustjanauskas, A.E., Harris, J.L. and Schwartz, M.B. (2014) Food and beverage advertising on children's web sites. *Pediatric Obesity*, **9**, 362–372.

Utter, J., Scragg, R., Mhurchu, C.N. *et al.* (2007) At-home breakfast consumption among New Zealand children: associations with body mass index and related nutrition behaviors. *Journal of the American Dietetic Association*, **107**, 570–576.

Wang, Y.C., Bleich, S.N. and Gortmaker, S.L. (2008) Increasing caloric contribution from sugar-sweetened beverages and 100% fruit juices among US children and adolescents, 1988–2004. *Pediatrics*, **121**, e1604–e1614.

Wardle, J., Carnell, S., Haworth, C.M. *et al.* (2008) Evidence for a strong genetic influence on childhood adiposity despite the force of the obesogenic environment. *American Journal of Clinical Nutrition*, **87**, 398–404.

Waters, E., de Silva-Sanigorski, A., Hall, B.J. *et al.* (2011) Interventions for preventing obesity in children. *Cochrane Database of Systematic Reviews*, **7** (12), CD001871.

Wesnes, K.A., Pincock, C. and Scholey, A. (2012) Breakfast is associated with enhanced cognitive function in schoolchildren. An internet based study. *Appetite*, **59**, 646–649.

World Health Organization. (2011) *Reducing the marketing of unhealthy foods to children*, http://www.who.int/chp/media/news/releases/2011_1_marketing/en/ (accessed 20 May 2014).

Wright, C.M., Parker, L., Lamont, D. *et al.* (2001) Implications of childhood obesity for adult health: findings from thousand families cohort study. *British Medical Journal*, **323**, 1280–1284.

Wright, C.M., Parkinson, K.N., Shipton, D. *et al.* (2007) How do toddler eating problems relate to their eating behavior, food preferences, and growth? *Pediatrics*, **120**, e1069–e1075.

Additional reading

If you would like to find out more about the material discussed in this chapter, the following sources may be of interest.

Morgan, J.B. and Dickerson, J.W.T. (2002) *Nutrition in Early Life*, Wiley Blackwell.

O'Dea, J.A. and Eriksen, M. (eds) (2010) *Childhood Obesity Prevention: International Research, Controversies and Interventions*, Oxford University Press.

Parizkova, J. (1996) *Nutrition, Physical Activity, and Health in Early Life: Studies in Preschool Children*, CRC Press.

Poskitt, E. and Edmonds, L. (2008) *Management of Childhood Obesity*, Cambridge University Press.

CHAPTER 7
Nutrition and adolescence

LEARNING OBJECTIVES

This chapter will enable the reader to:
- Describe the patterns of growth that are seen during the adolescent period
- Discuss the changes in body composition that are associated with the pubertal phase of growth
- Show an appreciation of the relationship between endocrine factors and nutritional status as determinants of bone growth and sexual maturation
- Describe the processes that allow the growth of bone and how they are sensitive to micronutrient intake, physical activity and overweight
- Discuss the physiological processes that determine requirements for energy, macronutrients and micronutrients during adolescence

- Describe how the increasing independence that is associated with adolescence is a major factor that determines food choices during this life stage
- Identify behaviours that may promote problems with nutritional status among adolescents. These will include restrictive dietary practices, excessive physical activity, disordered eating and the use of alcohol and tobacco products
- Discuss the main features of anorexia nervosa and bulimia nervosa and identify key risk factors for the development of these eating disorders in adolescence
- Describe the particular nutritional concerns that are associated with pregnancy during adolescence

7.1 Introduction

Adolescence is the transitional stage that lies between childhood and adulthood. This stage of life is dominated by the physiological processes that surround puberty, which are accompanied by rapid growth and maturation. Alongside these biological processes, there are psychological changes as the child attains an adult capacity for cognitive processes and acquires the ability to take on adult responsibilities. The impact that the adolescent period has upon nutritional status is not only influenced by these biological and psychological changes but is also strongly modulated by the sociocultural aspects of adolescence. In many of the developing countries, the transition from child to adult is mostly a physiological issue, and culturally, the child becomes an adult by passing through a coming-of-age ceremony. Thereafter, the boys take on the roles of adult men, and the girls marry and have children. In industrialized countries, the social construct of the 'teenager' is the dominant cultural pattern. This serves to extend the transition from child to adult, and in effect, the young adult lives for a longer period under the guidance of their parents. The teenager is culturally expected to undergo emotional trauma and erratic and occasionally rebellious behaviour. This chapter will consider how these issues and behaviours, coupled with the biological demands of adolescence, impact upon nutritional requirements and status.

7.2 Physical development

7.2.1 Growth rate

During childhood, growth occurs at a rate of 5–6 cm/year, with a steady decline in growth velocity from infancy through to the onset of puberty. With puberty, both girls and boys go through a 'growth spurt' that lasts for approximately 2–3 years. In terms of height, the gain associated with the growth spurt is a significant proportion of final adult stature (15–20%). During this growth phase, girls

---

Nutrition, Health and Disease: A Lifespan Approach, Second Edition. Simon Langley-Evans.
© 2015 John Wiley & Sons, Ltd. Published 2015 by John Wiley & Sons, Ltd.
Companion website: www.wiley.com/go/langleyevans/lifespan

gain approximately 20 cm (range 5–25 cm), while in boys, the gain is slightly greater at 23 cm (10–30 cm). Peak height velocities achieved during the growth spurt are 9 and 10.5 cm/year for girls and boys, respectively (Tanner, 1989). Timing of the growth spurt is earlier in girls than in boys, occurring at around the time the breasts begin to grow (thelarche, one of the earliest indicators of female puberty). In boys, sexual maturation has generally advanced to a relatively late stage before the onset of the growth spurt. The increase in rates of height gain is matched by increases in weight. In boys, height and weight gains occur together, but in girls, weight gain lags behind height gain by 3–6 months. In both sexes, weight gain is proportionally greater than height gain (e.g. girls gain 20% of adult height and 50% of adult weight during the growth spurt), leading to an increased body mass index.

Although the pubertal growth spurt is a phase of major height and weight gain, it is not the main determinant of final adult height. Indeed, it is estimated that only 30% of the variation in adult height is explained by the rate of growth during its maximal phase during puberty (Tanner, 1989). Growth before puberty is in fact the main determinant of adult stature, and the height and weight gained during the growth spurt are simply superimposed upon the prepubertal growth rate. Boys tend to grow taller than girls because they enter puberty at a later stage. Indeed, prior to puberty, boys and girls tend to be of similar stature (average height of Europeans at age 9 for boys is 132 cm and for girls 131 cm), but by adulthood, males are typically 12–13 cm taller. Similarly, girls who are 'late developers' and enter puberty at an older age will generally attain a greater than average height due to their extended prepubertal growth phase.

The growth spurt impacts upon all parts of the body, but the timing of regional growth is uneven. Limb growth precedes the growth of the trunk by 6–9 months, for example. Thickening of the skull and remodelling of tissues of the scalp, widening of the jaws and growth of the facial musculature are all events associated with the growth spurt and are more pronounced in boys than in girls, particularly later in puberty. Growth ceases in males between the ages of 18 and 20, which is usually 2–3 years after the end of the growth spurt. In females, growth usually ceases within 2–3 years of menarche, and on average, girls attain final adult height by the age of 16.5 years. In some cases, later sexual maturation allows growth to continue until 19 years.

Growth is sexually dimorphic, in terms of the timing and final achieved heights and the distribution of increasing mass. Males exhibit characteristic increases in size across the shoulders during puberty, while in females, there is greater growth at the hips. These differences in skeletal growth occur due to hormone

sensitivity of cartilage cells at these sites. At the hip, cells respond to oestrogen and this leads to greater pelvic girth to accommodate reproductive functions. Androgen sensitivity at the shoulders produces the characteristic male body shape and upper body strength.

7.2.2 Body composition

The rapid growth of adolescence is accompanied by remodelling of body composition in both sexes. In boys and girls, the larger body mass associated with greater stature is associated with an increase in muscle mass and hence the fat-free mass of the body (Figure 7.1). The growth spurt for muscle lags slightly behind the peak in linear growth, and as it is triggered by the events of puberty, it tends to occur earlier in females than in males. In fact, for a period between 12 and 14 years of age, girls will tend to be more muscular than boys (Tanner, 1989). However, there are significant differences between the

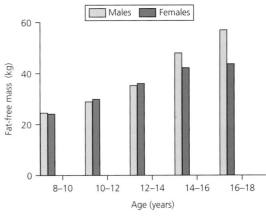

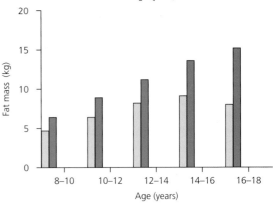

Figure 7.1 Accrual of lean and fat mass during the prepubertal and pubertal periods. During adolescence, there is a rapid increase in the lean body mass of males and females, coinciding with the pubertal growth spurt. Fat mass also increases but to a greater extent in females.
Data source: Guo *et al.* (1997).

sexes in terms of fat deposition, which is greater in girls than in boys. As a result, while fat-free mass as a proportion of body weight increases from 80 to 90% in boys across the period of adolescence, this declines from 80 to 75% in girls.

As shown in Figure 7.1, the absolute mass of body fat in boys increases slightly between the ages of 8 and the onset of the pubertal growth spurt and then declines. As a proportion of body mass, body fat increases from 15% at age 8 to 17.5% at 12–14 years, but by the end of puberty, it is only 11% (Guo *et al.*, 1997). In girls, puberty is associated with a steady increase in the amount of adipose tissue, as fat is deposited in the pelvic region, breasts, upper back, and arms and subcutaneously. As a proportion of body mass, fat increases from 20 to 25% in females over the adolescent years.

7.2.3 Puberty and sexual maturation

It should be clear from the sections earlier that sexual maturation and the events surrounding puberty are the principal processes that determine many of the requirements for nutrients and changes in body composition that are associated with the adolescent period. Puberty has its onset earlier in girls (8–13 years of age) than in boys (9.5–13.5 years of age) and is typically of 3–4 years in duration. There are wide variations in timing and speed of maturation between individuals. In boys, the growth of the penis, for example, on average begins at the age of 12.5 years. However, in some boys, this will occur much earlier (10.5 years) and in others as late as 14.5 years. Thus, among a population of boys aged 13–15 years, the level of sexual maturation will show huge variation. Although the timings are variable, in boys, the sequence of maturational events is well conserved. Testicular enlargement is always the first event, and with the ensuing increase in hormone secretion, this drives penile growth, the appearance of pubic hair, and the pubertal growth spurt.

As a result of the variability in timing of pubertal growth and maturation, it is more practical to consider adolescents in terms of their pubertal milestones than in terms of chronological age when reviewing influences of nutrition upon physiology. For this purpose, it is common to consider either skeletal age (see Section 7.2.4) or the sexual maturation rating (SMR, Tanner stage of development; Table 7.1). In girls, there is variability in terms of timing and sequencing of these stages. Breast stage 2 is often the first indicator of puberty and occurs on average at 10.8 years (range 8.8–12.8 years). In two-thirds of girls, this will precede other events, but a significant proportion of girls will develop pubic hair ahead of breast budding (Tanner, 1989). Timing of menarche also varies, and while most girls have their first

menstrual period at breast stage 4, around 25% will do so at stage 3. The SMR ratings generally map well against growth rates. In girls, the pubertal growth spurt begins at around stage 2. In boys, the growth spurt is delayed and coincides with SMR4 (Figure 7.2).

The major changes in body composition that are described in Section 7.2.2 are partly features of growth during adolescence. They are also driven by the actions of sex steroids that are secreted as the hypothalamic–pituitary–gonadal and hypothalamic–pituitary–adrenal axes mature. The independent and parallel processes of puberty and adrenarche result in the development of the secondary sexual characteristics and produce endocrine changes that remodel body composition in a gender-specific manner (Figure 7.3).

Table 7.1 Sexual maturation ratings (Tanner stages).

Both sexes	
Pubic hair	
Stage 1	None
Stage 2	Small amounts of long downy hair with little pigment
Stage 3	Coarse and curly extending across pubis
Stage 4	Adult-like features but not yet spreading to thighs
Stage 5	Adult pattern and features
Male genitals*	
Stage 1	Prepubertal appearance
Stage 2	Testes enlarging and scrotum reddening and thinning
Stage 3	Further enlargement of scrotum and testes. Penis lengthening
Stage 4	Penis increasing in length and scrotum darkening further
Stage 5	Adult characteristics
Female breasts	
Stage 1	Prepubertal appearance
Stage 2	Breast bud formation and growth of areola
Stage 3	Areola continuing expansion. Breast elevating and extending beyond areola
Stage 4	Breast size and elevation increasing. Nipple and areola extending as a secondary mound
Stage 5	Adult characteristics

*In males, staging based upon genital growth may be referred to as stages G1–G5.

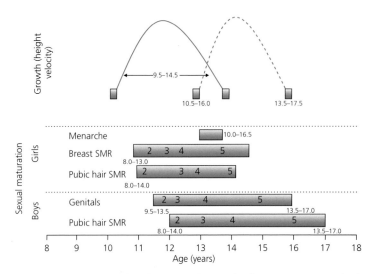

Figure 7.2 The relationship of growth velocity to pubertal staging in boys and girls. Average timings of pubertal (Tanner) staging are shown in the lower half of the figure. Age ranges beneath the pubertal staging boxes indicate the spread of values over which sexual maturation begins and ends. Height velocity curves at the top of the figure show the timings of the pubertal growth spurt in girls (——) and boys (– – – –) and the average age of maximal growth velocity. It is clear from the figure that in girls, acceleration of growth precedes pubertal development, while in boys, this acceleration occurs at a more advanced stage. Adapted from Tanner (1989). Reproduced with permission from Castlemead Publications.

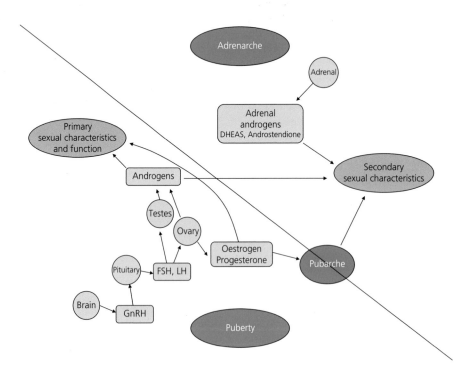

Figure 7.3 The key endocrine events of adolescence. Adrenarche and puberty are separate processes that promote endocrine maturation. Development of the adrenal gland increases secretion of androgens in both males and females. The adrenal androgens stimulate development of secondary sexual characteristics. Puberty begins with the maturation of the hypothalamus and the stable rhythm of production of GnRH. FSH, follicle-stimulating hormone; LH, luteinizing hormone.

Adrenarche usually occurs between the ages of 6 and 10 years. In boys, it is therefore a forerunner of puberty, but in girls, it may occur alongside pubertal changes. During adrenarche, the adrenal cortex expands and completes differentiation into three separate zones, the zona glomerulosa, the zona fasciculata and the zona reticularis. The zona reticularis synthesizes androgens, including androstenedione and dehydroepiandrosterone sulphate. These initiate the appearance of the secondary sexual characteristics and symptoms that are associated with puberty, including acne, body odour, changes to the vocal cords and deepening of the voice and appearance of pubic hair and axillary hair.

The appearance of pubic hair is termed pubarche and is also driven by the endocrine signals that develop with the onset of puberty (Figure 7.3). True puberty begins with the hypothalamus achieving a regular pulsatile pattern of gonadotrophin-releasing hormone (GnRH) release. This is partly achieved as a response to leptin signalling of body fatness in both girls and boys (see Chapter 2) and is also driven by the maturation of glutaminergic neurones within the hypothalamus. Stimulation of the gonads by luteinizing hormone and follicle-stimulating hormone has characteristic effects in boys and girls. In boys, the testes enlarge and produce testosterone and androstenedione. These further stimulate the appearance of the secondary sexual characteristics and the growth of the penis and testes. Production of androgens promotes both linear growth and the growth of muscular tissue. The greater activity of these hormones in males results in the development of a larger body with a greater proportion of lean body mass. In girls, ovarian synthesis of oestrogen and progesterone also contributes to the secondary sexual characteristics but more importantly leads to the establishment of reproductive cycling and thelarche. Oestrogens stimulate the deposition of body fat, and hence, with advancing pubertal stages, the female body contains a greater proportion of fat than that of the male. Menarche is an indicator that the uterus and ovaries are fully mature, but this does not mark the end of the events of puberty. In girls, growth will continue for a short period, allowing a further increase in height of approximately 6 cm, beyond menarche.

7.2.4 Bone growth

The mature skeleton is a complex tissue that comprises two main forms of bone, spongy trabecular bone and more dense cortical bone. Bones in different sites around the body differ in the relative amounts of the two forms that are present, and within bones, there are different layers of cortical and trabecular bone, with the latter being more prominent in and around joints (see also Section 9.6.1.1). During adolescent growth, all of the bones within the skeleton are increasing in size, but for the purposes of this text, the process will be described for the long bones (e.g. the femur or humerus).

Bones initially form from cartilaginous structures during the fetal period. The process of endochondral ossification converts these structures into mineralized (ossified) bone structures that are innervated and invaded by the cardiovascular system. Endochondral ossification ends in the first few years of life, and bone is then able to increase in size by virtue of the distribution of different zones of bone. As shown in Figure 7.4, the long bones in childhood comprise three regions. The shaft of the bone is called the diaphysis. This is mostly cortical bone surrounded by an external layer of connective tissue (the periosteum). This tissue is important in the growth process, as it allows an increase in bone girth. In mature bone, it is the point of connection for tendons and ligaments. There is also an internal layer of connective tissue (the endosteum), which surrounds the central medullary cavity, where the bone marrow is located. The end of the bone is called the epiphysis, which is mostly trabecular bone, with thin layers of cortical bone. In the growing bone, there is a layer between these two zones called the epiphyseal plate, which is composed of cartilage and partially calcified cartilage. It is this that allows linear growth to take place.

Within the epiphyseal plate, there are four layers of cells. Closest to the epiphysis lies a layer of resting chondrocytes (cartilage cells). The function of these cells is to anchor the epiphyseal bone to the growth zone. Beneath this layer, the chondrocytes are in a state of active multiplication by mitosis. Moving closer to the diaphysis, the cartilage of the plate begins to calcify. Within this zone are chondrocytes that are maturing and enlarging, and along the border of the epiphyseal plate and the diaphysis lies the fourth cell layer, comprising chondrocytes that are dying and becoming calcified. In effect, the process pushes the epiphysis out from the diaphysis by depositing strips of bone over the top of the diaphysis and new cartilage cells just below the epiphysis, hence elongating the bone. The newly formed bone may be remodelled through the action of osteoblasts, and other cells, and will be invaded by blood vessels. At the point of skeletal maturation, the cartilage is fully calcified and the epiphysis and diaphysis fuse together.

The same process occurs in all growing bones. While in the long bones the process relies on growth plates at the ends of the shaft, in other bones, the growth plates exist as concentric rings, with growth progressing from the outside, in towards the centre. Bone maturity can be assessed by x-ray and is often used as a marker of pubertal development to supplement Tanner staging based on

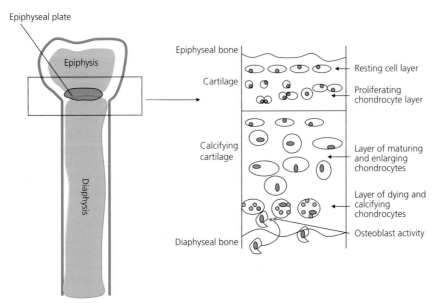

Epiphyseal plate

Epiphysis

Diaphysis

Epiphyseal bone

Cartilage

Calcifying cartilage

Diaphyseal bone

Resting cell layer

Proliferating chondrocyte layer

Layer of maturing and enlarging chondrocytes

Layer of dying and calcifying chondrocytes

Osteoblast activity

Figure 7.4 The growth of long bones. Long bones expand through activity within the epiphyseal growth plate, which lies at the interface of the bone shaft (diaphysis) and end (epiphysis). New cartilage cells (chondrocytes) are formed at the epiphyseal end of the growth plate, while mature cells on the diaphyseal end die and become calcified. The bone extends by virtue of this zone pushing the epiphysis away from the diaphysis.

breast or genital maturation. In bones that are still growing, the epiphyses are imaged as less radiographically dense than the ossified bone, while in mature bones, the fused epiphyses show as clear epiphyseal lines. Staging of maturity through skeletal ageing usually employs x-rays of the wrist or hand. These are then compared to atlases of images that consider the size and shape of bones, along with the degree of ossification (Tanner, 1989). Bone age is then graded using the Tanner–Whitehouse or Greulich and Pyle scales.

Bone growth occurs throughout childhood but is most rapid during adolescence, when approximately half of the eventual mass of the skeleton is laid down. As shown in Figure 7.5, there is a short continuation of the accrual of bone mass beyond the attainment of final height. In girls, the most rapid period of bone mineralization is between 12 and 15 years, while in boys, the peak lies between 14 and 17. During these brief periods, approximately 25% of adult bone mass is deposited, which is equivalent to the amount of bone mass which will be ultimately lost during late adulthood (Boreham and McKay, 2011). Peak bone mass, the point where bone mineral content and density are at its greatest, occurs between 25 and 35 years of age (Davies *et al.*, 2004).

Bone growth is strongly under the influence of genetic factors, which are believed to determine around 80% of the variation in adult bone mass. Many genes

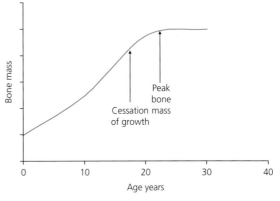

Figure 7.5 The accrual of bone mass. Much of the mass of the adult skeleton is deposited during the adolescent growth phase. The most rapid rate of bone mineralization coincides with the pubertal growth spurt. Deposition of bone continues beyond the cessation of growth, and peak bone mass is achieved in the third decade of life.

are important in formation, growth and maintenance of the skeleton, but those that appear to be of greatest importance during childhood and adolescent growth include the vitamin D receptor, type 1 collagen, the oestrogen receptor (ERβ), leptin, insulin-like growth factor 1 (IGF-1), interleukin-6, low-density lipoprotein receptor-related protein 5 and osteocalcin (Davies *et al.*, 2004). Endocrine signals are also the major factors that drive bone growth. Growth hormone and IGF-1, for example, stimulate accrual of bone mass by promoting the proliferation of osteoblasts. The secretion of these hormones is increased during puberty through the actions of the sex steroids. The sex steroids exert direct effects on bone also. Adrenal-derived androgens increase the overall strength of bone, while estradiol increases bone thickness.

While genetics determine most of the variation in rates of bone growth and accrual of mineral, diet and lifestyle factors are also of importance. Physical activity stimulates bone mineralization, particularly if comprising high-impact sports (e.g. basketball, volleyball, rugby and gymnastics) or weight-bearing activities. Optimal bone mineralization is driven by activities of short and intense nature with frequent rest periods (Boreham and McKay, 2011). Activity-induced bone growth is greatest at the skeletal sites that bear the greatest load (Daly, 2007). In other words, bone tends to accrue at the greatest rate along lines of stress. This structural response to exercise is seen in both boys and girls, but once puberty is initiated, it differs slightly. In boys, exercise stimulates bone thickening by expansion of the periosteum, while in girls, there is a contraction of the endosteum layer. Interventions of more than 6-month duration that involve 3 or more periods of activity can increase bone mass by up to 6% (Boreham and McKay, 2011), and the benefits of activity in terms of bone mineral accrual are greatest in children who are active in the prepubertal and early pubertal stages (Davies *et al.*, 2004). A study of elite Finnish tennis female players showed that those who started their careers before puberty achieved two to fourfold greater benefits from exercise-induced bone mineralization than those who started post-menarche (Kannus *et al.*, 1995). Welten and colleagues (1994) performed a longitudinal study of 13-year-old boys and girls with a follow-up to 27 years of age. Levels of physical activity in adolescence explained 17% of the variation in adult bone mineral density and were the main predictor of adult bone mass. Excessive exercise in adolescent girls can, however, be detrimental to bone health if it impacts upon menstrual cycle function (see Section 7.6.3).

Nutrition-related factors are known to be of importance in determining adolescent bone growth. Girls who have suffered from anorexia nervosa (AN) generally have reduced bone mineral density into adulthood and are therefore at risk of bone disorders such as osteoporosis later in life. Eating disorders or excessive underweight is associated with reduced production of sex steroids and expression of IGF-1, hence limiting bone growth. Interestingly, overweight may also limit bone growth. Ducy *et al.* (2000) used mutant mouse strains to demonstrate that leptin is a negative regulator of skeletal growth. The *ob/ob* mouse, which lacks a functional leptin gene, and the *db/db* mouse, which does not express leptin receptors, have almost threefold greater bone volume than wild-type mice. Skeletal development can be normalized by administration of exogenous leptin. Overweight children will secrete more leptin and this may therefore reduce bone mineralization. As obese individuals tend to be leptin resistant, it might be argued that obesity in adolescence could provide some benefits for skeletal growth. However, as discussed in Chapter 6, excessive obesity in childhood can lead to deformation of the skeleton or damage to the epiphyses of the hip, associated with the need to bear a heavier load. The complex relationship between obesity and bone growth in adolescents is explored in more detail in Research Highlight 7.1.

The major nutrient associated with skeletal growth is calcium, with increased intakes promoting accrual of bone mass, provided that vitamin D status is adequate. Most but not all studies of adolescents and prepubescent children show positive associations between bone mineralization and calcium intake (Davies *et al.*, 2004). Fiorito *et al.* (2006), for example, showed that the habitual calcium intakes of 9-year-olds were predictive of bone mineral content at age 11. Supplementation with calcium, with and without vitamin D, invariably demonstrates increases in bone mineralization. A randomized controlled trial in identical twins aged 9–13 showed that 800 mg/day calcium with 400 IU/day vitamin D produced significant gains in bone mass and strength over a 6-month period (Greene and Naughton, 2011). A number of studies in boys (Prentice *et al.*, 2005) and girls (Stear *et al.*, 2003) have shown that provision of calcium supplements to adolescents can increase whole-body bone mineral density and have specific benefits at the hip, spine, and wrist. A study of Chinese 12–15-year-olds (Yin *et al.*, 2010) reported that supplementation of calcium at doses over 230 mg/day over a 2-year period was sufficient to improve accretion of bone mineral. Given the importance of attained peak bone mass in determining long-term bone health, optimizing calcium and vitamin D status in adolescence would appear to be a high priority. The poor calcium intakes and high prevalence of vitamin D deficiency identified in surveys (Baker *et al.*, 2009; CDC, 2012; Bates *et al.*, 2014) are therefore of major concern.

It is unclear whether the benefits associated with increased calcium intake in adolescence are carried through to the adult years. Certainly, the study of Welten *et al.* (1994) found no relationship between

Research Highlight 7.1 Obesity and bone health.

The relationship between obesity and bone health is complex. The main outcome of low bone mineral deposition is a diagnosis of osteoporosis, a condition that generally affects older adults. Osteoporosis is diagnosed on the basis of low bone mineral density (BMD). In adults, low BMI is seen as a risk factor for low BMD and for fracture, while a high BMI is associated with higher BMD (De Laet *et al.*, 2005). It is thought that this is a response to the greater mechanical load on the skeleton that is associated with excess weight, which will stimulate bone deposition (Ribot *et al.*, 1994). However, obesity is not protective against fractures, which are the key clinical outcomes of osteoporosis. Ong *et al.* (2014) surveyed female patients over the age of 50, who were attending a fracture clinic, and found that although obese women were less likely to have a diagnosis of osteoporosis, they were more likely to suffer fractures.

The effects of excess adiposity upon the skeletal development of adolescents appear to be different to what are observed in adults, with higher BMI generally associated with lower bone mineralization and impaired growth. The main predictor of bone mass before puberty is lean mass, but beyond puberty, fat mass becomes more strongly associated with bone growth (Mosca *et al.*, 2013). El Hage *et al.* (2013) reported a lower whole-body bone mineral content in obese boys compared to those of healthy weight. Distribution of body fat may also play a key role, with central adiposity being associated with impaired bone growth at weight-bearing sites (Laddu *et al.*, 2013). Goulding and colleagues (2000) noted that obese children aged 3–19 had greater bone mineral content for their age, compared to those with lower body fat, but when bone mineral and area were expressed relative to body weight, they were lower. This suggests that there may be a mismatch between bone growth and rapidly increasing weight in obese children.

The mechanisms that link obesity to bone growth are still not fully understood and may be complex. Adiposity may disrupt the endocrine signals that drive bone growth and maturation and is known to impact upon production of growth hormone (Perotti *et al.*, 2013) and sex hormones (Vandewalle *et al.*, 2014). Bone is also responsive to adipokines (including leptin and adiponectin) and pro-inflammatory cytokines (tumour necrosis factor α) that are produced by adipose tissue, and these agents may impact upon activity of osteoblasts and osteoclasts, resulting in altered rates of bone deposition (Campos *et al.*, 2013; Mosca *et al.*, 2013).

bone mineral density at 27 years and habitual calcium intake at 13. Lambert and colleagues (2008) reported that 18 months of calcium supplements (792 mg/day) to 12-year-old girls with low habitual calcium intakes boosted whole-body bone mineral density in the short term, but had no lasting effect when followed-up 2 years beyond the end of the supplementation period.

7.3 Psychosocial development

Adolescence is a period of intense cognitive, emotional and social development. Over the period from 11 to 21 years of age, the individual undergoes a transition from a childlike way of thinking and interacting with others to a mature, adult level of functioning (Story *et al.*, 2002). These changes can impact significantly upon nutrition, as the transition process generates attitudes, beliefs and ways of thinking that can strongly influence food choices.

In the earliest stages of adolescence, children find it difficult to think in abstract terms. The average 11–14-year-old is able to only focus upon present realities and thinks in concrete terms. The ability to process abstract concepts and make associations between current actions and later consequences is poorly developed. This can make health promotion at this stage very challenging, as these adolescents are unable to perceive that their current eating behaviours might impact upon their health three or more decades into the future. On a social and emotional level, the young adolescent increasingly strives to establish independence from parents and family. The peer group becomes overwhelmingly important and influential, and this can be a cause of conflict in the home as acceptance by peers often dictates a degree of rebellion against authority.

Between 15 and 17 years, the adolescent acquires a more advanced range of cognitive skills and begins to be able to think about abstract scenarios and consider the possibilities and intangible consequences that may stem from their actions. At this age, the individual can begin to grasp multiple viewpoints of a given situation or argument, and as a result, conflicts within families will reduce. The peer group remains hugely important, and the desire to be accepted by peers and to conform with the expectations of the social network can lead to the adolescent being very self-conscious about their appearance, behaviours and how they might be perceived by others. By the age of 18–21, the individual is capable of all advanced cognitive processes and will have established a firm view of their personal identity and their overall place within society and local culture. These young adults may still show immature behaviour and decision making, particularly under pressure, and will retain strong links with a wide social group of like-minded individuals of similar age.

7.4 Nutritional requirements in adolescence

The high rates of growth during adolescence carry significant increments in nutritional requirements over and above those seen in earlier childhood. Indeed, this stage of life has requirements for energy and nutrients that are greater than seen in adulthood, both in absolute terms and when expressed per body weight (Table 7.2). It is recognized that adolescence increases nutrient requirements, mostly due to growth. The remodelling of body shape and body composition and the maturation of organ systems also contribute to adolescence being a peak time in terms of nutrient requirements. Precise guidelines and recommendations for nutrient intakes in adolescence are, however, largely undefined. This is due to a lack of relevant research and due to the difficulties of reconciling chronological age and physiological stage of development. For some nutrients, it is more useful to set dietary reference values based upon height, body weight or energy intake, rather than age.

7.4.1 Macronutrients and energy

Estimating the energy requirements of adolescents represents a particular challenge, as the true energy requirement is more closely related to body size and the growth velocity than to age. The pubertal period sees an increase in height of 15–20% and a gain in weight that corresponds to approximately 50% of the final attained adult weight. The bulk of the height gain and weight gain is through accrual of skeletal mass and lean body mass and therefore requires an anabolic state and hence a high demand for energy (Giovannini *et al.*, 2000). As shown in Table 7.3, the energy requirements of boys are greater than for girls at any given body weight, by virtue of their larger bulk of metabolically active tissue (lean body mass). With the onset of puberty, therefore, the difference in energy requirements of males and females begins to diverge sharply. Adolescents often have higher levels of physical activity than seen in adults, and these can contribute significantly to energy requirements.

To deliver the energy needs of growth, the appetite of adolescents increases markedly. One of the challenges of this period is to manage intake such that optimal growth can be sustained, without excessive weight gain. As described in Chapter 6, the emergence of overweight and obesity during the adolescent years is an indicator of increased risk of obesity during adulthood. The major sources of energy within the diet are carbohydrate (which in adolescence should provide up to 55% of daily energy) and fat (no more than 35% of energy). There are no specific recommendations for these macronutrients in adolescence, but intakes need to be sufficient in order to spare protein for growth.

There are major requirements for protein in order to sustain growth. Protein demands reach their peak during the pubertal growth spurt (11–14 years in girls, 15–18 years in boys). In addition to growth, protein is required for the maintenance of existing tissues and the

Table 7.2 A comparison of nutrient requirements* between adults and children aged 11–18 years.

Nutrient	Age					
	11–14		15–18		19–50	19–50
	Male	Female	Male	Female	Male	Female
Energy (kcal/day)	2220	1845	2755	2110	2550	1940
Protein (g/day)	42.1	41.2	55.2	45.4	55.5	45.0
Riboflavin (mg/day)	1.2	1.1	1.3	1.1	1.3	1.1
Vitamin A (retinol equiv./day)	600	600	700	600	700	600
Folate (µg/day)	200	200	200	200	200	200
Ascorbate (mg/day)	35	35	40	40	40	40
Cobalamin (µg/day)	1.2	1.2	1.5	1.5	1.5	1.5
Iron (mg/day)	11.3	14.8	11.3	14.8	8.7	14.8
Zinc (mg/day)	9.0	9.0	9.5	7.0	9.5	7.0
Calcium (g/day)	1.0	0.8	1.0	0.8	0.7	0.7
Selenium (µg/day)	45	45	70	60	75	60
Magnesium (mg/day)	280	280	300	300	300	270

Data shown are UK, Estimated Average Requirements for energy, and Reference Nutrient Intakes for protein and micronutrients (DoH, 1998).
*Selected nutrients.

Table 7.3 Energy requirements of adolescents are dependent upon physiological development and physical activity level (PAL).

Body weight (kg)	Basal metabolic rate (kcal/day)	Estimated average requirement (kcal/day)				
		Physical activity level				
		1.4	1.5	1.6	1.8	2.0
Boys						
30	1186	1670	1789	1909	2148	2363
40	1362	1909	2052	2172	2458	2720
50	1539	2148	2315	2458	2768	3078
60	1715	2410	2578	2744	3078	3437
Girls						
30	1093	1527	1646	1742	1957	2195
40	1227	1718	1837	1957	2195	2458
50	1360	1909	2028	2172	2458	2720
60	1494	2100	2243	2386	2697	2983

Data from DoH (1998). PAL of 1.0 corresponds to sleeping (basal rate); 1.2–1.4, lying or sitting at rest, reading, eating or watching television; 1.5–1.8, moderately active seated, for example, driving, playing piano or operating computer, and moderate standing activities; 1.9–2.4, walking 3–4 km/h and low-intensity sports. High-intensity sports and exercise will have PAL of 4.5–7.9. Average PAL for boys aged 10–18 years is 1.56 and for girls is 1.48 calculated from estimates of time spent sleeping, at school and engaged in light-, moderate- or high-intensity activities.

deposition of new lean mass. To maintain nitrogen balance in the face of growth and deposition of lean body mass, protein intake should be at a level corresponding to 12–14% of energy intake (Table 7.2). Most adolescents in the developed countries consume protein at a level beyond requirements. Excessive intakes have been suggested as potentially detrimental to calcium homeostasis and bone growth.

7.4.2 Micronutrients

Micronutrients are essential during adolescence in order to ensure that the major physiological processes and functions can be maintained during the period of maximal growth (Olmedilla and Granado, 2000). Generally speaking, the demands for vitamins and minerals increase in proportion to energy requirements. For vitamins, there are little available data on which to base specific recommendations for adolescents. It is assumed that growth and the increased rates of energy utilization will increase requirements for riboflavin, thiamin and niacin. Protein metabolism and the synthesis of DNA and RNA will increase the demand for vitamin B6 and cobalamin. Folate is also required for these important synthetic processes, and it is a key nutrient in the synthesis of red blood cells. The pubertal growth spurt sees a major (25%) increase in blood volume.

Most minerals and trace elements accumulate within the body in large amounts during adolescence due to increasing body mass and stature. For most of these, there are physiological adaptations in place to maximize absorption and bioavailability. Among the minerals, those of particular significance during the adolescent years are calcium, iron and zinc. Zinc is an essential nutrient for protein and nucleic acid synthesis and is a cofactor for many metabolically important enzymes. In adults, most zinc within the body is locked into muscle and bone. As these tissues gain in mass during adolescence, the accrual of zinc is at a maximal rate, and the biochemical measurements of zinc status in body fluids or hair often show declines as it is redistributed to bone and muscle. Poor zinc status can have important consequences, as zinc deficiency is associated with impaired growth, reduced appetite and delayed skeletal and sexual maturation.

The absorption of calcium from the diet (~35–40%) during adolescence does not appear to be markedly greater than that at other stages of life. As described earlier in this chapter, bone mineralization is at a maximal rate during puberty, and hence, this is a peak period in terms of calcium requirements. The high RNI set for the adolescent years (Table 7.2) reflects this accrual of bone mineral. Optimal utilization of calcium obtained within the diet is dependent upon the supply of other nutrients, including vitamin D, phosphorus, protein, magnesium and ascorbate. Magnesium and phosphorus are also important skeletal minerals. The ratio of calcium to phosphorus in the diet becomes important at low intakes of calcium, when excessive intake of phosphorus leads to oversecretion of parathyroid hormone. This promotes release of calcium from bone. Ascorbate is an essential cofactor for the action of prolyl hydroxylase, which converts proline to hydroxyproline. This uncommon amino acid is incorporated into collagen, which is the major protein within bone, providing the basic fibrous structure into which calcium and other minerals are deposited.

Adolescence sees an increase in requirements for iron. This is driven partly by the increase in blood volume but mainly by the increase in lean body mass and the synthesis of the muscle protein myoglobin. The increase in lean mass is greater in boys than in girls, but the iron requirements of girls increase to a greater extent (Table 7.2) in order to compensate for blood losses associated with the onset of menstruation. Poor iron status is associated with iron deficiency anaemia, reduced ability to exercise and impaired cognitive abilities. Iron status is influenced by a variety of other nutrients and components of food (Table 7.4). Phenolic compounds and phytates reduce absorption of non-haem iron, while ascorbate enhances absorption. It is desirable for adolescents to maintain high intakes of dairy products as a rich source of calcium, but as calcium inhibits uptake of iron, this can have a negative impact upon iron status. Individuals with poor vitamin A intakes will tend to develop problems with iron status. Vitamin A deficiency increases the occurrence of infectious disease, and the acute-phase response results in the sequestration of iron within the liver, reducing availability for the physiological processes associated with puberty.

7.5 Nutritional intakes in adolescence

Adolescents are frequently identified as being at risk of undernutrition, largely because their very high nutrient demands often appear incompatible with their range of preferred foods and patterns of eating. Surveys from all over the developed world identify high levels of potential nutrient deficiency, as will be described later. Interpretation of such surveys should, however, be very cautious. Nutritional surveys carried out at a national level often use estimates of intakes carried out over just a 24 or 48 h period. These will rarely provide an accurate picture of nutritional status in the population and will be particularly misleading if the intention is to estimate the prevalence of low micronutrient intakes (Mackerras and Rutishauser, 2005). Even the well-designed National Diet and Nutrition Surveys (NDNS) carried out periodically in the United Kingdom (collects data over a 4 day period) may have problems with the validity and reliability of the data that are generated due to issues of under-reporting. The disparity between estimates of intake and actual prevalence of nutrient deficiency disease perhaps best illustrates the perils and pitfalls of such survey data. Forty-six per cent of British girls aged 11–14 and 50% of girls aged 15–18 years were shown to consume iron at a level below the lower reference nutrient intake (LRNI; Bates *et al.*, 2014). However, assessment of iron status from blood samples showed the prevalence of iron deficiency anaemia (based on low haemoglobin and plasma ferritin) to be only 4.9%. Accurate estimation of the intakes of some micronutrients requires food records gathered over several weeks (iron, 6–7 days; calcium, 7–10 days; thiamin, 13–16 days; ascorbate, 19–33 days; vitamin A, 39–44 days; Basiotis *et al.*, 1987).

Table 7.4 Vegetarian dietary practices.

Vegetarian diet	Practice defined as
Semi-vegetarian	Diet based on plant material but including some meat products
Pollotarian	A semi-vegetarian practice in which poultry but no mammalian meat is consumed
Pescetarian	A semi-vegetarian practice in which fish and shellfish are consumed
Pollo-pescetarian	A semi-vegetarian practice in which poultry, fish and shellfish are consumed. No mammalian meat is consumed
Ovo-vegetarian	All meat and dairy products are avoided but eggs are consumed
Lacto-vegetarian	All meat and eggs are avoided but dairy products are consumed
Ovo-lacto vegetarian	All meat is avoided but eggs and dairy products are consumed
Macrobiotic	Only whole grains and beans are consumed
Vegan	No animal products (including honey) or refined foods that might have been tested or processed with animal material are consumed
Fruitarian	Only fruit, nuts and seeds or material that can be obtained without harming plants are consumed
Raw vegan	Only fresh and uncooked fruit, nuts, seeds and vegetables are consumed
Jain vegetarian	No meat, eggs, honey or root vegetables are consumed, but dairy products are acceptable

In most of the developed countries, surveys indicate that adolescents consume adequate amounts of energy but that this is generally delivered through excessive consumption of fat and sugar. The UK NDNS (Bates *et al.*, 2014) reported that mean energy intake of adolescents was below the EAR but this age group were the lowest consumers of fruit and the highest consumers of chocolate, sweets, pasta, rice and pizza. In the NDNS sample, 78% of the adolescents reported having consumed soft drinks within the 4-day period and sweetened beverages provided 40% of non-milk extrinsic sugars. The HELENA study, which considered the diets of over 3000 adolescents in 10 European cities, also reported that energy intakes were in line with recommendations but that energy requirements were not met through fruit and vegetables, milk or dairy products (Diethelm *et al.*, 2012). While these foods were consumed well below population recommendations, intakes of saturated fats were high and PUFA intakes were considerably below age-specific references (Diethelm *et al.*, 2014).

Micronutrient intakes of adolescents are most frequently identified as being below dietary reference values or population guidelines. This concern is illustrated by the UK NDNS, which showed high prevalence of intake below the LRNI for vitamin A, riboflavin, folate, iron, calcium, magnesium, potassium, zinc, selenium and iodine (Bates *et al.*, 2014). The diets of 11–18-year-old girls appeared particularly poor with more than 20% being at risk of deficiency of iron, riboflavin, magnesium, selenium and zinc. Similar concerns have been raised by surveys in Australia (Gallagher *et al.*, 2014) and the United States (CDC, 2012) and HELENA (Diethelm *et al.*, 2014), with low intakes of iron, vitamin A, folate, iodine, calcium and magnesium emerging as a consistent theme.

7.5.1 Factors that influence food choice

Although reliable estimates of the prevalence of undernutrition with respect to specific micronutrients may be difficult to establish, it is clear that the diet of the typical adolescent does not comply with guidelines for healthy eating and may not deliver the full profile of nutrient requirements. This is of concern at a life stage when optimal nutrition is necessary for rapid growth and development. The reasons contributing to poor nutrition need to be explored. Suboptimal nutrition partly stems from the preferred range of foods that are consumed by adolescents and by the, sometimes erratic, meal patterns that are followed by this increasingly independent group of young people.

The range of influences upon adolescents' food choices is broad and varied (Figure 7.6). While current health status and other health behaviours are influential, food choices and eating behaviours are also determined by environmental factors and personal factors. Environmental factors include the influences of parents and family, socio-economic factors, the influence of peers and exposure to media and sociocultural expectations. Personal factors include the values and beliefs of the individual (e.g. religious or ethical viewpoints), emotional and physiological needs and

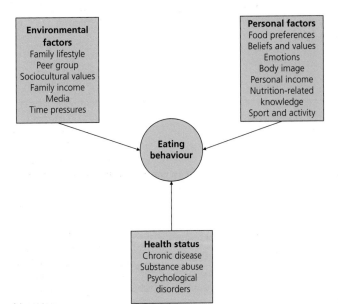

Figure 7.6 Factors that influence the food choices and eating behaviours of adolescents.

perceptions of body image. Several of these factors may interact with each other to influence behaviour. For example, dissatisfaction with appearance and body weight is common among adolescents (50% of girls and 20% of boys; Hill, 2002). Part of this dissatisfaction comes from the exposure of adolescents to images in magazines and television programmes that depict thinness as the epitome of beauty and a state to aspire to. Girls in their mid-teens are particularly influenced by reported material depicting celebrities who are praised for weight loss and thinness and ridiculed for overweight or physical flaws. Thus, society shapes adolescents views of their own body size and shape and may prompt engagement in restrictive dietary practices (Hill, 2006).

Adolescence is in all ways a period of transition, both physically and emotionally. Food becomes an element of the developing autonomy of adolescents, and young people increasingly take control over the purchasing and preparation of meals. This can become embroiled in the general rebellion associated with the adolescent years, and poor food choices (fast convenience foods) may be particularly pleasurable because of their labelling as 'bad' foods by parents and other authorities (Hill, 2002). The main influences on the food choices of adolescents are, however, obvious ones. With appetite drives high in order to meet physiological demands, adolescents are strongly influenced by feelings of hunger and select foods that taste good, have favourable aroma and appearance and are familiar to them from earlier childhood exposures (Neumark-Sztainer et al., 1999).

Adolescents tend to feel constrained in terms of time, as they have to integrate their strong desire to sleep in late in the mornings with heavy workloads at school, busy social programmes, part-time jobs and sporting activities. This promotes preferences for foods that are readily available and that are easy and fast to prepare (Neumark-Sztainer et al., 1999). Adolescents who are taking responsibility for finding their own food for at least part of the day often find it hard to access more healthful alternatives (O'Dea, 2003). Outlets that sell high-fat, high-sugar, fast foods can act as focal points for adolescents to meet with friends. There are some claims that poor food selections may be an element of achieving integration with the peer group and fulfilling social expectations, but the evidence to support this is not strong. Correlations of adolescents' food choices with parental preferences are considerably stronger than correlations with preferences of best friends (Hill, 2002).

While convenience and hedonic factors are strong factors that determine food choices, there are other factors that are of low importance to adolescents as a population group, but those may be major influences for some individuals with the population. These include the desire to enhance health or sporting performance, compliance with religious or family rules pertaining to food and issues relating to body image and influences of the media (Neumark-Sztainer et al., 1999).

7.5.2 Food consumed out of the home

While younger children will predominantly consume food in a supervised environment such as home or school, where food is purchased and prepared by adults, adolescents increasingly take responsibility for this themselves. Generally speaking, adolescents have some income that they can spend on food, and they begin to consume a considerable proportion of their daily energy and nutrient intakes in school or college, from vending machines, in snack bars, in fast-food restaurants, in sandwich shops or in the homes of their friends. Although school meals are increasingly being formulated to comply with nationally set standards (see Section 6.3.2), foods purchased from other sources tend to be of lower nutritional quality and of higher energy density. The HELENA study found that 7% of adolescents in their European sample bought lunches out of school, in shops and fast-food restaurants. These children had higher intakes of sweets and bread (Müller et al., 2013). The autonomy of adolescents in selection and preparation of foods may therefore be a determining factor leading to low micronutrient intakes.

Fast-food restaurants aim much of their marketing at adolescents, and indeed, a high proportion of their workforces tend to be within this age group. Sometimes, these workers receive some of their remuneration in the form of free food (French et al., 2001). Intakes of foods from fast-food restaurants increased rapidly over the last decades of the twentieth century and remain high in the early twenty-first century despite growing awareness of the importance of nutrition for health. Estimates of access to such establishments by adolescents vary considerably. Among teenagers in the United States, estimates of the proportion who purchase fast food several times a week have been put at between 39 and 50% (Paeratakul et al., 2003; Bowman et al., 2004). Bauer et al. (2009) found that only 21% of US teenagers reported not having consumed fast food in the week preceding their survey and that a third had consumed fast food three or more times in that week. Seventy per cent of Canadian adolescents reported consumption at least once a week (Lillico et al., 2014). A study of teenagers living in an impoverished London community found 10% consumed fast food daily and 50% twice or more per week (Patterson et al., 2012). Consumption of food from such outlets greatly increases the energy density of the diet and intakes of fat, sugar and sodium. Good sources of micronutrients such as grains, fruit, vegetables, legumes, seeds, milk and dairy products are displaced from the diet by fast foods (Paeratakul *et al.*, 2003). Although having a high personal income is strongly related to consuming less healthy foods outside the home (Bowman *et al.*, 2004), the main predictors of external food sources displacing home-prepared foods are having low socio-economic status, having a part-time job, and being active in sport (French *et al.*, 2001).

The convenience and time-saving attributes of snack foods and items from fast-food restaurants are a major attraction to busy adolescents, but the drivers of a fast-food-rich diet are more complex. The ease of access to fast-food restaurants is an important factor with several studies showing greater consumption by children who live in areas with a high density of outlets (Laxer and Janssen, 2014). Lower socio-economic status and personal food preferences increase the likelihood of regular consumption, as does an unhealthy home eating environment (Bauer *et al.*, 2009). Strong maternal support for healthy eating and concerns about health and weight reduce consumption.

7.5.3 Meal skipping and snacking

In keeping with their increasing income and access to food outside the home, adolescents are the population group who are most likely to have erratic eating habits, with missed meals and high intakes of snack foods. Adolescents have strong appetites and tend to eat outside meal times in order to fulfil feelings of hunger and cravings for specific snack items (Neumark-Sztainer *et al.*, 1999). Skipping meals can impact significantly upon nutrient intakes, particularly as the meal that is most frequently missed is breakfast. Where the normal breakfast foods are fortified cereals with milk, this can produce marked reductions in micronutrient intakes. Some studies have estimated that up to one-third of adolescents regularly miss breakfast. The major reason underpinning this behaviour appears to be a lack of time and low levels of hunger on rising in the morning (Shaw, 1998).

Breakfast is not the only meal that may be missed. In some families, adolescents either opt out of family meals or, if in the position of providing their own meals for at least some part of the day, will choose to adopt a 'grazing' pattern of snacking throughout the day. van Den Bulck and Eggermont (2006) reported that this kind of behaviour is more prevalent among adolescents who watch television for more than 5 h/day and who play computer games four times a week or more. They postulated that in these children, these activities were displacing time that would otherwise be spent on meals.

Skipping of meals is more common among adolescents who are high consumers of snacks (Savige *et al.*, 2007). Adolescents generally consume two to three snacks per day, with greatest frequency in those who are sedentary. Snacks are consumed in a variety of settings and at all times of the day, including in front of the television, while doing homework, with friends, and in transit to school or other activities. Snacks provide between a quarter and a third of total daily energy intake for adolescents (Kerr *et al.*, 2009). The selection of snack foods is usually reported to be biased towards foods that are rich in salty or sweet taste rather than healthy foods.

Foods of high-energy density have been linked to overweight and obesity and would displace micronutrients from the diet. However, the literature suggests that not all aspects of adolescent snacking are negative. Sebastian and colleagues (2008) reported that among US adolescents, snacking contributed 35% of the daily energy intake and 43% of added sugar intake and was associated with greater total energy intake and higher intakes of carbohydrate (Figure 7.7). However, high snack consumers also consumed more ascorbate and less protein and fat than adolescents with lower snack consumption. Intakes of milk and fruit were actually increased by snacking, suggesting that awareness of healthy eating messages may influence some aspects of snacking behaviour. This agrees with the findings of Kerr *et al.* (2009), who reported that though the favoured snack foods of British adolescents included chocolate, carbonated drinks and cakes and biscuits, bread, fruit and breakfast cereals were also widely consumed as snack items.

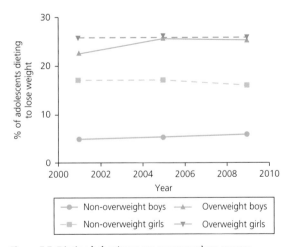

Figure 7.7 Dieting behaviours are commonplace among adolescents, including those who are not overweight. Reproduced with permission from Quick *et al.* (2014). © Nature Publishing Group.

7.6 Potential problems with nutrition

7.6.1 Dieting and weight control

Restriction of dietary intake or other actions that can promote weight loss is commonplace behaviours among some groups of adolescents. Most surveys show that girls are more likely to indulge in such behaviours than boys but that between 20 and 50% of adolescents of either sex will attempt some sort of weight loss behaviour (Neumark-Sztainer and Hannan, 2000), although the WHO Collaborative Health Behaviours in School-Aged Children Study (Quick *et al.*, 2014) of 40 countries suggested a lower prevalence (Figure 7.8). Adolescents are prone to adopting dieting behaviour as a response to the major changes in body size and shape associated with puberty. Other influences include exposure to media items about body weight and dieting, parental concerns about weight gain, teasing from other children about weight and aspiration to share the dieting experiences of peers.

Some restrictive practices may improve the quality of the diet, for example, increasing intakes of fruits and vegetables in place of energy-dense snacks. These behaviours are more the norm for younger adolescents. Later in puberty, girls, in particular, develop increased concerns about their body image and become more likely to restrict weight gain in an unhealthy manner (Abraham, 2003). Unhealthy practices related to weight loss include meal skipping, use of dieting drugs, fasting, consumption of food substitutes (e.g. slimming shakes) and smoking. These can impact in a negative way upon nutritional status, particularly with respect to calcium and other micronutrients, and are associated with slower rates of growth, psychological disorders, and poor physical health (Neumark-Sztainer and Hannan, 2000). Longer-term health may also be compromised. Reduced bone mineralization and lower attained peak bone mass may, for example, increase risk of osteoporosis later in life. Interestingly, adolescents who dieted were shown by Neumark-Sztainer and colleagues (2006) to have threefold greater risk of overweight at a 5-year follow-up. Adolescents who indulge in dieting behaviours may be eight times more likely to go on to develop eating disorders than those who do not diet (Neumark-Sztainer and Hannan, 2000).

Dissatisfaction with body size and shape or fatness is believed to be a major driver of dieting behaviour in adolescents. Many researchers report lower levels of self-esteem and greater prevalence of depression among adolescents who attempt to lose weight. Isomaa *et al.* (2010) described four distinct groups of dieting adolescents: 'vanity dieters' (aspiring to an ideal body image), 'overweight dieters' (recognize their overweight and seek better health), 'depressed dieters' (seeking to overcome emotional issues through control over food and weight) and 'feeling fat dieters' (seeking to addressed misperceived overweight). Strategies adopted to try to improve body image vary between boys and girls. While girls are more likely to restrict food intake in order to reduce weight, boys are more likely to attempt to remodel their bodies to more muscular forms through changes in diet and exercise (Lawrie *et al.*, 2007). The reasons for dieting will also influence the approach taken to weight loss. Among the overweight dieters of the Isomaa study (2010), sensible, healthy approaches based upon exercise and dietary change were adopted, while depressed dieters and feeling fat dieters were more likely to exhibit disordered eating, meal skipping and purging behaviours (use of laxatives or inducing vomiting).

The body image of both sexes is unquestionably influenced by media images, as described in Section 7.5.1, and is often inaccurate. A study of US 12–15-year-olds from the 2005–2010 NHANES cohort found that only half of overweight children recognized their overweight and that 8% of girls of appropriate weight perceived themselves to be overweight (Chung *et al.*, 2013). In this latter group, 68% were trying to lose weight. The thin-ideal image portrayed by the media influences the eating behaviours of adolescent girls, who are exposed to the idea of thin as beauty through advertising, television and magazines. The latter has the greatest influence on perception of body image and behaviour (Hill, 2006). Van den Berg *et al.* (2007) reported that girls who were the most frequent readers of magazine articles on dieting and weight loss were twice as likely as non-readers

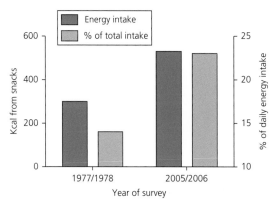

Figure 7.8 Snack foods comprise a significant proportion of daily intakes of energy, sugars and total and saturated fats among adolescents. This proportion increased between the 1977/1978 and 2005/2006 NHANES surveys in the United States. Reproduced with permission from Sebastian *et al.* (2008). © Elsevier.

to lose weight through unhealthy means (fasting, meal skipping and smoking) and three times more likely to use extreme measures such as purging. It should be noted, however, that these associations are not necessarily causal and that girls with unhealthy and restrictive dietary practices will show a greater interest in articles about dieting.

7.6.2 The vegetarian teenager

Vegetarianism is a pattern of diet that has increased in popularity in most developed countries since the 1960s. There are many forms of vegetarian diet ranging from the semi-vegetarian to variations on the lacto-ovo vegetarian dietary pattern and to the more restrictive vegan patterns (Table 7.5). Adolescents are the population group most likely to make the switch from a mixed diet to a vegetarian diet. Girls are significantly more likely than boys to become vegetarians and estimates from the United Kingdom, Canada and Australia suggest that while veganism is extremely rare, around 8–10% of adolescent girls and 1–2% of boys (15–18 years) follow a lacto-ovo vegetarian diet. Pollo-vegetarianism and semi-vegetarianism may be considerably more common. Worsley and Skrzypiec (1998) noted that up to 37% of Australian girls and 11–17% of boys reported a semi-vegetarian pattern of diet.

There is little research on the long-term health benefits of adopting a vegetarian diet during adolescence. As expected, given the lower energy density of the diet, vegetarian adolescents typically have a lower body mass index and waist circumference, with lower LDL-cholesterol concentrations (Grant et al., 2008). There are no long-term follow-up studies to confirm the future benefit of this, but being leaner during adolescence makes it less likely that the individual will be overweight in adult life (see Section 6.4.3.2). Dos Santos Silva et al. (2002) reported that among Asian migrants to the United Kingdom, risk of breast cancer was lower among those who had been lifelong vegetarians, but the study was unable to determine whether childhood and adolescence had a specific, independent benefit, as opposed to there being a cumulative effect of prolonged meat avoidance. As with all forms of restrictive dietary practice

in adolescence, there are concerns that vegetarianism could have a negative impact upon nutritional status and the capacity to maintain optimal rates of growth and development. Adolescents are likely to experiment with diets and to make unplanned and abrupt shifts from a diet including meat to some form of vegetarianism, without any informed guidance. This can increase the risk that the dietary pattern adopted will fail to deliver an adequate balance of nutrients (Research Highlight 7.2).

7.6.3 Sport and physical activity

The impact of physical activity upon health and well-being is overwhelmingly positive at any stage of life. Adolescence is no exception to this, and adolescents who are more active will be protected against overweight and obesity and will have enhanced skeletal growth. Exercise benefits bone mineralization, for example, with particularly strong effects in trabecular regions (Specker, 2006). Often, the diets of adolescents who are involved in sports are of higher quality than those of less active peers (D'Alessandro et al., 2007). However, where levels of physical activity become more intense over longer and more frequent periods, such as in adolescents who become involved in organized sports or dance activities, this can impact upon energy balance, nutritional status, growth and development in an adverse manner.

Intense physical activity will, by definition, increase demands for energy, and the sporting teenager will need to consume more energy sources than a sedentary individual in order to maintain growth and sustain their performance. Requirements for protein may also be increased as physical activity will promote the deposition of muscle mass over and above that, which normally occurs in growth. This is most marked in adolescents who partake in events that are weight-class dependent, that is, where the optimal performance is associated with a highly muscular but lightweight body (e.g. martial arts and gymnastics) and endurance sports (swimming, long-distance running). Swimmers, for example, may increase their protein requirements from 0.73 (girls) to between 1.2 and 2.32 g/kg body weight

Table 7.5 Enhancers and inhibitors of iron absorption.

Inhibit iron absorption	Promote iron absorption
Phytates (bran and seeds)	Ascorbic acid
Polyphenols, especially catechols and galloyls (tea, coffee, wine)	Cysteine-rich peptides (meat)
	Vitamin A (overcomes effect of phytates)
Calcium	
High-dose zinc, manganese or copper	

Research Highlight 7.2 Concerns surrounding nutrition and health in vegetarian adolescents.

Nutritional status

Vegetarian adolescents appear to be at greater risk of having inadequate intakes of a number of nutrients. The low digestibility of plant foods and the poor bioavailability of minerals from plant sources (particularly with high phytate intake) mean that intakes of protein, zinc and iron may be of concern in vegetarians (Amit, 2010). This is of major importance at a time of rapid growth. Plant foods are rich in phytic acid, which inhibits absorption of iron and calcium, and oxalates, which inhibit calcium uptake. The bioavailability of iron from a vegetarian diet is only 10% compared to 18% from a mixed diet (Hunt, 2003). An 80% increase in intake is therefore required to meet requirements (Amit, 2010), which is challenging without supplementation or careful dietary planning. Vegetarian girls are six times more likely than omnivores to have low haemoglobin concentrations and three times more likely to have reduced iron stores (Thane *et al.*, 2003). Calcium uptake is poor from many plant sources, but some such as soya beans, broccoli and kale have relatively high bioavailability (Weaver *et al.*, 1999). Inclusion of dairy produce alongside such foods in the vegetarian diet should maintain healthy calcium status. In the absence of dairy produce, the vegan adolescent will need to take supplements of calcium and vitamin B12 (Amit, 2010).

Overall health and health behaviours

Notwithstanding the previous concerns, the dietary intakes of vegetarian adolescents are considered healthier by virtue of their greater consumption of fruit and vegetables and complex carbohydrates. It is also reported that vegetarian adolescents are less likely to smoke, consume alcohol or use drugs (Robinson-O'Brien *et al.*, 2009). In adolescence, vegetarianism may be associated with a number of negative health behaviours. Vegetarians are less likely than omnivores to be smokers, consume less alcohol and are less likely to be overweight and obese. However, there is a greater prevalence of underweight, and vegetarian girls are more likely to suffer mental health disturbances and require medication for depression (Baines *et al.*, 2007). A vegetarian diet can be used as a cover to hide more serious restriction of the diet and disordered eating by both girls and boys (Martins *et al.*, 1999). Forestell *et al.* (2012) reported that vegetarians have less food neophobia and experiment with a wider range of new food experiences than omnivores. However, their dietary choices were more motivated by weight control, and they were more likely to restrict their diet in an unhealthy manner. Vegetarian adolescents are also more likely to engage in binge eating with loss of control, supporting the idea that the vegetarian diet is a proxy for increased risk of disordered eating (Robinson-O'Brien *et al.*, 2009).

Fertility and reproductive function

Vegetarian girls may exhibit a number of problems with reproductive function. Vegetarianism is associated with longer cycle length, greater prevalence of amenorrhoea, anovulation and luteal phase defects. This may be partly explained by reduced body fatness and leptin secretion but may also relate to hypothalamic control over sex hormone secretion (Griffith and Omar, 2003). Vegetarians secrete lower levels of luteinizing hormone, even if cycles are regular. Diets rich in fibre and low in fat alter the profile of sex steroids that are synthesized within the ovary and increase cycle length (Goldin *et al.*, 1994). Baines *et al.* (2007) also noted that vegetarians were less likely than omnivorous teenagers to use the contraceptive pill.

---

per day (Petrie *et al.*, 2004). High-level physical activity also increases demands for micronutrients. Demand for most vitamins follows energy intake and utilization. Mineral requirements will increase as calcium, iron, magnesium, sodium, phosphorus and trace elements are incorporated into lean tissues and the skeleton as they grow under the influence of activity. Electrolyte and fluid status may also be perturbed by participation in sports.

Where physical activity is at a level that does not exert consistently high nutritional demands, there is unlikely to be any adverse impact upon physiological processes. Certain sports, however, particularly gymnastics, dance and the weight-class sports, can lead to delayed maturation. These activities often result in negative energy balance as individuals attempt to develop a lighter physique with greater muscular strength (Roemmich *et al.*, 2001). Energy deficit, poor nutritional status and reduced body

fatness are particularly associated with amenorrhoea and menstrual cycle abnormalities in adolescent girls involved in intense sport, with up to 25% of US high school athletes being affected (Misra, 2008). The loss of the permissive effects of leptin on the hypothalamic–pituitary–ovarian axis as body fat declines may largely explain these problems. Hormones such as cortisol, which is secreted at higher levels during activity, may also suppress hypothalamic production of GnRH. Failure to produce oestrogen can impact upon growth, particularly of the skeleton, as oestrogen normally increases secretion of growth hormone and IGF-1. Only regular, intense activity will produce these effects. Lower levels of activity actually promote growth by stimulating growth hormone production (Borer, 1995).

The worst-case scenario associated with high-level sport in adolescence has become known as the 'female athlete triad' (Figure 7.9). This is noted where

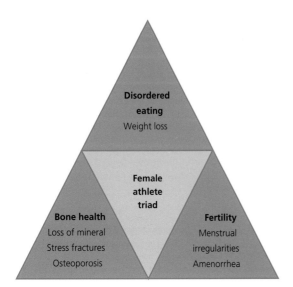

Figure 7.9 The female athlete triad is a syndrome of disordered eating resulting in reproductive and skeletal abnormalities. The syndrome is associated with high-level participation in sports that emphasize body size and appearance.

involvement in sport and exercise is at a high or elite level, particularly if the activity is associated with having a strictly controlled body weight that stems predominantly from a high proportion of lean body mass (Brunet, 2005). Aesthetic athletes (gymnasts, dancers, cheerleaders) are particularly at risk as their activity is in part judged on appearance. Long-distance runners are also at risk as an exceptionally lean body is advantageous for performance. A lean physique is generally achieved and maintained through the combination of activity itself and controlled eating. If the control over diet tips into disordered eating (see Section 7.6.4), the first element of the triad is in place. This can also occur due to an individual's lack of awareness of energy requirements (Thein-Nissenbaum, 2013). The second element is amenorrhoea, which is a direct consequence of low body fat and loss of the stimulatory effect of leptin upon the hypothalamic–pituitary–ovarian axis. While amenorrhoea is seen in less than 5% of the general population during adolescence, 28% of aesthetic athletes and 65% of long-distance runners report menstrual irregularity (Thein-Nissenbaum, 2013). The third element is osteoporosis or osteopenia, which stems from inadequate bone mineralization. This will not only be mainly a result of the endocrine immaturity and suppressed reproductive cycling of the individual but can also be related to calcium intake. Avoidance of dairy products as a means of weight control is a common feature of this condition. While exercise is known to

increase bone mineral density in adolescents (see Section 7.4), young high-level female athletes have been reported to have low bone mineral and are prone to stress fractures. Emerging evidence suggests that this persists into adulthood as the lost bone mass cannot be replaced (Thein-Nissenbaum, 2013).

7.6.4 Eating disorders

Eating disorders are psychiatric conditions that manifest as extremely abnormal patterns of food intake and weight control. A number of such conditions have been identified, of which the best characterized are AN and bulimia nervosa (BN). These conditions, along with binge eating disorder and the spectrum of conditions that fail to meet the diagnostic criteria for AN and BN (partial eating disorders or eating disorders not otherwise specified), are believed to lie on a broad continuum of eating behaviours extending from normal eating to behaviours promoting underweight (including normal dieting) and to behaviours promoting severe overweight (Chamay-Weber *et al.*, 2005). All of the eating disorders are most common in young women and often first manifest during the adolescent years. Eating disorders, particularly AN, are among the major causes of death among adolescents in developed countries.

7.6.4.1 AN

AN is characterized by the adoption of a pattern of eating and physical activity that promotes severe weight loss. Individuals with AN generally have a highly distorted image of their own body size and shape and an intense fear of becoming fat or gaining weight. As a consequence, they impose a starvation regime upon themselves. The full diagnostic criteria used for assessment of AN are shown in Table 7.6. Individuals with AN may adopt a purely restrictive dietary pattern, with minimal food intake, or may be of a bingeing–purging type whereby occasional episodes of excessive food intake are compensated through the use of laxatives, diuretics, extreme exercise or techniques to induce vomiting. All of these behaviours surrounding food are often compounded by the presence of obsessions with food, ritualistic calorie counting, food hoarding and collection of food recipes (Abraham, 2003).

Individuals with AN undergo extreme weight loss and, if in adolescence, a failure of growth and delay of sexual maturation. Muscle wasting occurs, along with loss of subcutaneous fat. The body often grows a layer of downy hair (lanugo), and the individual develops gastrointestinal and renal disturbances. Electrolyte imbalances are common and result from dehydration and losses associated with purging behaviours. Treatment of AN involves hospitalization and nutritional

Table 7.6 Diagnostic criteria for eating disorders.

Anorexia Nervosa

A Refusal to maintain body weight at or above minimally normal for age and height (<85% of expected weight)
B Intense fear of gaining weight or becoming fat, even though underweight
C Disturbance of the perception of body weight or shape. Denial of seriousness of current underweight
D Amenorrhoea (absence of three consecutive menstrual periods)

Bulimia Nervosa

A Recurrent episodes of binge eating characterized by both of the following:
  1 Eating an amount of food in a discrete period of time that is larger than most people would achieve in the same time, under similar circumstances
  2 A sense of lack of control over eating during the bingeing episode
B Recurrent inappropriate behaviour to compensate for eating in order to control weight gain (e.g. use of laxatives, enemas or diuretics or excessive exercise)
C Binge eating and compensatory behaviour occurring at least twice a week for 3 months
D No undue influence of body shape and weight on behaviour
E The disturbance does not occur excessively during periods of anorexia nervosa

From Diagnostic and statistical manual of mental disorders (APA, 2000).

support to promote weight gain and metabolic stabilization. Psychotherapy is necessary to resolve the underlying condition. Getting individuals to treatment is challenging as AN sufferers will often deny that they have a problem. As a result, mortality rates can be as high as 20%.

AN is most common in women and is generally seen between the ages of 15 and 23 years. The average age of onset is around 17 years. AN is also seen in males, who account for around 10% of cases. Estimates of the prevalence of the condition vary considerably, but between 0.3 and 0.5% of the young female population are likely to be affected (Hoek and van Hoeken, 2003). The incidence of AN has not varied significantly since the 1930s in the United States, but in European countries, it appeared to increase between 1935 and the early 1980s. Risk may be higher among girls and young women who engage in particular activities. Arcelus *et al.* (2014) reported that AN occurs in 4% of ballet dancers.

The causes of AN are complex and not fully understood. The condition has always been more common in girls, particularly white Caucasians from middle or high socio-economic status. The key features of AN are very low self-esteem and a poor view of body image, and these psychological traits often stem from unhappiness in the home life of the individual. Common indicators of risk include having conflicts in the home (Felker and Stivers, 1994), a passive father and domineering mother, lack of independence for the adolescent or sexual or physical abuse. AN may therefore be perceived as a failure of the individual to respond adequately to the growing emotional challenges of adulthood (Baluch *et al.*, 1997). It is also argued that AN is a response to the pressures of a modern culture and society that idealizes a thin body shape and equates dieting and thinness with beauty and success. The marketing of this ideal to adolescent girls (and boys) is known to be highly effective (Hill, 2006). Field and colleagues (2008) reported that purging behaviour was associated with a desire to look like women in the media.

The main driver for AN may, in fact, be a genetic predisposition, which produces the eating disorder when coupled to sociocultural stimuli and/or emotional and psychological disturbance. Studies of extended families and twins have indicated that an excess of the risk of AN (48–88%) is determined by genetic factors (Klump and Gobrogge, 2005; Hinney and Volckmar, 2013). Engaging in purging behaviours among girls under the age of 14 is more common where there is a history of maternal eating disorders (Field *et al.*, 2008), and there are reports of 10-fold greater risk of AN where there are first-degree relatives with the condition (Hinney and Volckmar, 2013). The basis of the genetic links is, as yet, poorly understood, but there is considerable interest in the potential role of the serotonergic system and the oestrogen receptor (ESR1). The neurotransmitter serotonin (5HT) plays a role in determining mood, and central defects of serotonin action are a common cause of anxiety and depression. Serotonin is also a component of the appetite regulation system, hence linking together eating behaviour and psychological states. Genome-wide association studies which systematically analyse the relationship between gene polymorphisms and disease suggest that several components of the serotonergic system may be involved in AN (the serotonin transporter 5HTTLPR, the receptor 5HT2a and tryptophan hydroxylase which is a key step in 5HT synthesis; Hinney and Volckmar, 2013) along with the closely related dopaminergic system (controls food intake and body weight; Bergen *et al.*, 2005). A role for oestrogen is also attractive as AN often manifests during puberty. ESR1 mediates many of the effects of oestrogen and can regulate the expression of genes with oestrogen-response elements. 5-HT2a is one such gene.

7.6.4.2 BN

BN shares the same basic psychopathology as AN, namely, a distorted view of body size and shape, but despite this, it manifests in a different way and impacts upon a slightly different population (Fairburn and Harrison, 2003). While AN can begin to appear as early as 8 years of age and reaches a peak of incidence in adolescence, development of BN prior to 13 years of age is unusual, and most sufferers are young adults (Gowers, 2008). BN is estimated to affect approximately 1% of young women, although claims of prevalence rates of up to 3.2% in school girls have been reported and 4.4% in dancers (Arcelus *et al.*, 2014). The prevalence is 10 times higher in women than in men (Hoek and van Hoeken, 2003).

BN is more challenging to identify than AN if working purely from physical symptoms. It is characterized by episodes of binge eating that occur on a frequent basis (Table 7.6). Usually, these binges involve the ingestion of between 1000 and 2000 kcal in a single 2 h session (Fairburn and Harrison, 2003), but there are reports that bulimics can take in 15 000 kcal during a binge. Sufferers sometimes report that during a binge, they lose all control and will eat raw food and food straight from tins and packets, stopping only when they are overcome by pain, fatigue or vomiting. The ability to take in larger binges is likely to develop over time as the normal signals from the gut that indicate satiety become suppressed.

Following binge sessions, the BN sufferer will take compensatory action to prevent weight gain. This can involve excessive exercising but more commonly utilizes techniques to purge the food from the body. Laxative substances or emetics are widely abused for this purpose. In between binges, there may be periods of intense food restriction to maintain control over body weight, but physically, the BN sufferer will often appear to be of normal or even slightly above average weight. Physiologically, however, there is an accrual of damage related to bingeing–purging cycles including loss of gut peristalsis and associated colonic problems, electrolyte imbalances and dehydration, damage to the salivary glands, malabsorption of fat soluble vitamins leading to deficiency of vitamin A and vitamin D, oesophagitis and erosion of dental enamel due to contact with stomach acid during vomiting.

As with AN, the development of BN is strongly linked to genetic factors and probably involves disturbances of the serotonergic system (Hinney and Volckmar, 2013). The profile of sufferers is similar to AN, with girls from home situations that create anxiety and depression being at greatest risk. Concerns about overweight that lead to dieting are also associated with greater risk, and in boys, negative paternal comments about weight are predictive of bingeing behaviours (Field *et al.*, 2008). Early menarche is also seen as a risk factor for BN in adolescent girls (Fairburn and Harrison, 2003). In the case of BN, the means of coping with emotional problems is to binge, which either provides a feeling of taking control over matters in an otherwise out of control life or a means of temporarily escaping from negative thoughts and feelings (Abraham, 2003). However, as shown in Figure 7.10, the bulimic individual falls into a negative cycle as the process of bingeing and purging creates feelings of shame, self-loathing and revulsion that exacerbate the initiating negative feelings.

Treatment for BN involves similar approaches to those used for AN sufferers. Hospitalization and the need for intense nutritional support are less likely as BN sufferers become malnourished less frequently. In adults, the prescribing of antidepressant medication can serve to reduce the frequency of bingeing and purging, but this benefit is often short lived and has not been reported in adolescents (Gowers, 2008).

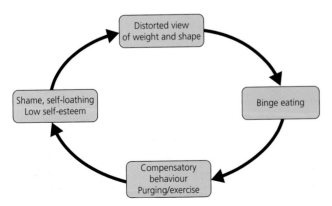

Figure 7.10 BN as a cycle of behaviour driven by poor self-esteem. Individuals with BN go through frequent episodes of binge eating followed by use of laxatives and emetics or excessive exercise to compensate for ingested energy. The bingeing is seen as a way of dealing with anxiety and depression linked to poor self-esteem and feelings of low self-worth. Feelings of shame that follow the binge–purge episode actually serve to reinforce the initial problem and hence maintain the bulimic behaviour.

7.6.5 The pregnant teenager

Adolescent pregnancies account for up to 20% of all births (16 million/year) on a global scale (WHO, 2012). While in developed countries they are unusual and are generally considered socially unacceptable, in the developing countries where early marriage is the norm, pregnancy under the age of 20 is commonplace. Indeed, 95% of all such births are seen in the poorer nations, and adolescent pregnancy rates are as high as 100–143 births per 1000 women aged 15–19 in Africa and 70–119 births per 1000 women in the Indian subcontinent. Some of the highest rates of adolescent pregnancy in developed nations are seen in the United States. Although rates here have declined considerably from the 107 per 1000 women aged 15–19 in the late 1980s, the US adolescent pregnancy rate remains at 34.3 per 1000 women. In Western Europe, adolescent pregnancy rates are low due to high standards of sex education and are typically between 3 and 10 pregnancies per 1000 women aged 15–19. The United Kingdom is the exception to this (26.4 adolescent pregnancies per 1000 women) as the rate has not changed appreciably in over a decade. Eastern Europe has high rates of adolescent pregnancy at 30–40 per 1000 women.

In developed countries, adolescent pregnancies are more likely among girls of lower socio-economic status. In the United Kingdom, for example, more than half of adolescent pregnancies are seen in girls from socially deprived backgrounds, and pregnancy rates are six times more likely in socially deprived areas (Wallace *et al.*, 2006). Most adolescent pregnancies are unplanned and are the consequence of either poor knowledge of, or restricted access to, contraception. Among the developing countries, pregnancy rates among teenagers are highest in the poorest nations, for example, those of sub-Saharan Africa. Pregnancy rates are higher in the rural populations of such countries than in the urban areas.

The risks associated with pregnancy that were described in Chapter 3, for example, miscarriage, fetal death and maternal death, are considerably greater in adolescents than in older mothers. Adolescents have a fourfold greater risk of death during pregnancy than women over the age of 20 years. Post-partum haemorrhage (often related to iron deficiency anaemia) or obstructive labour due to the pelvis being too narrow for the passage of the baby is the major cause of maternal death among 15–19-year-old girls in developing countries.

Adolescent pregnancies, particularly where the mother is under the age of 16 years, are significantly more likely to end in miscarriage, premature labour or low birth weight (Wallace *et al.*, 2006). As shown in Figure 7.11, risk of adverse outcomes of pregnancy for

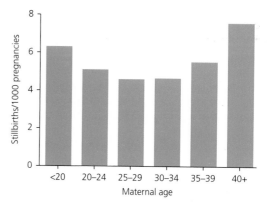

Figure 7.11 Adolescent pregnancy is associated with a number of adverse outcomes including stillbirth. Mothers under the age of 20 are 1.4 (95% CI 1.2–1.6) times more likely to have a stillbirth than 25–29-year-olds.
Data source: CMACE (2011).

babies is also markedly higher. Stillbirth and neonatal death (infant death in the first 28 days post-partum) are significantly more common where mothers are below the age of 20 (CMACE, 2011). Girls aged 15–16 are significantly more likely (OR 1.42, 95% CI 1.06–1.89) to have low-birth-weight infants and to deliver prematurely (OR 1.87, 95% CI 1.51–2.31; Gibbs *et al.*, 2012). Risks are higher in younger mothers. These observations were made in populations with good antenatal care, suggesting that factors related to biological immaturity drive many of the observed outcomes. Indeed, for adolescents in the developing world, antenatal care and medical supervision are likely to be poor. Teenagers in developed countries will often conceal their pregnancies until later in gestation due to the associated social stigma. This makes antenatal care, particularly strategies aimed at optimizing nutrition, extremely challenging. In addition to these immediate threats to health associated with pregnancy, the offspring of adolescent mothers are at risk in the long term. Low birth weight is associated with increased risk of cardiovascular disease and metabolic syndrome (Barker, 1998). Children of adolescent mothers tend to remain socially disadvantaged, are less likely to succeed educationally and are more likely to have behavioural problems (Wallace *et al.*, 2006).

Nutritional status may be a critical element of the greater risk associated with adolescent pregnancy. The relationship between the nutritional status of adolescents and pregnancy outcomes is complex and poorly understood. It is clear however that there is major competition between maternal growth and the growth of the fetus and placenta. Growth generally continues during pregnancy and produces the apparently paradoxical situation of greater pregnancy weight gain than that seen in adult women but with lower eventual birth weights (Wallace *et al.*, 2006). Growth of adolescent girls continues for up to 4 years after menarche and is maximal between 13 and 15 years. The energy utilization to sustain growth appears to have priority over requirements for pregnancy, and as a result, adolescent mothers fail to deposit reserves of fat in early pregnancy and cannot sustain rapid rates of fetal growth in the second and third trimesters.

Adolescent mothers are more likely to consume alcohol, smoke tobacco and engage in other high-risk behaviours than older women. These factors may also contribute to the greater prevalence of adverse outcomes. These women are less likely to optimize nutritional status prior to conception, for example, they are unlikely to take folate supplements in the periconceptual period (Langley-Evans and Langley-Evans, 2002) and often enter pregnancy with low micronutrient reserves. Adolescent mothers are more likely to have low intakes of calcium, iron, zinc, riboflavin and folate than adults during pregnancy (Moran, 2007). A study of 500 British adolescent pregnancies found that 52% had iron deficiency anaemia, 30% had circulating 25-hydroxy-vitamin D below the threshold for deficiency (25 nmol/l) and 10–20% showed biochemical evidence of poor folate and vitamin B12 status (Baker *et al.*, 2009). Biochemical evidence of iron deficiency has been reported to have a high prevalence in adolescent pregnancies, reaching 70–80% in some populations. Allen (1993) reported that likelihood of iron deficiency anaemia increased with advancing pregnancy. Eleven per cent of pregnant teenagers were anaemic in the first trimester of pregnancy, but this rose to 37% by the third trimester. Iannotti *et al.* (2005) reported that 61% of adolescent mothers had low serum ferritin in the third trimester, and the high vulnerability of adolescents to late gestation anaemia was confirmed by the systematic review of Moran (2007). Micronutrient deficiency is endemic in the developing countries, and supplementation of young mothers with iron and folate is a commonly used strategy to combat low birth weight and other poor pregnancy outcomes (Mishra *et al.*, 2005).

In developed countries, it is often assumed that poor nutritional status in pregnant adolescents is a product of poor dietary habits (e.g. missed meals and snacking) both prior to and during pregnancy (Gutierrez and King, 1993). This may be an overly simplistic view as this does not explain the greater risks associated with pregnancy in adolescence, which are seen in developing countries. Nor do all surveys of nutrition in pregnancy indicate problems with dietary intake. Giddens *et al.* (2000) found no differences in nutrient intakes between pregnant teenagers and adults in a US population.

Competition for nutrients between the pregnancy and maternal growth and poorly understood issues related to how the placenta partitions nutrients between the mother and fetus are likely to play the major role in determining the relationship between maternal nutritional status and pregnancy outcomes.

7.6.6 Alcohol

Adolescence is a time when individuals attempt to assert their individuality and independence from parents and family. This transition to adulthood can manifest in a variety of ways, but in many cultures, the rebellion of adolescence is heavily focused upon the misuse of alcohol. In the countries of northern Europe (the United Kingdom, Scandinavia, Ireland and the Netherlands), teenagers are the population group that is most likely drink excessively, focusing mostly on the intoxicating properties of alcoholic beverages, rather than on drinking as one aspect of social interaction. Among these countries, 17–32% of 16-year-olds report being intoxicated more than 10 times in a given year (Engels and Knibbe, 2000), and binge drinking (more than five alcoholic drinks in a session) is widespread, particularly among girls (McArdle, 2008). In contrast, in the countries of southern Europe (France, Spain, Italy and Portugal), cultural attitudes differ and alcohol is mostly consumed with meals. Drunkenness among adolescents is relatively uncommon in this region (Engels and Knibbe, 2000). However, even in these countries, alcohol is consumed in large quantities by teenagers, and this may impact upon development, disease risk and nutritional status. There is growing evidence that adolescents are beginning to heed public health messages about alcohol. Among Australian 14–17-year-olds, the proportion who reported having abstained from alcohol over a 12-month period increased from 35.7% in boys and 29.9% in girls in 2001 to 51.4% in boys and 48.8% in girls in 2011 (Livingston, 2014). Similarly, the YRBSS survey (CDC, 2011) in the United States found that between 1999 and 2011, the prevalence of alcohol consumption and binge drinking behaviour among adolescents declined markedly.

The metabolism of alcohol (Figure 7.12) occurs primarily within the liver, where it can be cleared by several pathways. Most metabolism is mediated by the cytosolic pathway in which alcohol dehydrogenase converts ethanol to acetaldehyde. This can then be cleared to acetate through the action of aldehyde dehydrogenases in the cytosol (ALDH1) or mitochondria (ALDH2). If alcohol consumption is excessive, these processes will have a number of effects upon nutritional status, primarily through increases in demand for thiamin, riboflavin and nicotinic acid. Alcohol dehydrogenase is also

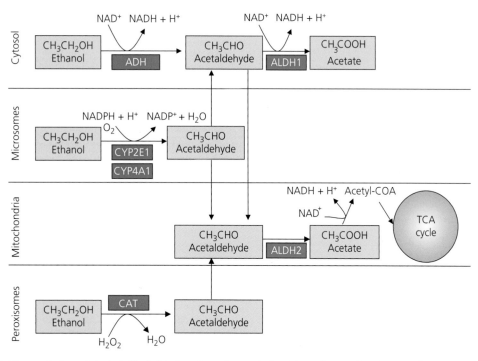

Figure 7.12 The metabolism of alcohol. Alcohol (ethanol) can be metabolized through cytosolic, microsomal or peroxisomal pathways. Cytosolic metabolism involves the enzymes alcohol dehydrogenase (ADH) and acetaldehyde dehydrogenase 1 (ALDH1). Where the cytosolic capacity is exceeded, microsomal metabolism utilizes the cytochrome P450 enzymes (CYP2E1 and CYP4A1). Acetaldehyde products of microsomal ethanol metabolism are cleared by acetaldehyde dehydrogenase 2 (ALDH2). Peroxisomal catalase (CAT) can also contribute to alcohol clearance.

responsible for the conversion of retinol to retinaldehyde. Regular consumption of excessive alcohol will competitively inhibit retinol metabolism and hence impact upon vitamin A status.

If the capacity of the alcohol dehydrogenase pathway is exceeded, either due to the quantity of alcohol consumed or due to B vitamins being limiting nutrients, then detoxification follows the microsomal ethanol oxidation pathway. Cytochrome P450 enzymes catalyze the conversion of ethanol to acetaldehyde. As the expression of these enzymes is induced by ethanol, metabolism via this pathway has different consequences in individuals who consume frequently to those seen in irregular drinkers. Regular consumption increases the formation of free radical and carcinogenic intermediates. Clearance of xenobiotics, retinoids and steroids is more rapid, and as a consequence, hepatic vitamin D metabolism is disrupted. Damage to cells within the liver promotes cirrhosis. Specific damage to hepatic stellate cells further impacts on vitamin A status as these are the sites of liver storage. Acetaldehyde is itself a toxic intermediate and can cause injury to the liver and form adducts that promote cell death or carcinogenesis.

Accumulation of lipid within the liver is commonly seen in alcohol abusers, and this stems from excess production of NADH from the alcohol dehydrogenase pathway and also from the actions of CYP4A1.

The effects of alcohol upon physiology and metabolism depend upon the nature and frequency of the exposure. In the short term, alcohol is associated with stimulation of the appetite and the consumption of energy-dense snacks. Berkey and colleagues (2008) reported that even moderate consumption (two or more servings per week) of alcohol by teenaged girls was associated with greater increases in body mass index over a 12-month follow-up, although other studies show that effects of alcohol on body weight are confined to younger teenagers (Croezen et al., 2009; Figure 7.13). More frequent and excessive consumption has contrasting effects and may be extremely harmful to health and social development. While alcohol dependency (alcoholism) may be rare among adolescents, alcohol abuse (a pattern of alcohol use in which the individual drinks in a manner that is hazardous to physical well-being and is likely to suffer problems with meeting obligations at home and at school) is increasingly a cause for concern. Alcoholics and alcohol abusers are often malnourished.

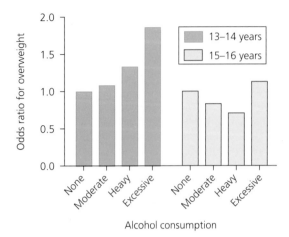

Figure 7.13 There is a weak association between alcohol consumption and BMI in adolescents. In younger Dutch adolescents, heavy or excessive intake was associated with greater risk of overweight, but the effect was absent in older adolescents. Moderate intake, 1–3 glasses per occasion per week for girls and 1–5 for boys; heavy, 4–6 glasses for girls and 6–10 for boys; excessive >7 glasses for girls and >10 for boys. Reproduced with permission from Croezen *et al.* (2009). © Nature Publishing Group.

This can stem from reduced nutrient intakes (alcoholic beverages displacing food intake), hyperexcretion of nutrients or reductions in bioavailability. Given the often marginal micronutrient intakes of adolescents, even moderate alcohol consumption may impact significantly upon nutritional status (Alonso-Aperte and Varela-Moreiras, 2000). Individuals who abuse alcohol are more likely to self-harm, suffer from attention deficit hyperactivity disorder, have learning difficulties and have problems with their behaviour and conduct. Adolescence is a critical period of development for the brain, during which regions in the hippocampus are rewired. These are centres that are responsible for memory. The adolescent brain appears more sensitive to alcohol than the adult, so excessive consumption during this stage may be particularly damaging (White and Swartzwelder, 2005).

7.6.7 Tobacco smoking

Among adult populations, the prevalence of smoking is in decline as awareness of the links between smoking and cancer, cardiovascular disease and pulmonary disease grows. The age group of 20–34-year-olds is the group in the population that is most likely to be smokers, but adolescence represents the life stage at which smoking is most likely to be initiated. Up to 75% of adolescents will experiment with cigarette smoking, and over 90% of adult smokers begin smoking in their teenage years (Hampl and Betts, 1999). The recent years

have seen a reduction in the numbers of adolescents taking up smoking. In the United Kingdom, the proportion of 16–19-year-olds who smoke declined markedly between 1998 (31%) and 2012 (15%; ASH, 2013). A similar decline occurred in the United States (36% 1997 20% 2007) and in Western Europe. The highest rates of smoking among adolescents are seen in Central Europe (29% of Austrian girls) and the Baltic States (34% of Lithuanian boys). Smoking rates among adolescent girls are generally slightly higher than in boys.

As with alcohol consumption, cigarette smoking is often an act of rebellion among adolescents, and the habit is most commonly initiated in order to achieve social acceptance among peers. There are suggestions that adolescents may also begin smoking as a means of addressing concerns about body weight or body image. Smoking is known to suppress weight gain, and typically, smoking males weigh 5 kg less than non-smokers (Hampl and Betts, 1999). Jensen and colleagues (1995) reported that hip circumference in young men was inversely correlated with excretion of cotinine (a breakdown product of nicotine). Awareness of the association between smoking and body weight appears to be greater among girls than boys, and there is evidence that this is an important influence on smoking behaviour in girls and young women (Potter *et al.*, 2004). French and colleagues (1994) noted that among teenaged girls, the odds of initiating smoking during a 12-month period were 1.44–2.15 times greater if individuals had expressed fear of weight gain and the desire to lose weight or indulged in restrictive dietary practices.

The effects of smoking upon the nutritional status of adults are well documented, but there have been few studies that have specifically addressed the issue in adolescents. As adolescent smokers are highly likely to have parents who smoke, it may be that their diets differ from non-smokers in the same respects as noted with adults. Indeed, Crawley and While (1996) reported that non-smoking teenagers' dietary intakes were similar to those of smokers if their parents were smokers. Typically, smokers have low circulating concentrations of folate, vitamin C, vitamin E and carotenoids, which may be explained by greater turnover due to oxidative stress (Tappia *et al.*, 1995). Dietary patterns also differ and smokers consume more meat, processed meat, eggs and fried foods. Adolescent boys who smoke tend to consume less fruit and fruit juices, while girls consume less fruit and vegetables (Hampl and Betts, 1999). Smoking among adolescents is associated with lower intakes of fibre, vitamin C, selenium, calcium and thiamin and greater intakes of fat, sugar and alcohol (Crawley and While, 1996).

Smoking clearly impacts upon eating behaviours, and a number of explanations for this have been advanced.

Primarily, the fact that an individual is a smoker indicates that they make less healthy choices in general. Poor dietary habits are therefore unsurprising. Indeed, individuals who cease smoking often also adopt very healthy dietary habits as an element of wholesale lifestyle changes. It is also proposed that food intake may be displaced by smoking and that cigarette smoking dulls the sense of taste, particularly for sweet foods (Hampl and Betts, 1999). The act of smoking may also determine meal frequency and duration. This might be particularly influential in adolescents, whose smoking habit is usually an illicit and furtive activity.

The health consequences of cigarette smoking are well established, and clearly, the initiation of smoking in adolescence will be a risk factor for disease at later stages of life. Smoking is one of a cluster of lifestyle factors in adolescence which may impact upon bone health (Research Highlight 7.3).

7.6.8 Drug abuse

While the majority of adolescents do not use illicit substances, this age group is the population subgroup that is most likely to experiment with abuse of hallucinogenic solvents, intravenous drugs, inhaled drugs and prescription drugs. Statistics from developed countries suggest that the numbers of adolescents using drugs increased significantly between the 1980s and the early part of the twenty-first century. In the United States, cannabis use was reported by 6.5% of 13–14-year-olds (8th grade at school) and 18.3% of 17–18-year-olds

Research Highlight 7.3 Bone health and substance use in adolescence.

Adolescence is a critical phase in the development of the skeleton. Puberty is the main phase for the accrual of bone mineral under the influence of sex steroids, so lifestyle factors during this stage of life that may have a detrimental effect on bone growth may result in lower peak bone mass and future bone health. Adolescents as a group are most likely to initiate cigarette smoking, begin consuming alcohol and experiment with recreational drugs and other substances.

Smoking

There is a well-established relationship between smoking and bone health in adults, with a 30% greater lifetime fracture risk in smokers compared to non-smokers. Reports of lower bone mineral density are common, with the hip, spine and femoral neck all exhibiting lower BMD in smokers (Wong *et al.*, 2007). The impact upon the skeleton during adolescence is less well documented, but Jones *et al.* (2004) found that girls who smoked were significantly more likely to suffer fractures before age 18 if they smoked (OR 1.43, 95% CI 1.05–1.95). Regular smoking was associated with lower BMD at the hip and femoral neck in the study of Dorn and colleagues (2011) and also slowed the accrual of bone at the hip between the ages of 13 and 19 (Dorn *et al.*, 2013). Välimäki and colleagues (1994) reported that men aged 20–29 had lower bone mineral density if they had smoked in adolescence. Similar findings were noted in a comparison of 18–19-year-old men who smoked with non-smokers (Lorentzon *et al.*, 2007). The mechanistic basis of these effects upon bone may lie in the metabolism of vitamin D and hence the availability of calcium for deposition of bone mineral. Serum 1,25 dihydroxycholecalciferol concentrations are lower in smokers compared to non-smokers, and this will inhibit intestinal uptake of calcium.

Alcohol

Alcohol has known effects upon the skeleton, specifically the inhibition of osteoblast activity, which slows bone healing and turnover. However, there is evidence that in adults the relationship between alcohol and BMD is J-shaped, with low-to-moderate intakes actually stimulating accrual of greater bone mass (Wosje and Kalkwarf, 2007). This benefit of alcohol appears to be absent, however, with chronically excessive consumption or episodic binge drinking. In adolescents, the impact of alcohol is not well documented. While there is evidence that alcohol consumption does not alter the rate of accrual of bone between the ages of 13 and 19 (Dorn *et al.*, 2013), adolescents who are regular consumers of alcohol have lower BMD at the hip and femoral neck (Dorn *et al.*, 2011). Korkor *et al.* (2009) found no significant effect of alcohol or smoking in a small cohort of US high school students.

Other substances

Adolescents are experimental by nature and can be drawn to use of recreational drugs and abuse of toxic substances. Dündaröz *et al.* (2002) found that a group of young people who abused solvents had lower bone mineral density than an age-matched control group, but could not dissect the possible confounding effects of cigarettes and alcohol. There are several reports that abuse of opioids is also associated with loss of bone (Milos *et al.*, 2011). Although there are no reports in the literature of the effects of cannabis use on bone health, it is known that bone contains cannabinoid receptors. These allow the tissue to respond to endocannabinoids which regulate the activity of osteoclasts (Idris and Ralston, 2012). Blockade or genetic knockout of these receptors stimulates bone growth, so there is the possibility that use of cannabis during adolescence could impact negatively on future bone health.

(12th grade). Cocaine use was reported by 2.5% of the older adolescents (CDC, 2006). In the United Kingdom, cannabis is the most commonly used drug among teenagers. Thirteen per cent of girls and 15% of boys aged 11–15 years reported use of cannabis, with these figures rising to 24 and 31%, respectively, for 16–19-year-olds. Among Australian adolescents, cannabis is also the main drug of choice, being used by up to 35% of 14–19-year-olds.

Abuse of drugs and other substances is often associated with undernutrition. This effect can be direct, by virtue of effects of drugs upon food intake, absorption of nutrients, urinary and faecal losses of nutrients and metabolic rate. The latter will often be elevated by substance abuse due to requirements to metabolize xenobiotics in the liver. In adolescents, there may be problems with micronutrient status that can potentiate the effects of drugs (both illicit and those administered for therapeutic purposes), and the enzyme systems needed for xenobiotic detoxification are not fully matured (Alonso-Aperte and Varela-Moreiras, 2000). Indirect effects on nutritional status may be more important. For example, substance addiction will lead to crime and social exclusion, and this limits normal access to a healthy diet. Disordered eating is also often linked to drug abuse. Herzog and colleagues (2006) reported that 20% of women with AN or BN had a history of drug use, with amphetamines, cocaine and cannabis most frequently used. Pisetsky *et al.* (2008) also noted strong associations between abuse of anabolic steroids or cannabis and extreme dieting and the use of vomiting and laxatives for weight control among male high school students.

Drug use is also associated with other unhealthy behaviours and factors that can impact upon nutritional status. Cannabis use is positively correlated with alcohol consumption and tobacco smoking (Rodondi *et al.*, 2006). Consumption of snack foods tends to be greater, and drug users are more frequently from lower-income families or ethnic minority groups. Overall, drug use is one manifestation of a wider spectrum of behaviours and influences that promote undernutrition. There are few studies that have been able to quantify the impact upon nutritional status, mainly because drug users are an unreliable group to survey accurately. Knight *et al.* (1994) were able to relate drug use to biochemical measures of nutritional status in a group of socially deprived, pregnant women. Use of cannabis, cocaine or phencyclidine was associated with reduced serum ferritin and poor ascorbate, folate and vitamin B12 status. This would be consistent with the imbalanced meals, erratic eating patterns and increased alcohol consumption that are associated with substance abuse.

SUMMARY

- Adolescence is a life stage that is dominated by rapid rates of growth, remodelling of body shape and composition and sexual maturation. These physiological processes may be vulnerable if nutritional status is compromised.
- Puberty is associated with gains in lean body mass, rising fat mass in girls and rapid increases in bone mineralization.
- Requirements for energy and nutrients are higher during adolescence than at any other stage of life.
- Intakes of nutrients may be compromised by poor food choices that are related to the growing emotional and social independence of adolescents. Low iron, zinc, calcium and folate status is a concern in this sub-population.
- Nutrient status in adolescents may be impaired by experimentation with restrictive dietary practices such as vegetarianism or weight loss diets.
- Adolescents are a high-risk group for eating disorders. These conditions have a strong genetic component, but risk is increased by emotional disturbance, anxiety and depression.
- Adolescent pregnancy is a major challenge from a nutritional perspective. The competition for nutrients between fetal and ongoing maternal growth increases the risk of poor pregnancy outcomes.
- Use of tobacco, alcohol and drugs can negatively impact upon nutritional status and normal growth and development in adolescents.

References

Abraham, S.F. (2003) Dieting, body weight, body image and self-esteem in young women: doctors' dilemmas. *Medical Journal of Australia*, **178**, 607–611.

Action on Smoking and Health (ASH) (2013) *Smoking Statistics. Who Smokes and How Much?* http://ash.org.uk/files/documents/ASH_106.pdf (accessed 2 June 2014).

Allen, L.H. (1993) Iron-deficiency anemia increases risk of preterm delivery. *Nutrition Reviews*, **51**, 49–52.

Alonso-Aperte E and Varela-Moreiras G (2000) Drugs-nutrient interactions: a potential problem during adolescence. *European Journal of Clinical Nutrition* **54**(Suppl.), S69–S74.

American Psychiatric Association (APA) (2000) *Diagnostic and Statistical Manual of Mental Disorders*, 4th edn, APA, Washington DC.

Amit, M. (2010) Vegetarian diets in children and adolescents. *Paediatrics and Child Health*, **15**, 303–314.

Arcelus, J., Witcomb, G.L. and Mitchell, A. (2014) Prevalence of eating disorders amongst dancers: a systemic review and meta-analysis. *European Eating Disorders Review*, **22**, 92–101.

Baines, S., Powers, J. and Brown, W.J. (2007) How does the health and well-being of young Australian vegetarian and semi-vegetarian women compare with non-vegetarians? *Public Health Nutrition*, **10**, 436–442.

Baker, P.N., Wheeler, S.J., Sanders, T.A. *et al.* (2009) A prospective study of micronutrient status in adolescent pregnancy. *American Journal of Clinical Nutrition*, **89**, 1114–1124.

Baluch, B., Furnham, A. and Huszcza, A. (1997) Perception of body shapes by anorexics and mature and teenage females. *Journal of Clinical Psychology*, **53**, 167–175.

Barker, D.J.P. (1998) *Mothers, Babies and Health in Later Life*, Churchill Livingstone, Edinburgh.

Basiotis, P.P., Welsh, S.O., Cronin, F.J. *et al.* (1987) Number of days of food intake records required to estimate individual and group nutrient intakes with defined confidence. *Journal of Nutrition*, **117**, 1638–1641.

Bates, B., Lennox, A., Prentice, A. *et al.* (2014) *National Diet and Nutrition Survey: Results from Years 1–4 (combined) of the Rolling Programme (2008/2009 – 2011/12)*, Public Health England, London.

Bauer, K.W., Larson, N.I., Nelson, M.C. *et al.* (2009) Fast food intake among adolescents: secular and longitudinal trends from 1999 to 2004. *Preventive Medicine*, **48**, 284–287.

Bergen, A.W., Yeager, M., Welch, R.A. *et al.* (2005) Association of multiple DRD2 polymorphisms with anorexia nervosa. *Neuropsychopharmacology*, **30**, 1703–1710.

Berkey, C.S., Rockett, H.R. and Colditz, G.A. (2008) Weight gain in older adolescent females: the internet, sleep, coffee, and alcohol. *Journal of Pediatrics*, **153**, 635–639.

Boreham, C.A. and McKay, H.A. (2011) Physical activity in childhood and bone health. *British Journal of Sports Medicine*, **45**, 877–879.

Borer, K.T. (1995) The effects of exercise on growth. *Sports Medicine*, **20**, 375–397.

Bowman, S.A., Gortmaker, S.L., Ebbeling, C.B. *et al.* (2004) Effects of fast-food consumption on energy intake and diet quality among children in a national household survey. *Pediatrics*, **113**, 112–118.

Brunet, M. (2005) Female athlete triad. *Clinical Sports Medicine*, **24**, 623–636.

Campos, R.M., de Mello, M.T., Tock, L. *et al.* (2013) Interaction of bone mineral density, adipokines and hormones in obese adolescents girls submitted in an interdisciplinary therapy. *Journal of Pediatric Endocrinology and Metabolism*, **26**, 663–668.

Centers for Disease Control and Prevention (CDC) (2006) Youth risk behavior surveillance-United States, 2005. *Morbidity and Mortality Weekly Report*, **55**, SS-5.

Centers for Disease Control and Prevention (CDC) (2011) *YRBSS: Youth Risk Behavior Surveillance System*, http://www.cdc.gov/HealthyYouth/yrbs/ (accessed June 2014).

Centers for Disease Control and Prevention (CDC) (2012) *Second National Report on Biochemical Indicators of Diet and Nutrition in the U.S. Population*, http://www.cdc.gov/nutrition report/pdf/Nutrition_Book_complete508_final. pdf#zoom=100 (accessed June 2014).

Centre for Maternal and Child Enquiries (CMACE) (2011) *Perinatal Mortality 2009*, http://www.hqip.org.uk/assets/ NCAPOP-Library/CMACE-Reports/35.-March-2011-Perinatal-Mortality-2009.pdf (accessed June 2014).

Chamay-Weber, C., Narring, F. and Michaud, P.A. (2005) Partial eating disorders among adolescents: a review. *Journal of Adolescent Health*, **37**, 417–427.

Chung, A.E., Perrin, E.M. and Skinner, A.C. (2013) Accuracy of child and adolescent weight perceptions and their relationships to dieting and exercise behaviors: a NHANES study. *Academy of Pediatrics*, **13**, 371–378.

Crawley, H.F. and While, D. (1996) Parental smoking and the nutrient intake and food choice of British teenagers aged 16–17 years. *Journal of Epidemiology and Community Health*, **50**, 306–312.

Croezen, S., Visscher, T.L., Ter Bogt, N.C. *et al.* (2009) Skipping breakfast, alcohol consumption and physical inactivity as risk factors for overweight and obesity in adolescents: results of the E-MOVO project. *European Journal of Clinical Nutrition*, **63**, 405–412.

D'Alessandro, C., Morelli, E., Evangelisti, I. *et al.* (2007) Profiling the diet and body composition of subelite adolescent rhythmic gymnasts. *Pediatric Exercise Science*, **19**, 215–227.

Daly, R.M. (2007) The effect of exercise on bone mass and structural geometry during growth. *Medicine and Sport Science*, **51**, 33–49.

Davies, J.H., Evans, B.A. and Gregory, J.W. (2004) Bone mass acquisition in healthy children. *Archives of Disease in Childhood*, **90**, 373–378.

De Laet, C., Kanis, J.A., Odén, A. *et al.* (2005) Body mass index as a predictor of fracture risk: a meta-analysis. *Osteoporosis International*, **16**, 1330–1338.

Department of Health (DoH) (1998) *Dietary Reference Values for Energy and Nutrients for the United Kingdom*, Stationery Office, London.

Diethelm, K., Jankovic, N., Moreno, L.A. *et al.* (2012) Food intake of European adolescents in the light of different food-based dietary guidelines: results of the HELENA (Healthy Lifestyle in Europe by Nutrition in Adolescence) Study. *Public Health Nutrition*, **15**, 386–398.

Diethelm, K., Huybrechts, I., Moreno, L. *et al.* (2014) Nutrient intake of European adolescents: results of the HELENA (Healthy Lifestyle in Europe by Nutrition in Adolescence) Study. *Public Health Nutrition*, **17**, 486–497.

Dorn, L.D., Pabst, S., Sontag, L.M. *et al.* (2011) Bone mass, depressive, and anxiety symptoms in adolescent girls: variation by smoking and alcohol use. *Journal of Adolescent Health*, **49**, 498–504.

Dorn, L.D., Beal, S.J., Kalkwarf, H.J. *et al.* (2013) Longitudinal impact of substance use and depressive symptoms on bone accrual among girls aged 11–19 years. *Journal of Adolescent Health*, **52**, 393–399.

Dos Santos Silva, I., Mangtani, P., McCormack, V. *et al* (2002) Lifelong vegetarianism and risk of breast cancer: a population-based case-control study among South Asian migrant women living in England. *International Journal of Cancer*, **99**, 238–244.

Ducy, P., Amling, M., Takeda, S. *et al.* (2000) Leptin inhibits bone formation through a hypothalamic relay: a central control of bone mass. *Cell*, **100**, 197–207.

Dündaröz, M.R., Sarici, S.U., Türkbay, T. *et al.* (2002) Evaluation of bone mineral density in chronic glue sniffers. *Turkish Journal of Pediatrics*, **44**, 326–329.

El Hage, Z., Theunynck, D., Jacob, C. *et al* (2013) Bone mineral content and density in obese, overweight and normal weight adolescent boys. *Lebanese Medical Journal*, **61**, 148–154.

Engels, R.C. and Knibbe, R.A. (2000) Young people's alcohol consumption from a European perspective: risks and benefits. *European Journal of Clinical Nutrition*, **54** (Suppl. 1), S52–S55.

Fairburn, C.G. and Harrison, P.J. (2003) Eating disorders. *Lancet*, **361**, 407–416.

Felker, K.R. and Stivers, C. (1994) The relationship of gender and family environment to eating disorder risk in adolescents. *Adolescence*, **29**, 821–834.

Field, A.E., Javaras, K.M., Aneja, P. *et al.* (2008) Family, peer, and media predictors of becoming eating disordered. *Archives of Pediatric and Adolescent Medicine*, **162**, 574–579.

Fiorito, L.M., Mitchell, D.C., Smiciklas-Wright, H. *et al.* (2006) Girls' calcium intake is associated with bone mineral content during middle childhood. *Journal of Nutrition*, **136**, 1281–1286.

Forestell, C.A., Spaeth, A.M. and Kane, S.A. (2012) To eat or not to eat red meat. A closer look at the relationship between restrained eating and vegetarianism in college females. *Appetite*, **58**, 319–325.

French, S.A., Perry, C.L., Leon, G.R. *et al.* (1994) Weight concerns, dieting behavior, and smoking initiation among adolescents: a prospective study. *American Journal of Public Health*, **84**, 1818–1820.

French, S.A., Story, M., Neumark-Sztainer, D. *et al* (2001) Fast food restaurant use among adolescents: associations with nutrient intake, food choices and behavioral and psychosocial variables. *International Journal of Obesity*, **25**, 1823–1833.

Gallagher, C.M., Black, L.J. and Oddy, W.H. (2014) Micronutrient intakes from food and supplements in Australian adolescents. *Nutrients*, **6**, 342–354.

Gibbs, C.M., Wendt, A., Peters, S. *et al.* (2012) The impact of early age at first childbirth on maternal and infant health. *Paediatric Perinatology and Epidemiology*, **26** (Suppl 1), 259–284.

Giddens, J.B., Krug, S.K., Tsang, R.C. *et al.* (2000) Pregnant adolescent and adult women have similarly low intakes of selected nutrients. *Journal of the American Dietetic Association*, **100**, 1334–1340.

Giovannini, M., Agostoni, C., Gianní, M. *et al.* (2000) Adolescence: macronutrient needs. *European Journal of Clinical Nutrition*, **54** (Suppl. 1), S7–S10.

Goldin, B.R., Woods, M.N., Spiegelman, D.L. *et al.* (1994) The effect of dietary fat and fiber on serum estrogen concentrations in premenopausal women under controlled dietary conditions. *Cancer*, **74**, 1125–1131.

Goulding, A., Taylor, R.W., Jones, I.E. *et al.* (2000) Overweight and obese children have low bone mass and area for their weight. *International Journal of Obesity*, **24**, 627–632.

Gowers, S.G. (2008) Management of eating disorders in children and adolescents. *Archives of Disease in Childhood*, **93**, 331–334.

Grant, R., Bilgin, A., Zeuschner, C. *et al.* (2008) The relative impact of a vegetable-rich diet on key markers of health in a cohort of Australian adolescents. *Asia Pacific Journal of Clinical Nutrition*, **17** (1), 107–115.

Greene, D.A. and Naughton, G.A. (2011) Calcium and vitamin-D supplementation on bone structural properties in peripubertal female identical twins: a randomised controlled trial. *Osteoporosis International*, **22**, 489–498.

Griffith, J. and Omar, H. (2003) Association between vegetarian diet and menstrual problems in young women: a case presentation and brief review. *Journal of Pediatric and Adolescent Gynecology*, **16**, 319–323.

Guo, S.S., Chumlea, W.C., Roche, A.F. *et al.* (1997) Age- and maturity-related changes in body composition during adolescence into adulthood: the Fels Longitudinal Study. *International Journal of Obesity*, **21**, 1167–1175.

Gutierrez, Y. and King, J.C. (1993) Nutrition during teenage pregnancy. *Pediatric Annals*, **22**, 99–108.

Hampl, J.S. and Betts, N.M. (1999) Cigarette use during adolescence: effects on nutritional status. *Nutrition Reviews*, **57**, 215–221.

Herzog, D.B., Franko, D.L., Dorer, D.J. *et al.* (2006) Drug abuse in women with eating disorders. *International Journal of Eating Disorders*, **39**, 364–368.

Hill, A.J. (2002) Developmental issues in attitudes to food and diet. *Proceedings of the Nutrition Society*, **61**, 259–266.

Hill, A.J. (2006) Motivation for eating behaviour in adolescent girls: the body beautiful. *Proceedings of the Nutrition Society*, **65**, 376–384.

Hinney, A. and Volckmar, A.L. (2013) Genetics of eating disorders. *Current Psychiatry Reports*, **15**, 423.

Hoek, H.W. and van Hoeken, D. (2003) Review of the prevalence and incidence of eating disorders. *International Journal of Eating Disorders*, **34**, 383–396.

Hunt, J.R. (2003) Bioavailability of iron, zinc, and other trace minerals from vegetarian diets. *American Journal of Clinical Nutrition*, **78**, 633S–639S.

Jensen, E.X., Fusch, C., Jaeger, P. *et al.* (1995) Impact of chronic cigarette smoking on body composition and fuel metabolism. *Journal of Clinical Endocrinology and Metabolism*, **80**, 2181–2185.

Iannotti, L.L., O'Brien, K.O., Chang, S.C. *et al.* (2005) Iron deficiency anemia and depleted body iron reserves are prevalent among pregnant African-American adolescents. *Journal of Nutrition*, **135**, 2572–2577.

Idris, A.I. and Ralston, S.H. (2012) Role of cannabinoids in the regulation of bone remodeling. *Frontiers in Endocrinology*, **16**, 136.

Isomaa, R., Isomaa, A.L., Marttunen, M. *et al.* (2010) Psychological distress and risk for eating disorders in subgroups of dieters. *European Eating Disorders Review*, **18**, 296–303.

Jones, I.E., Williams, S.M. and Goulding, A. (2004) Associations of birth weight and length, childhood size, and smoking with bone fractures during growth: evidence from a birth cohort study. *American Journal of Epidemiology*, **159**, 343–350.

Kannus, P., Haapasalo, H., Sankelo, M. *et al.* (1995) Effect of starting age of physical activity on bone mass in the dominant arm of tennis and squash players. *Annals of Internal Medicine*, **123**, 27–31.

Kerr, M.A., Rennie, K.L., McCaffrey, T.A. *et al.* (2009) Snacking patterns among adolescents: a comparison of type, frequency and portion size between Britain in 1997 and Northern Ireland in 2005. *British Journal of Nutrition*, **101**, 122–131.

Klump, K.L. and Gobrogge, K.L. (2005) A review and primer of molecular genetic studies of anorexia nervosa. *International Journal of Eating Disorders*, **37**, S43–S48.

Knight, E.M., James, H., Edwards, C.H. *et al.* (1994) Relationships of serum illicit drug concentrations during pregnancy to maternal nutritional status. *Journal of Nutrition*, **124**, 973S–980S.

Korkor, A.B., Eastwood, D. and Bretzmann, C. (2009) Effects of gender, alcohol, smoking, and dairy consumption on bone mass in Wisconsin adolescents. *Wisconsin Medical Journal*, **108**, 181–188.

Laddu, D.R., Farr, J.N., Laudermilk, M.J. *et al.* (2013) Longitudinal relationships between whole body and central adiposity on weight-bearing bone geometry, density, and bone strength: a pQCT study in young girls. *Archives of Osteoporosis*, **8**, 156.

Lambert, H.L., Eastell, R., Karnik, K. *et al.* (2008) Calcium supplementation and bone mineral accretion in adolescent girls: an 18-mo randomized controlled trial with 2-y follow-up. *American Journal Clinical Nutrition*, **87**, 455–462.

Langley-Evans, S.C. and Langley-Evans, A.J. (2002) Use of folic acid supplements in the first trimester of pregnancy. *Journal of the Royal Society of Health*, **122**, 181–186.

Lawrie, Z., Sullivan, E.A., Davies, P.S. *et al.* (2007) Body change strategies in children: relationship to age and gender. *Eating Behaviour*, **8**, 357–363.

Laxer, R.E. and Janssen, I. (2014) The proportion of excessive fast-food consumption attributable to the neighbourhood food environment among youth living within 1 km of their school. *Applied Physiology Nutrition and Metabolism*, **39**, 480–486.

Lillico, H.G., Hammond, D., Manske, S. *et al.* (2014) The prevalence of eating behaviors among Canadian youth using cross-sectional school-based surveys. *BMC Public Health*, **14**, 323.

Livingston, M. (2014) Trends in non-drinking among Australian adolescents. *Addiction*, **109**, 922–929.

Lorentzon, M., Mellström, D., Haug, E. *et al.* (2007) Smoking is associated with lower bone mineral density and reduced cortical thickness in young men. *Journal of Clinical Endocrinology and Metabolism*, **92**, 497–503.

Mackerras, D. and Rutishauser, I. (2005) 24-Hour national dietary survey data: how do we interpret them most effectively? *Public Health Nutrition*, **8**, 657–665.

Martins, Y., Pliner, P. and O'Connor, R. (1999) Restrained eating among vegetarians: does a vegetarian eating style mask concerns about weight? *Appetite*, **32**, 145–154.

McArdle, P. (2008) Use and misuse of drugs and alcohol in adolescence. *British Medical Journal*, **337**, a306.

Milos, G., Gallo, L.M., Sosic, B. *et al.* (2011) Bone mineral density in young women on methadone substitution. *Calcified Tissue International*, **89**, 228–233.

Mishra, V., Thapa, S., Retherford, R.D. *et al.* (2005) Effect of iron supplementation during pregnancy on birthweight: evidence from Zimbabwe. *Food and Nutrition Bulletin*, **26**, 338–347.

Misra, M. (2008) Bone density in the adolescent athlete. *Reviews in Endocrine and Metabolic Disorders*, **9**, 139–144.

Moran, V.H. (2007) Nutritional status in pregnant adolescents: a systematic review of biochemical markers. *Maternal and Child Nutrition*, **3**, 74–93.

Mosca, L.N., da Silva, V.N. and Goldberg, T.B. (2013) Does excess weight interfere with bone mass accumulation during adolescence? *Nutrients*, **5**, 2047–2061.

Müller, K., Libuda, L., Diethelm, K. *et al.* (2013) Lunch at school, at home or elsewhere. Where do adolescents usually get it and what do they eat? Results of the HELENA Study. *Appetite*, **71**, 332–339.

Neumark-Sztainer, D. and Hannan, P.J. (2000) Weight-related behaviors among adolescent girls and boys: results from a national survey. *Archives of Pediatric and Adolescent Medicine*, **154**, 569–577.

Neumark-Sztainer, D., Story, M., Perry, C. *et al.* (1999) Factors influencing food choices of adolescents: findings from focus-group discussions with adolescents. *Journal of the American Dietetic Association*, **99**, 929–937.

Neumark-Sztainer, D., Wall, M., Guo, J. *et al.* (2006) Obesity, disordered eating, and eating disorders in a longitudinal study of adolescents: how do dieters fare 5 years later? *Journal of the American Dietetic Association*, **106**, 559–568.

O'Dea, J.A. (2003) Why do kids eat healthful food? Perceived benefits of and barriers to healthful eating and physical activity among children and adolescents. *Journal of the American Dietetic Association*, **103**, 497–501.

Olmedilla, B. and Granado, F. (2000) Growth and micronutrient needs of adolescents. *European Journal of Clinical Nutrition*, **54** (Suppl. 1), S11–S15.

Ong, T., Sahota, O., Tan, W. *et al.* (2014) A United Kingdom perspective on the relationship between body mass index (BMI) and bone health: a cross sectional analysis of data from the Nottingham Fracture Liaison Service. *Bone*, **59**, 207–210.

Paeratakul, S., Ferdinand, D.P., Champagne, C.M. *et al.* (2003) Fast-food consumption among US adults and children: dietary and nutrient intake profile. *Journal of the American Dietetic Association*, **103**, 1332–1338.

Patterson, R., Risby, A. and Chan, M.Y. (2012) Consumption of takeaway and fast food in a deprived inner London Borough: are they associated with childhood obesity? *BMJ Open*, **2**, e000402.

Perotti, M., Perra, S., Saluzzi, A. *et al.* (2013) Body fat mass is a strong and negative predictor of peak stimulated growth hormone and bone mineral density in healthy adolescents during transition period. *Hormone and Metabolic Research*, **45**, 748–753.

Petrie, H.J., Stover, E.A. and Horswill, C.A. (2004) Nutritional concerns for the child and adolescent competitor. *Nutrition*, **20**, 620–631.

Pisetsky, E.M., Chao, Y.M., Dierker, L.C. *et al.* (2008) Disordered eating and substance use in high-school students: results from the Youth Risk Behavior Surveillance System. *International Journal of Eating Disorders*, **41**, 464–470.

Potter, B.K., Pederson, L.L., Chan, S.S. *et al.* (2004) Does a relationship exist between body weight, concerns about weight, and smoking among adolescents? An integration of the literature with an emphasis on gender. *Nicotine and Tobacco Research*, **6**, 397–425.

Prentice, A., Ginty, F., Stear, S.J. *et al.* (2005) Calcium supplementation increases stature and bone mineral mass of 16- to 18-year-old boys. *Journal of Clinical Endocrinology and Metabolism*, **90**, 3153–3161.

Quick, V., Nansel, T.R., Liu, D. *et al.* (2014) Body size perception and weight control in youth: 9-year international trends from 24 countries. *International Journal of Obesity*, **38**, 988–994.

Ribot, C., Trémollières, F. and Pouillès, J.M. (1994) The effect of obesity on postmenopausal bone loss and the risk of osteoporosis. *Advances in Nutrition Research*, **9**, 257–271.

Robinson-O'Brien, R., Perry, C.L., Wall, M.M. *et al.* (2009) Adolescent and young adult vegetarianism: better dietary intake and weight outcomes but increased risk of disordered eating behaviors. *Journal of the American Dietetic Association*, **109**, 648–655.

Rodondi, N., Pletcher, M.J., Liu, K. *et al.* (2006) Coronary artery risk development in young adults (CARDIA) study. Marijuana use, diet, body mass index, and cardiovascular risk factors (from the CARDIA study). *American Journal of Cardiology*, **98**, 478–484.

Roemmich, J.N., Richmond, R.J. and Rogol, A.D. (2001) Consequences of sport training during puberty. *Journal of Endocrinological Investigation*, **24**, 708–715.

Savige, G., Macfarlane, A., Ball, K. *et al.* (2007) Snacking behaviours of adolescents and their association with skipping meals. *International Journal of Behavioural Nutrition and Physical Activity*, **4**, 36.

Sebastian, R.S., Cleveland, L.E. and Goldman, J.D. (2008) Effect of snacking frequency on adolescents' dietary intakes and meeting national recommendations. *Journal of Adolescent Health*, **42**, 503–511.

Shaw, M.E. (1998) Adolescent breakfast skipping: an Australian study. *Adolescence*, **33**, 851–861.

Specker, B.L. (2006) Influence of rapid growth on skeletal adaptation to exercise. *Journal of Musculoskeletal and Neuronal Interactions*, **6**, 147–153.

Stear, S.J., Prentice, A., Jones, S.C. *et al.* (2003) Effect of a calcium and exercise intervention on the bone mineral status of 16–18-y-old adolescent girls. *American Journal of Clinical Nutrition*, **77**, 985–992.

Story, M., Holt, K. and Softka, A. (2002) *Bright Futures in Practice: Nutrition*, National Center for Education in Maternal and Child Health, Arlington, VA.

Tanner, J.M. (1989) *Foetus into Man*, Castlemead Publications, Ware.

Tappia, P.S., Troughton, K.L., Langley-Evans, S.C. *et al.* (1995) Cigarette smoking influences cytokine production and antioxidant defences. *Clinical Science*, **88**, 485–489.

Thane, C.W., Bates, C.J. and Prentice, A. (2003) Risk factors for low iron intake and poor iron status in a national sample of British young people aged 4–18 years. *Public Health Nutrition*, **6**, 485–496.

Thein-Nissenbaum, J. (2013) Long term consequences of the female athlete triad. *Maturitas*, **75**, 107–112.

Välimäki, M.J., Kärkkäinen, M., Lamberg-Allardt, C. *et al.* (1994) Exercise, smoking, and calcium intake during adolescence and early adulthood as determinants of peak bone mass. Cardiovascular Risk in Young Finns Study Group. *British Medical Journal*, **309**, 230–235.

van den Berg, P., Neumark-Sztainer, D., Hannan, P.J. *et al.* (2007) Is dieting advice from magazines helpful or harmful? Five-year associations with weight-control behaviors and psychological outcomes in adolescents. *Pediatrics*, **119**, e30–e37.

van Den Bulck, J. and Eggermont, S. (2006) Media use as a reason for meal skipping and fast eating in secondary school children. *Journal of Human Nutrition and Dietetics*, **19**, 91–100.

Vandewalle, S., Taes, Y., Fiers, T. *et al.* (2014) Sex steroids in relation to sexual and skeletal maturation in obese male adolescents. *Journal of Clinical Endocrinology and Metabolism*, **99**, 2977–2985.

Wallace, J.M., Luther, J.S., Milne, J.S. *et al.* (2006) Nutritional modulation of adolescent pregnancy outcome – a review. *Placenta*, **27**, S61–S68.

Weaver, C.M., Proulx, W.R. and Heaney, R. (1999) Choices for achieving adequate dietary calcium with a vegetarian diet. *American Journal of Clinical Nutrition*, **70**, 543S–548S.

Welten, D.C., Kemper, H.C., Post, G.B. *et al.* (1994) Weight-bearing activity during youth is a more important factor for peak bone mass than calcium intake. *Journal of Bone and Mineral Research*, **9**, 1089–1096.

White, A.M. and Swartzwelder, H.S. (2005) Age-related effects of alcohol on memory and memory-related brain function in adolescents and adults. *Recent Developments in Alcohol*, **17**, 161–176.

Wong, P.K., Christie, J.J. and Wark, J.D. (2007) The effects of smoking on bone health. *Clinical Science*, **113**, 233–241.

World Health Organization (WHO) (2012) *Adolescent Pregnancy*. http://www.who.int/mediacentre/factsheets/fs364/en/ (accessed June 2014).

Worsley, A. and Skrzypiec, G. (1998) Teenage vegetarianism: prevalence, social and cognitive contexts. *Appetite*, **30**, 151–170.

Wosje, K.S. and Kalkwarf, H.J. (2007) Bone density in relation to alcohol intake among men and women in the United States. *Osteoporosis International*, **18**, 391–400.

Yin, J., Zhang, Q., Liu, A. *et al.* (2010) Calcium supplementation for 2 years improves bone mineral accretion and lean body mass in Chinese adolescents. *Asia Pacific Journal of Clinical Nutrition*, **19**, 152–160.

Additional reading

If you would like to find out more about the material discussed in this chapter, the following sources may be of interest:

Jaffa, T. and McDermott, B. (eds) (2006) *Eating Disorders in Children and Adolescents*, Cambridge University Press, Cambridge/New York.

More, J. (ed) (2013) *Infant, Child and Adolescent Nutrition. A Practical Handbook*, Taylor and Francis Ltd, Boca Raton.

CHAPTER 8
The adult years

LEARNING OBJECTIVES

This chapter will enable the reader to:
- Show an awareness of the need to adjust diet and lifestyle during the adult years in order to promote maintenance of a healthy weight and avoid major disease states including cardiovascular disease, cancer and type 2 diabetes
- Describe some of the different approaches taken by governments to promote healthy diet and lifestyle in populations
- Describe the global trends in the prevalence of overweight and obesity
- Demonstrate an understanding of the relationship between obesity, insulin resistance and risk of cardiovascular disease and diabetes
- Describe optimal strategies for the management and treatment of obesity and related disorders
- Discuss the diet-related risk factors for cardiovascular disease, including the classical risk factors (e.g. high-sodium and high-fat diets) and emerging risk factors (e.g. hyperhomocysteinaemia)
- Critically review different approaches to nutritional epidemiology, showing an understanding of the limitations of observational and intervention studies
- Describe the relationship between diet and cancer, showing an awareness of the elements of human diets that may drive the processes of carcinogenesis and metastasis, and the factors that may play a role in cancer prevention

8.1 Introduction

All of the preceding chapters in this book have considered the relationships between diet and health during periods of major physiological change. Demanding life stages and processes, such as development, growth, maturation and reproduction, all increase requirements for nutrients. Failure to deliver those nutrient demands can result in rapid onset of potentially disastrous outcomes for the individual or may set in place an increased risk of disease later in life. In contrast to this, the adult years from 19 to 65 are therefore relatively 'quiet' from a nutritional perspective, but do represent the stage of life at which most of the adverse consequences of poor nutrition and acquisition of unhealthy lifestyle behaviours at earlier life stages begin to manifest as major disease states. The main focus of this chapter will be on these nutrition-related diseases of adulthood and how diet and lifestyle change might offset risk of ill health and mortality.

8.2 Changing needs for nutrients

With the completion of growth at the end of the adolescent years, adult physiology becomes stable, with no further changes of a major nature until the degenerative processes associated with ageing begin to impact on organ functions (see Chapter 9). The peak of performance for most systems is achieved at around the age of 30 years, but with demand for most nutrients simply meeting the need for maintenance of function and repair processes, there is little variation in the need for nutrients across the earlier adult years. As there is no longer a demand associated with growth and maturation, requirements for most nutrients are lower in adulthood than were seen in adolescence.

Beyond the change in demands associated with attainment of mature physique, protein and micronutrient requirements are unchanging across the earlier adult years. The requirements for protein are stable at 0.8 g/day/kg protein, and the requirements for vitamins

Nutrition, Health and Disease: A Lifespan Approach, Second Edition. Simon Langley-Evans.
© 2015 John Wiley & Sons, Ltd. Published 2015 by John Wiley & Sons, Ltd.
Companion website: www.wiley.com/go/langleyevans/lifespan

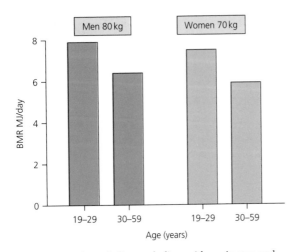

Figure 8.1 Basal metabolic rate declines with age in men and women. Data show basal metabolic rate (BMR) estimates for men and women of average weight, derived from the Schofield equations: Males aged 18–29 years:
BMR = 0.063 × body weight + 2.869.
Males aged 30–59 years: BMR = 0.048 × body weight + 3.653.
Females aged 18–29 years: BMR = 0.062 × body weight + 2.036.
Females aged 30–59 years: BMR = 0.034 × body weight + 3.538.

and minerals are essentially similar at age 19 and age 60. However, this lack of change in demands masks the major change that is required in terms of the quality of diet across this time span. With ageing comes a need for the diet to become more nutrient dense (i.e. for the concentration of protein and micronutrients per unit of energy to increase). This reflects a downward shift in energy requirements with ageing.

Energy requirements of adults are lower than those of adolescents partly due to the loss of requirement for growth, but mainly due to typically lower levels of expenditure through physical activity. Actual energy requirements of individual adults will vary widely with gender, activity level, state of health and body size, all contributing to this variation. For most adults, engaged in sedentary occupations, energy requirements will fall not only relative to the adolescent years, but across the middle years of adulthood also. This is due to a decline in the resting metabolic rate (Figure 8.1).

Making adjustments to this protracted change in nutrient requirements can often be problematic, and overnutrition leading to overweight and obesity is commonplace among adults in Westernized and, increasingly, the developing countries. Most of the major disease states – diabetes, cardiovascular disease (CVD) and cancer – which are reviewed later in this chapter are the consequence of this overnutrition. However, it is important to bear in mind that the undernutrition described earlier in this book in relation to children

remains a significant problem among adult populations. Adult undernutrition will be observed in developing countries and in the developed countries of the world among particular subgroups in the population. Those at risk of malnutrition include the homeless, alcoholics, intravenous drug users, institutionalized individuals, the chronically ill, the elderly (see Chapter 9) and those infected with HIV. Whereas in children malnutrition rapidly becomes a life-threatening factor, among adults undernutrition in these circumstances will generally be present over a longer term. Malnutrition in adults reduces the capacity to do physical work, which in many countries will impact on the ability to provide food and care for whole families. Undernutrition will also reduce the capacity of individuals to respond to metabolic trauma, triggered by infection, injury or surgery. Ultimately, the undernourished adult is as much at risk of premature death as the overweight or obese adult.

8.3 Guidelines for healthy nutrition

Decades of research that has considered the relationships between diet and disease have left no doubt that defining the optimal diet for a population is a complex process and that communicating dietary advice clearly to the population is a major challenge. Individuals respond metabolically to variation in the composition of the diet in different ways, and this variation will depend upon often poorly understood genetic factors, early life programming influences and lifestyle factors. However, it is clear that in general terms a healthier diet should be a varied diet in which carbohydrate provides the basic staple, with energy intakes from fat and protein providing lesser components of intake (Table 8.1). In most circumstances, healthy adults are advised to base meals on starchy foods, to consume five portions of fruit and vegetables per day, to consume two portions of fish per week (including one of oily fish) and to have low intakes of fats and sugars. Food intakes should be well spaced throughout the day, and breakfast remains an essential meal of the day, as in childhood.

Engagement of the public with healthy eating messages is variable and understanding is often poor. To a large extent, this results from the way in which the media portrays nutritional science. The reporting of studies of nutrition, health and disease is often overly simplistic and selective and fails to cover the limitations of studies. Reporting rarely describes an overview of a large body of evidence and instead represents single, isolated studies. Mixed messages and inappropriate reporting can induce scepticism and resentment, leading to rejection of

Table 8.1 General guidelines for intake of sugars, fats and salt by adults.

Nutrient	Maximum recommended intake*
Fats	
Saturated fatty acids	10% of daily energy
Polyunsaturated fatty acids	10% of daily energy
Monounsaturated fatty acids	12% of daily energy
Total fats	35% of daily energy
Sugars	
Milk sugars and starch	39% of daily energy
Non-milk extrinsic sugars	11% of daily energy[†]
Total carbohydrate	50% of daily energy
Salt	6 g/day

Data Source: Department of Health (1999). Reproduced with permission of Crown copyright.
*Also referred to as population averages.
[†]Also referred to as free sugars. Changes in recommendations are expected following expert review and consultation in 2014.

established healthy eating guidelines by the public. For example, a report by Oyebode *et al.* (2014) demonstrating that consumption of seven or more portions of fruit and vegetables per day reduced all-cause mortality in the Health Survey for England prompted media reporting that existing guidelines should change and tabloid pronouncements about 'food police' and unreasonable demands for dietary change. However, the original paper had done no more than confirm well-established observations. Similarly, reporting of a meta-analysis on fats and CVD (Chowdhury *et al.*, 2014) that concluded that there was little evidence to back up current advice to replace saturated fats with polyunsaturated fats prompted a media outcry about the merits of butter and further public misunderstanding of science. The media highlights disagreement and controversy, and as a result, the public struggle to understand how scientific evidence accumulates slowly and that the overall balance of data is more important than single studies. UK reporting of a call from Action on Sugar for aggressive action to reduce sugar consumption in 2014 (Action on Sugar 2014) suggested to the public that single nutrients or classes of nutrients were drivers of disease, which, as will be described later in this chapter, is a viewpoint that most nutritional scientists now reject. This view was reinforced by reports that the World Health Organization (WHO) had changed their stance on sugar, calling for a reduction of intake to 5% of energy intake. This was, in fact, untrue as the WHO guidance is still that non-milk extrinsic (free) sugar intake should be less than 10% of daily energy (World Health Organization, 2014).

Despite these contradictions in the media and associated confusion among consumers, highly successful health promotion campaigns across the Westernized countries, such as the five-a-day campaign (National Health Service, 2007), mean that many general messages about healthy nutrition are now widely recognized, but are not necessarily fully understood. Communicating information such as that shown in Table 8.1 to the population presents a sizeable problem. Concepts such as percentage of daily energy intake are complex and mean nothing within the context of individuals' daily dietary choices. Even with successful campaigns such as five-a-day, understanding of the detail behind the generalized message is often weak. The need to consume five portions of fruit and vegetables per day is simple to remember, but defining a 'portion' (actually 80 g of fresh, frozen, canned or dried fruit, vegetables, salad, fruit juice) is beyond most people. As a result, most governments in the Westernized nations have sought to develop simple pictorial models to act as a guide to healthy adults, showing what comprises a healthy and well-balanced diet. In the United Kingdom, the Balance of Good Health plate model was introduced in the mid-1990s for this purpose (Health Education Authority, 1995). The Food Standards Agency redesigned this model in 2007, producing the new Eatwell plate (Figure 8.2).

The Eatwell model works on a principle that is common to similar models that are used in other countries, for example, the US Food Pyramid (USDA, 2005). Foods are divided into food groups. Within the Eatwell model, there are fruits and vegetables, breads, cereals and potatoes, milk and dairy, meat, fish and alternatives and foods containing fat and sugar. The sectors on the plate (Figure 8.2) are supposed to reflect the relative amount of food intake that should come from each group; hence, breads, cereals and potatoes, fruits and vegetables should provide approximately two-thirds of intake. There are variations on this model (e.g. Japanese Spinning Top Food Guide, Swedish Food Circle), and within the US Food Pyramid, for example, fruits and vegetables are in their own separate food groups, and it is suggested that intakes of foods from the breads, cereals, pasta and rice group outweigh intakes of the fruit and vegetable groups. The Swedish Food Circle is similar in design to the Eatwell plate but crucially lacks the foods containing fat and sugar food group (hence discouraging their intake altogether) and separates vegetables into 'root vegetables' (starchy roots such as carrots and potatoes) and 'essential vegetables' (green leafy vegetables that are important micronutrient sources). The US Food Pyramid was first introduced in 1992 and was widely taken up by other countries in Europe, Australasia, Africa and Asia. An updated version of the pyramid model, MyPyramid,

The eatwell plate

Use the eatwell plate to help you get the balance right. It shows how much of what you eat should come from each food group

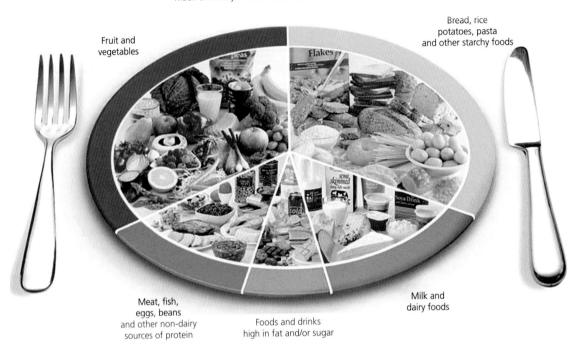

Figure 8.2 The Eatwell plate. This pictorial representation of the relative proportions of foods from each of five groups that should be included in a healthy diet is used as one of the key aids in health education in the United Kingdom. *Data Source*: Public Health England.

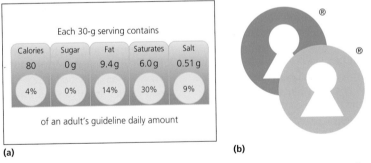

(a)   (b)

Figure 8.3 Symbols used in food labelling. **a)** A guideline daily amount (GDA)-based food label. GDAs on food labels represent the average requirements of an adult woman. Presenting front-of-pack GDA information on energy, sugar, fats and salt is intended to enable consumers to make healthy choices. **b)** The Swedish National Food Administration Keyhole symbol. Only foods that are low in fat, sugar and salt can carry this logo, which allows consumers to identify the foods that comprise a healthy diet, both in shops and when eating out.

was introduced in the United States in 2005 to reflect some of the factors, including age, weight and ethnicity, that shape nutrient demands. This provides a more personalized format for nutrition advice but requires positive engagement with users who should ideally input data to the MyPyramid web pages.

This latter point emphasizes the major problem with all such pictorial guidance schemes, as they can educate but are of little practical use to individuals in daily life. When confronted with the infinite variety of food products in supermarkets, individuals either forget or become confused by healthy eating messages. This has prompted many countries to promote improved food labelling schemes that provide clear and simple nutritional messages at the point of sale. In the United Kingdom, attempts to introduce a food traffic light scheme in which foodstuffs would bear a label showing content of fat, saturated fat, sugar and salt highlighted as red for high, amber for medium and green for low have largely failed due to lack of commitment from supermarkets. It is now common practice for foods to be labelled with the less informative 'guideline daily amounts' (Figure 8.3). Consumers in Norway, Sweden and Denmark have a simplified guide to healthy options when buying food in shops or eating out. The Livsmedelsverket Keyhole (Figure 8.3) symbol is a voluntary label, and food producers take responsibility for ensuring that foods bearing the symbol conform to regulations and are low in fat, sugar and salt and high in dietary fibre.

8.4 Disease states associated with unhealthy nutrition and lifestyle

8.4.1 Obesity

8.4.1.1 Classification of overweight and obesity

Obesity is normally defined on the basis of body mass index (BMI) as shown in Table 8.2. This anthropometric measurement based on height and weight is actually a poor indicator of body fatness, so its usefulness in studying or managing obesity (which is essentially the presence of excess body fat) has been questioned. BMI cannot discriminate between lean tissue mass and fat mass and so will often misclassify individuals who are particularly muscular. However, for most clinical purposes and for epidemiological studies at the population level, BMI is a measurement that is fit for purpose. The BMI classifications shown in Table 8.2 are a generalization, and many obesity researchers argue that specific cut-offs should be used for different ethnic groups and should be age specific. South Asians, for example, have more body fat than Caucasians at any given level of BMI, when this is measured using robust methods such as computed tomography. A BMI of 27.0 may therefore be a more appropriate cut-off to define obesity in this ethnic group (Weisell, 2002).

Fat is distributed in different regions of the body and will be found in a subcutaneous layer, in depots with the abdomen and in depots around organs such as the heart and kidneys and present within tissues such as the liver and skeletal muscle. The fat stored in

Table 8.2 Classifying obesity using body mass index or waist circumference.

	Body mass index (kg/m²)	
Underweight	<18.5	
Desirable weight	18.5–24.9	
Overweight	25.0–29.9	
Obese	>30.0	
	Waist circumference (cm)	
	Men	**Women**
Action level* 1	94	80
Action level 2	102	88

Data Source: Lean *et al.* (1995).
*Action levels 1 and 2 correspond to overweight and obese classifications and indicate the waist circumferences at which action to reduce weight would be beneficial to health.

locations other than subcutaneously is termed visceral fat. The patterns of fat deposition within an individual may be critical determinants of their disease risk (see Sections 8.4.4.3.1 and 8.4.5.4.1) and will vary between the sexes. Males typically store fat in an *android* pattern, where most visceral fat accumulates in the abdomen. Women store fat in a *gynoid* pattern, with the buttocks and hips providing the main depots. In obesity, however, women will tend to adopt an android shape, as fat is stored centrally.

BMI cannot determine the patterns of fat distribution within the body, so other anthropometric tools are necessary. Historically, the waist–hip ratio, which simply required measurements of the circumference of the body around the waist and the hips, was viewed as a measure of abdominal fat deposition. Lean *et al.* (1995), however, suggested that waist circumference alone serves as a robust marker of central obesity, and this measure is now widely accepted (Table 8.2).

8.4.1.2 Prevalence and trends in obesity

The rise in the prevalence of obesity across the globe is well documented and widely reported. In most countries of the world, the proportion of obese adults increased by 40–50% between the mid-1990s and the first few years of the twenty-first century. In Westernized countries, this increase in prevalence coincided with a decrease in overall energy intake, which strongly suggests that the rising trend was related to sedentary lifestyle.

The WHO (2013a) estimates that globally there are 1.4 billion overweight and 500 million obese adults over the age of 20, representing 35% and 11% of world population, respectively. As increasing economic prosperity brings about changes in diet and lifestyle in the

Table 8.3 Global distribution of obesity in adults.

Region	Obesity in men	Obesity in women
Europe	Greece, 27.9%	Scotland, 28.8%
	Scotland, 26.6%	England, 26.1%
	Cyprus, 26.6%	Turkey, 29.4%
Eastern	Kuwait, 36%	Kuwait, 48%
Mediterranean	Qatar, 35%	Qatar, 45%
	Saudi Arabia, 26%	Saudi Arabia, 44%
North America	United States, 35%	United States, 33%
	Canada, 28%	Mexico, 35%
	Mexico, 24%	Barbados, 31%
South and Central	Panama, 28%	Panama, 36%
America	Venezuela, 25%	Paraguay, 36%
Africa	Seychelles, 14.7%	Seychelles, 34.2%
	Algeria, 8.8%	South Africa, 27.4%
	South Africa, 8.8%	Lesotho, 23.2%
Southeast Asia	Nauru, 56%	Tonga, 56%
Pacific	Tonga, 47%	Samoa, 63%
	Cook Islands, 41%	Nauru, 61%

Data from World Obesity Federation (2012).
The table shows the countries within each region with the highest prevalence of obesity, with prevalence figures for the period 2001–2006.

developing countries, overweight and obesity have become a greater driver of disease and mortality than underweight. Among the 27 countries of the European Union, it is estimated that 60% of adults are overweight or obese. Table 8.3 shows data from the World Obesity Federation (2012), which highlights the countries with the greatest adult obesity problems, in different regions of the world.

The United Kingdom and the United States are among the most closely studied countries with regard to increasing obesity prevalence in both adults and children. In England (Health and Social Care Information Centre, 2014), the prevalence of obesity (BMI >30 kg/m^2) increased from 6% in men and 8% in women in 1980 to 24.4% in men and 25.1% in women by 2012. This represents an overall increase of two- to threefold over 30 years, with most of that increase occurring in the last two decades of the twentieth century. In the United States, similar increases have been noted. Kim *et al.* (2007) reported that among women of childbearing age, the prevalence of obesity rose by 69% between 1993 (13% of women obese) and 2003 (22% of women obese). The NHANES survey 2011–2012 (Ogden *et al.*, 2013) reported that 34.9 of US adults were obese, with the highest prevalence seen in the 40–59 age group (men 39.4%, women 395%). Although no increase from the 2009 to 2010 NHANES study was

observed, prevalence in males was markedly higher than reported by Flegal *et al.* (2002), who found that 28.8% of men and 34.2% of women aged 40–59 were obese.

8.4.1.3 Causes of obesity in adulthood

While some associations between body fatness in childhood and early life experience may explain the development of obesity in adulthood (see earlier chapters), the adult lifestyle is the primary driver of weight gain and body fatness.

The combination of an excessive nutrient intake and a sedentary lifestyle promotes positive energy balance and adiposity. Positive energy balance will also be driven by genetic factors, and polymorphisms in genes that contribute to the regulation of appetite, energy metabolism and adipokine release may well predispose individuals to obesity. However, single locus mutations that contribute to obesity are extremely rare, and most obesity-promoting genotypes are dependent on lifestyle factors to be fully expressed.

The rising prevalence of obesity across the globe over the last decades of the twentieth and first decade of the twenty-first centuries is almost wholly explained by changes in lifestyle over the same period. The availability and consumption of energy increased hugely relative to the 1970s and 1980s, and while intakes of sugars tended to decrease, fat consumption increased markedly (Prentice and Jebb, 1995). Food processing technology generated an infinite variety of inexpensive and attractive products. The low cost of this food contributed to increased portion sizes, and with changing patterns of family life, greater proportions of people chose to consume pre-packaged foods that were energy dense and nutrient poor. The increased use of cars in preference to walking and cycling, even over relatively short distances, contributed to a slump in physical activity and associated energy expenditure. Occupations that involved manual labour and heavy industry were replaced with desk-based jobs, and leisure activities reinforced the sedentary way of living, by becoming focused on television and the Internet.

8.4.1.4 Treatment of obesity

Obesity is associated with significantly greater risk of major illness and premature death due to a variety of causes. Greenberg and colleagues (2007) estimated that BMI greater than 30 kg/m^2 increased risk of death from any cause by 170% in a US population aged between 51 and 70 years. Banegas *et al.* (2003) estimated that in European countries 7.7% of all deaths were related to obesity, of which 70% were CVD deaths and 20% cancer related. The association of obesity with diabetes,

CVD and certain cancers is discussed in greater depth later in this chapter.

Given the importance of obesity and overweight as risk factors for life-threatening disease, the treatment and management of obesity is a major priority. Weight loss can be achieved through a wide variety of different approaches that utilize dietary change, increases in physical activity, pharmacological agents and bariatric surgery. Short-term weight loss carries no real health benefits, and there are some suggestions that weight cycling, in which individuals continually lose and then regain body weight, may actually increase risk of major disease. If the goal for obese individuals in the population is to lose weight for a sustained period, none of the approaches indicated above will be successful in isolation. Sustained weight loss depends upon wholesale lifestyle and behavioural changes that incorporate strategies for reducing energy intake while increasing expenditure through activity.

Dietary approaches to losing weight are legion, and a massive multibillion-pound industry has grown up around the global obesity pandemic. Most, if not all, of the restrictive diet practices that are advocated will be effective in the short term but are unlikely to produce sustained weight loss (Figure 8.4). The more bizarre and difficult it is to follow the commercial/fad diet programmes, the harder the users will find the process. This reduces the likelihood that the new eating pattern will be successfully incorporated into a permanent lifestyle change. The most effective strategies for reducing energy intake will be those that require less willpower to follow. In this respect, reducing energy intake by

limiting snacking (which may contribute in excess of 300 kcal/day to the typical diet) or reducing portion sizes may be a helpful strategy (Jebb, 2005). Reductions of energy intake of approximately 500 kcal/day would be expected to produce weight loss of around 0.25 kg/ week. This slow gradual weight loss is more likely to be successful in the longer term. Intermittent fasting is one approach to reducing energy intake without the problem of sustaining a continual restraint on food intake (Varady, 2011). Typically, this involves 2 days a week of severe caloric restriction (<200 kcal/day) and 5 days of ad libitum intake. In the short term, this brings about weight loss that is equivalent to continuous restriction (Klempel *et al.*, 2012, Kroeger *et al.* 2012), and this loss may be sustained to 1 year (Arguin *et al.*, 2012).

Many weight loss diets have been designed to reduce fat intake, working on the assumption that if obesity is increased body fatness, then consuming less fat will promote weight loss. This is of course overly simplistic, and most studies show that decreasing fat intake has only short-term effects on body weight and that these are almost certainly the result of reducing the energy density of the diet (Jebb, 2005).

There is major interest in diets that limit carbohydrate intake. These have been shown to be as effective as low-fat diets in terms of weight loss but confer more metabolic benefits (Frigolet *et al.*, 2011). The Atkins diet, for example, reduces intake of carbohydrates to just 10–30% of daily energy intake and allows unlimited consumption of protein and fat. Weight loss is supposed to occur as the lower blood sugar resulting from carbohydrate restriction promotes ketosis and lowers insulin concentrations. This is proposed to stimulate lipolysis and inhibit lipogenesis. However, it is far more likely that the greater protein intakes associated with such diets promote satiety and simply reduce overall energy intake. Consumption of high-protein–low-carbohydrate diets results in the body entering a ketogenic state, and the resulting increase in β-hydroxybutyrate concentrations will suppress appetite and increase gluconeogenesis. The latter is proposed to increase energy expenditure (Veldhorst *et al.*, 2009). A high-protein diet will also favour the deposition of fat-free mass over fat mass, where weight regain occurs (Westerterp-Plantenga *et al.*, 2012).

Another approach to modifying the diet is to restrict intake of carbohydrates to those with a lower glycaemic index (GI). GI is a ranking system that rates different carbohydrate sources according to their impact upon blood glucose and insulin concentrations. Simple sugars that are rapidly absorbed, producing a large spike in blood glucose, have high GI, while complex carbohydrates that require greater digestion and release glucose

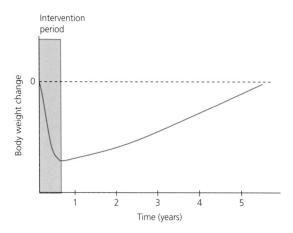

Figure 8.4 Weight loss is often followed by regain. Weight loss interventions generally result in weight loss for their duration in compliant individuals. Weight regain will begin once the intervention is complete, and full regain of lost weight will usually occur within a 5-year period.

into the blood in a slow sustained fashion have low GI. True GI will vary between individuals due to variation in the response to different foodstuffs. Low-GI diets appear to promote weight loss in animal studies, but data from human trials remains controversial. Miller and colleagues (2011) reported that an intervention to increase consumption of low-GI foods resulted in weight loss and a reduction in waist circumference, but this study only considered short-term weight loss and did not have a control group. In contrast, Papadaki *et al.* (2014) found no significant benefits of a low-GI diet upon weight or symptoms of the metabolic syndrome, and Ajala *et al.* (2013) concluded from a meta-analysis that low-GI diets had no significant benefits over other dietary approaches for weight loss in subjects with type 2 diabetes. Although some studies suggest that low-GI diets promote weight loss of 5% or more over a 12-month period, this may occur simply because subjects seeking lower-GI foods consume more fruits and vegetables and less processed, refined foods, which tend to be more energy dense (Jebb, 2005).

Individuals with higher-grade obesity (BMI over $35\,kg/m^2$) may be advised to follow a very-low-calorie diet (VLCD). This type of diet focuses on severely reducing energy intake to approximately $800–1200\,kcal/$ day. This often promotes rapid weight loss of around $1\,kg/week$. However, VLCD is largely ineffective as a tool for achieving longer-term weight loss. Vogels and Westerterp-Plantenga (2007) reported that in a group that followed a VLCD for 6 weeks, achieving an average weight loss of $7.2\,kg$, 87% of the individuals regained the lost weight within 2 years.

Mild-to-moderate exercise such as walking or housework is sufficient to increase energy expenditure, and even with no change in dietary intakes, sedentary individuals taking on such activities in addition to normal activity should experience some weight loss. However, weight loss associated with physical activity alone will be minor, and exercise is most effective when coupled to a change in diet (Shaw *et al.*, 2006). Higher-intensity exercise produces greater improvements in weight profile than mild–moderate activity, but for any individual to succeed, it is important that exercise and weight loss goals are realistic and achievable.

Pharmacological agents are considered appropriate for patients who either cannot or do not lose weight using conventional approaches. They are a suitable adjunct to lifestyle advice and change but should only be used for the short term since all carry some form of undesirable side effects. Typically, anti-obesity drugs have their maximum effect over a period of 7–8 months, beyond which users will tend to start regaining weight unless adequate lifestyle changes have also been implemented.

Orlistat is a widely used anti-obesity drug that works by inhibiting lipase activities and hence reducing the absorption of fat across the gut. On a diet that provides 30% of energy in the form of fat, approximately one-third of the fat will be lost in the faeces (Bray and Ryan, 2007). Orlistat has been shown to promote loss of approximately 7% of body weight in obese individuals over a 2-year period. Similar effects are noted with sibutramine, which is a central inhibitor of serotonin, noradrenaline and dopamine reuptake. This drug inhibits appetite and also promotes energy expenditure by activating thermogenesis. Apfelbaum and colleagues (1999) showed that sibutramine was highly effective alongside VLCD, allowing patients to maintain weight loss associated with their initial dietary change, for at least 1 year. The most recently licensed anti-obesity drug is rimonabant, which is an antagonist of the CB1 cannabinoid receptor. This receptor, which binds the active constituents of marijuana, promotes appetite for sweet and high-fat foods. Rimonabant selectively reduces appetite for these foods and is capable of producing a 9% weight loss in obese patients over a 2-year period (Pi-Sunyer *et al.*, 2006).

Bariatric surgery is an extreme approach to treating obesity and would normally be reserved only for the morbidly obese (BMI over $40\,kg/m^2$). There are a number of different surgical approaches, which include gastric banding or surgery to form a gastric pouch. These interventions promote major weight loss, with maximal effects over the first 12–24 months after surgery (up to 70% of excess weight lost). Although the impact on satiety may be reduced over time as the gastric bands stretch or the pouch capacity increases, studies considering follow-up of patients for 10 years or more suggest that around 60% of excess weight will be permanently lost (Kral and Naslund, 2007). The efficacy of bariatric surgery is described in more detail in Research Highlight 8.1.

8.4.2 Type 2 diabetes

Diabetes mellitus is a condition in which control over blood glucose homeostasis is lost through impairment of either the production of insulin by the pancreas or through impairment of the actions of insulin in the main target tissues (liver, skeletal muscle). Type 1 diabetes mellitus (formerly described as insulin-dependent diabetes) is the result of destruction of the β-cells of the pancreas, leading to either an absence of or low production of insulin. Type 1 diabetes is generally of early onset, and most sufferers will be diagnosed in childhood. Type 2 diabetes mellitus (T2DM, non-insulin-dependent diabetes) is characterized by either blunted insulin production in response to ingestion of carbohydrates or, more commonly, extremely high plasma insulin concentrations

Research Highlight 8.1 The efficacy of bariatric surgery.

The term bariatric surgery collectively describes procedures that are designed to induce major weight loss in morbidly obese individuals. These procedures work either by restricting food intake or limiting absorption of nutrients, or both factors combined. Restrictive surgeries typically reduce stomach size and hence the capacity to ingest food through placement of a gastric band or an intragastric balloon or by removing a portion of the stomach (sleeve gastrectomy). Malabsorption can be induced through techniques such as the duodenal switch, where most of the stomach is removed and the small remnant is joined directly to the ileum, bypassing the jejunum and duodenum. Roux-en-Y bypass surgery limits stomach capacity and induces malabsorption by creating a pouch within the stomach, which empties directly into the ileum.

Bariatric surgery is significantly more effective in affecting weight loss in morbidly obese patients than non-surgical methods. Sjöström *et al.* (2007) reported that over the first 2 years post-surgery, weight loss was between 20% and 32% of initial weight, dependent upon the surgical procedure. This weight loss was largely sustained at 10 years post-surgery (14–23% weight loss from baseline). The meta-analysis of Gloy *et al.* (2013) considered 11 randomized controlled trials of bariatric surgery versus non-surgical approaches and found that mean weight loss with surgery was 26 kg.

There are clear health benefits associated with surgically induced weight loss. Sjöström *et al.* (2007) reported a 24% reduction in 10-year mortality among surgical patients. The meta-analysis of Kwok *et al.* (2014) reported a more marked effect on mortality with a 50% reduction. Lower death rates are associated with remission of diabetes and metabolic syndrome (Gloy *et al.*, 2013), leading to lower risk of myocardial infarction (HR 0.46, 95% CI 0.30–0.69) and stroke (HR 0.49, 95% CI 0.32–0.75; Kwok *et al.*, 2014). There is also evidence that patients who have undergone bariatric surgery are less likely to develop cancer (Sjöström *et al.*, 2009).

Bariatric surgery is not a risk-free procedure, particularly given the general complications of anaesthesia and surgery with morbidly obese subjects. The mortality rate for Roux-en Y bypass surgery is between 0.1% and 0.27% (Benotti *et al.*, 2014; Stroh *et al.*, 2014). Around 5% of patients suffer other complications such as post-operative infection and leakage of the anastomosis (surgical junction of the stomach and small intestine). Complications with sleeve gastrectomy are far more frequent (Stroh *et al.*, 2014). Patients who have undergone bariatric surgery may also develop iron deficiency anaemia and other manifestations of malnutrition (Gloy *et al.*, 2013).

with a blunted response to insulin (insulin resistance; see following text). T2DM generally first appears in the middle years of adulthood.

The simplest diagnostic tools used to identify individuals with T2DM are the presence of symptoms such as thirst and polyuria or the observation of a raised fasting plasma glucose concentration (>126 mg/dl glucose in venous blood). However, the fasting plasma glucose method is less reliable and will tend to underdiagnose T2DM in the population. The oral glucose tolerance test is a more robust method, which should always be used to confirm any provisional diagnosis. In an oral glucose tolerance test, the patient is fasted overnight and then provided with a solution of glucose (usually a 75 g load) to drink. As shown in Figure 8.5, this promotes a rapid increase in blood glucose concentrations. In healthy individuals, this promotes a release of insulin, which drives the excess blood glucose into the liver and skeletal muscle and brings blood glucose back to the baseline concentration within 2 h of loading. Among individuals with glucose intolerance (a prediabetic state), the peak in plasma glucose will tend to be greater than in healthy individuals, and concentrations will remain elevated (>140 mg/dl) after 2 h. In individuals with T2DM, the peak in blood glucose will be over 200 mg/dl and the return to baseline concentrations greatly delayed (Figure 8.5).

The risk of developing T2DM is strongly influenced by genetic factors. Individuals with a sibling with T2DM are

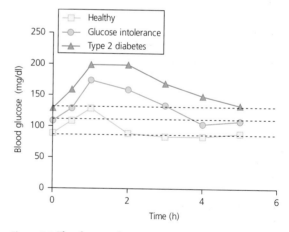

Figure 8.5 The glucose tolerance test. Subjects consume an oral load of 75 g glucose. This promotes a rise in blood glucose concentrations. Blood samples at 2 h into the test can discriminate between healthy subjects (glucose should have returned to the baseline, normal range of below 110 mg/dl), subjects who are glucose intolerant (glucose will remain above 140 mg/dl) and subjects with frank diabetes (glucose will remain above 200 mg/dl).

four times more likely to develop T2DM than individuals with no family history (Rich, 1990). There are some rare forms of T2DM that are attributable to defects of specific genes. These maturity-onset diabetes of the young (MODY) variants of T2DM are associated with defects of hepatocyte nuclear factor 4α (MODY1), glucokinase (MODY2), hepatocyte nuclear factor 1α (MODY3), insulin promoter factor 1 (MODY4), hepatocyte nuclear factor 1β (MODY5) and neurogenic differentiation factor 1 (MODY6). It has proven difficult however to firmly identify genes that drive T2DM risk in the rest of the population, as it is clear that several genes or polymorphisms of genes are likely to play a role and, more importantly, that these genetic influences are modified by environmental factors (McIntyre and Walker, 2002). Candidate genes that may contribute to risk of T2DM include the insulin gene itself, sulphonylurea receptor (SUR)-1, insulin receptor substrate 1 (IRS-1), peroxisome proliferator-activated receptor gamma and glycogen synthase. All of these show polymorphisms in humans that have variants that appear to predispose to T2DM. Obesity is the main diet- and lifestyle-related risk factor for T2DM. Storage of fat in adipose tissue impairs insulin sensitivity in target tissues by promoting the delivery of fat in the form of triacylglycerides to peripheral tissues and by direct production of antagonists of insulin action by the adipocytes (Roche *et al.*, 2005).

The prevalence of T2DM is rapidly increasing all over the world, in line with the increasing levels of obesity and overweight. It is estimated by the WHO that global prevalence will be 45% greater in 2025 than in 1995 (Alberti and Zimmet, 1998), with most of the increase accounted for by soaring prevalence rates in China, India and other developing countries. While much of this increase will be occurring in the adult population, there is growing concern in the Westernized countries that T2DM is increasingly manifesting in childhood and adolescents.

The migration of certain ethnic minorities to Westernized countries has resulted in greater prevalence of T2DM in those migrant populations. As reported by Patel *et al.* (2006), Asian Indians in the United Kingdom exhibit greater prevalence of obesity and T2DM than the Caucasian population of the United Kingdom and considerably higher prevalence than non-migrant Indians. Similar observations are noted in migrant Indians living in South Africa, where the association between migrant status and T2DM is more marked if the migrants retain their traditional diet and lifestyle (Misra and Ganda, 2007). The finding that migration promotes an increase in prevalence rates adds weight to the argument that T2DM risk is strongly associated with a thrifty genotype (Neel, 1962) or thrifty phenotype (Hales and Barker, 2001). Generations of undernutrition and regular famine will either program traits or select for genetic traits that promote the most efficient use of metabolic substrates. On encountering an environment where energy is widely

available, this metabolic thrift will drive development of obesity and associated disorders.

The concept of thrift, whether acquired through programming or through genetic selection, is also supported by studies of the two populations with the highest global prevalence of T2DM. The Pima Indians of Arizona and the Nauruan islanders exhibit T2DM rates of 40–50%, and in both populations, the shift to endemic diabetes was associated with a rapid shift in availability of high-energy foods and adoption of sedentary patterns of work and physical activity. However, the situation with migrant populations may be less clear-cut, as migration brings social inequalities, stress and greater prevalence of unhealthy behaviours such as smoking and alcohol consumption in addition to a nutritional transition (Misra and Ganda, 2007).

T2DM is a major risk factor for CVD (see following text) but is also associated with a range of other complications that arise due to the damaging effects of chronically high blood glucose concentrations upon the vasculature and nerves. Within the eye, glucose causes damage to the vessels that supply the retina (non-proliferative diabetic retinopathy), and this causes leakage of plasma into the retina, blurring vision. In more severe diabetes, abnormal blood vessels develop on the face of the retina (proliferative diabetic retinopathy). This reduces normal blood flow to the tissue and can cause blindness. Within the kidneys, high glucose concentrations cause loss of nephrons, and this can lead to chronic renal failure in diabetic subjects. The legs and feet of diabetic subjects are vulnerable as nerve damage (diabetic neuropathy) numbs sensation and leads to greater risk of physical injury. With lower blood flow to the limbs (a further consequence of diabetes), these injuries are prone to infection and ulceration. Amputation of feet and lower limbs can be a consequence of failure to heal these ulcers successfully.

The treatment and management of T2DM relies upon a mixture of dietary and lifestyle change and medication. Monitoring of blood glucose concentrations by diabetic patients is an essential element of management of the condition, as this allows carbohydrate intakes to be tailored to fluctuations in blood glucose, which may be influenced by the time since the last food consumption or by levels of physical activity. Clinical monitoring is also recommended (NICE, 2008), with regular screening of the glycosylated haemoglobin (HbA1c) concentration providing a good indicator of the quality of glycaemic control (target HbA1c concentration is 6.5–7.5%; Figure 8.6).

Patients with T2DM who are of optimal body weight may be able to maintain good control over blood glucose concentrations through relatively simple management of the carbohydrate content of their diet. In overweight or obese individuals, the priorities will shift so as to couple

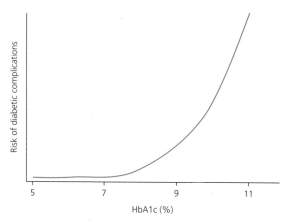

Figure 8.6 HbA1c percentage is a measure of the degree of glycation of haemoglobin and as such serves as a marker for longer-term blood glucose concentration. Relatively small increases in HbA1c are associated with significant increases in risk of cardiovascular disease and nephropathy. Risk of complications increases sharply with values of 7.5% or greater.

weight loss to glycaemic control. There is no 'diabetic diet' as such, and the guidelines given to diabetic patients are broadly in line with the healthy eating guidelines for adults that were outlined earlier in this chapter. T2DM patients are advised to increase intakes of complex carbohydrates and reduce intakes of simple sugars, in effect taking on a low-GI diet. Intakes of dietary fibre should be high, and it is suggested that complex carbohydrates should be consumed with every meal or snack to delay absorption of glucose into the circulation. Meals should be regular and low-fat options should be the mainstay of intake. Special foods aimed at diabetics are not necessary and often have a high-fat content to maintain palatability, so should be avoided. Diabetic patients should be given individualized advice and health education from an appropriate specialist, such as a dietitian, so that a lifestyle change incorporating both diet modification and increased physical activity can be tailored to the individuals' needs (NICE, 2007). Surprisingly, while T2DM is a common condition and dietary change is the main element used in the management of the condition, Nield and colleagues (2007) suggested that there was no high-quality data available to allow assessment of the efficacy of diet in management of T2DM. This is in contrast to other analyses that suggest that low-carbohydrate or low-GI diets can improve glycaemic control and fasting glucose concentrations (Kirk *et al.*, 2008; Ajala *et al.*, 2013). Diabetes UK maintains the position that in addition to weight loss, management of carbohydrate intake is a central element of T2DM management (Dyson *et al.*, 2011).

Where T2DM patients are overweight or obese and have difficulties in maintaining satisfactory glycaemic

control, pharmacological agents are widely used. These include metformin, sulphonylurea derivatives and the glitazones (thiazolidinediones). Metformin increases sensitivity to insulin and also helps to control blood glucose by inhibiting the absorption of glucose across the gut and inhibiting hepatic gluconeogenesis. Sulphonylureas promote uptake of calcium by the pancreas, and this elicits increased secretion of insulin, hence promoting reduction of blood glucose concentrations. Glitazones are agonists of peroxisome proliferator-activated receptor gamma and work by increasing sensitivity to insulin in peripheral tissues. Often, the glitazones are used in combination with metformin.

8.4.3 The metabolic syndrome

The metabolic syndrome, also called the insulin resistance syndrome or syndrome X, is a cluster of metabolic and physiological disturbances that all stem from the occurrence of insulin resistance in an individual. Insulin resistance is the state in which the response to insulin is blunted, and hence, insulin-resistant individuals need to produce more insulin to regulate their blood glucose concentrations. Insulin is a powerful metabolic regulator and has effects in skeletal muscle, the liver, the brain, the kidney and vascular tissues. As a result, insulin resistance will impact upon multiple organ systems, producing a broad spectrum of effects (Figure 8.7). The metabolic syndrome is strongly linked to CVD as most of the functional defects that accompany insulin resistance are all independent risk factors for coronary heart disease (CHD) and stroke (see later sections in this chapter). Lakka and colleagues (2002) estimated that metabolic syndrome increases risk of CVD mortality by threefold.

Insulin resistance can be measured in individuals using a variety of different techniques, but mostly, the homeostasis model assessment – insulin resistance (HOMA-IR) scale is applied. HOMA-IR is determined using the calculation (plasma insulin concentration x plasma glucose concentration)/22.5. An alternative is the quantitative insulin sensitivity check index (QUICKI), which is calculated as 1/(log fasting insulin concentration+log fasting glucose concentration). These results can be used alongside other diagnostic criteria to confirm the presence of the metabolic syndrome. A number of diagnostic definitions are in use, and that used by the WHO is shown in Table 8.4.

The basic actions of insulin are to stimulate glucose uptake by the muscle and liver and to inhibit lipolysis. In insulin-resistant individuals, these functions will be impaired, and hence, blood glucose clearance is reduced and circulating lipid concentrations rise. However, some other functions of insulin are not impaired, and the high circulating insulin concentrations that are associated with insulin resistance will

increase these. For example, insulin promotes eleva-
tions of blood pressure, and this function is not lost in
the insulin-resistant individual.

The origins of metabolic syndrome may vary considerably between individuals. Certainly, obesity promotes

Table 8.4 World Health Organization diagnostic criteria
for the metabolic syndrome.

Criteria	Defined by
Insulin resistance	Measure of resistance in top 25% for population
Impaired glucose tolerance	Raised fasting glucose, impaired glucose tolerance
	Test or type 2 diabetes
Hypertension	Systolic pressure >159, diastolic pressure >89
Central obesity	BMI>30 kg/m². Waist–hip ratio >0.9 in men or 0.8 in women
Raised triglycerides	Serum triglycerides >2.0 mmol/l
Reduced HDL-cholesterol	HDL-cholesterol <1.0 mmol/l
Microalbuminuria	Urinary albumin excretion >30 mg/day

Data Source: Alberti and Zimmet (1998). Reproduced with
permission of Wiley.
Individuals manifesting one of the first two criteria and two of
the remaining criteria should receive a diagnosis of metabolic
syndrome.

insulin resistance, possibly because factors such as
cytokines produced from adipose tissue act as antagonists
of insulin action. Insulin resistance itself will promote
deposition of lipid in adipose tissue, as adipocytes often
retain greater sensitivity to insulin than other tissues.
This promotes storage of energy in the adipose tissue in
preference to the liver or muscle. Obesity should therefore be regarded as both a cause and a consequence of
insulin resistance. Concentrations of hormones such as
cortisol also become elevated in obese individuals, and
these may oppose the actions of insulin. There are a
number of genetic defects that may also contribute to
risk. Loss or impairment of insulin-responsive elements
in a number of different pathways that control lipid or
carbohydrate metabolism would be expected to promote
the development of an insulin-resistant phenotype.

8.4.4 Cardiovascular disease
8.4.4.1 What is CVD?
CVD is a term that collectively describes a number of different conditions, which include CHD, cerebrovascular
disease and peripheral artery disease. All of these conditions stem from the same basic pathology, which is the
development of atherosclerosis within major arteries.

8.4.4.1.1 Atherosclerosis
Atherosclerosis is the process through which deposits of
cholesterol, collagen and calcium accumulate within the
intimal layer of arteries, resulting in the occlusion of the

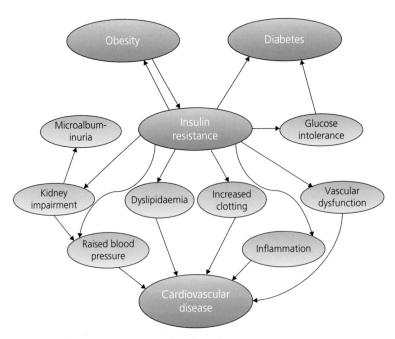

Figure 8.7 Schematic representation of the consequences of insulin resistance.

arterial lumen and a focus for the formation of clots (thrombosis). Atherosclerotic plaques can form in any of the arterial vessels of the body, and each individual may potentially have tens or hundreds of plaques. The main feature of plaques is the accumulated mass of cholesterol-bearing foam cells and vascular smooth muscle cells (VSMC) (see Figure 8.8). Most plaques are stable as they are covered in a fibrous crust. Should this crust split, then the resultant release of collagen and other material will provide the focus for thrombosis, which can trigger potentially fatal consequences.

There are two prerequisites for the initiation of plaque formation. The first requires the accumulation of oxidized low-density lipoprotein (LDL)-cholesterol within the arterial intima. LDL is responsible for the transport of cholesterol away from the liver to deliver it to sites that require it for metabolism, for example, the adrenal glands where it is used to manufacture steroid hormones. Some of this circulating LDL-cholesterol can be deposited in the arterial wall. Cholesterol may be transferred from LDL to high-density lipoprotein (HDL), which carries it back to the liver. However, the conditions within the intimal layer will also tend to favour the oxidation of LDL-cholesterol by reactive oxygen species (ROS). The LDL-cholesterol complex is vulnerable to

ROS attack, despite having antioxidant defences, due to the high polyunsaturated fatty acid (PUFA) density present within the phospholipid shell. Oxidative damage will spread from the lipids to the key apolipoprotein B100, which is required to recognize the LDL receptor on target tissues.

The second key event in atherosclerosis is damage to the endothelial lining of the intima. This is generally due to inflammation, which can be triggered by local injury, infection or raised circulating concentrations of inflammatory cytokines, as is seen in obese individuals. Endothelial inflammation attracts monocytes, a class of undifferentiated white blood cell. Monocytes bind to vascular cell adhesion molecule (VCAM) on the endothelial surface, allowing movement through to the underlying intimal zone. Here, the presence of cytokines associated with endothelial inflammation drives differentiation of the monocytes to macrophages.

Macrophages bear a scavenger receptor that is able to recognize and bind oxidized LDL-cholesterol. Macrophages that have taken up oxidized LDL will remain in the intima and steadily accumulate this oxidized material, eventually becoming foam cells. The first sign of atherosclerosis in blood vessels is the appearance of a yellowish spot, termed a fatty streak. The accumulated foam cells promote the

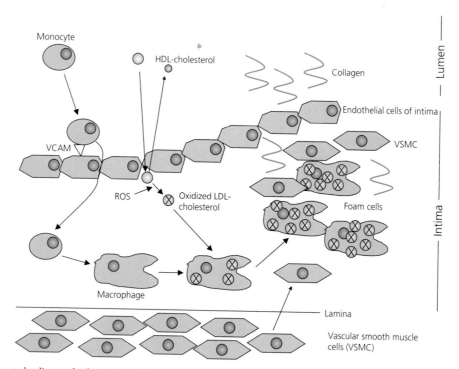

Figure 8.8 Events leading to the formation of the fatty streak and atherosclerotic plaque. ROS, reactive oxygen species; VCAM, vascular cell adhesion molecule.

proliferation of VSMC in the intima, and thus, the plaque becomes established. VSMC secrete collagen into the plaque, providing the associated protein accumulation. Established plaques will also accrue calcium and this causes stiffening of the arteries.

8.4.4.1.2 CHD

CHD is also referred to as ischaemic heart disease. It is the result of atherosclerotic plaque formation within the coronary arteries, which supply the heart muscle with oxygen and nutrients. Formation of plaques will occlude these arteries causing chest pain, termed angina pectoris. The potentially life-threatening aspect of atherosclerosis in the coronary arteries results from thrombosis, causing full occlusion of the vessels. The heart muscle, starved of oxygen, will then begin to die, forming a damaged area called an infarct. In individuals surviving this injury (myocardial infarction (MI)), future heart function will be impaired, and they may suffer from arrhythmias and other cardiac problems.

Although deaths from CHD have generally been in decline in the Westernized countries throughout the 1990s and the early twenty-first century, CHD remains the leading cause of death in the western hemisphere. Alongside this, the disease has increased in prevalence in the developing countries, as they enter economic and nutritional transition. Figure 8.9 shows the prevalence rates for CHD in selected countries and highlights the fact that the disease is most prevalent in countries of the former Soviet Union (e.g. Ukraine and Belarus) and has the lowest prevalence in Southern Europe (e.g. Spain, Portugal, Greece, France). There can be considerable variation within countries. For example, in the United Kingdom, the lowest rates of CHD are seen among men and women in the south and eastern parts of England. CHD rates among the male population of Scotland are at a level 60% above those in southern England. This variation largely reflects regional differences in diet and lifestyle.

8.4.4.1.3 Cerebrovascular disease

Cerebrovascular disease manifests itself when individuals suffer a cerebrovascular accident, or stroke. Strokes occur when the blood supply to the brain is interrupted, which can lead to reversible or irreversible damage. Strokes may be haemorrhagic, in which case blood leaks from vessels into the brain tissue. These strokes are unrelated to atherosclerosis and are the product of raised blood pressure. Ischaemic strokes are caused by blockage of the arterial supply to the brain due to atherosclerosis and thrombosis. Strokes are the second most common cause of death in the United Kingdom and other European countries.

8.4.4.1.4 Peripheral artery disease

Peripheral artery disease stems from the formation of atherosclerotic plaques in arteries other than those supplying the heart or brain. Typically, these problems affect the legs. Often, peripheral artery disease will manifest as pain during exercise, which is termed claudication. In severe cases, these plaques will lead to ischaemic injury to the limbs, resulting in amputation.

8.4.4.1.5 Hypertension

Hypertension, or raised blood pressure, is often included as one of the CVDs. However, raised blood pressure is not truly a disease state and should instead be regarded as a risk factor or clinical indicator for other CVDs. High

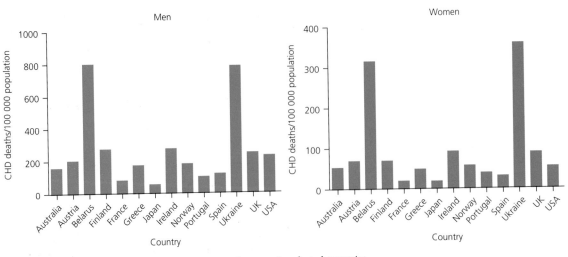

Figure 8.9 Coronary heart disease mortality in men and women in selected countries.

blood pressure is associated with increased risk of both CHD and stroke. In the case of CHD, it may be that atherosclerosis impairs the ability of the major vessels to contract or dilate to maintain normal pressure, but it is also the case that raised pressure causes a form of arterial damage, called shear stress, that can act as the focus for plaque formation. Higher blood pressures will also make atherosclerotic plaques less stable.

8.4.4.2 Risk factors for CVD

The classical risk factors for CVD are generally defined as modifiable or non-modifiable characteristics. Non-modifiable risk factors include age, gender and ethnicity. The strong association of risk with gender can be clearly seen in Figure 8.9, which shows death rates from CHD to be lower in women than men in all countries. Much of the protection associated with female gender disappears after the menopause, and it is suggested that this is due to postmenopausal women adopting an android pattern of abdominal fat deposition. Risks of CHD and stroke both increase with increasing age and this may, at least in part, be explained by rising blood pressure that typically occurs with ageing.

Certain ethnic groups exhibit increased risk of CVD within Westernized nations. Individuals of South Asian descent (i.e. populations from India, Bangladesh and Pakistan) have increased risk of CHD, which appears to be related to a greater propensity to develop abdominal obesity. Patel *et al.* (2006) compared a population of Gujarati migrants in the United Kingdom with a non-migrant Gujarati population in India. The UK population had considerably greater BMI, raised circulating lipids and other CVD risk factors compared to the Indian group. Thus, the combination of a South Asian heritage with a Westernized lifestyle appeared to increase CVD risk. Afro-Caribbean populations are at greater risk of stroke-related death than other ethnic groups, and this appears to be due to a genetic predisposition to hypertension.

Aspects of lifestyle that increase CVD risk are generally considered to be modifiable risk factors. Lower socio-economic status (SES) can be included in this category. Lower SES is an indicator of a number of different factors that include lower income, poor health behaviours such as smoking and a diet of lower quality. Ramsay *et al.* (2007) reported that lower SES in adulthood was a risk factor for CHD in men aged 52–74. Men who had manual occupations were significantly more likely to suffer from fatal or nonfatal CHD and were more likely to be smokers, to be overweight and to be physically inactive, when compared to those in non-manual occupations.

Smoking increases risk of CVD through a number of mechanisms, including increasing concentrations of clotting factors and thereby increasing risk of thrombosis, by promoting endothelial dysfunction and by increasing oxidative stress. Obesity and related disorders, including type 2 diabetes, are major risk factors for CHD and other cardiovascular conditions. Abdominal obesity in particular will increase risk. Factors that contribute to development of obesity, such as physical inactivity, are independently associated with greater risk of CVD. The nutrition-related risk factors for CVD, including obesity, will be described in more detail in the next section.

8.4.4.3 Nutrition-related factors and risk of CVD
8.4.4.3.1 Obesity

The major lifestyle-related risk factors for CVD are cigarette smoking and obesity. At a time when the prevalence of smoking is declining in most Westernized populations, the secular trend for increasing prevalence of obesity is reducing the beneficial impact of smoking reduction (Hu *et al.*, 2000) and is rapidly becoming the main contributor to CHD and stroke-related death. Bender and colleagues (2006) reported that obesity increased risk of CVD death by 2.2-fold in men and 1.6-fold in women (comparing BMI of over $30\,kg/m^2$ to BMI in the ideal range).

Determining the influence of obesity upon CVD risk, independent of all other risk factors, is almost impossible. Obese individuals will also tend to be the individuals who are least physically active and who have raised blood pressure, type 2 diabetes, insulin resistance and dyslipidaemia, all of which are associated with greater risk of atherosclerosis. However, it is clear that all anthropometric measures of overweight and obesity, whether considering BMI, waist–hip ratio or total percentage body fat, determined by bioimpedance, are powerful indicators of increased CVD risk. Abdominal fat deposition is most strongly related to risk, presumably because fat stored centrally either triggers or is a marker of metabolic events that impact upon mechanisms that drive atherosclerotic plaque formation. Leander *et al.* (2007) reported that the presence of excess central fat was also strongly predictive of risk of a further nonfatal or fatal MI in individuals who had undergone treatment for a first MI.

Obesity clearly increases CVD risk via a number of different routes. Blood pressure becomes elevated in obesity, as the blood volume increases in proportion to the greater body size. Obese individuals also become hypertensive because the homeostatic regulation of blood pressure is abnormal. Factors produced from the adipose tissue, including leptin, will also contribute to elevated blood pressure. Obesity is associated with increased circulating concentrations of a number of clotting factors including fibrinogen, factor VII and factor VIII. This increases the likelihood of thrombosis in subjects with established atherosclerosis. Morbid obesity is a major risk factor for death from acute pulmonary thromboembolism (Blaszyk *et al.*, 1999).

Adipose tissue is a source of a wide range of adipokines, cytokines and other factors that can modulate the process of atherosclerosis. Adiponectin, for example, suppresses inflammation and tends to accumulate in the vascular wall following local trauma. Adiponectin will block atherosclerosis as it prevents the transformation of macrophages to foam cells at an early stage in the formation of the fatty streak. However, in obesity, concentrations of adiponectin tend to be low, and so this protective mechanism is less effective. The pro-inflammatory cytokines tumour necrosis factor-α (TNFα) and interleukin-6 (IL-6) are also produced by adipose tissue, and with obesity, their secretion is increased. IL-6, in particular, appears to drive atherosclerosis and thrombosis as it induces the production of C-reactive protein and fibrinogen, increasing blood viscosity. IL-6 suppresses the activity of lipoprotein lipase in macrophages, and this promotes the uptake of lipids by the fatty streak. IL-6 has also been linked to development of hypertension and promotes endothelial cell dysfunction.

Interventions that promote weight loss and increase physical activity produce clear benefits in terms of CVD risk factors. In hypertensive patients, for example, weight loss is associated with a lowering of blood pressure (Siebenhofer *et al.*, 2011). Reducing adiposity will reverse the insulin resistance associated with obesity and hence reduce risk of diabetes. The Look AHEAD Research Group (2007) reported that an intensive lifestyle intervention over a 12-month period in over 5000 obese or overweight adults with type 2 diabetes reduced body weight by an average of 8.9%. This weight loss was associated with lowered blood pressure, reduced use of diabetes and hypertension medication, increased physical fitness, raised HDL-cholesterol and lowered LDL-cholesterol concentrations. However, the longer-term follow-up of this intervention found that despite improvements in HbA1c and blood pressure, there was no effect upon cardiovascular mortality (Look Ahead Research Group, 2013). A lack of effect of weight loss upon mortality in healthy obese subjects was also reported by Harrington *et al.* (2009), although the same study found that in the 'unhealthy' obese population, weight loss reduced mortality (HR 0.87, 95% CI 0.77–0.99). Romeo *et al.* (2012) showed that among subjects who had undergone bariatric surgery (initial BMI over 40 kg/m², weight loss reduced the risk of MI over 14 years post-surgery by 44%.

8.4.4.3.2 Diabetes

Type 2 diabetics are at significantly greater risk of CVD and of fatal outcomes associated with CVD events than the non-diabetic population. Men with T2DM have two- to threefold greater CVD mortality, and in women, the risk is even greater (three- to fourfold; Goff *et al.*, 2007). Twice as many type 2 diabetics as non-diabetics show clinical evidence of atherosclerosis, and death rates following MI are 2–3 times higher where diabetes is present. Diabetes tends to be associated with other classical risk factors for CVD, including obesity, hypertension and dyslipidaemia, and this undoubtedly explains some of the increased risk. However, insulin resistance is the main driver of CVD risk in T2DM.

Insulin resistance impacts upon atherosclerosis and the associated disease outcomes (MI and stroke) at several different levels (Bansilal *et al.*, 2007). The processes that drive endothelial cell dysfunction, the uptake of oxidized lipid by macrophages to form foam cells and the development of a chronic inflammatory state that favours plaque formation are all consequences of insulin resistance and the associated hyperglycaemia and dyslipidaemia. The cytokines and adipokines that are the products of adipocytes are major players in mediating these effects, as described earlier, in the context of obesity. Insulin resistance is associated with elevated leptin, IL-6 and TNFα and lower concentrations of adiponectin, all of which will contribute to the development of atherosclerosis and a hypercoagulant state that promotes thrombosis. In addition to these factors, insulin resistance favours the production of angiotensinogen by the adipocytes. This is the precursor of angiotensin II, which promotes vasoconstriction and elevated blood pressure and also increases the vascular expression of monocyte chemoattractant protein 1 (MCP-1), vascular cell adhesion molecule 1 (VCAM-1) and intracellular adhesion molecule 1 (ICAM-1), all of which drive the recruitment and binding of monocytes to the intima in the early stages of atherosclerosis. Plasminogen activation inhibitor-1 is also over-expressed by the adipocytes in insulin resistance, and this promotes the formation of clots around existing, unstable atherosclerotic plaques.

Interventions that target T2DM, either through improved control over blood glucose or through improving other associated metabolic abnormalities (e.g. dyslipidaemia in diabetic subjects), generally show that cardiovascular risk declines with successful management. An intensive programme to manage glycaemia, blood pressure, microalbuminuria and dyslipidaemia in the Steno-2 Study (Gaede *et al.*, 2003) showed that over an 8-year period CVD risk was reduced by 53% in patients with type 2 diabetes. The United Kingdom Prospective Diabetes Study (UKPDS, 1998) showed that intensive

Table 8.5 Reference ranges for plasma lipids in adults.

	Reference range (mmol/l)	Healthy range (mmol/l)
Triglycerides	0.70–1.80	0.70–1.70
Total cholesterol	3.50–7.80	<5.20
HDL-cholesterol	0.80–1.70	>1.15
LDL-cholesterol	2.30–6.10	<4.0

The reference range is the range of values that would be within the normal distribution for the population. There are sex differences in these ranges, with triglyceride concentrations tending to be higher in men and HDL-cholesterol higher in women.

control of blood glucose using oral drugs or insulin reduced risk of MI by 39%.

8.4.4.3.3 Dietary fat and cholesterol transport

Risk of CVD is strongly related to circulating concentrations of total cholesterol, lipoproteins and triglycerides. Reference ranges for these lipids are shown in Table 8.5. High total cholesterol, hypertriglyceridaemia, raised LDL-cholesterol and low HDL-cholesterol are all risk factors for atherosclerosis. The main basis for this risk stems from the fact that cholesterol uptake by macrophages as they become foam cells is an essential process in plaque formation. HDL-cholesterol reduces risk as it is responsible for carrying excess cholesterol away from the arterial wall to the liver. Concentrations of triglycerides tend to be inversely correlated with HDL-cholesterol.

The strong association between dyslipidaemia (an abnormal lipid profile) and CVD risk has made manipulation of cholesterol and triglycerides a primary target for interventions designed to prevent disease, both in individuals and at the population level. Statins are a class of drug that are designed specifically to lower LDL-cholesterol concentrations. These agents, such as lovastatin, are inhibitors of 3-hydroxy-3-methyl-glutaryl-CoA reductase (HMG-CoA reductase), which is the rate-limiting step in the pathway of cholesterol biosynthesis. Statins effectively lower cholesterol concentrations, and this in turn leads to up-regulation of LDL receptors in the liver, which causes LDL to be more rapidly cleared from circulation. Gould and colleagues' (2007) analyses of interventions using statins found that they reduced total cholesterol concentrations by between 4% and 34% and LDL-cholesterol concentrations by up to 52%, with no effect on HDL-cholesterol. 1 mmol/l reductions in total cholesterol were shown to reduce prevalence of CHD events by 29.5% and CHD death rates by 24.5%. One millimole per litre reductions in serum LDL-cholesterol produced similar changes in risk. The meta-analysis of

Naci and colleagues (2013) found that statins reduced coronary events (31% reduction) and mortality (18% reduction). The most effective statins were atorvastatin and fluvastatin, and differences in efficacy between drugs were not related to their effects upon LDL-cholesterol.

Dietary change provides the alternative strategy for minimizing the prevalence of dyslipidaemia and the associated burden of CVD. For several decades, the public health message has been to reduce total intakes of fat, to consume less saturated fat and to consume more starchy carbohydrates as an alternative energy source (see Section 8.3). This is a message familiar to most people in Westernized countries, but it is now becoming clear that this may not be the most effective strategy.

Saturated fats (Figure A2; Appendix) increase total cholesterol concentrations in circulation and elevate LDL-cholesterol. PUFA have the opposite effect. HDL-cholesterol concentrations are increased by all classes of fatty acids (saturates, PUFA and monounsaturated fatty acids (MUFA)), if these fats replace carbohydrate in the diet. Interestingly, saturated fatty acids may be more effective than PUFA and MUFA in this respect. Replacing fats in the diet with carbohydrates actually increases serum triglyceride concentrations. This means that following advice to replace saturated fats in the diet with carbohydrate is likely to have little cardiovascular benefit, since this will effectively lower both LDL-cholesterol and HDL-cholesterol and increase triglyceride concentrations (Hu and Willett, 2002). A more effective strategy may be to replace the saturated fats in the diet with alternative fats. MUFA and PUFA in place of saturates would lower LDL-cholesterol, and although there would be no increase in HDL-cholesterol, the HDL–LDL ratio would be improved. It is though that substitution of saturated fatty acids with MUFA and PUFA would carry additional benefits as the unsaturated fatty acids improve insulin sensitivity and risk of diabetes, which effectively reduces CVD risk independently of direct effects on the process of atherosclerosis. However, the meta-analysis of Chowdhury et al. (2014) found that there was no significant reduction in CHD events associated with increased saturated fat intake or higher intakes of MUFA or n-6 PUFA.

There has been considerable concern over the high levels of trans-fatty acids present in the processed foods consumed in the Westernized nations. Trans-fatty acids (Figure A2; Appendix) are derived from both MUFA and PUFA and are formed during the processing of vegetable oils to convert them to solids. The majority of trans-fatty acids in the human food chain are associated with the hydrogenation of vegetable oils, and they are primarily consumed in margarines and in deep-fried foods. Trans-fatty acids formed in food processing generally have similar effects to saturated fatty acids and will increase LDL-cholesterol concentrations (Hu and Willett, 2002). The trans-fatty acids inhibit the enzyme delta 6 desaturase and therefore disrupt the metabolism of essential fatty acids and the generation of prostaglandins and inflammatory mediators. This contributes to endothelial cell dysfunction. Chowdhury *et al.* (2014) found that risk of CHD events was increased by 16% when comparing the highest and lowest thirds of trans-fatty acid consumption. Naturally occurring trans-fatty acids are found in dairy products and include vaccenic acid and conjugated linoleic acid. Some isomers of these fatty acids have been shown to protect against atherosclerosis and even cause regression of existing atherosclerotic lesions in mice (Toomey *et al.*, 2003), but beneficial effects in humans have not been convincingly demonstrated. These ruminant-derived trans-fatty acids make up less than 0.5% of total fatty acid intake from food, and there is no robust evidence of cardiovascular benefit in humans (Bendsen *et al.*, 2011). Intake may be significant in individuals who consume conjugated linoleic acid supplements. Studies of such supplements suggest that the impact of conjugated linoleic acid upon LDL-cholesterol is essentially the same as industrially generated trans-fatty acids (Brouwer *et al.*, 2013).

A number of intervention trials have suggested that greater intakes of n-3 fatty acids are protective against CVD. Bucher *et al.* (2002) noted that eicosapentaenoic acid and docosahexaenoic acid were associated with significantly lower CVD mortality, whether consumed as part of the normal diet or if taken as supplements.

The greatest benefits were noted in individuals with established CVD. Dietary n-3 PUFA are associated with a small but significant reduction in coronary events (RR 0.87, 0.78–0.97) when comparing upper and lower thirds of consumption, and high circulating concentrations of n-3 fatty acids are similarly associated with low cardiovascular risk (Chowdhury *et al.*, 2014). In contrast, supplemental n-3 PUFA were found by Rizos *et al.* (2012) to have no significant cardiovascular benefit. The n-3 fatty acids may work by a number of mechanisms as they have been shown to lower serum triglyceride concentrations, improve endothelial cell function and inhibit platelet aggregation.

A number of food products have been developed to reduce total cholesterol through the inclusion of plant stanols and stanol esters. There is a large global market for low-fat spreads containing these agents, which block the absorption of exogenous dietary cholesterol and endogenous biliary cholesterol in the small intestine. This has the effect of reducing circulating cholesterol and increasing expression of hepatic LDL receptors (Figure 8.10). Raitakari and colleagues (2007) showed that regular consumption of margarine containing stanol esters over a 2-year period significantly improved carotid artery compliance (reduced stiffness) in healthy non-smokers with normal blood lipid profiles. Castro Cabezas *et al.* (2006) demonstrated that combining stanol ester margarine with statin treatment in patients with primary hyperlipidaemia enhanced the impact of the statin treatment, producing declines in serum

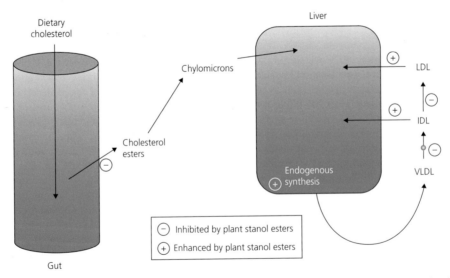

Figure 8.10 Plant stanol esters lower circulating LDL-cholesterol concentrations. This is partially achieved through inhibition of cholesterol ester (CE) uptake from the gut. This increases endogenous synthesis, but production of LDL is inhibited, and the reuptake from circulation is enhanced. As a result, circulating LDL falls.

cholesterol and LDL-cholesterol that were double those observed with statins alone. Although effective in lowering LDL-cholesterol concentrations, there is little evidence that these products impact upon cardiovascular outcomes in humans. Raitakari *et al.* (2008) reported no effect of plant stanol esters upon arterial function.

8.4.4.3.4 Folic acid and plasma homocysteine

Homocysteine is a sulphur-containing amino acid, which is found in circulation bound to proteins (70%) and other sulphates (5%) or as homocysteine dimers (25%). Elevated plasma homocysteine is recognized as a risk factor for CVD. Risk associated with elevated concentrations of homocysteine is independent of all other CVD risk factors and appears to be graded and linear, that is, as plasma homocysteine concentration increases, the increase in CVD risk is directly proportional.

The normal range of homocysteine concentrations in human plasma is considered to be 5–15 μmol/l. The range 16–100 μmol/l represents mild-to-moderate hyperhomocysteinaemia, and concentrations over 100 μmol/l represent severe hyperhomocysteinaemia. Hyperhomocysteinaemia is reported in up to half of patients with atherosclerosis. Concentrations of homocysteine are determined by the flux through two biochemical pathways, both of which are subject to regulation by micronutrients (Figure 8.11).

The methionine cycle involves reactions that either demethylate or remethylate methionine and homocysteine,

respectively. This cycling is critical in determining the availability of methyl groups for a variety of processes, including synthesis of phosphatidylcholine and the methylation of DNA in epigenetic gene silencing. When methionine is in excess, concentrations of homocysteine will increase unless it can be converted to cysteine via the trans-sulphuration pathway. The rate-limiting step in this pathway, catalysed by cystathionine-β-synthase, requires vitamin B6 as a cofactor. If methionine is limiting, then homocysteine will be remethylated by methionine synthase. This step requires vitamin B12 and an adequate supply of methyltetrahydrofolate, which is derived from folate in the folate cycle. Thus, the metabolism and circulating concentration of homocysteine are controlled by the B vitamins, of which folic acid appears to be the most important.

There are well-described inborn errors of metabolism that impact upon the three key enzyme steps in the methionine–homocysteine cycle identified in Figure 8.11. Individuals with these inherited disorders share the characteristics of having severe hyperhomocysteinaemia and premature atherosclerotic disease. This emphasizes the potential importance of homocysteine as a risk factor for CVD. In addition to these inborn errors of metabolism, a relatively common polymorphism of methylenetetrahydrofolate reductase (MTHFR C677T) is associated with increased CVD risk. The TT variant of MTHFR C677T leads to enzyme activity being two-thirds lower than in individuals with the CC variant. Individuals with TT are therefore predisposed to a higher circulating

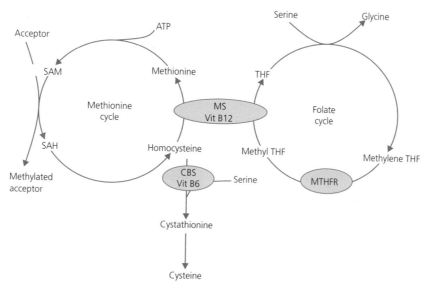

Figure 8.11 The methionine and folate cycles. CBS, cystathionine-β-synthase; MS, methionine synthase; MTHFR, methylenetetrahydrofolate reductase; SAH, *S*-adenosylhomocysteine; SAM, *S*-adenosylmethionine; THF, tetrahydrofolate.

homocysteine concentration as their capacity to form MTHF for the methionine synthase step of the methionine cycle is impaired. Holmes and colleagues (2011) reported that homocysteine concentrations were up to 4 µmol/l higher in the TT population than in CC, but that the effect was only seen where folate intake was habitually low.

The Homocysteine Studies Collaboration (2002) reviewed evidence from 30 studies that had considered homocysteine in relation to CVD, following on from some smaller meta-analyses that suggested hyperhomocysteinaemia increased CHD risk by 70%. The aim of the Homocysteine Studies Collaboration was to assess the likely impact of a 25% reduction in populations' plasma homocysteine concentrations. It was suggested that such a reduction would reduce risk of both CHD (OR 0.73, 95% confidence intervals 0.64–0.83) and stroke (OR 0.77, 0.66–0.90). For CHD, at least, this reduction in risk would be dependent on the MTHFR genotype of individuals. Klerk et al. (2002) also noted that MTHFR genotype modified CHD risk, but found that other factors could modify this risk. In European populations, carrying the TT genotype increased CHD risk (OR 1.16, 1.05–1.28), but in North America, where folate status is better due to fortification, there was no evidence that TT impacted significantly on CHD risk. In Asian countries with low folate status, the TT genotype was associated with 68% greater risk of stroke (Holmes et al. 2011).

A variety of mechanisms have been proposed to explain the association of hyperhomocysteinaemia with CVD risk. Homocysteine may initiate atherosclerosis through oxidative processes and by causing endothelial cell injury. In the presence of ferric or cupric ions, homocysteine will auto-oxidize, and the ensuing production of hydrogen peroxide could be an early step in LDL-cholesterol oxidation. In particular, this process inhibits the formation of nitric oxide, which normally serves to protect LDL-cholesterol from oxidation within the vessel wall. Animal studies indicate that experimentally induced hyperhomocysteinaemia promotes changes in the arterial wall that are early stages in the process of atherosclerosis, including endothelial cell dysfunction, activation of thrombosis and increased adhesion of monocytes.

Given the epidemiological findings that hyperhomocysteinaemia increases CVD risk and the presence of apparently robust biological mechanisms to explain the association, there is considerable interest in the use of B vitamins, and particularly folate, to modify this risk factor. A number of studies have shown that supplements of folate, vitamin B12 and vitamin B6 at doses up to 20 times normal intakes could reduce plasma homocysteine by up to 32%, with folate providing the strongest

effect. Malinow and colleagues (1998) studied the impact of supplementing breakfast cereals with folate at doses ranging from 127 to 665 µg/day. All doses were effective in reducing plasma homocysteine, and the effect of folate was dose dependent. Since 1998, staple foods in the United States have been fortified with folic acid. In that time, there have been a 50% decrease in the prevalence of hyperhomocysteinaemia and a significant decrease in stroke-related death rates.

The HOPE 2 (Lonn et al., 2006) trial was a prospective cohort study that aimed to investigate whether folate and other B vitamins might be effective in preventing CVD. Over 5500 patients with established CVD or diabetes were randomly assigned to either placebo or a supplement containing 2.5 mg folate, 50 mg vitamin B6 and 1 mg vitamin B12 over a 5-year period. This supplement regimen decreased the homocysteine concentration of the population by 2.4 µmol/l, but had no effect on overall CVD death rates or the prevalence of MIs. However, significant benefit was seen with respect to stroke risk, with a reduction in the number of strokes in the patients taking supplements (OR 0.75, 0.59–0.97). In contrast, the VITATOPS trial (2010) found no significant cardiovascular benefit associated with 3.4 years of supplementation (2 mg folate, 25 mg vitamin B6, 0.5 mg vitamin B12) of men and women who had previously suffered a stroke. A meta-analysis of 19 randomized controlled trials (Huang et al., 2012) found that while folate-based interventions had no effect upon risk of CHD or MI, supplementation significantly reduced risk of stroke (RR 0.88, 0.82–0.95).

Taken overall, the available evidence supports the view that folate status determines homocysteine concentrations and risk of stroke. However, the evidence that reduction in stroke is associated with folate does not always fit the hypothesis that the mechanism of action is related to homocysteine. Durga et al. (2005) reported that in 820 subjects with normal homocysteine concentrations, folate status was associated with arterial stiffness (a marker of atherosclerosis), independently of homocysteine. Folate may therefore be protective in other ways. For example, it lowers production of superoxide radicals in the vessel wall preventing oxidative damage to LDL-cholesterol. Endothelial function is enhanced as folic acid increases nitric oxide production by inducing nitric oxide synthase. This also dampens oxidative stress within the vessels (Förstermann, 2010). Interventions that aim to prevent CVD by targeting homocysteine may therefore be ineffective and should be redesigned with cardiovascular outcome as the primary focus (Moat et al., 2004). The efficacy of folic acid supplements will be strongly dependent upon MTHFR genotype, and the habitual intake of folate and benefits may be substantially greater in populations that are not exposed to fortification (Holmes *et al.*, 2011).

8.4.4.3.5 Antioxidant nutrients

Given the importance of LDL oxidation and uptake of the oxidized complex by macrophages in the etiology of atherosclerosis, it is suggested that antioxidant nutrients present within the diet may be protective against CVD. LDL is a rich target for ROS attack as each LDL complex comprises a spherical arrangement of approximately 2700 phospholipids around a hydrophobic core of cholesterol and cholesterol esters. Around 50% of the fatty acids in the phospholipid shell are polyunsaturated, and the presence of a high density of double bonds serves to increase the likelihood of reaction with free radicals. Oxidation of these fatty acids can establish chain reactions that will spread through the phospholipid shell, eventually leading to oxidation of apoprotein B100. Antioxidant protection within LDL is provided primarily by vitamin E (α-tocopherol), with between 5 and 9 molecules inserted into the phospholipid shell of each LDL complex. In addition to vitamin E, the core of the LDL will contain other fat-soluble antioxidants, including β-carotene, lycopene, ubiquinone and polyphenolics.

Increased consumption of foods that are rich in antioxidants has been shown in epidemiological studies to provide protection against CVD. Law and Morris (1998) showed that higher levels of consumption of fruits and vegetables could significantly reduce CHD risk. In general, studies that have considered the impact of specific antioxidant nutrients upon risk provide results that are consistent with the hypothesis that consumption of antioxidants will oppose LDL oxidation and protect against atherosclerosis. Abbey (1995) and colleagues performed a series of studies that showed that vitamin E could inhibit LDL oxidation *in vitro* and that LDL obtained from volunteers who had taken vitamin E supplements was also protected from copper-induced oxidation. The CHAOS intervention study (Stephens *et al.*, 1996) evaluated the impact of supplementing patients with established atherosclerosis with vitamin E at doses of 400 or 800 IU/day over a period of over 500 days. The study found that supplements led to a 47% reduction in risk of nonfatal MI. Nagao *et al.* (2012) found that stroke mortality was lower in subjects with the highest circulating concentrations of α- and γ-tocopherol in a Japanese population. Similarly, the Finnish ATBC trial found lower cardiovascular mortality in subjects with higher α-tocopherol intake (Wright *et al.*, 2006). The EURAMIC study (Kardinaal *et al.*, 1993) compared fat-soluble antioxidant status in fat biopsies from men who had suffered an MI event

and healthy controls. No difference in vitamin E status was reported, but there was evidence that the MI patients had consumed less β-carotene and less fat-soluble antioxidants in total. Other studies suggest a protective role for carotenoids, with β-cryptoxanthin and lutein emerging as cardioprotective in the study of Koh and colleagues (2011).

The overall effectiveness of vitamin E and other antioxidant nutrients in lowering CVD risk appears to depend upon their source. Knekt *et al.* (2004) performed a meta-analysis of nine major cohort studies, comprising over 290 000 people that had considered the impact of dietary sources of vitamin E, vitamin C and the carotenoids, and the impact of supplements of these nutrients, upon risk of CHD. Within the normal diet, comparing the highest quintile of vitamin E intake, with the lowest quintile of intake, showed a reduced risk of CHD (OR 0.77, 0.64–0.92). Carotenoids had a similar protective effect (OR 0.83, 0.73–0.95), with α-carotene, β-carotene, β-cryptoxanthin and lutein, but not lycopene, all contributing to this effect. In contrast, vitamin C within the normal diet had no significant impact upon CHD risk. This evidence argues in favour of supplementation as a strategy for CVD prevention. To attain the doses of fat-soluble antioxidant vitamins required to obtain significant cardiovascular protection through diet alone would necessitate sizeable increases in consumption of fats and oils that would probably offset any benefit. However, the Knekt analysis also evaluated the impact of antioxidant supplements and concluded that while supplemental vitamin C produced a dose-dependent reduction in CHD risk (500 mg/day ascorbate reduced risk by 25%), vitamin E supplements were ineffective. It is likely therefore that the benefits associated with increased intakes of vitamin E and carotenoids may be, at least in part, explained by other components present in the foods that are their richest sources. This view would be supported by the meta-analysis of Ye *et al.* (2013) which considered 19 randomized controlled trials of antioxidant supplementation and found no beneficial effect upon MI, angina, CHD, stroke or cardiovascular mortality.

Tea is regarded as a major source of dietary antioxidants, with some studies estimating that 40–50% of the daily intake of scavenging antioxidants is derived from this source. There is an extensive literature on tea in relation to both CHD and stroke risk, which is briefly reviewed in Research Highlight 8.2. The general balance of opinion is that green and black teas both confer cardiovascular benefits. Although their mode of action is generally regarded as involving antioxidant protection of LDL, anti-inflammatory and other properties of tea polyphenols may also be of importance.

Research Highlight 8.2 Tea and cardiovascular disease.

Tea is the most commonly consumed beverage, other than water, on a global scale. In the Eastern countries, green tea is favoured and is prepared by infusion of dried leaves of *Camellia sinensis*. Black tea, favoured in Western countries, is prepared from leaves that have been macerated prior to drying. Both teas are rich sources of polyphenolic compounds, providing a significant proportion of daily intakes in the populations where they are consumed. The oxidation that accompanies the production of black tea alters the profile of polyphenolics present, effectively reducing the quantity of catechins in the drink and introducing more complex theaflavins and thearubigins.

Tea is regarded as a potential source of antioxidants in the diet, and consumption of both green (Leenen *et al.*, 2000) and black tea (Langley-Evans, 2000) increases plasma antioxidant status in healthy volunteers. Both drinks are associated with lower CVD risk. There is a graded and linear relationship between black tea consumption and CHD risk, with every three cup (711 ml) increment in consumption reducing risk of MI by 11% (Peters *et al.*, 2001). Some studies suggest that high levels of consumption could reduce risk by up to 70% (Gardner *et al.*, 2007). Risk of stroke is also reduced by higher consumption of black tea (Keli *et al.*, 1996) and green tea (Fraser *et al.*, 2007). A Chinese study that compared habitual green tea drinkers with non-consumers showed OR of 0.6 (95% confidence intervals 0.42–0.85) for stroke-related death. The most recent meta-analysis (Arab *et al.*, 2013) reported that consumption of 3 or more cups of tea per day reduces risk of stroke incidence and mortality by 21%.

A variety of plausible biological mechanisms have been proposed to explain the protective effects of tea drinking:
- The polyphenolics in green and black tea are potent fat-soluble antioxidants that are readily incorporated into the LDL complex and prevent oxidation. Experimental studies show that tea consumption by healthy volunteers increases the concentration of tea flavonoids present in LDL and inhibits LDL oxidation *in vitro*.
- Tea-derived flavonoids are vasodilators that are capable of lowering blood pressure.
- The polyphenolic compounds in tea inhibit clotting by suppressing platelet aggregation.
- Polyphenolic compounds may down-regulate genes and transcription factors that are involved in the inflammatory process and thereby reduce the impact of pro-inflammatory cytokines upon endothelial cell function.

There is also evidence that tea consumption may impact upon other risk factors for cardiovascular disease. Intervention trials where green or black tea have been used as vehicles for cardiovascular disease prevention have reported lower blood pressure and LDL-cholesterol as outcomes (Hartley *et al.*, 2013).

8.4.4.3.6 Sodium and blood pressure

Blood pressure is the pressure generated within the vascular tree when blood pushes against the arterial walls. In measurement of blood pressure, two components are determined. The systolic pressure is the pressure generated when blood is ejected from the left ventricle of the heart, while the diastolic pressure is the pressure between heartbeats. Table 8.6 shows the normal ranges of values for systolic and diastolic pressures and the different classifications of prehypertension and hypertension. From a clinical perspective, the cut-off points generally used in treatment of hypertension are systolic blood pressure (SBP) of 140 mmHg and diastolic blood pressure (DBP) of 90 mmHg.

In Westernized countries, blood pressure will generally increase with age in both men and women, and systolic pressure is 20–30 mmHg higher at age 75 than at age 24. Men have higher blood pressure than women. Rising blood pressure is associated with increased risk of stroke death in both sexes. In men, comparing the highest decile of the blood pressure distribution (SBP 151, DBP 98 mmHg) with the lowest decile (SBP < 112, DBP < 71 mmHg) indicates an eightfold greater risk of stroke death with the higher pressure. In women, a fourfold greater risk is noted. The association between stroke risk and blood pressure applies across the whole of the population distribution of blood pressures, and so men who may not be considered for antihypertensive treatment (SBP 137–142, DBP 89–92 mmHg) have fourfold greater risk of stroke death than those in the population who have the lowest blood pressures.

High blood pressure is driven by a number of non-modifiable risk factors, which, in addition to increasing age, includes male gender, ethnicity and a number of genetically determined disorders of renal and vascular function. For example, the syndrome of apparent mineralocorticoid excess is a genetic disorder of the renal form of 11β-hydroxysteroid dehydrogenase, which allows cortisol to bind to the aldosterone receptor. This leads to sodium retention and hypertension. Modifiable factors that increase blood pressure include lower SES, physical inactivity, high intakes of alcohol and dietary factors.

Within diet, sodium intake is the major concern in relation to blood pressure. On a low-salt (sodium chloride) diet, homeostatic mechanisms ensure that the kidneys will excrete any excess sodium via the urine. Acute and modest changes in sodium intake will be comfortably accommodated by these mechanisms. In salt-sensitive individuals (Figure 8.12) and with age-related declines in renal function, the capacity of the kidneys to clear excess sodium may be exceeded with high intakes of salt. As a result, sodium will be retained necessitating a movement of water from the intracellular compartment to the extracellular compartment. Effectively, the required dilution of circulating sodium will produce an increase in blood volume. With more blood to be pumped by the heart, blood pressure increases. Over a relatively short period of time, these blood pressure changes can become fixed as the vessels accommodate to the raised pressure by reducing their elasticity. Greater resistance to flow will push blood pressure still higher.

Animal studies clearly show the relationship between sodium intake and blood pressure. Rats, for example, provided with a solution of 1.5% sodium chloride instead of water to drink, show increases of SBP of around 40 mmHg within 3–5 days of treatment. Experiments with chimpanzees showed that increasing salt intake from 5 to 15 g/day led to a rise in blood pressure of 30 mmHg SBP and 10 mmHg DBP over a

period of 16 months. As in the rodent studies, this effect was reversible.

Epidemiological studies of the association between sodium and blood pressure in humans have been rather controversial due to concerns regarding the analytic methods used and potential confounding factors. However, that such a relationship exists is irrefutable. One of the first major studies to consider this issue was INTERSALT (Elliott et al., 1989), which considered 10 000 people in 52 populations across 32 different countries. The full analysis showed that blood pressure was related to sodium excretion, which provides the most robust marker of intake. Every 100 mmol sodium greater excretion predicted an 11.3 mmHg rise in SBP and 6.4 mmHg rise in DBP. Moreover, when considering 4 rural populations in INTERSALT, with the lowest salt intakes, blood pressure was lower than in Westernized populations, and there was no age-related rise in blood pressure, unlike all other populations in the study.

The findings of INTERSALT were reproduced by the more recent European Prospective Investigation into Cancer and Nutrition (EPIC)-Norfolk study (Khaw et al., 2004), which studied 23 104 men and women aged 45–79. Comparing the lowest to the highest quintile of sodium excretion, there were a 7.2 mmHg SBP difference in men and a 3.0 mmHg difference in women. These differences appear to be very small in the context of Table 8.6, but at the whole population level would be highly

Table 8.6 Normal and hypertensive blood pressure references.

Category	Systolic blood pressure (mmHg)	Diastolic blood pressure (mmHg)
Normotensive	<120	<80
Pre-hypertensive	120–139	80–89
Hypertensive		
Stage 1	140–159	90–99
Stage 2	160+	100+

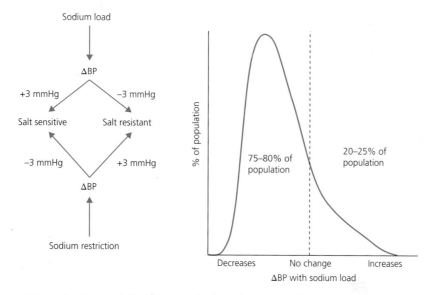

Figure 8.12 Salt sensitivity and resistance. Individuals are defined as salt sensitive if the ingestion of a sodium load induces an increase in blood pressure and if the adoption of sodium restriction leads to a corresponding decrease in blood pressure. Individuals with the opposite response are termed salt resistant. Salt resistance is seen in a minority of individuals (20–25% of the population), while most humans exhibit a degree of salt sensitivity.

significant. In the United Kingdom, a 5 mmHg reduction of SBP for the whole population would halve the number of hypertensive individuals, reducing stroke-related deaths by 14% and CHD deaths by 9%.

Given this potentially very powerful impact of minor shifts in the population blood pressure profile, it is of major importance to develop and evaluate interventions that could reduce sodium intake. The Trials of Hypertension Prevention study (Cook *et al.*, 1998), which included 2382 participants, evaluated the effectiveness of counselling to reduce sodium intake and promote weight loss over a 4-year period. At the end of the trial, sodium reduction alone had reduced the prevalence of hypertension by 18%. Similarly, the Dietary Approaches to Stop Hypertension (DASH) study showed that a diet low in fat, high in fibre, low in sodium and rich in magnesium and potassium could reduce SBP and DBP in hypertensive individuals by 11 and 5.5 mmHg, respectively, over just an 8-week period (Sacks *et al.*, 2001). He and MacGregor (2003) performed a meta-analysis of the largest and longest intervention trials that have applied sodium reduction in human populations. Reducing sodium intakes was shown to provide proportionate changes in populations' blood pressure, with the greatest effects noted in hypertensives. For example, a 9.0 g/day reduction in salt intake would be expected to reduce SBP by 5.4 mmHg in normotensive subjects and by 10.7 mmHg in hypertensive subjects. Reductions of this magnitude would be sufficient to prevent 150 000 cardiovascular events and 50 000 deaths per year in the United Kingdom alone. Average intakes of salt in the United Kingdom are estimated to be 9.3 g/day in men and 6.8 g/day in women (Department of Health, 2002). Despite a decline of approximately 1.4 g/day since 2001, 80% of men and 58% of women in the United Kingdom exceed the current advice to consume no more than 6 g/day.

Progress in reducing the salt intake of the population represents a public health nutrition success in the United Kingdom, but new evidence from the GenSalt trial in China suggests that the response to salt reduction may not be beneficial in all individuals (Chen 2010). GenSalt considered the blood pressure response to 7 days of low-salt (3 g/day) or high-salt (18 g/day) diets. On average, salt reduction decreased blood pressure by 7–8 mmHg (systolic), and high salt increased pressure by 5–6 mmHg. Responses were slightly greater in women than in men and were greatest in older subjects (Figure 8.13). Importantly, the blood pressure response to variation in salt intake followed a normal distribution around the mean changes, with approximately 23% of subjects *increasing* blood pressure in response to salt reduction and *reducing* blood pressure with a high-salt diet. GenSalt is now considering genetic variants

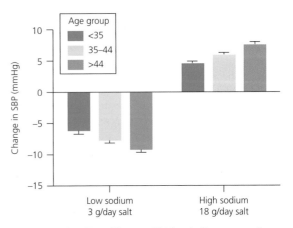

Figure 8.13 The effect of low- and high-salt diets on systolic blood pressure in a Chinese population; the GenSalt study. *Data Source*: Chen (2010).

that may explain the variability in response to salt, and this will enable more targeted and tailored advice on salt in the future. A region on chromosome 2 (Mei *et al.*, 2012) and the oestrogen receptor (Kelly *et al.*, 2013) have been identified as potential mediators of salt sensitivity.

Other minerals may play a role in determining blood pressure. Calcium, for example, is believed to lower blood pressure, but studies with supplements show that even megadoses (twice normal daily intake) produce only minor changes. Similarly, magnesium is believed to be of importance as hypertensives often manifest low serum magnesium concentrations. However, supplemental magnesium has no significant effect upon blood pressure in humans. Increasing potassium intakes will lower blood pressure. INTERSALT suggested that a 50 mmol/day increase in potassium excretion would be associated with 3 mmHg lower SBP and 2 mmHg lower DBP.

8.4.5 Cancer
8.4.5.1 What is cancer?
Cancers, or tumours, can arise in any of the tissues of the body. They develop through a process termed carcinogenesis and are essentially the products of uncontrolled cell division. All mammalian cells have a limited capacity for cell division, termed the Hayflick limit. In humans, differentiated cells can divide only 52 times before undergoing apoptosis (programmed cell death), but in cancer, the processes that control cell division are lost through genetic mutation. Prevention of cell division beyond the Hayflick limit is achieved by action of the products of genes called proto-oncogenes and anti-oncogenes.

Proto-oncogenes are genes whose protein products participate in cell–cell signalling and signal transduction pathways. Under normal circumstances, these proteins are expressed at levels that do not allow cell division to occur and are represented as the c-forms of the gene, for example, c-ras or c-myc. Mutations of the proto-oncogenes render them oncogenes (cancer genes), which actively drive unregulated mitotic cell division. The oncogenic forms are given the 'v-' prefix, for example, v-ras. A large number of proto-oncogenes have now been identified, and all are known components of signal transduction pathways. Ras, for example, is a membrane-associated G protein and in the mutated form is frequently found in colorectal tumours. The Trk genes are tyrosine kinases and Raf is a threonine kinase.

Anti-oncogenes are also called tumour suppressor genes. Most of their protein products are factors that prevent cell division. For example, the p53 protein is a transcription factor that promotes the expression of other genes that suppress mitosis. Mutations of p53 will therefore allow unregulated cell division to occur. p53 mutations are among the most common found in human tumours. Some other tumour suppressors have roles in repairing DNA damage that might lead to mutations of anti-oncogenes or proto-oncogenes. For example, mutations of BRCA1 are known to greatly increase risk of breast cancer. BRCA1 and the related BRCA2 gene encode enzymes that have a role in repairing double-stranded DNA breaks.

The process of developing cancer follows three defined stages, as shown in Figure 8.14. Carcinogenesis is *initiated* with damage to either proto-oncogenes or anti-oncogenes, resulting in cells that are actively expressing oncogenes or have the inhibitory affectors of the cell cycle silenced. Such mutations are commonplace within cells and tissues and are generally repaired without any adverse consequences. However, should a mutated oncogene not undergo repair and should the cell be stable and able to survive in the mutated form, then it becomes transformed. A transformed cell dedifferentiates, essentially losing all of its specialized structures and functions. In many cases, the transformed cell will not be viable and will be eliminated through apoptosis. If this does not occur, then the cell will *proliferate* through mitotic divisions to form a primary tumour. Many tumours are benign and grow only slowly, but others are more aggressive and will *invade* tissues rapidly. Often, these aggressive tumours will shed cells into the circulation, which then act as the focus for development of secondary tumours (metastases) in other organs.

The initiation phase of carcinogenesis depends upon contact between cells and carcinogenic agents. These include all factors that are capable of inducing genetic mutations through DNA damage. Thus, ionizing radiation, ultraviolet radiation, chemical agents and certain viruses (e.g. human papillomavirus) are all carcinogenic. Most carcinogen exposures are either lifestyle or occupation related. Occupations that involve exposure to hazardous chemicals, for example, asbestos or pesticides,

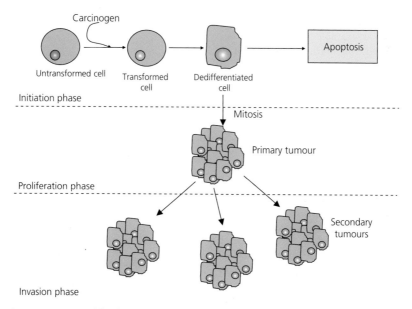

Figure 8.14 Schematic representation of the three stages of tumourigenesis: initiation, proliferation and invasion.

are associated with elevated cancer risk. Carcinogenic exposures also occur due to tobacco smoking, exposure to environmental pollution, excessive sunlight exposure and the presence of carcinogenic chemicals in the food chain.

8.4.5.2 Diet is a modifiable determinant of cancer risk

While tobacco smoking and environmental or occupational exposures are most obviously viewed as risk factors for cancer, it is becoming clear that diet and lifestyle factors related to diet are major determinants of risk of cancer in all organs and tissues. Some estimates suggest that up to 70% of all cancer deaths may be attributable to diet-related factors (Doll and Peto, 1981), although it is more generally accepted that 30–40% of risk is diet related. The historic view that specific components of the diet (e.g. vitamin C, alcohol, fat, protein) are able to modify cancer risk is changing. It is now recognized that foods and their constituents influence cancer initiation and progression in many different ways. There is convincing evidence that some diet-related agents increase risk of cancer, while other dietary behaviours have a protective effect.

The most obvious way in which the diet can increase the risk of cancer is by directly delivering carcinogenic chemicals to the body. Later in this chapter, agents such as safrole will be discussed as carcinogens that are normally present within certain foodstuffs. Intakes of such agents at levels that are hazardous are unusual, and so they are not generally considered as a major threat to human health. Most carcinogens that are ingested as components of food at levels that pose risk will be present either as contaminants or as products of cooking. Nitrosamines are a good example of the latter. The nitrosamines are derived from nitrites combined with secondary amino groups on certain amino acids or proteins. The most commonly occurring dietary nitrosamine is *N*-nitrosodimethylamine. Such compounds are present in high quantities in cooked, processed meats and in salted foods and pickles and are formed as by-products of food processing. Nitrosamines can also be inhaled as components of tobacco smoke. Nitrosamines are associated with a range of different cancers, particularly within the digestive tract. Larsson *et al.* (2006) reported that stomach cancer risk was elevated twofold in women consuming high levels of *N*-nitrosodimethylamine derived from salami, ham and sausages. Similarly, high intakes of nitrosamines and foods rich in nitrosamines are associated with risk of rectal and oesophageal cancers (Le Marchand *et al.*, 2002). A case–control study of bladder cancer found that cancer patients were more likely to have had high consumption of amine- and nitrosamine-rich foods (salami, pastrami, corned beef,

liver) than controls in the 2 years prior to diagnosis (Catsburg *et al.* 2014).

Some foods may also deliver compounds to the body that themselves may be only weakly carcinogenic but which when processed through phase I metabolism in the liver generate potent carcinogenic forms (Figure 8.15). A good example of this is benzo(a)pyrene (B(a)P), which is a polycyclic aromatic hydrocarbon formed during combustion. B(a)P can be present on grains and cereals as an environmental pollutant but is more likely to enter the body during the cooking of meats, particularly if the meat is charred on the outside. B(a)P is metabolized by aryl hydrocarbon hydroxylase (cytochrome P450 1B1) to form a series of hydroxyl and diol intermediates. These products, and most notably the B(a)P diol epoxides, are able to form adducts with DNA, leading to damage and mutation.

The metabolism of nitrosamines may also determine their ultimate carcinogenicity. Nitrosamines are metabolized by the cytochrome P450, CYP2E1. This can exist in different forms as there is a polymorphism of the *CYP2E1* gene, with some individuals having a gene with 96 bp 5′ insert. In a study of a Hawaiian population, individuals with the 5′ insert had 60% greater risk of rectal cancer (Le Marchand *et al.*, 2002). This increased risk may be further elevated by consumption of a nitrosamine-rich diet. Individuals carrying the gene with the 5′ insert were noted to have up to threefold greater risk of rectal cancer if consuming a diet rich in processed meats.

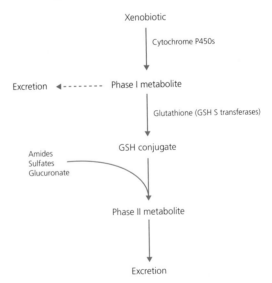

Figure 8.15 Xenobiotics (chemicals that are not components of normal mammalian biochemistry) are metabolized via phase I and phase II systems. Phase I metabolism generates metabolites that are conjugated with glutathione (phase II) and further compounds that enable urinary excretion.

Components of the diet may also interact with each other or with other cancer risk factors to modify risk of cancer. Stomach cancer is generally preceded by inflammatory disorders of the stomach lining, which permit infection with bacteria that promote carcinogenesis, for example, *Helicobacter pylori*, or which increase the likelihood of cell transformation occurring in the presence of carcinogens (Figure 8.16). A high-sodium diet is proposed to irritate the stomach mucosa and promote localized inflammation (gastritis). In addition to promoting infection, high salt concentrations appear to alter expression of certain *H. pylori* genes, and this may contribute to tumour initiation (Loh *et al.*, 2007). Nitrosamines may also promote development of gastric carcinomas once gastritis is established.

Once within the body, the ability of carcinogens to drive the formation of tumours, or for tumours to become established, may be modulated by other components of the diet. Antioxidant nutrients have an anticarcinogenic function as they have the capacity to neutralize free radicals such as the hydroxyl radical, which unquenched can cause DNA strand scission or modify base sequences. It is also proposed that some components of the diet can modulate the access of carcinogens to their sites of action. For example, certain non-nutrient components of plant foodstuffs may bind carcinogenic compounds

and prevent their absorption across the gut and therefore have anti-tumour properties (see Section 8.4.5.5, 'Nonnutrient components of plant foodstuffs'). Other antitumour agents are active postabsorption and bind carcinogens to prevent their interaction with DNA. As described in Research Highlight 8.3, the actions of nutrients may differ according to stage of tumourigenesis, and while they may be protective against initiation, they may promote proliferation and invasion.

8.4.5.3 Nutritional epidemiology and cancer
The study of the relationship between diet and cancer has been one of the main areas of focus for nutritional epidemiologists over the last four decades. A wide range of different methodological approaches have been adopted, each yielding data that is suggestive of associations between particular components of the diet and either increased or decreased risk of cancers at different sites of the body.

8.4.5.3.1 Ecological studies
Ecological studies involve comparing prevalence rates for specific diseases between different regions of a country or between different countries. They can also look at changes in prevalence rates within a population over an extended period of time. To uncover the underlying

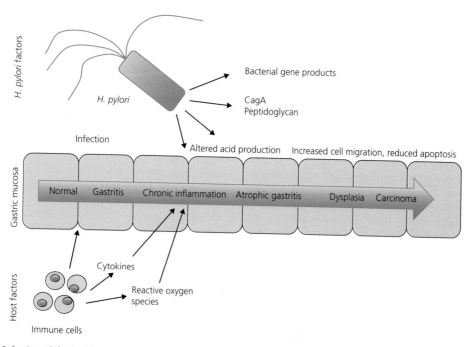

Figure 8.16 Infection of the gastric mucosa with *Helicobacter pylori* is a risk factor for cancer. The host response to infection promotes inflammation and cell damage. Bacterial products change the nature of the gastric mucosa and can prevent apoptosis and inhibit tumour suppressor functions.

Research Highlight 8.3 Micronutrients and cancer: the importance of timing.

Evidence gathered from case–control studies and cohort studies in the cancer field has often been shown to differ from randomized controlled trials that have been developed to test the anti-cancer properties of specific micronutrients. This disparity is well demonstrated by trials involving β-carotene and folic acid. Animal studies and observational studies indicate that foods that are rich in both nutrients have a strong potential to prevent cancer (World Cancer Research Fund, 2007; Giovannucci, 2002). For example, in a US population, serum carotenoid concentrations were associated with lower lung cancer mortality, particularly among smokers (Min and Min, 2014).

Randomized controlled trials yield strongly divergent findings. In the case of β-carotene, the best-documented trials were CARET (Omenn et al., 1996) and ATBC (Albanes et al., 1996) which both found that β-carotene supplementation increased lung cancer incidence and mortality among smokers. The meta-analysis of Druesne-Pecollo et al. (2014) estimated that β-carotene supplements increased risk of stomach and lung cancers by up to 34% in non-smokers and up to 54% in smokers and asbestos workers. For folic acid, the story is similar, with reports of a 67% increase in the incidence of advanced colorectal adenocarcinoma and a twofold increase in the occurrence of multiple carcinomas (Cole et al., 2007).

Much of the divergence between randomized controlled trials and observational studies may be explained by timing of supplementation in relation to the progression from a transformed cell to a cancerous lesion. Folic acid is well documented to prevent the early stages of cancer, and it does so by maintaining normal patterns of DNA methylation and gene silencing and by providing a precursor for nucleotides that are required for DNA repair following damage. However, folic acid will promote the replication of established tumour cells through the same mechanisms – a plentiful supply of nucleotides is required for tumour growth. Chemotherapy using methotrexate or 5-fluorouracil targets folate metabolism, limiting cell division by blocking nucleotide synthesis and inducing apoptosis as tumour cells accumulate unrepaired DNA damage (Kamen, 1997). Similarly, β-carotene will prevent DNA damage through antioxidant properties but may act as a mitogen that enhances replication of transformed cells through interference with retinoid metabolism and associated signalling pathways (Goralczyk, 2009).

The design of randomized controlled trials is generally flawed for evaluation of the efficacy and safety of micronutrients in prevention of cancer. The Cole et al. (2007) trial, for example, recruited elderly subjects with a prior occurrence of colorectal adenoma in order to evaluate the effects of folate. Such subjects would have carried precancerous polyps and lesions whose progression to tumours may be accelerated by folate supplementation. The impact of increased intakes on low-risk populations is more complex to model and may require longer duration trials and integration with other epidemiological data (Mason et al., 2007). The lesson may be that micronutrients have differential effects upon cancer at different stages of disease and that future therapeutic use will have to be carefully assessed based upon pre-screening for cells at an early stage of precancerous potential, genotype and overall dietary patterns.

reasons between temporal or geographical variation in disease rates, the ecological studies explore variation in putative exposures that might explain the patterns of disease. For example, it is widely reported that there is a strong correlation between risk of breast cancer in women and total fat intake. This assertion is based on the observation that on a global scale, the nations with the highest breast cancer death rates (e.g. the United Kingdom, Netherlands, New Zealand, Canada, Denmark and the United States) are those with the highest per capita fat intakes. The nations with the lowest death rates from breast cancer (Thailand, Japan, Taiwan, El Salvador) are those with the lowest fat intakes. This example typifies the limitations of ecological studies, which at best can only be suggestive of a diet–cancer relationship. In the example described earlier, it is not possible to establish whether the women dying of breast cancer are the same women who were exposed to high fat intake, nor is it possible to exclude important confounding factors that are known to impact upon breast cancer risk and that vary between these nations (e.g. age at menarche and menopause, age at first pregnancy, number of pregnancies, use of oral contraceptives).

All ecological studies must be followed up with studies using more reliable methodologies. In the case of the putative relationship between fat and breast cancer, there is little reliable evidence to suggest a major risk (Hunter et al., 1996; Mazhar and Waxman, 2006).

8.4.5.3.2 Migrant studies

Migrant populations, that is, groups of people who have moved from a country where they have been established for many generations to a new country, were widely used in early studies of diet and cancer. Migrant populations provide the ability to discriminate between influences of genetics and influences of the environment in the etiology of disease. Genetic changes in migrant populations occur slowly as they often require three or more generations to mix significantly with the indigenous peoples of their new homeland. Environmental changes such as exposure to pollutants or background radiation will exert effects immediately. Dietary changes often occur within two generations as younger people, in particular, will take on the dietary patterns of the new country very readily.

Studies of Japanese migrants to the United States in the period following the Second World War provided

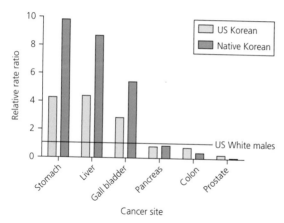

Figure 8.17 Cancer rates in male Korean migrants to the United States compared to the native South Korean population. Migration is associated with significantly decreased prevalence of cancers of the stomach, liver and gall bladder, but these cancers still remain more common than in the full US population. Migration increased risk of colon and prostate cancers. *Data Source*: Lee *et al.* (2007).

some of the first clues to the dietary basis of cancers of the stomach and colon. Over three generations, the US Japanese developed colon cancer rates fivefold above those seen in Japan, while stomach cancer rates fell by 80%. These observations were taken as evidence that high salt intake was a risk factor for stomach cancer, while a high-red-meat, low-fibre diet could increase risk of colon cancer. More recently, Lee *et al.* (2007) have reported on changes in prevalence of cancers among Korean migrants to the United States. In South Korea, rates of certain cancers are very high, and this has been attributed to high intakes of salted foods and foods rich in nitrosamines. As shown in Figure 8.17, among the male population of US Koreans, migration decreased prevalence rates of stomach, liver and gall bladder cancers, while risk of cancers of the colon and prostate appeared to increase. This illustrates that the shift to a more Westernized lifestyle produces profound changes in cancer risk and investigation of the nature of those lifestyle changes could inform understanding of the diet–cancer relationship.

8.4.5.3.3 Studies of populations with unique characteristics

There are some groups of individuals living among national or continental populations, whose beliefs and lifestyles set them apart. Through comparisons of such groups with the broader population, it may be possible to elucidate nutritional factors that could explain variance in cancer risk. For example, some orders of English nuns who follow a vegetarian diet have been useful in exploring relationships between meat consumption and breast cancer risk. The nuns are celibate and therefore not reproductively active, so they represent a high-risk group for these tumours. As they also abstain from alcohol and tobacco smoking, the influence of diet can be studied in the absence of these other risk factors (Willett, 1990).

One group that has been extensively studied in this context is the Seventh Day Adventist population in the United States. This religious group is notable in that dietary practices are very varied. While some Adventists are omnivores, a high proportion are vegetarians, with many following a vegan lifestyle. The very wide range of intakes of many different nutrients, coupled to low rates of smoking and other risk exposures, makes the Adventists an attractive group to consider the dietary determinants of cancer (Willett, 2003). Adventists have low rates of colon and lung cancers but higher rates of breast and prostate cancers than the broader US population, and this has promoted interest in the contribution of red meat consumption to tumours at these sites. Some Adventists are prodigious consumers of milk and dairy products and so are a useful group to study when considering relationships between these foods and cancer risk. The Adventist Health Study 2 prospective cohort study reported cancer incidence rates among 69 120 Adventists with varying dietary habits (Tantamango-Bartley *et al.*, 2013). In this low-risk group for cancer, it was found that a lacto-ovo vegetarian diet was associated with lower risk of gastrointestinal cancers (HR 0.72, 0.61–0.86).

8.4.5.3.4 Case–control studies

Case–control studies have been a valuable investigative tool for considering relationships between diet and cancer. Essentially, in a case–control study, researchers will recruit subjects who have been diagnosed with the disease of interest. These cases will then be compared to a suitably matched control group without the disease to ascertain the factors that could explain why the cases but not the controls developed the disease. For example, Taylor and colleagues (2007) studied 35 372 women, of whom 1750 developed malignant breast cancers. Using a case–control analysis, it was shown that after adjustment for known confounding factors, postmenopausal women who consumed the highest amounts of meat had significantly greater risk of breast cancer than those who consumed no meat at all (HR 1.10, 95% CI 1.01–1.20).

There are a number of important problems with this approach that can undermine confidence in any findings. Firstly, the recruiting of suitable control populations is often fraught with difficulty, and case–control studies are highly vulnerable to influences of confounding factors. It is impossible to exclude the possibility that control subjects are undiagnosed cases or cases waiting to happen. Finally, all exposure data (i.e. data relating to diet) is either collected well after the period during which carcinogenesis was initiated or has to be collected retrospectively. Asking subjects to recall their typical diet from a decade previously is bound to introduce considerable bias to a study.

8.4.5.3.5 Cohort studies

Prospective cohort studies that are able to follow a population over an extended period of time provide a very powerful tool for examining relationships between diet and cancer. Prospective cohorts require very large populations (tens of thousands of people) to be recruited to allow for the fact that specific cancers are actually uncommon events. Baseline data on diet and other exposures can be collected at the start of the study and at intervals thereafter. These data can then be related to the occurrence of disease over the duration of the study. Although many prospective studies are plagued by inaccurate estimation of the exposure data in the initial stages, there are several major prospective cohorts that have informed much of what we know about diet–cancer relationships.

The US Nurses' Health Study (Colditz and Hankinson, 2005) began to collect data on diet and alcohol consumption among US women in 1980 and has included over 80 000 subjects. By sustaining the follow-up of these women over three decades, it has proved possible to investigate the role of diet in the etiology of many cancers and other disease states. The Nurses' Health Study is one of the key studies that have shown the proposed relationship between fat intake and risk of breast cancer to be fallacious. The EPIC cohort was established in 1992 and by 2006 had recruited 521 448 individuals across 23 centres in 10 European countries (Gonzalez, 2006). The chief advantage of such a large study is that the actual number of cancer cases will be high, which greatly increases the chances of observing diet–cancer relationships. EPIC used a range of dietary assessment methods to obtain baseline data from participants and was designed to follow-up for at least 20 years.

8.4.5.3.6 Intervention studies

Intervention studies are arguably the most effective tool for studying the relationship between any dietary component and cancer risk. Typically, an intervention will seek to provide volunteers with a diet that is either supplemented with a putative protective factor or which has a reduced content of a suspected harmful agent. The volunteers can then be followed up over a period of time to assess the impact on cancer risk. Many of these very expensive intervention trials have been performed to assess efficacy of antioxidants, dietary fibre and other

agents in cancer prevention, but despite their power, many of the trials have proven inconclusive or have yielded results of an unexpected nature. For example, the CARET trial was an intervention trial in which supplements of β-carotene were provided to smokers and other individuals at high risk of lung cancer. The trial was abandoned at an early stage when it was noted that the supplements actually increased rather than decreased cancer mortality (Omenn *et al.*, 1996). It is thought that this occurred because although vitamin A may block carcinogenesis at the initiation stage, it may accelerate the progression of tumours at the proliferation and invasion stages (Research Highlight 8.3).

The CARET experience highlights some of the main drawbacks of almost all diet–cancer intervention trials. Most trials, for reasons of good scientific method, seek to only manipulate subjects' intakes of a single nutrient. This instantly renders them unrepresentative of a typical human diet. Moreover, selected doses are often ill considered. As cancer will generally develop very slowly, perhaps taking decades to progress from actual critical exposure to clinically significant stages, most intervention studies will save time and cost in following up volunteers who are at high risk. It is commonplace, for example, to recruit individuals who have previously been treated for a cancer and who are at high risk of recurrence. Again, this is not representative of the population and their risk in relation to diet.

8.4.5.3.7 Cancer risk is a product of the whole diet

All of the approaches to the study of diet–cancer relationships outlined earlier suffer from a common limitation in that they generally fail to take into account the ways in which nutrients interact with each other, with the genes carried by individuals and with other risk factors in the environment (Figure 8.17). Humans consume foods with mixed and variable components, not single nutrients in isolation. It is therefore overly simplistic to assume that intakes of a single nutrient are representative of the whole range of dietary and environmental exposures experienced by individuals. The CARET study described earlier typifies this and highlights the fact that nutritional factors impact on cancer risk at all stages of the development and progression of the disease. As shown in Figure 8.18, just the progression from a damaged cell to a cell with cancerous potential during the initiation phase of cancer is influenced by interactions of genetics and lifestyle. These can be both pro-cancer and anti-cancer in nature.

The human diet comprises varied mixtures of foods, each providing different combinations of nutrients, prepared in a variety of different ways. This means that within each food and within each meal, there is

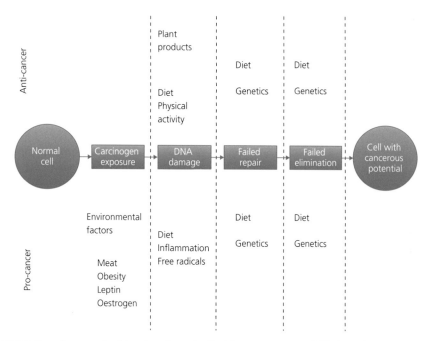

Figure 8.18 The progression of a normal cell to a transformed cell with cancerous potential is dependent upon DNA damage, a failure to repair that damage and the evasion of systems that eliminate damaged cells. Environmental factors, including diet, interact with genetic factors at all stages of the process.

considerable scope for interactions between nutrients and between nutrients and the non-nutrient components of foodstuffs (Gerber, 2001). Having a varied diet is desirable as it increases the chances that a broad array of protective agents will be ingested and minimizes the risk of repetitive exposure to harmful factors. As such, it will be the combinations of factors in the habitual diet of any individual that confer cancer risk, rather than intakes of specific nutrients or foods. For example, in relation to colon cancer risk, a diet high in processed and red meats, high in refined sugars and high in fat carries significantly greater risk than one high in fish, legumes, vegetables and fresh fruits (Gerber, 2001). These are complex dietary patterns, and it is challenging to ascertain where the difference lies. Is the reduced risk associated with the latter diet due to the lower intake of meat or saturated fats, or could it be explained by greater intakes of antioxidants from plant materials? Almost certainly it is a combination of these factors that provides the observed benefit.

Despite these concerns about methodology and the limitations of considering single nutrients as risk factors, it still remains tempting and desirable to pick out the contributions of different components of the overall diet to cancer risk. Clear identification of factors, or combinations of factors, that may increase or decrease risk will

help to refine dietary guidelines given to populations and will inform the design of future dietary interventions. There is now a new approach to thinking about diet and cancer relationships, moving the focus away from specific micro- or macronutrients towards broader classes of foodstuffs. As shown in Table 8.7, the 2007 World Cancer Research Fund (WCRF) report on food, nutrition and cancer indicates that the main risk factors for cancer are obesity, alcohol consumption and meat consumption, while physical activity and a prudent diet based upon fruits, vegetables and foods rich in dietary fibre reduce risk.

8.4.5.4 Dietary factors that may promote cancer
8.4.5.4.1 Obesity
Excessive weight gain and body fatness, whether attributable to poor diet, low physical activity levels or both, are firmly associated with cancers at all sites around the body. The 2007 WCRF report on food, nutrition and cancer linked low levels of physical activity, higher BMI and greater waist–hip ratio (proxy for abdominal obesity) to postmenopausal breast cancer cancers of the colon, oesophagus, pancreas, endometrium and kidney (Table 8.8). Findings from EPIC indicated a greater risk of colon cancer in both men and women associated with greater waist circumference or waist–hip ratio

Table 8.7 Associations between diet and lifestyle factors and specific cancers.

Tumour site	Decreased risk	Increased risk
Mouth/pharynx/ larynx	Non-starchy vegetables, fruit, foods rich in carotenoids	Alcoholic beverages
Nasopharynx		Cantonese-style salted fish
Oesophagus	Non-starchy vegetables, fruit, foods rich in beta-carotene or vitamin C	Alcoholic beverages, body fatness
Lung	Fruits, foods rich in carotenoids	Beta-carotene supplements
Stomach	Allium vegetables, non-starchy vegetables	Salted foods
	Fruit	Salt
Pancreas	Foods rich in folate	Body fatness, abdominal fatness
Liver		Alcoholic beverages, aflatoxins
Colorectal	Physical activity, foods containing dietary fibre, milk, garlic	Alcoholic beverages, red meat, processed meat, body fatness
Kidney		Body fatness
Prostate	Foods containing lycopene or selenium	Diets high in calcium
Endometrium	Physical activity	Body fatness and abdominal fatness
Premenopausal breast	Body fatness	Alcoholic beverages
Postmenopausal breast	Physical activity	Alcohol, body fatness

World Cancer Research Fund (2007) report considers evidence for these factors being associated with cancer to be convincing or probable.

(Pischon *et al.*, 2006). Risk was increased in men when comparing the highest and lowest quintiles of BMI (HR 1.55, 1.12–2.15). The American Cancer Society Prospective Cohort (Calle *et al.*, 2003) showed, in a population of 900 000 men and women, that risk of death from cancer at all sites was increased by almost twofold by obesity, with the greatest effects noted for kidney and uterine cancers in women and for liver cancer in men. Risk of breast cancer was reported to be reduced by up to 80% in highly active women compared to sedentary women in the study of Cerhan *et al.* (1998), and similarly, Zhang *et al.* (2006) found lower risk of colon cancer in men and women with high occupational or recreational activity. As shown in Figure 8.19, Bergstrom *et al.* (2001) estimated that 6.4% of all female and 3.4% of all male cancer cases in Europe were attributable to overweight and obesity. Given the shifts in prevalence of obesity occurring around the world as developing countries

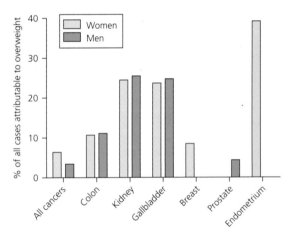

Figure 8.19 Contribution of obesity and overweight to cancer risk in European men and women. *Data Source*: Bergstrom *et al.* (2001).

Table 8.8 Estimates of risk of cancer associated with high BMI.

Cancer site	Summary estimate RR (95%CI) per 1 kg/m²	Summary estimate RR (95%CI) per 2 kg/m²	Summary estimate RR (95%CI) per 5 kg/m²
Oesophageal	1.11 (1.07–1.15)		
Colon	1.03 (1.02–1.04)		
Breast (premenopause)		0.94 (0.92–0.95)	
Breast (postmenopause)		1.05 (1.05–1.06)	
Endometrium			1.56 (1.45–1.66)
Kidney			1.31 (1.24–1.39)
Gall bladder			1.23 (1.15–1.32)

Data Source: World Cancer Research Fund (2007).

take on Westernized patterns of food intake, leisure and employment, there is likely to be a large rise in the prevalence of these cancers on a global scale (Popkin, 2007).

The mechanisms through which obesity increases cancer risk are varied and largely unidentified and may be specific to each tumour site. Obese individuals produce greater background concentrations of pro-inflammatory cytokines, and in tissues such as the colon, the presence of a persistent, low-level inflammation will increase risk of tumour growth. Obesity is also associated with insulin resistance and raised concentrations of sex steroids and insulin-like growth factor 1. All of these factors will promote the growth and metabolic activity of tumour cells and hence drive the proliferative and invasion phases of cancer.

Breast cancer risk is strongly related to the duration of production of oestrogens. As described in Chapter 2, obesity in childhood is associated with an earlier menarche and hence a longer phase of oestrogen production, while obesity beyond the menopause will allow for oestrogen production beyond the phase of normal ovarian function. The association between female BMI and breast cancer risk is dependent on stage of life. Premenopausal women of greater BMI are apparently protected against breast cancer (WCRF, 2007), with some studies suggesting that BMI of 30 or greater may halve risk. However, in postmenopausal women, there is a significant increase in risk, particularly with central adiposity. Oestrogens are produced beyond the menopause through the action of aromatases in adipose tissue that convert androgens to a range of oestrogen metabolites. Insulin resistance associated with obesity increases the production of androgens and hence drives this process. Oestrogens are mitogenic and will promote tumour growth. It is suggested that before the menopause, the actions of oestrogens are opposed by progesterone, but following the menopause, this protective action of progesterone will be lost. The association of obesity with breast cancer mortality may also be explained by delays in recognizing symptoms and detecting breast lumps at an early stage of cancer due to the accumulation of fatty tissue in the breasts.

Effects of body fatness upon cancer risk may vary within a tissue. Organs and tissues are not homogenous and comprise varied cell types that may give rise to different types of tumour with differing origins and risk factors. Oesophageal cancers, for example, may be squamous cell carcinomas (derived from epithelial cells) or adenocarcinomas (derived from glandular cells). Both types of tumour are related to direct exposures to carcinogens entering the gastrointestinal tract (e.g. alcohol, tobacco smoke). While squamous carcinomas of the oesophagus are related to infection by the human papillomavirus,

adenocarcinomas are associated with obesity. This may be driven through greater gastric reflux with greater abdominal fat deposition.

8.4.5.4.2 Fat intake

Ecological studies generally show that in populations with higher intakes of fat, there is greater prevalence of cancers of the breast, colon and lung. These studies typically support findings from animal studies that consistently show that high-fat diets increase susceptibility to chemically induced carcinogenesis in the colon and mammary glands. However, these experimental and ecological observations do not stand up to robust analytical approaches in nutritional epidemiology, and the balance of opinion is that dietary fat has little impact on cancer risk in humans. There is no basis for any advice to reduce fat intake in order to prevent cancer, nor to modify the profile of fats consumed. Avoidance of obesity should be a higher priority (Kushi and Giovannucci, 2002).

The breast was one site at which possible links between cancer and fat intake were identified in early studies (WCRF, 1997). To some extent, the meta-analysis of case–control studies performed by Howe and colleagues (1990) supported this view, as it found that increasing intakes of total fat by 100 g/day would increase risk of breast cancer by approximately 40%. Given that typical daily intakes among Western populations are only of the order of 70–80 g/day, the benefits of a modest reduction in fat intake are likely to be minor. Willett (2001) reviewed the findings of prospective cohort studies with follow-ups of up to 8 years' duration. No evidence of risk was observed in relation to either total fat or saturated fat intakes. The 14-year follow-up of the US Nurses' Health Study (Holmes *et al.*, 1999) found that there was no evidence of any risk of breast cancer associated with four different measures of fat intake. Even at very low intakes of fat (less than 20% of energy intake), there was no evidence of benefit, and in fact, a slightly higher risk of breast cancer was noted in such women.

Some animal studies have identified MUFA and n–3 fatty acids derived from fish oils as possibly having a protective role in breast and colorectal cancers (CRC). Although some studies from Southern Europe support the concept that olive oils may reduce risk of breast cancer, the evidence is insufficient to make a definitive statement on this. Engeset *et al.* (2006) considered the impact of fish consumption on breast cancer risk in women from the EPIC cohort. Highest intakes of fatty fish, that is, the fish with the greatest n–3 content, were associated with an increased risk of breast cancer. The WCRF expert report (2007) concluded that there is only limited evidence that intake of fats and oils is associated with postmenopausal breast cancer and lung cancer or that animal fat is associated with CRC. High fat intakes are only of relevance to cancer in terms of their impact upon body weight and fatness.

8.4.5.4.3 Meat

The initial interest in meat consumption as a risk factor for cancer stemmed from observational studies that suggested that high intakes of animal protein and saturated fat increased risk. However, it is now believed that formation of nitrosamines and heterocyclic amines during the cooking and preservation of meats is the main vehicle through which meat products contribute to cancer risk. Although there is some limited evidence that meat intake is associated with risk of cancers of the lung, oesophagus, endometrium, stomach and prostate, the main association is with CRC when there is convincing evidence that high intakes of red meat and processed meat play a causal role (WCRF, 2007). Processed meats include all products that are preserved either by curing, salting, smoking or the addition of nitrates and nitrites.

Several cohort studies have shown an increased risk of CRC associated with meat consumption. A large study of male health professionals in the United States (Giovannucci *et al.*, 2004) found that regular consumption of meat increased risk (relative risk (RR) 3.6) compared to rare or infrequent consumption of meat. Processed meat and red meats are generally identified as the main contributor to risk, with white meat (poultry) apparently having little or no impact. The meta-analysis of the WCRF (2007) found that the RR for CRC for every 100 g/day red meat intake was 1.29 (95% CI

1.05–1.59) and for processed meat was 1.21 for every 50 g/day intake (95% CI 1.04–1.44). Current advice is that intakes of red meat should be limited to 500 g/week (cooked weight) with avoidance of processed meats (WCRF, 2008).There is no convincing evidence that poultry, fish or egg intake is related to cancer risk.

As stated earlier, red and processed meat may directly deliver carcinogens formed during preservation and cooking to the body, and these are believed to play a major role in CRC. As shown in Figure 8.20, the high iron content of red meat may also play a role as iron has the potential to drive the generation of ROS. Meat is also an energy-dense food, so high consumption can lead to weight gain.

Heterocyclic amines are formed in the cooking of all meats, including poultry, so the lack of evidence linking consumption of white meats to cancer is perplexing. The explanation may be that peptides derived from red, but not white, meats undergo metabolism in the colon, greatly increasing their mutagenicity. *N*-nitrosation generates *N*-methyl-*N*-nitroso compounds that form adducts with DNA. Many of these adducts are excised during DNA repair processes and can be detected in the colon as a marker of carcinogenic processes. Lewin *et al.* (2007) studied healthy volunteers who were allocated to consume either a vegetarian diet or a diet rich in red meat. In a third element of the study, the high meat intake was supplemented with fibre. Shedding of cells containing the adduct O^6-carboxymethyl guanine was determined in faecal samples. As shown in Figure 8.21, the high-meat diet greatly increased this marker of

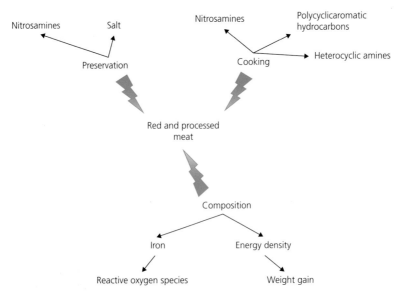

Figure 8.20 Possible routes from meat intake to colorectal cancer.

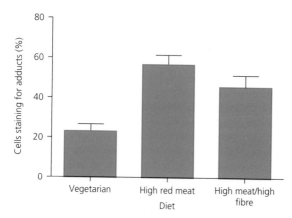

Figure 8.21 Healthy volunteers consumed vegetarian, high-meat or high-meat/high-fibre diets for periods of 10 days. Exfoliated colonic cells shed in faecal matter were stained for 0^6-carboxymethyl guanine. Meat increased appearance of these positive cells and fibre partially offset this effect. *Data Source*: Lewin *et al.* (2007).

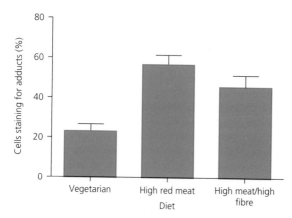
(y-axis) Cells staining for adducts (%)
(x-axis) Vegetarian | High red meat | High meat/high fibre
Diet

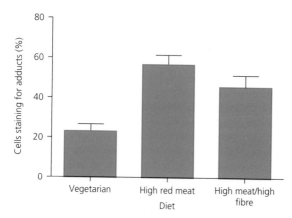

carcinogenic processes, and high-fibre intake partially offset this effect. Thus, delivery of N-nitroso compounds to the colon may be an important means through which red meat increases risk of CRC.

8.4.5.4.4 Alcohol

Levels of alcohol consumption are extremely varied both across and within global populations. While some groups never consume alcoholic beverages, there are others where around 10% of energy is consumed as alcohol. Consumption is increasing steadily in many Westernized countries. Across Europe, the estimated per capita intake is over 12.5 l of pure alcohol per annum (World Health Organization, 2013b), with lower consumption (10–12.49 l in Australia and 7.5–9.99 l in North America). In the United Kingdom, for example, overall alcohol consumption in women increased by 16% between 1992 and 2005 (General Household Survey, 2006), and the proportion of women consuming more than the recommended 14 units per week increased by 50% over a similar period. Thirty-six percent of English adults reported consuming more than the recommended limits (21 units per week for men, 14 units per week for women) in 2013 (Health and Social Care Information Centre, 2013). These trends are a major concern as globally alcohol consumption is associated with 2.5 million deaths per annum (World Health Organization, 2013b) and alcohol has been positively identified as a carcinogen in humans.

There is convincing evidence that alcohol consumption is a risk factor for cancers of the mouth, pharynx, larynx, oesophagus, breast (pre- and postmenopause)

and colon and rectum (in men), and it is probably causally associated with cancers of the liver, colon and rectum (in women; WCRF, 2007). The mechanisms of action proposed include direct DNA damage by ethanol and acetaldehyde, the main product of alcohol degradation in the liver; activation of microsomal phase I metabolism; and delivery of other carcinogens that may be present in alcoholic beverages, such as nitrosamines. Alcohol is associated with generation of ROS. It is also suggested that alcohol in drinks may increase the bioavailability of ethanol-soluble carcinogens across the digestive tract.

Most epidemiological studies suggest that risk of breast cancer increases with alcohol consumption although care has to be taken in adjusting analysis for tobacco smoking as a confounder and consumption of alcoholic beverages is often under-reported. Meta-analysis of well-designed cohort studies (Smith-Warner *et al.*, 1998) showed that for every 10 g/day increase in alcohol consumption, risk of breast cancer rose by 9%. Risk of oesophageal and other head and neck cancers is increased by up to tenfold in heavy drinkers (over 80 g alcohol per day), a hazard that is further increased by cigarette smoking. Analyses compiled for the WCRF (2007) indicated dose–response relationships between consumption of alcoholic beverages and risk of cancers of the mouth, pharynx and larynx (RR 1.03, 1.02–1.06 per drink per week) and oesophagus (RR 1.04, 1.03–1.05 per drink per week). In men, risk of CRC increased over a threshold of 30 g alcohol per week (RR 1.09, 1.03–1.14 per 10 g alcohol per week). Analyses suggest that all alcoholic beverages (beer, wine, spirits) carry equal risk for all cancer sites where data are available.

Rehm *et al.* (2007) performed a systematic review of the literature that examined whether this risk could be ameliorated through cessation of drinking. As shown in Figure 8.22, alcohol consumption increased risk of oesophageal cancer by 2.7-fold compared to subjects who never consumed alcohol. Cessation of drinking produced an initial increase in risk, which is also seen in relation to breast cancer (Willett, 2001), but by 5 years postcessation of drinking significant health benefits became apparent.

8.4.5.4.5 Specific carcinogens in food

Foodstuffs deliver a huge range of chemical agents that are not normally regarded as nutrients to the body. Some of these are present as contaminants, entering the food chain during production and preparation; others are generated during the process of cooking. In addition, there is a vast array of agents that are the products of the complex secondary metabolism of plants. As will be described in the following, some of the non-nutrient

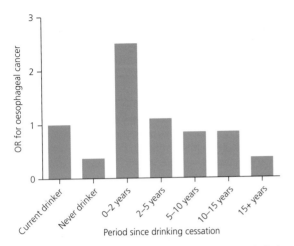

Figure 8.22 Risk of oesophageal cancer associated with alcohol consumption is significantly higher when comparing current drinkers to individuals who have never consumed alcohol. Cessation of alcohol drinking initially increases risk of cancer but over the longer term restores risk to the equivalent of never drinking.
Data Source: Rehm *et al.* (2007).

components of food may have anti-cancer properties. It is also the case that some of these factors are directly carcinogenic and if consumed in excess may directly promote the development of primary tumours.

A simple test was developed by Bruce Ames and colleagues in the 1970s to screen potential carcinogenic agents from food or from other sources. The Ames Test assesses the mutagenic capacity of compounds and works on the assumption that any agent capable of damaging DNA will have the potential to have carcinogenic effects. The test involves growing mutant strains of *Salmonella typhimurium* that lack genes for key enzymes involved in amino acid metabolism, on media lacking those amino acids (Figure 8.23). Any colonies that grow in the presence of a suspected carcinogen must have undergone mutation to be able to utilize the limiting medium and therefore signal that the test chemical is a mutagen. The number of colonies that grow will provide an index of how potent a mutagen, the agent, is. Many compounds that are not carcinogens could produce a positive Ames Test result, and some carcinogens that only become active when

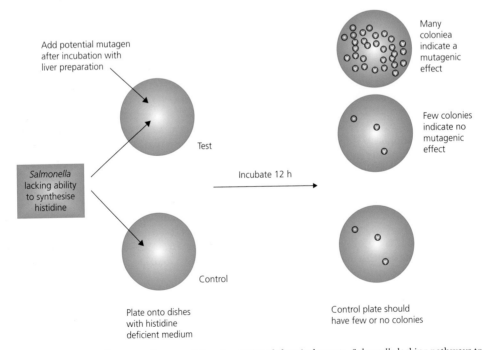

Figure 8.23 The Ames Test is used to assess the potential mutagenicity of chemical agents. *Salmonella* lacking pathways to synthesize histidine are plated onto histidine-free medium. Bacterial growth can only occur if mutation reinstates the synthetic pathway. Refinements of the Ames Test include a pre-incubation of suspected mutagens with mammalian liver in order to generate phase I metabolites, which may be mutagenic in their own right.

metabolized within the human body (e.g. B(a)P) give a negative Ames Test result. The main disadvantage of the Ames Test is that the test organism is a prokaryote, and thus, it is a poor model for studying potential harm to humans. The test can be improved by using eukaryotic yeast cells instead of bacteria and by adding extracts of rodent liver to the test medium to introduce hepatic phase I and phase II xenobiotic metabolism (Figure 8.23).

There are some important Ames Test-positive agents that can regularly appear in the human food chain and promote carcinogenesis. Several such agents are present in commonly consumed herbs. Basil and tarragon, for example, deliver estragole, while comfrey contains carcinogenic alkaloids. Generally speaking, however, these agents are not consumed in significantly large amounts and risk is negligible. The same is true of safrole – a compound found in cinnamon and nutmeg. In Taiwan, however, the habit of chewing betel is associated with oesophageal cancer. Betel is essentially ground areca nut mixed with leaves and lime to form a chewable quid that has a high safrole content. Safrole is also present in peppercorns, which are used to produce the pepper used in cooking and as a condiment in most Western cuisines. Red peppers and chilli peppers have their characteristic flavour due to the presence of capsaicin. Capsaicin is mutagenic when subjected to the Ames Test and has been shown to be carcinogenic in animal studies. Archer and Jones (2002) studied different ethnic groups in the United States, where capsaicin-containing peppers are widely used in Mexican, Creole and Cajun cooking. Evidence was found to relate high consumption of capsaicin to increased risk of stomach cancer.

A variety of fungal toxins are known to be potent carcinogens, providing a concern over some foods grown in the tropics. Peanuts, for example, can be a source of aflatoxins, which are highly active liver carcinogens (WCRF, 2007). Ochratoxins are also fungal contaminants, arising through development of mildews on cereal crops. While controls over the quality of imported peanuts and other foods from at-risk areas minimize aflatoxin and ochratoxin exposures of Western populations, in the developing world, contamination of staple foods is widespread. Most contamination occurs after harvest due to storage in unventilated, hot and humid conditions with poor hygiene. Maize and groundnut crops are particularly at risk, and consumption of these staples in West Africa is associated with high circulating concentrations of aflatoxin–albumin adducts in both children and adults (Egal et al., 2005). Simple procedures to reduce contamination such as sun-drying of crops and storage in natural-fibre bags can reduce exposure in affected areas (Turner et al., 2005).

8.4.5.5 Dietary factors that may reduce cancer risk
8.4.5.5.1 Complex carbohydrates

Much of the literature that discusses the associations between complex carbohydrates and risk of cancer will refer to the influence of dietary fibre. Dietary fibre is a term that is perhaps better replaced, as it is more appropriate to discuss the influence of non-starch polysaccharides and insoluble starches. The complex carbohydrates within the human diet are a diverse group of materials that share the common property of resisting digestion and hence are able to pass through the digestive tract to the colon relatively unchanged. The complex carbohydrates include cellulose from plant materials, insoluble starches (largely of vegetable or cereal origin), lignans (of vegetable origin), phytoestrogens and chitin (from fungal cell walls and shellfish). 'Fibre' is therefore not a single substance, and the effects of fibre reported in the literature should be expected to vary according to the source of the material in the diet, as the composition of fruit, vegetable or cereal-derived fibre will differ considerably. There is an extensive literature that links higher consumption of complex carbohydrates to lower risk of cancer at several sites. It is difficult to isolate dietary fibre as a beneficial component of the diet, as individuals who have higher intakes of these complex carbohydrates from plant materials will also tend to have lower intakes of meat and the associated putative carcinogenic agents described earlier.

It is widely reported that complex carbohydrate consumption reduces the risk of cancers of the breast and ovary in women. These cancers are largely driven by hormonal factors, which implies that complex carbohydrates may somehow modify the production of oestrogens beyond the menopause, which is the major risk factor for these cancers. Certainly, feeding high-fibre diets to rodents protects the animals against development of chemically induced mammary tumours, and the meta-analyses of case–control studies in human populations suggests that a 20g/day increase in fibre intake would reduce risk of breast cancer by approximately 15% (Howe et al., 1990). However, large prospective cohort studies, including the US Nurses' Health Study, have suggested that there is little benefit associated with increased intakes of complex carbohydrates with respect to breast cancer (Willett, 2001). Interventions in which women have made lifestyle changes favouring a low-fat–high-fibre diet have produced small reductions in risk of breast cancer over follow-up periods of around

8–10 years, but these may be attributed more to the associated weight and body fat loss than to specific effects of complex carbohydrates (Forman, 2007).

Case–control studies spanning more than 40 years have suggested that higher intakes of complex carbohydrates, particularly those of vegetable rather than cereal origin, are associated with lower risk of CRC. However, these observations are not supported by all large prospective cohort studies performed in European and US settings. The Nurses' Health Study, for example, found that there was no difference in CRC risk between groups with the highest compared to the lowest intakes of dietary fibre (Fuchs *et al.*, 1999), and in fact, the highest intakes of vegetable fibre were actually associated with a 35% increase in CRC risk. Kato *et al.* (1997) reported no association between dietary fibre intake and CRC, a finding echoed by the Netherlands Cohort Study (Wark *et al.*, 2005). This prospective study of 120 852 people found that dietary fibre intake was not associated with risk of two types of colon tumour. A pooled analysis of 13 prospective cohorts concluded that an inverse association between fibre intake and CRC risk was present, but that this was explained by other dietary risk factors. In addition to this apparent indication that the case–control data were misleading, a number of intervention trials of dietary fibre supplementation found that administration of fibre to individuals with previous history of CRC failed to prevent either tumour recurrence or short-/medium-term survival (Alberts *et al.*, 2000).

Support for a protective effect of complex carbohydrates against CRC has been provided by the EPIC study. With over half a million participants across 10 different countries, EPIC had unprecedented power to consider any putative diet–cancer association. The heterogeneity of diets between European countries means that the range of nutrient intakes is extremely broad, which enhances the prospects of detecting significant influences. As reviewed by Bingham (2006), EPIC found that when comparing dietary fibre intakes in the highest quintile (mean 35 g/day) with the lowest quintile (15 g/day), the RR for CRC was 0.58 (95% CI 0.41–0.85), with beneficial effects of fibre becoming apparent at intakes of around 20 g/day. The main benefit in this study appeared to be associated with intakes of cereal fibre. Risk of CRC is obviously determined by complex interactions of nutrients and other factors. The EPIC study was able to assess some of these interactions and noted that the greatest CRC risk was associated with the highest intakes of meat and lowest intakes of fibre, when compared to the lowest intakes of meat and highest intakes of fibre (Bingham, 2006). The WCRF (2007) analysis concluded that there is a probable benefit associated with higher intakes of fibre, with an RR of 0.90 (0.84–0.97) for each 10 g/day increment of intake.

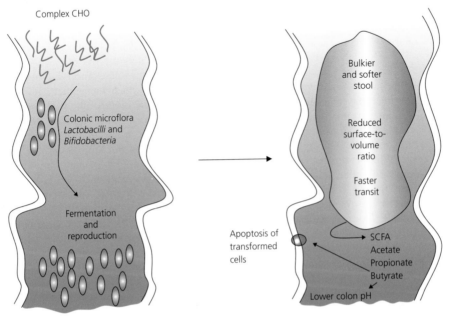

Figure 8.24 Proposed mechanism to explain the protective influence of complex carbohydrate in colorectal cancer. CHO, carbohydrate.

The mechanism through which complex carbohydrates are proposed to protect the colon from tumourigenesis is shown in Figure 8.24. Entry of complex carbohydrates into the large intestine provides substrates for the growth of the bacterial species that make up the colonic microflora. Fermentation of complex carbohydrates is associated with reproduction and metabolism of these organisms and has several beneficial side effects for the human host. Firstly, the presence of fibre itself within the faecal material has the effect of bulking up the stool, but this is further enhanced by accumulation of bacteria and retention of water. The larger and softer stool that results is more rapidly moved through the colon, and this reduced transit time minimizes the length of time that potential carcinogens will be present within the colon. The larger stool also has a reduced surface area to volume ratio, which effectively means that any carcinogenic agents are more likely to be buried within the faecal material rather than on an exterior surface that might come into contact with the colonic mucosal cells. The fermentation of the complex carbohydrates by the microflora will also generate short-chain fatty acids (SCFA), which include butyrate, propionate and acetate. This reduces the pH of the colon, which reduces the likelihood of inflammation of the mucosa. More importantly, butyrate is an inducer of apoptosis and inhibits the transformation of cells in the colonic epithelium (Chai *et al.*, 2000). Thus, utilization of complex carbohydrate by bacteria generates potent anti-tumour agents within the human colon. The nature of the carbohydrates reaching the colon may determine the profile of bacterial species present, and some of the more soluble complex carbohydrates have been proposed to favour the growth of beneficial *Bifidobacteria* over other species such as *Escherichia coli* or *Bacteroides* (Slavin, 2003).

The functional food industry exploits the fibre–CRC relationship and markets two classes of product on the basis of their potential protective properties. Probiotic foods supply bacterial species such as *Lactobacilli* directly to the gut with the intention of boosting fermentation by species that generate SCFA. Prebiotics are complex carbohydrates such as inulin or fructooligosaccharides that are intended to enter the colon and selectively stimulate the reproduction of *Lactobacilli* and *Bifidobacteria*.

Another explanation of the protective effects of complex carbohydrates in the colon is that foods that are rich in fibre will also deliver other cancer-preventive compounds. Folate, for example, will tend to be consumed in greater quantities with fibre-rich foods. There is also a wide range of non-nutrient compounds present in plants that have anti-tumour and tumour-suppressing properties, and these could confound the apparent relationship between CRC and fibre.

8.4.5.5.2 Milk and dairy produce

Milk and dairy produce represent the main source of bioavailable calcium within the human diet and play an important role in maintaining bone health (see Chapter 9). There is now sufficient evidence to conclude that higher intakes are associated with lower risk of CRC. Meta-analysis of 10 cohort studies indicated a substantial reduction in CRC risk when comparing the highest and lowest intakes (RR 0.78, 0.69–0.88; WCRF, 2007). This reduction in risk appears to be largely attributable to calcium intake. Slob *et al.* (1993) reported that in a 28-year follow-up of a Dutch cohort, calcium intakes were significantly lower in men and women who subsequently died of CRC. Similarly, Garland and colleagues (1985) reported that risk of CRC was more than doubled in men in the lowest quartile of calcium intake compared to the highest quartile. It is estimated that increasing calcium intake by 200 mg/day reduces CRC risk by 5% (WCRF, 2007).

There is strong evidence, however, that in men high intakes of calcium significantly increase risk of prostate cancer and, in particular, aggressive metastatic prostate cancers. An 8-year prospective cohort study (Giovannucci *et al.*, 1998) found that intakes of more than 2 g calcium/day (from supplements and food) were associated with almost threefold greater risk of prostate cancer relative to intakes of 500 mg/day or less.

8.4.5.5.3 Antioxidant nutrients

There is a very robust literature relating to the cancer-preventive properties of agents present in fruits and vegetables, and in fact, some of the most convincing evidence in cancer epidemiology relates to the strong inverse relationship between consuming diets rich in fruits and vegetables and risk of cancers at all sites. Ames and Wakimoto (2002) combined evidence from two major reviews of the evidence and concluded that 75% of all studies showed clear protective effects. Generally, a higher intake of fruits and vegetables had the potential to halve the risk of cancer, with most of the convincing data relating to squamous cell cancers of the digestive tract, lung and liver. Greatest benefits were noted for pancreatic and stomach cancers, while the only cancer showing little associated benefit was prostate cancer. The WCRF (2007) reported probable anti-cancer effects of non-starchy vegetables (mouth, pharynx and larynx, oesophagus and stomach cancer), fruit (mouth, pharynx and larynx, oesophagus, lung and stomach cancer), foods containing folate (pancreatic cancer), foods containing carotenoids (mouth, pharynx and larynx and lung cancer), foods containing beta-carotene (oesophageal cancer), foods containing lycopene (prostate cancer), foods containing vitamin C (oesophageal cancer) and foods containing selenium (prostate cancer). Fruits and vegetables are foodstuffs that deliver a very broad range of putative cancer-preventing nutrients and agents, including dietary fibre and folic acid. Most attention has focused on the possible impact of the antioxidant nutrients they deliver, most notably the vitamins A, C and E and selenium. These are proposed to primarily act through protection of DNA from oxidative damage mediated by ROS but may also prevent tumour formation and proliferation by other mechanisms. Quenching of ROS action will prevent some conversion of inactive precursors to active carcinogens. There is also some evidence that vitamin C and retinol have the capacity to induce apoptosis in tumour cells.

Foods rich in antioxidant nutrients are clearly beneficial in protecting against cancer at many sites. For example, fruit reduces risk of mouth, pharynx and laryngeal cancer by 28% for every 100 g/day intake (RR 0.72, 0.59–0.87), and consumption of raw vegetables is associated with lower risk of oesophageal cancer (RR 0.69, 0.58–0.83 per 50 g/day increment; WCRF, 2007). Green and yellow vegetable intakes are associated with substantial decreases in risk of stomach cancer. A 24-year follow-up of Norwegian men found that risk of mouth, pharynx and laryngeal cancer was reduced by 50% in those with the higher intakes of oranges (Kjaerheim *et al.*, 1998). Although it is now recognized that the benefits of these foods go beyond the delivery of the classical antioxidant nutrients (see 'Non-nutrient components of plant foodstuffs'), much of the literature has focused on these nutrients in an attempt to isolate factors that could be used as cancer-preventive supplements. In considering the associations between the antioxidant nutrients and cancer risk, it is necessary to dissociate the evidence from observational studies at the population level, based upon intake of food, and intervention trials using supplements, as these frequently yield widely contrasting results (Research Highlight 8.3). Vitamin E, for example, was first identified as potentially beneficial when rodent studies showed that it could prevent mammary tumour formation. However, in humans, there is no evidence of protection against breast cancer associated with normal ranges of intake. Higher vitamin C intakes are associated with lower prevalence of oesophageal cancer (WCRF, 2007), but there is no convincing evidence that there is any benefit at other sites or that the protection is present when vitamin C is taken as a supplement. Eighteen out of 19 case–control studies have shown that there is

reduced risk of adenocarcinoma of the oesophagus with higher intakes of citrus fruits, with the summary estimate of a 30% reduction in risk for each 50 g/day increment in intake.

The most effective specific antioxidant nutrients in relation to cancer risk are the carotenoids, notably those which are precursors of retinol (β-carotene, α-carotene and β-cryptoxanthin). Carotenoid-rich foods appear to provide protection against cancer of the lung, mouth, pharynx and larynx and oesophagus (WCRF, 2007). Intake of all carotenoids reduces risk of mouth, pharynx and larynx cancers and cuts risk of lung cancer by approximately 2% for every 1 mg increment of intake.

Higher intakes of foods containing β-carotene have been suggested to reduce risk of oesophageal cancer. Six out of 10 case–control studies showed significant beneficial effects. Valsecchi (1992), for example, reported a threefold difference in risk in subjects with an intake equivalent to less than 60 mg/month compared to 90 mg/month or more. Mayne and colleagues (2001) found that higher intakes of β-carotene were associated with around 50% reduction in risk of adenocarcinoma but not squamous cell carcinoma of the oesophagus in a US population of 743 oesophageal cancer cases and 687 controls.

Following on from the wealth of studies that suggest that the antioxidant components of fruit and vegetables account for at least some of the protective effects that accompany consumption of these foods, there have been a multitude of cancer intervention trials designed around supplementation with vitamins A, C and E and with selenium. The CARET trial mentioned earlier in this chapter typifies the null or often negative outcomes of such trials, with unexpectedly increased cancer mortality associated with supplementation. Almost all studies that have administered single antioxidant nutrients or combinations of antioxidant nutrients have failed to show the benefits predicted by case–control or other observational studies. The WCRF now lists β-carotene supplements as a causative factor for lung cancer (WCRF, 2007).

Bjelakovic *et al.* (2004) performed a meta-analysis of intervention trials performed to prevent gastrointestinal and liver cancers using antioxidants. Fourteen large randomized trials of over 170 000 individuals were considered, and no benefits of vitamins A, C and E or selenium were noted, regardless of whether they were given alone or in combination. In fact, there was evidence of an increase in death rates associated with supplementation (RR of death 1.06, 95% CI 1.02–1.10). This latter finding was supported by the work of Lawson *et al.* (2007) who considered risk of prostate cancer in a population of almost 300 000 US men. Men consuming seven doses of multivitamin supplements per week were at greater risk of fatal cancers (RR 1.98, 95% CI 1.07–3.66) than men who did not take supplements. Clearly, the benefits of fruit and vegetable intake cannot be solely attributed to their antioxidant content, and the promise of antioxidant supplement therapy in cancer prevention strategies cannot be realistically delivered.

One of the main reasons why antioxidant supplements fail to prevent cancer is most likely to be an arbitrary dose selection that may be considerably higher than required. At high concentrations, some antioxidants take on a pro-oxidant activity that would promote oxidative processes. Providing supplements of single nutrients shows a lack of consideration of the interactions between antioxidant nutrients and between the antioxidants and other components of the diet such as fibre, which may be critical in mediating the protective effects of plant-derived foodstuffs. It is also important to appreciate that ROS play a normal role in several processes, including the destruction of precancerous or cancerous cells. Inhibiting these processes may allow tumours to progress beyond the initiation stage of carcinogenesis (Bjelakovic and Gluud, 2007).

8.4.5.5.4 Folic acid

As with complex carbohydrates, a large proportion of the early cancer epidemiology literature identified that poor dietary intakes of folic acid were associated with increased risk of cancers at many sites, particularly the colon, lung, cervix and breast. Closer scrutiny of the data is, however, less convincing. With respect to cervical cancer, most of the evidence comes from case–control studies that have inadequately adjusted for other risk factors, and so there is no consensus on the role of folate (Powers, 2005). Meta-analyses suggest that while folate does not significantly impact on breast cancer risk, it may ameliorate the risk associated with high alcohol consumption. However, the mechanism for this effect is unclear as folate has been shown to have no effect on development of benign proliferative epithelial disorders of the breast, which are precursors of cancer (Cui *et al.*, 2007).

The epidemiological data appears more slightly robust with respect to CRC, and there are inverse relationships between both intakes and red blood cell concentrations of folate and CRC risk (Duthie *et al.*, 2004). Konings *et al.* (2002) followed up over 120 000 men and women in the Netherlands for 7 years and found that CRC risk was 34% lower for the highest quintile of folic acid intake compared to the lowest quintile of intake, but in men only. Porcelli *et al.* (1996) reported that the concentrations of plasma and red cell folate were lower in patients with existing CRC compared to healthy controls. There have also been a number of small intervention trials using folate that have provided suggestive, if not convincing, evidence of protective effects. Lashner *et al.* (1997), for example, studied a group of 98 individuals with ulcerative colitis, a condition that increases risk of neoplastic changes in the colon and of CRC. Folate supplements in this group reduced risk of neoplasia in a dose-dependent manner and appeared to reduce risk of CRC by 55%, although the effect was not statistically significant. WCRF (2007) stated that the data on folate and CRC was suggested but limited.

A small number of case–control and cohort studies have evaluated the relationship of folate-containing foods and pancreatic cancer. Meta-analysis of the cohorts suggested that folate may be beneficial when consumed from rich food sources including foods which have been fortified with folic acid. Each 100 µg increment reduced risk by 14% (WCRF, 2007).

Folate status is extensively determined by genotype for a number of polymorphisms of genes in the folic acid cycle, for example, the MTHFR C677T polymorphism described earlier in this chapter. Surprisingly, the TT variant of this polymorphism, which is associated with the lowest concentrations of folate in circulation, actually appears to be protective against CRC (Sharp and Little, 2004). The explanation for this paradox lies in the fact that two mechanisms may underlie the association between folate and cancer risk.

Both of the putative mechanisms of protection involve folate increasing the stability of DNA. Folate is critical in the synthesis of nucleotides, and poor folate status is associated with limited synthesis of thymine, and so instead, uracil is incorporated into DNA during cell replication or DNA repair processes. Uracil misincorporation promotes DNA strand breaks and is associated with cell transformation. Some regions of DNA may be more susceptible than others to uracil misincorporation, and rodent studies have suggested that the p53 tumour suppressor gene is especially sensitive to this misrepair (Kim *et al.*, 1996).

The other protective mechanism depends upon the role of folate in determining levels of DNA methylation. Methylation of DNA at CpG islands in promoter regions effectively silences the expression of key genes. Low folate status results in hypomethylation and activation of gene expression, and it is proposed that in susceptible individuals, this will result in the expression of normally silenced proto-oncogenes. While the TT polymorphism of MTHFR, which is associated with lower folate concentrations, may promote hypomethylation, individuals with this gene variant appear to be more effective at synthesizing nucleotides for DNA repair and therefore have lower levels of uracil misincorporation. This would explain why there are lower rates of CRC among the TT-carrying population (Duthie *et al.*, 2004).

8.4.5.5.5 Non-nutrient components of plant foodstuffs

As described earlier, non-starchy vegetables and fruits are recognized as having a cancer-preventive role within the diet. It is becoming clear that these benefits are not associated with compounds that are traditionally classed as nutrients. A wide range of putative cancer-preventive bioactive compounds are present within foods of plant origin. There is evidence from *in vitro* studies and animal models that these may be protective either against specific cancers or possibly all cancers, but as yet, little evidence exists to firmly support claims made regarding human disease.

The strongest evidence from human trials using specific plant compounds as opposed to whole foods relates to the protective role of allium vegetables in stomach cancer. The principal allium vegetables in the human diet are onions, garlic and chives, which have a distinctive flavour due to the presence of allicin and allyl sulphides. Higher consumption of these has been shown in many case–control studies to be associated with lower risk of stomach cancer. For example, De Stefani and colleagues (2001) reported that allium consumption was beneficial in a Uruguayan population (OR 0.56, 95% CI 0.34–0.92). It is estimated that the risk of stomach cancer

decreases with each 50 g increment in allium vegetable intake (WCRF, 2007). You *et al.* (2006), however, found no benefit associated with garlic extract supplementation over a 7-year follow-up in China. The mode of action for allium extracts remains unclear. As allicin has antimicrobial activity, it has been proposed that it protects against stomach cancer by limiting infection by *H. pylori*. There is, as yet, little evidence to support this assertion, and it has been noted that allicin also has direct antiproliferative activity in cell culture (Tyagi *et al.*, 2014).

Phytoestrogens such as the soy isoflavones are proposed to confer protection against breast cancer by modifying circulating oestrogen concentrations after the menopause. However, there is no convincing evidence of benefit seen in human populations (Willett, 2001), and phytoestrogens in the diet may simply contribute to the overall bulk of antioxidants that are delivered by plant foodstuffs. These antioxidants also include polyphenolic compounds, terpenoids (such as limonene) and the flavonoids (including quercetin and myricetin). These potent antioxidants may provide some protection against cancer by reducing oxidative damage to DNA. There are other modes of action though, and many of these compounds are known to inhibit mutagenicity in the Ames

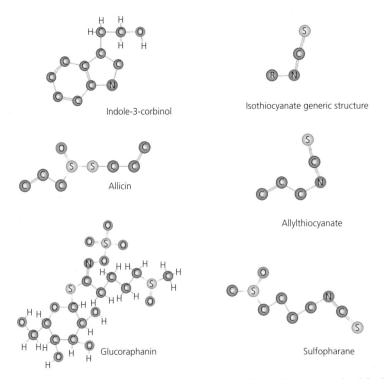

Figure 8.25 Plant-derived anti-cancer agents include a number of chemicals of the isothiocyanate and indole classes. Many of these are delivered in the diet as glucuronides (e.g. glucoraphanin) which are subsequently converted to isothiocyanates (sulphopharane).

Test, although curiously some of the flavonoids such as quercetin appear to be mutagens according to this test. Quercetin can act as conjugator of carcinogens within the digestive tract and hence reduce the bioavailability of harmful agents. Some phenolics also have the capacity to inhibit angiogenesis, thereby restricting the formation of new blood vessels around primary tumours and limiting the capacity for metastasis (Fresco *et al.*, 2006). Polyphenols have not been specifically studied in relation to human cancer, so the actual efficacy of such agents in cancer prevention is largely unknown.

Cruciferous vegetables (broccoli, Brussels sprouts, cauliflower, cabbage, cress, bok choy) in the diet are strongly associated with lower risk of cancer. These foods are rich in glucosinolates which are precursors of a range of compounds that have anti-cancer activity (Figure 8.25). Two major classes of glucosinolate derivatives have been identified: the isothiocyanates (e.g. sulphopharane) and the indoles (e.g. indole-3-carbinol). Isothiocyanates and indoles are present in plants as their glucosinolate conjugates, but chopping or chewing releases myrosinase which cleaves off the bioactive compounds (Houghton *et al.*, 2013; Razis and Noor, 2013). Sulphopharane is the product of glucoraphanin, while glucobrassicin is the precursor for indole-3-carbinol. Once ingested, the indoles and isothiocyanates undergo further transformation in the acid environment of the stomach, yielding many derivatives. The principal anti-cancer activity of the indoles and isothiocyanates derives from their effects upon xenobiotic metabolism. Isothiocyanates are potent inducers of glutathione-*S*-transferases and therefore activate phase II metabolism, while the indoles activate both phase I and phase II pathways. These compounds therefore increase the potential for cells to detoxify and eliminate xenobiotics prior to tumour initiation. There is also evidence of anti-tumour activity post-initiation. The indole-3-carbinol derivative diindolylmethane and sulphopharane have both been shown to induce apoptosis and limit cancer cell proliferation *in vitro*.

SUMMARY

- The adult years (19–65) are associated with decreasing energy requirements and therefore adjustment to a more nutrient-dense pattern of dietary intake. Undernutrition remains a significant issue among sub-populations, but for the majority of adults, a healthy diet and lifestyle aimed at preventing obesity and related metabolic disorders are a high priority.
- Obesity and overweight are increasing in prevalence all over the world due to greater availability of food and declining physical activity levels.
- Risk of type 2 diabetes is the product of an interaction between genetic factors and environmental influences. Obesity-related insulin resistance is the main feature of this condition.
- The metabolic syndrome represents a complex cluster of disorders including hypertension, renal dysfunction and disordered lipid and glucose metabolism. All of these disorders are driven by insulin resistance. The metabolic syndrome is a major risk factor for development of cardiovascular disease.
- Atherosclerosis is the process through which deposits of cholesterol and collagen in the arterial wall promote occlusion of blood flow and clot formation. This provides the fundamental basis of coronary heart disease, cerebrovascular disease and peripheral artery disease.
- The major dietary risk factors for CVD are high intakes of saturated fats, trans-fatty acids and sodium and obesity and related metabolic disorders. Increasing intakes of n-3 fatty acids, folic acid and plant-derived antioxidant nutrients may reduce risk.
- Cancer risk is strongly related to the overall quality of the diet. Risk is greatest with obesity and high intakes of red or processed meats and low intakes of fruits and vegetables.
- Attempts to identify specific dietary components that may be cancer preventive have been largely unsuccessful, and attention is now strongly focused upon the putative anti-tumour agents that are present in fruits and vegetables.

References

Abbey, M. (1995) The importance of vitamin E in reducing cardiovascular risk. *Nutrition Reviews*, **53**, S28–S32.

Action on Sugar (2014) Action on sugar http://www.actiononsugar. org (accessed May 2014).

Ajala, O., English, P. and Pinkney, J. (2013) Systematic review and meta-analysis of different dietary approaches to the management of type 2 diabetes. *American Journal of Clinical Nutrition*, **97**, 505–516.

Albanes, D., Heinonen, O.P., Taylor, P.R. *et al.* (1996) Alpha-Tocopherol and beta-carotene supplements and lung cancer incidence in the alpha-tocopherol, beta-carotene cancer prevention study: effects of base-line characteristics and study compliance. *Journal of the National Cancer Institute*, **88**, 1560–1570.

Alberti, K.G.M.M. and Zimmet, P.Z. (1998) Definition, diagnosis and classification of diabetes mellitus and its complications. Part 1: Diagnosis and classification of diabetes mellitus. Provisional report of a WHO consultation. *Diabetic Medicine*, **15**, 539–553.

Alberts, D.S., Martinez, M.E., Roe, D.J. *et al.* (2000) Lack of effect of a high-fiber cereal supplement on the recurrence of colorectal adenomas. Phoenix colon cancer prevention physicians' network. *New England Journal of Medicine*, **342**, 1156–1162.

Ames, B.N. and Wakimoto, P. (2002) Are vitamin and mineral deficiencies a major cancer risk? *Nature Reviews Cancer*, **2**, 694–704.

Apfelbaum, M., Vague, P., Ziegler, O. *et al.* (1999) Long-term maintenance of weight loss after a very-low-calorie diet: a randomized blinded trial of the efficacy and tolerability of sibutramine. *American Journal of Medicine*, **106**, 179–184.

Arab, L., Khan, F. and Lam, H. (2013) Tea consumption and cardiovascular disease risk. *American Journal of Clinical Nutrition*, **98** (6 Suppl), 1651S–1659S.

Archer, V.E. and Jones, D.W. (2002) Capsaicin pepper, cancer and ethnicity. *Medical Hypotheses*, **59**, 450–457.

Arguin, H., Dionne, I.J., Sénéchal, M. *et al.* (2012) Short- and long-term effects of continuous versus intermittent restrictive diet approaches on body composition and the metabolic profile in overweight and obese postmenopausal women: a pilot study. *Menopause*, **19**, 870–876.

Banegas, J.R., Lopez-Garcia, E., Gutierrez-Fisac, J.L. *et al.* (2003) A simple estimate of mortality attributable to excess weight in the European Union. *European Journal of Clinical Nutrition*, **57**, 201–208.

Bansilal, S., Farkouh, M.E. and Fuster, V. (2007) Role of insulin resistance and hyperglycemia in the development of atherosclerosis. *American Journal of Cardiology*, **99**, 6B–14B.

Bender, R., Zeeb, H., Schwarz, M. *et al.* (2006) Causes of death in obesity: relevant increase in cardiovascular but not in all-cancer mortality. *Journal of Clinical Epidemiology*, **59**, 1064–1071.

Bendsen, N.T., Christensen, R., Bartels, E.M. *et al.* (2011) Consumption of industrial and ruminant trans fatty acids and risk of coronary heart disease: a systematic review and meta-analysis of cohort studies. *European Journal of Clinical Nutrition*, **65**, 773–783.

Benotti, P., Wood, G.C., Winegar, D.A. *et al.* (2014) Risk factors associated with mortality after Roux-en-Y gastric bypass surgery. *Annals of Surgery*, **259**, 123–130.

Bergstrom, A., Pisani, P., Tenet, V. *et al.* (2001) Overweight as an avoidable cause of cancer in Europe. *International Journal of Cancer*, **91**, 421–430.

Bingham, S. (2006) The fibre-folate debate in colo-rectal cancer. *Proceedings of the Nutrition Society*, **65**, 19–23.

Bjelakovic, G. and Gluud, C. (2007) Surviving antioxidant supplements. *Journal of the National Cancer Institute*, **99**, 742–743.

Bjelakovic, G., Nikolova, D., Simonetti, R.G. *et al.* (2004) Antioxidant supplements for prevention of gastrointestinal cancers: a systematic review and meta-analysis. *Lancet*, **364**, 1219–1228.

Blaszyk, H., Wollan, P.C., Witkiewicz, A.K. *et al.* (1999) Death from pulmonary thromboembolism in severe obesity: lack of association with established genetic and clinical risk factors. *Virchows Archive*, **434**, 529–532.

Bray, G.A. and Ryan, D.H. (2007) Drug treatment of the overweight patient. *Gastroenterology*, **132**, 2239–2252.

Brouwer, I.A., Wanders, A.J. and Katan, M.B. (2013) Trans fatty acids and cardiovascular health: research completed? *European Journal of Clinical Nutrition*, **67**, 541–547.

Bucher, H.C., Hengstler, P., Schindler, C. *et al.* (2002) N-3 polyunsaturated fatty acids in coronary heart disease: a meta-analysis of randomized controlled trials. *American Journal of Medicine*, **112**, 298–304.

Calle, E.E., Rodriguez, C., Walker-Thurmond, K. *et al.* (2003) Overweight, obesity, and mortality from cancer in a prospectively studied cohort of U.S. adults. *New England Journal of Medicine*, **348**, 1625–1638.

Castro Cabezas, M., de Vries, J.H., van Oostrom, A.J. *et al.* (2006) Effects of a stanol-enriched diet on plasma cholesterol and triglycerides in patients treated with statins. *Journal of the American Dietetic Association*, **106**, 1564–1569.

Catsburg, C.E., Gago-Dominguez, M., Yuan, J.M. *et al.* (2014) Dietary sources of N-nitroso compounds and bladder cancer risk: findings from the Los Angeles bladder cancer study. *International Journal of Cancer*, **134**, 125–135.

Cerhan, J.R., Chiu, B.C., Wallace, R.B. *et al.* (1998) Physical activity, physical function, and the risk of breast cancer in a prospective study among elderly women. *Journal of Gerontology Series A. Biological Science and Medical Science*, **53**, M251–M2566.

Chai, F., Evdokiou, A., Young, G.P. *et al.* (2000) Involvement of p21(Waf1/Cip1) and its cleavage by DEVD-caspase during apoptosis of colorectal cancer cells induced by butyrate. *Carcinogenesis*, **21**, 7–14.

Chen, J. (2010) Sodium sensitivity of blood pressure in Chinese populations. *Current Hypertension Reports*, **12**, 127–134.

Chowdhury, R., Warnakula, S., Kunutsor, S. *et al.* (2014) Association of dietary, circulating, and supplement fatty acids with coronary risk: a systematic review and meta-analysis. *Annals of Internal Medicine*, **160**, 398–406.

Colditz, G.A. and Hankinson, S.E. (2005) The nurses' health study: lifestyle and health among women. *Nature Reviews Cancer*, **5**, 388–396.

Cole, B.F., Baron, J.A., Sandler, R.S. *et al.* (2007) Folic acid for the prevention of colorectal adenomas: a randomized clinical trial. *Journal of the American Medical Association*, **297**, 2351–2359.

Cook, N.R., Kumanyika, S.K. and Cutler, J.A. (1998) Effect of change in sodium excretion on change in blood pressure corrected for measurement error. The trials of hypertension prevention, phase I. *American Journal of Epidemiology*, **148**, 431–444.

Cui, Y., Page, D.L., Chlebowski, R.T. *et al.* (2007) Alcohol and folate consumption and risk of benign proliferative epithelial disorders of the breast. *International Journal of Cancer*, **121**, 1346–1351.

De Stefani, E., Correa, P., Boffetta, P. *et al.* (2001) Plant foods and risk of gastric cancer: a case-control study in Uruguay. *European Journal of Cancer Prevention*, **10**, 357–364.

Department of Health (1999) *Dietary Reference Values for Energy and Nutrients for the United Kingdom*, Stationary Office, London.

Department of Health (2002) *National Service Framework for Diabetes: Delivery Strategy*, Stationery Office, London.

Doll, R. and Peto, R. (1981) The causes of cancer: quantitative estimates of avoidable risks of cancer in the United States today. *Journal of the National Cancer Institute*, **66**, 1191–1308.

Druesne-Pecollo, N., Keita, Y., Touvier, M. *et al.* (2014) Alcohol drinking and second primary cancer risk in patients with upper aerodigestive tract cancers: a systematic review and meta-analysis of observational studies. *Cancer Epidemiology, Biomarkers and Prevention*, **23**, 324–331.

Durga, J., Bots, M.L., Schouten, E.G. *et al.* (2005) Low concentrations of folate, not hyperhomocysteinemia, are associated with carotid intima-media thickness. *Atherosclerosis*, **179**, 285–292.

Duthie, S.J., Narayanan, S., Sharp, L. *et al.* (2004) Folate, DNA stability and colo-rectal neoplasia. *Proceedings of the Nutrition Society*, **63**, 571–578.

Dyson, P.A., Kelly, T., Deakin, T. *et al.* (2011) Diabetes UK evidence-based nutrition guidelines for the prevention and management of diabetes. *Diabetic Medicine*, **28**, 1282–1288.

Egal, S., Hounsa, A., Gong, Y.Y. *et al.* (2005) Dietary exposure to aflatoxin from maize and groundnut in young children from Benin and Togo, West Africa. *International Journal of Food Microbiology*, **104**, 215–224.

Elliott, P., Marmot, M., Dyer, A. *et al.* (1989) The INTERSALT study: main results, conclusions and some implications. *Clinical and Experimental Hypertension*, **11**, 1025–1034.

Engeset, D., Alsaker, E., Lund, E. *et al.* (2006) Fish consumption and breast cancer risk. The European prospective investigation into cancer and nutrition (EPIC). *International Journal of Cancer*, **119**, 175–182.

Flegal, K.M., Carroll, M.D., Ogden, C.L. *et al.* (2002) Prevalence and trends in obesity among US adults, 1999–2000. *Journal of the American Medical Association*, **288**, 1723–1727.

Forman, M.R. (2007) Changes in dietary fat and fiber and serum hormone concentrations: nutritional strategies for breast cancer prevention over the life course. *Journal of Nutrition*, **137**, 170S–174S.

Förstermann, U. (2010) Nitric oxide and oxidative stress in vascular disease. *Pflügers Archiv*, **459**, 923–939.

Fraser, M.L., Mok, G.S. and Lee, A.H. (2007) Green tea and stroke prevention: emerging evidence. *Complementary Therapies in Medicine*, **15**, 46–53.

Fresco, P., Borges, F., Diniz, C. *et al.* (2006) New insights on the anticancer properties of dietary polyphenols. *Medicinal Research Reviews*, **26**, 747–766.

Frigolet, M.E., Ramos Barragán, V.E. and Tamez González, M. (2011) Low-carbohydrate diets: a matter of love or hate. *Annals of Nutrition and Metabolism*, **58**, 320–334.

Fuchs, C.S., Giovannucci, E.L., Colditz, G.A. *et al.* (1999) Dietary fiber and the risk of colorectal cancer and adenoma in women. *New England Journal of Medicine*, **340**, 169–176.

Gaede, P.H., Jepsen, P.V., Larsen, J.N. *et al.* (2003) The Steno-2 study. Intensive multifactorial intervention reduces the occurrence of cardiovascular disease in patients with type 2 diabetes. *Ugeskrift for Laeger*, **165**, 2658–2661.

Gardner, E.J., Ruxton, C.H.S. and Leeds, A.R. (2007) Black tea-helpful or harmful? A review of the evidence. *European Journal of Clinical Nutrition*, **61**, 3–18.

Garland, C., Shekelle, R.B., Barrett-Connor, E. *et al.* (1985) Dietary vitamin D and calcium and risk of colorectal cancer: a 19-year prospective study in men. *Lancet*, **1**, 307–309.

General Household Survey (2006) *General Household Survey*, Office for National Statistics, Lagos.

Gerber, M. (2001) The comprehensive approach to diet: a critical review. *Journal of Nutrition*, **131**, 3051S–3055S.

Giovannucci, E. (2002) Epidemiologic studies of folate and colorectal neoplasia: a review. *Journal of Nutrition*, **132** (8 Suppl), 2350S–2355S.

Giovannucci, E., Rimm, E.B., Wolk, A. *et al.* (1998) Calcium and fructose intake in relation to risk of prostate cancer. *Cancer Research*, **58**, 442–447.

Giovannucci, E., Rimm, E.B., Stampfer, M.J. *et al.* (2004) Intake of fat, meat, and fiber in relation to risk of colon cancer in men. *Cancer Research*, **54**, 2390–2397.

Gloy, V.L., Briel, M., Bhatt, D.L. *et al.* (2013) Bariatric surgery versus non-surgical treatment for obesity: a systematic review and meta-analysis of randomised controlled trials. *British Medical Journal*, **347**, f5934.

Goff, D.C., Jr, Gerstein, H.C., Ginsberg, H.N. *et al.* (2007) Prevention of cardiovascular disease in persons with type 2 diabetes mellitus: current knowledge and rationale for the Action to Control Cardiovascular Risk in Diabetes (ACCORD) trial. *American Journal of Cardiology*, **99**, 4i–20i.

Gonzalez, C.A. (2006) The European prospective investigation into cancer and nutrition (EPIC). *Public Health Nutrition*, **9**, 124–126.

Goralczyk, R. (2009) Beta-carotene and lung cancer in smokers: review of hypotheses and status of research. *Nutrition and Cancer*, **61**, 767–774.

Gould, A.L., Davies, G.M., Alemao, E. *et al.* (2007) Cholesterol reduction yields clinical benefits: meta-analysis including recent trials. *Clinical Therapeutics*, **29**, 778–794.

Graham, S., Hellmann, R., Marshall, J. *et al.* (1991) Nutritional epidemiology of postmenopausal breast cancer in western New York. *American Journal of Epidemiology*, **134**, 552–566.

Greenberg, J.A., Fontaine, K. and Allison, D.B. (2007) Putative biases in estimating mortality attributable to obesity in the US population. *International Journal of Obesity*, **31**, 1449–1455.

Hales, C.N. and Barker, D.J. (2001) The thrifty phenotype hypothesis. *British Medical Bulletin*, **60**, 5–20.

Harrington, M., Gibson, S. and Cottrell, R.C. (2009) A review and meta-analysis of the effect of weight loss on all-cause mortality risk. *Nutrition Research Reviews*, **22**, 93–108.

Hartley, L., Flowers, N., Holmes, J. *et al.* (2013) Green and black tea for the primary prevention of cardiovascular disease. *Cochrane Database of Systematic Reviews*, **6**, CD009934.

He, F.J. and MacGregor, G.A. (2003) How far should salt intake be reduced? *Hypertension*, **42**, 1093–1099.

Health and Social Care Information Centre (2013) *Statistics on Alcohol-England, 2013*, http://www.hscic.gov.uk/catalogue/PUB10932 (accessed May 2014).

Health and Social Care Information Centre (2014) *Statistics on Obesity, Physical Activity and Diet-England, 2014*, http://www.hscic.gov.uk/catalogue/PUB13648 (accessed May 2014).

Health Education Authority (1995) *Enjoy Healthy Eating. The Balance of Good Health*, HEA, London.

Holmes, M.D., Hunter, D.J., Colditz, G.A. *et al.* (1999) Association of dietary intake of fat and fatty acids with risk of breast cancer. *Journal of the American Medical Association*, **281**, 914–920.

Holmes, M.V., Newcombe, P., Hubacek, J.A. *et al.* (2011) Effect modification by population dietary folate on the association between MTHFR genotype, homocysteine, and stroke risk: a meta-analysis of genetic studies and randomised trials. *Lancet*, **378**, 584–594.

Homocysteine Studies Collaboration (2002) Homocysteine and risk of ischemic heart disease and stroke: a meta-analysis. *Journal of the American Medical Association*, **288**, 2015–2022.

Houghton, C.A., Fassett, R.G. and Coombes, J.S. (2013) Sulforaphane: translational research from laboratory bench to clinic. *Nutrition Reviews*, **71**, 709–726.

Howe, G.R., Hirohata, T., Hislop, T.G. *et al.* (1990) Dietary factors and risk of breast cancer: combined analysis of 12 case-control studies. *Journal of the National Cancer Institute*, **82**, 561–569.

Hu, F.B. and Willett, W.C. (2002) Optimal diets for prevention of coronary heart disease. *Journal of the American Medical Association*, **288**, 2569–2578.

Hu, F.B., Stampfer, M.J., Manson, J.E. *et al.* (2000) Trends in the incidence of coronary heart disease and changes in diet and lifestyle in women. *New England Journal of Medicine*, **343**, 530–537.

Huang, T., Chen, Y., Yang, B. *et al.* (2012) Meta-analysis of B vitamin supplementation on plasma homocysteine, cardiovascular and all-cause mortality. *Clinical Nutrition*, **31**, 448–454.

Hunter, D.J., Spiegelman, D., Adami, H.O. *et al.* (1996) Cohort studies of fat intake and the risk of breast cancer–a pooled analysis. *New England Journal of Medicine*, **334**, 356–361.

Jebb, S.A. (2005) Dietary strategies for the prevention of obesity. *Proceedings of the Nutrition Society*, **64**, 217–227.

Kamen, B. (1997) Folate and antifolate pharmacology. *Seminars in Oncology*, **24** (5 Suppl 18), S18-30–S18-39.

Kardinaal, A.F., Kok, F.J., Ringstad, J. *et al.* (1993) Antioxidants in adipose tissue and risk of myocardial infarction: the EURAMIC Study. *Lancet*, **342**, 1379–1384.

Kato, I., Akhmedkhanov, A., Koenig, K. *et al.* (1997) Prospective study of diet and female colorectal cancer: the New York University Women's Health Study. *Nutrition and Cancer*, **28**, 276–281.

Keli, S.O., Hertog, M.G., Feskens, E.J. *et al.* (1996) Dietary flavonoids, antioxidant vitamins, and incidence of stroke: the Zutphen study. *Archives of Internal Medicine*, **156**, 637–642.

Kelly, T.N., Rebholz, C.M., Gu, D. *et al.* (2013) Analysis of sex hormone genes reveals gender differences in the genetic etiology of blood pressure salt sensitivity: the GenSalt study. *American Journal of Hypertension*, **26**, 191–200.

Khaw, K.T., Bingham, S., Welch, A. *et al.* (2004) Blood pressure and urinary sodium in men and women: the Norfolk cohort of the European prospective investigation into cancer (EPIC-Norfolk). *American Journal of Clinical Nutrition*, **80**, 1397–1403.

Kim, Y.I., Pogribny, L.P., Salomon, R.N. *et al.* (1996) Exon-specific DNA hypomethylation of the p53 gene of rat colon induced by dimethylhydrazine: modulation by dietary folate. *American Journal of Pathology*, **149**, 1129–1137.

Kim, S.Y., Dietz, P.M., England, L. *et al.* (2007) Trends in pre-pregnancy obesity in nine states, 1993–2003. *Obesity*, **15**, 986–993.

Kirk, J.K., Graves, D.E., Craven, T.E. *et al.* (2008) Restricted-carbohydrate diets in patients with type 2 diabetes: a meta-analysis. *Journal of the American Dietetic Association*, **108**, 91–100.

Kjaerheim, K., Gaard, M. and Andersen, A. (1998) The role of alcohol, tobacco, and dietary factors in upper aerogastric tract cancers: a prospective study of 10,900 Norwegian men. *Cancer Causes and Control*, **9**, 99–108.

Klempel, M.C., Kroeger, C.M., Bhutani, S. *et al.* (2012) Intermittent fasting combined with calorie restriction is effective for weight loss and cardio-protection in obese women. *Nutrition Journal*, **11**, 98.

Klerk, M., Verhoef, P., Clarke, R. *et al.* (2002) MTHFR 677C–>T polymorphism and risk of coronary heart disease: a meta-analysis. *Journal of the American Medical Association*, **288**, 2023–2031.

Knekt, P., Ritz, J., Pereira, M.A. *et al.* (2004) Antioxidant vitamins and coronary heart disease risk: a pooled analysis of 9 cohorts. *American Journal of Clinical Nutrition*, **80**, 1508–1520.

Koh, W.P., Yuan, J.M., Wang, R. *et al.* (2011) Plasma carotenoids and risk of acute myocardial infarction in the Singapore Chinese Health Study. *Nutrition, Metabolism and Cardiovascular Disease*, **21**, 685–690.

Konings, E.J., Goldbohm, R.A., Brants, H.A. *et al.* (2002) Intake of dietary folate vitamers and risk of colorectal carcinoma: results from The Netherlands Cohort Study. *Cancer*, **95**, 1421–1433.

Kral, J.G. and Naslund, E. (2007) Surgical treatment of obesity. *Nature Clinical Practice Endocrinology & Metabolism*, **3**, 574–583.

Kroeger, C.M., Klempel, M.C., Bhutani, S. *et al.* (2012) Improvement in coronary heart disease risk factors during an intermittent fasting/calorie restriction regimen: relationship to adipokine modulations. *Nutrition and Metabolism*, **9**, 98.

Kushi, L. and Giovannucci, E. (2002) Dietary fat and cancer. *American Journal of Medicine*, **113**, 63S–70S.

Kwok, C.S., Pradhan, A., Khan, M.A. *et al.* (2014) Bariatric surgery and its impact on cardiovascular disease and mortality: a systematic review and meta-analysis. *International Journal of Cardiology*, **173**, 20–28.

Lakka, H.M., Laaksonen, D.E., Lakka, T.A. *et al.* (2002) The metabolic syndrome and total and cardiovascular disease mortality in middle-aged men. *Journal of the American Medical Association*, **288**, 2709–2716.

Langley-Evans, S.C. (2000) Consumption of black tea elicits an increase in plasma antioxidant potential in humans. *International Journal of Food Science and Nutrition*, **51**, 309–315.

Larsson, S.C., Bergkvist, L. and Wolk, A. (2006) Processed meat consumption, dietary nitrosamines and stomach cancer risk in a cohort of Swedish women. *International Journal of Cancer*, **119**, 915–919.

Lashner, B.A., Provencher, K.S., Seidner, D.L. *et al.* (1997) The effect of folic acid supplementation on the risk for cancer or dysplasia in ulcerative colitis. *Gastroenterology*, **112**, 29–32.

Law, M.R. and Morris, J.K. (1998) By how much does fruit and vegetable consumption reduce the risk of ischaemic heart disease? *European Journal of Clinical Nutrition*, **52**, 549–556.

Lawson, K.A., Wright, M.E., Subar, A. *et al.* (2007) Multivitamin use and risk of prostate cancer in the National Institutes of Health-AARP Diet and Health Study. *Journal of the National Cancer Institute*, **99**, 754–764.

Le Marchand, L., Donlon, T., Seifried, A. *et al.* (2002) Red meat intake, CYP2E1 genetic polymorphisms, and colorectal cancer risk. *Cancer Epidemiology, Biomarkers and Prevention*, **11**, 1019–1024.

Lean, M.E., Han, T.S. and Morrison, C.E. (1995) Waist circumference as a measure for indicating need for weight management. *British Medical Journal*, **311**, 158–161.

Leander, K., Wiman, B., Hallqvist, J. *et al.* (2007) Primary risk factors influence risk of recurrent myocardial infarction/death from coronary heart disease: results from the Stockholm Heart Epidemiology Program (SHEEP). *European Journal Cardiovascular Preventive & Rehabilitation*, **14**, 532–537.

Lee, J., Demissie, K., Lu, S.E. *et al.* (2007) Cancer incidence among Korean-American immigrants in the United States and native Koreans in South Korea. *Cancer Control*, **14**, 78–85.

Leenen, R., Roodenburg, A.J., Tijburg, L.B. *et al.* (2000) A single dose of tea with or without milk increases plasma antioxidant activity in humans. *European Journal of Clinical Nutrition*, **54**, 87–92.

Lewin, M.H., Bailey, N., Bandaletova, T. *et al.* (2007) Red meat enhances the colonic formation of the DNA adduct O6-carboxymethyl guanine: implications for colorectal cancer risk. *Cancer Research*, **66**, 1859–1865.

Loh, J.T., Torres, V.J. and Cover, T.L. (2007) Regulation of Helicobacter pylori cagA expression in response to salt. *Cancer Research*, **67**, 4709–4715.

Lonn, E., Yusuf, S., Arnold, M.J. *et al.* (2006) Homocysteine lowering with folic acid and B vitamins in vascular disease. *New England Journal of Medicine*, **354**, 1567–1577.

Look AHEAD Research Group (2007) Reduction in weight and cardiovascular disease risk factors in individuals with type 2 diabetes: one-year results of the look AHEAD trial. *Diabetes Care*, **30**, 1374–1383.

Look AHEAD Research Group (2013) Cardiovascular effects of intensive lifestyle intervention in type 2 diabetes. *New England Journal of Medicine*, **369**, 145–154.

Malinow, M.R., Duell, P.B., Hess, D.L. *et al.* (1998) Reduction of plasma homocyst(e)ine levels by breakfast cereal fortified with folic acid in patients with coronary heart disease. *New England Journal of Medicine*, **338**, 1009–1015.

Mason, J.B., Dickstein, A., Jacques, P.F. *et al.* (2007) A temporal association between folic acid fortification and an increase in colorectal cancer rates may be illuminating important biological principles: a hypothesis. *Cancer Epidemiology, Biomarkers and Prevention*, **16**, 1325–1329.

Mayne, S.T., Risch, H.A., Dubrow, R. *et al.* (2001) Nutrient intake and risk of subtypes of esophageal and gastric cancer. *Cancer Epidemiology, Biomarkers and Prevention*, **10**, 1055–1062.

Mazhar, D. and Waxman, J. (2006) Dietary fat and breast cancer. *Quarterly Journal of Medicine*, **99**, 469–473.

McIntyre, E.A. and Walker, M. (2002) Genetics of type 2 diabetes and insulin resistance: knowledge from human studies. *Clinical Endocrinology*, **57**, 303–311.

Mei, H., Gu, D., Hixson, J.E. *et al.* (2012) Genome-wide linkage and positional association study of blood pressure response to dietary sodium intervention: the GenSalt study. *American Journal of Epidemiology*, **176** (Suppl 7), S81–90.

Miller, C.K., Headings, A., Peyrot, M. *et al.* (2011) A behavioural intervention incorporating specific glycaemic index goals improves dietary quality, weight control and glycaemic control in adults with type 2 diabetes. *Public Health Nutrition*, **14**, 1303–1311.

Min, K.B. and Min, J.Y. (2014) Serum carotenoid levels and lung cancer mortality risk in US adults. *Cancer Science*, **105** (6), 736–743.

Misra, A. and Ganda, O.P. (2007) Migration and its impact on adiposity and type 2 diabetes. *Nutrition*, **23**, 696–708.

Moat, S.J., Lang, D., McDowell, I.F. *et al.* (2004) Folate, homocysteine, endothelial function and cardiovascular disease. *Journal of Nutritional Biochemistry*, **15**, 64–79.

Naci, H., Brugts, J.J., Fleurence, R. *et al.* (2013) Comparative benefits of statins in the primary and secondary prevention of major coronary events and all-cause mortality: a network meta-analysis of placebo-controlled and active-comparator trials. *European Journal of Preventive Cardiology*, **20**, 641–657.

Nagao, M., Moriyama, Y., Yamagishi, K. *et al.* (2012) Relation of serum α- and γ-tocopherol levels to cardiovascular disease-related mortality among Japanese men and women. *Journal of Epidemiology*, **22**, 402–410.

National Health Service (2007) *Five-a-Day Campaign*, http://www.nhs.uk/Livewell/5ADAY/Pages/5ADAYhome.aspx (accessed May 2014).

Neel, J.V. (1962) Diabetes mellitus: a "thrifty" genotype rendered detrimental by "progress"? *American Journal of Human Genetics*, **14**, 353–362.

NICE (2007) *Clinical Guidelines for Type 2 Diabetes*, http://guidance.nice.org.uk/page.aspx?o=36881 (accessed September 2007).

NICE (2008) *Clinical Guideline 66. Type 2 Diabetes: National Clinical Guideline for Management in Primary and Secondary Care (Update)*, http://www.nice.org.uk (accessed January 19, 2009).

Nield, L., Moore, H., Hooper, L. *et al.* (2007) *Dietary advice for treatment of type 2 diabetes mellitus in adults.* Cochrane Database of Systematic Reviews, CD004097.

Ogden, C.L., Carroll, M.D., Kit, B.K. *et al.* (2013) Prevalence of obesity among adults: United States, 2011–2012. Centers for Disease Control and Prevention, USA.

Omenn, G.S., Goodman, G.E., Thornquist, M.D. *et al.* (1996) Risk factors for lung cancer and for intervention effects in CARET, the Beta-Carotene and Retinol Efficacy Trial. *Journal of the National Cancer Institute*, **88**, 1550–1559.

Oyebode, O., Gordon-Dseagu, V., Walker, A. *et al.* (2014) Fruit and vegetable consumption and all-cause, cancer and CVD mortality: analysis of Health Survey for England data. *Journal of Epidemiology and Community Health*, **68**, 856–862.

Papadaki, A., Linardakis, M., Plada, M. *et al.* (2014) Impact of weight loss and maintenance with ad libitum diets varying in protein and glycemic index content on metabolic syndrome. *Nutrition*, **30**, 410–417.

Patel, J.V., Vyas, A., Cruickshank, J.K. *et al.* (2006) Impact of migration on coronary heart disease risk factors: comparison of Gujaratis in Britain and their contemporaries in villages of origin in India. *Atherosclerosis*, **185**, 297–306.

Peters, U., Poole, C. and Arab, L. (2001) Does tea affect cardiovascular disease? A meta-analysis. *American Journal of Epidemiology*, **154**, 495–503.

Pi-Sunyer, F.X., Aronne, L.J., Heshmati, H.M. *et al.* and RIO-North America Study Group (2006) Effect of rimonabant, a cannabinoid-1 receptor blocker, on weight and cardiometabolic risk factors in overweight or obese patients: RIO-North America: a randomized controlled trial. *Journal of the American Medical Association*, **295**, 761–775.

Pischon, T., Lahmann, P.H., Boeing, H. *et al.* (2006) Body size and risk of colon and rectal cancer in the European Prospective Investigation Into Cancer and Nutrition (EPIC). *Journal of the National Cancer Institute*, **98**, 920–931.

Popkin, B.M. (2007) Understanding global nutrition dynamics as a step towards controlling cancer incidence. *Nature Reviews Cancer*, **7**, 61–67.

Porcelli, B., Frosi, B., Rosi, F. *et al.* (1996) Levels of folic acid in plasma and in red blood cells of colorectal cancer patients. *Biomedical Pharmacotherapeutics*, **50**, 303–305.

Powers, H.J. (2005) Interaction among folate, riboflavin, genotype, and cancer, with reference to colorectal and cervical cancer. *Journal of Nutrition*, **135**, 2960S–2966S.

Prentice, A.M. and Jebb, S.A. (1995) Obesity in Britain: gluttony or sloth? *British Medical Journal*, **311**, 437–439.

Raitakari, O.T., Salo, P. and Ahotupa, M. (2007) Carotid artery compliance in users of plant stanol ester margarine. *European Journal of Clinical Nutrition*, **62**, 218–224.

Raitakari, O.T., Salo, P., Gylling, H. *et al.* (2008) Plant stanol ester consumption and arterial elasticity and endothelial function. *British Journal of Nutrition*, **100**, 603–608.

Ramsay, S.E., Whincup, P.H., Morris, R.W. *et al.* (2007) Are childhood socio-economic circumstances related to coronary heart disease risk? Findings from a population-based study of older men. *International Journal of Epidemiology*, **36**, 560–566.

Razis, A.F. and Noor, N.M. (2013) Cruciferous vegetables: dietary phytochemicals for cancer prevention. *Asian Pacific Journal of Cancer Prevention*, **14**, 1565–1570.

Rehm, J., Patra, J. and Popova, S. (2007) Alcohol drinking cessation and its effect on esophageal and head and neck cancers: a pooled analysis. *International Journal of Cancer*, **121**, 1132–1137.

Rich, S.S. (1990) Mapping genes in diabetes. Genetic epidemiological perspective. *Diabetes*, **39**, 1315–1319.

Rizos, E.C., Ntzani, E.E., Bika, E. *et al.* (2012) Association between omega-3 fatty acid supplementation and risk of major cardiovascular disease events: a systematic review and meta-analysis. *Journal of the American Medical Association*, **308**, 1024–1033.

Roche, H.M., Phillips, C. and Gibney, M.J. (2005) The metabolic syndrome: the crossroads of diet and genetics. *Proceedings of the Nutrition Society*, **64**, 371–377.

Romeo, S., Maglio, C., Burza, M.A. *et al.* (2012) Cardiovascular events after bariatric surgery in obese subjects with type 2 diabetes. *Diabetes Care*, **35**, 2613–2617.

Sacks, F.M., Svetkey, L.P., Vollmer, W.M. *et al.* (2001) Effects on blood pressure of reduced dietary sodium and the Dietary Approaches to Stop Hypertension (DASH) diet. DASH-Sodium Collaborative Research Group. *New England Journal of Medicine*, **344**, 3–10.

Sharp, L. and Little, J. (2004) Polymorphisms in genes involved in folate metabolism and colorectal neoplasia: a HuGE review. *American Journal of Epidemiology*, **159**, 423–443.

Shaw, K., Gennat, H., O'Rourke, P. *et al.* (2006) *Exercise for overweight or obesity. Cochrane Database of Systematic Reviews*, CD003817.

Siebenhofer, A., Jeitler, K., Berghold, A. *et al.* (2011) *Long-term effects of weight-reducing diets in hypertensive patients. Cochrane Database of Systematic Reviews*, CD008274.

Sjöström, L., Narbro, K., Sjöström, C.D. *et al.* (2007) Effects of bariatric surgery on mortality in Swedish obese subjects. *New England Journal of Medicine*, **357**, 741–752.

Sjöström, L., Gummesson, A., Sjöström, C.D. *et al.* (2009) Effects of bariatric surgery on cancer incidence in obese patients in Sweden (Swedish Obese Subjects Study): a prospective, controlled intervention trial. *Lancet Oncology*, **10**, 653–662.

Slavin, J. (2003) Why whole grains are protective: biological mechanisms. *Proceedings of the Nutrition Society*, **62**, 129–134.

Slob, I.C., Lambregts, J.L., Schuit, A.J. *et al.* (1993) Calcium intake and 28-year gastro-intestinal cancer mortality in Dutch civil servants. *International Journal of Cancer*, **54**, 20–25.

Smith-Warner, S.A., Spiegelman, D., Yaun, F. *et al.* (1998) Alcohol and breast cancer in women: a pooled analysis of cohort studies. *Journal of the American Medical Association*, **279**, 535–540.

Stephens, N.G., Parsons, A., Schofield, P.M. *et al.* (1996) Randomised controlled trial of vitamin E in patients with coronary disease: Cambridge Heart Antioxidant Study (CHAOS). *Lancet*, **347**, 781–786.

Stroh, C., Weiner, R., Wolff, S. *et al.* (2014) Influences of gender on complication rate and outcome after Roux-en-Y gastric bypass: data analysis of more than 10,000 operations from the German Bariatric Surgery Registry. *Obesity Surgery*, **24** (10), 1625–1633.

Tantamango-Bartley, Y., Jaceldo-Siegl, K., Fan, J. *et al.* (2013) Vegetarian diets and the incidence of cancer in a low-risk population. *Cancer Epidemiology, Biomarkers and Prevention*, **22**, 286–94.

Taylor, E.F., Burley, V.J., Greenwood, D.C. *et al.* (2007) Meat consumption and risk of breast cancer in the UK Women's Cohort Study. *British Journal of Cancer*, **96**, 1139–1146.

Toomey, S., Roche, H., Fitzgerald, D. *et al.* (2003) Regression of pre-established atherosclerosis in the apoE-/-mouse by conjugated linoleic acid. *Biochemical Society Transactions*, **31**, 1075–1079.

Turner, P.C., Sylla, A., Gong, Y.Y. *et al.* (2005) Reduction in exposure to carcinogenic aflatoxins by postharvest intervention measures in West Africa: a community-based intervention study. *Lancet*, **365**, 1950–1956.

Tyagi, G., Pradhan, S., Srivastava, T. *et al.* (2014) Nucleic acid binding properties of allicin: spectroscopic analysis and estimation of anti-tumor potential. *Biochimica et Biophysica Acta*, **1840**, 350–356.

UKPDS (1998) Intensive blood-glucose control with sulphonylureas or insulin compared with conventional treatment and risk of complications in patients with type 2 diabetes (UKPDS 33). UK Prospective Diabetes Study (UKPDS) Group. *Lancet*, **352**, 837–853.

USDA (2005) *My Pyramid*, http://www.mypyramid.gov/ (accessed September 2007).

Valsecchi, M.G. (1992) Modelling the relative risk of esophageal cancer in a case-control study. *Journal of Clinical Epidemiology*, **45**, 347–355.

Varady, K.A. (2011) Intermittent versus daily calorie restriction: which diet regimen is more effective for weight loss? *Obesity Reviews*, **12**, e593–e601.

Veldhorst, M.A., Westerterp-Plantenga, M.S. and Westerterp, K.R. (2009) Gluconeogenesis and energy expenditure after a high-protein, carbohydrate-free diet. *American Journal of Clinical Nutrition*, **90**, 519–526.

VITATOPS Trial Study Group (2010). B vitamins in patients with recent transient ischaemic attack or stroke in the VITAmins TO Prevent Stroke (VITATOPS) trial: a randomised, double-blind, parallel, placebo-controlled trial. *Lancet Neurology*, **9**, 855–865.

Vogels, N. and Westerterp-Plantenga, M.S. (2007) Successful long-term weight maintenance: a 2-year follow-up. *Obesity*, **15**, 1258–1266.

Wark, P.A., Weijenberg, M.P., van't Veer, P. *et al.* (2005) Fruits, vegetables, and hMLH1 protein-deficient and -proficient colon cancer: The Netherlands cohort study. *Cancer Epidemiology, Biomarkers and Prevention*, **14**, 1619–1625.

Weisell, R.C. (2002) Body mass index as an indicator of obesity. *Asia Pacific Journal of Clinical Nutrition*, **11**, S681–S684.

Westerterp-Plantenga, M.S., Lemmens, S.G. and Westerterp, K.R. (2012) Dietary protein - its role in satiety, energetics, weight loss and health. *British Journal of Nutrition*, **108** (Suppl 2), S105–S112.

Willett, W.C. (1990) Epidemiologic studies of diet and cancer. *Progress in Clinical and Biological Research*, **346**, 159–168.

Willett, W.C. (2001) Diet and breast cancer. *Journal of Internal Medicine*, **249**, 395–411.

Willett, W.C. (2003) Lessons from dietary studies in Adventists and questions for the future. *American Journal of Clinical Nutrition*, **78**, 539S–543S.

World Cancer Research Fund (1997) *Food, Nutrition and the Prevention of Cancer: a Global Perspective*, American Institute for Cancer Research, Washington D.C.

World Cancer Research Fund (WCRF) (2007) *Food, Nutrition, Physical Activity, and the Prevention of Cancer: A Global Perspective*, American Institute for Cancer Research, Washington D.C.

WCRF (2008) *Red and Processed Meat: Finding the Balance for Cancer*, http://www.wcrf-uk.org/uk/preventing-cancer/ways-reduce-cancer-risk/red-and-processed-meat-and-cancer-prevention (accessed March 2015).

World Health Organization (2013a) *Obesity*, http://www.who.int/topics/obesity/en/ (accessed May 2014).

World Health Organization (2013b) *Alcohol*, http://www.who.int/mediacentre/factsheets/fs349/en/ (accessed May 2014).

World Health Organization (2014) *Draft Guideline: Sugars for Adults and Children*, http://www.who.int/nutrition/sugars_public_consultation/en/ (accessed May 2014).

World Obesity Federation (2012) *World Map of Obesity*, http://www.worldobesity.org/aboutobesity/world-map-obesity/ (accessed March 2015).

Wright, M.E., Lawson, K.A., Weinstein, S.J. *et al.* (2006) Higher baseline serum concentrations of vitamin E are associated with lower total and cause-specific mortality in the Alpha-Tocopherol, Beta-Carotene Cancer Prevention Study. *American Journal of Clinical Nutrition*, **84**, 1200–1207.

Ye, Y., Li, J. and Yuan, Z. (2013) Effect of antioxidant vitamin supplementation on cardiovascular outcomes: a meta-analysis of randomized controlled trials. *PLoS ONE*, **8**, e56803.

You, W.C., Brown, L.M., Zhang, L. *et al.* (2006) Randomized double-blind factorial trial of three treatments to reduce the prevalence of precancerous gastric lesions. *Journal of the National Cancer Institute*, **98**, 974–983.

Zhang, Y., Cantor, K.P., Dosemeci, M. *et al.* (2006) Occupational and leisure-time physical activity and risk of colon cancer by subsite. *Journal of Occupational and Environmental Medicine*, **48**, 236–243.

Additional reading

If you would like to find out more about the material discussed in this chapter, the following sources may be of interest:

Stanner, S. (ed) (2005) *Cardiovascular Disease: Diet, Nutrition and Emerging Risk Factors*, British Nutrition Foundation, Oxford, UK.

World Cancer Research Fund (2007) *Food, Nutrition, Physical Activity, and the Prevention of Cancer: A Global Perspective*, World Cancer Research Fund, Washington, DC.

CHAPTER 9
Nutrition, ageing and the elderly

LEARNING OBJECTIVES

This chapter will enable the reader to:
- Show an awareness of the changing demographic profile of the population and the impact that the ageing population will have on global trends in health and disease
- Describe the process of cellular ageing and how this contributes to physiological decline
- Appreciate the differing theories that explain the mechanistic basis of cellular senescence
- Describe how changes in nutrition, particularly caloric restriction, may impact upon ageing and longevity

- Discuss the energy, macronutrient and micronutrient requirements of the elderly population and how these differ with the younger adult population
- Show an appreciation of the fact that the elderly are at significant risk of malnutrition and the factors that contribute to this risk
- Describe the nutrition-related disorders of the elderly and the interrelationship between malnutrition and chronic disease
- Discuss the role of specific nutrients including vitamin D, calcium, folic acid and vitamin B12 in the aetiology and prevention of conditions including osteoporosis, anaemia and dementia

9.1 Introduction

The elderly population are generally considered to be those individuals who are aged 65 and over. As will be described in the following, the elderly population is rapidly growing in almost all parts of the world, and with the increase in the numbers of elderly people, the specific nutrition-related problems of the elderly years take on greater significance in terms of healthcare and health resources. It is important, however, to avoid stereotypes of elderly people as being frail, mentally incapable, dependent on others and plagued by chronic disease. Although elderly patients will make up a high proportion of the population in hospital and receiving long-term medical care, the vast majority of elderly people are healthy, free living and active. However, the elderly years are inevitably the years of decline and ultimately ageing. The development of disease and the loss of physiological functions will lead to death. This chapter will discuss the biological processes that are responsible for ageing and the degeneration of physiological systems that is associated with the elderly years. It will

consider the particular nutrient requirements that accompany this life stage and describe some of the main nutrition-related problems of the elderly.

9.2 The ageing population

Average life expectancy varies considerably between nations ranging from 44 years for men and 47 for women in the Central African Republic through to 79 years for men and 87 for women in Japan (World Health Organization, 2011). In the United Kingdom, average life expectancy at birth for men was 77 years in 2011 and 82 for women. This represents a remarkable shift, typical of all developed countries, as in 1900, life expectancy at birth was only 45.7 years for men and 49.6 years for women. Since 1840, life expectancy in the United Kingdom has increased by approximately 0.25 years every year.

As shown in Figure 9.1, the number of elderly people is increasing rapidly all over the world, and the United Nations estimate that almost two billion people will be

Nutrition, Health and Disease: A Lifespan Approach, Second Edition. Simon Langley-Evans.
© 2015 John Wiley & Sons, Ltd. Published 2015 by John Wiley & Sons, Ltd.
Companion website: www.wiley.com/go/langleyevans/lifespan

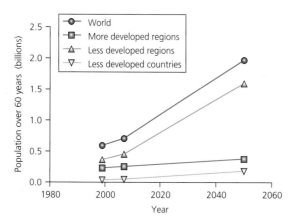

Figure 9.1 Global demographic trends show that the elderly population is rising. Increases in the proportion of the population over the age of 65 years in the developing world will drive a major demographic shift over the next four decades.

Table 9.1 Age-related decline in physiological functions.

Organ or system	Degenerative characteristics
Skeletal muscle	Loss of muscle mass and neuromuscular tone
Adipose tissue	Increasing fat deposition
Upper gastrointestinal tract	Loss of teeth, periodontal disease, reduced saliva production, gastric atrophy
Lower gastrointestinal tract	Bacterial overgrowth, reduced absorption, reduced colon motility
Respiratory	Declining vital capacity
Cardiovascular	Increasing blood pressure, reduced elasticity of arteries, left ventricular hypertrophy
Renal	Loss of nephrons, slower responses to salt load or other challenges
Bone	Declining bone mass leading to osteoporosis
Immunity	Impairment of cellular and passive immunity

aged over 60 by 2050. These increases are most marked in the developing regions, but even in developed countries such as the United Kingdom, significant demographic shifts are taking place. While the proportion of the UK population aged 65–74 has not changed markedly since the mid-1940s (~7.5% of the population), the overall proportion of elderly people in the population has increased greatly, as increasing numbers are living on beyond 75 years. In 1948, 8.5% of the UK population was over 65. The 2011 Census indicated this had increased to 15.9%, and by 2036, this figure is expected to have risen to 24.1%, with almost 5% of the population being 85 years or over. Shifts in the balance between younger and older members of the population have important implications for health and health resources. While UK men and women live for three decades longer than their counterparts a hundred years ago, the extra life is not necessarily healthy life, and for men, there are likely to be 14 years, and for women, 17 years of chronic illness in the final years of life.

9.3 The ageing process

9.3.1 Impact on physiological systems
Ageing brings about a progressive decline in the functioning of all organs and systems (Table 9.1). The function of the gastrointestinal tract is particularly vulnerable to the negative effects of ageing. Loss of teeth throughout life means that many elderly people will rely on dentures, which provide reduced power to masticate food. Periodontal disease afflicts many elderly people and contributes to further tooth loss. Reductions in

salivary flow impair the sense of taste and make it more difficult to swallow food. Production of stomach acid is reduced, and this impacts upon the bioavailability of several nutrients including folic acid, vitamin B6, vitamin B12 and iron. Lower down the tract, bacterial overgrowth of the small intestine limits nutrient uptake, and losses of colon motility lead to constipation and diverticular disease.

Some organs progressively lose function due to reductions in the numbers of functional units. For example, in the lungs, the alveolar numbers fall with ageing, and this reduces vital capacity and makes it harder for the elderly to partake in vigorous exercise. In the kidneys, loss of nephrons contributes to declining homeostatic functions, which can drive problems with fluid balance and lead to higher blood pressure. Skeletal mass is also lost with age, lean body mass declines, and fat mass tends to increase. These changes in body composition can increase the propensity of older people to fall and sustain injury, as the loss of lean body mass is generally a product of sarcopenia. Loss of skeletal muscle is not only partly driven by physical inactivity and decreased use of muscles but may also be attributable to impairments of the central nervous system innervation of muscles, to declining concentrations of sex steroids and growth hormone and to reduction in muscle contractility.

Immune function also declines in the elderly, with both cellular immunity and passive immunity (e.g. the skin barrier to infection) being compromised. The general level of chronic illness is also at its greatest within this group in the population, who are the most likely group in modern society to require long-term medication or to be hospitalized. In addition to these physical manifestations of ageing, there may also be psychological and cognitive changes, including depression and dementia. Sensory impairments also accumulate with ageing, including loss of taste, smell, sight and hearing.

9.3.2 Mechanisms of cellular senescence

The decline in physiological function and general degeneration of organs and systems that occurs during ageing is the physical manifestation of processes taking place at the cellular level. It is erroneous to believe that ageing is the product of programmed cell death (apoptosis), as in fact most cells enter a phase of senescence or quiescence and can remain in that state for a considerable period of time before their destruction via apoptotic pathways. The accumulation of senescent cells will impact upon the functions of organs and tissues with ageing, as generally these cells have altered phenotypes. Although

they retain their differentiated state, they will tend to under- or over-express the enzymes, receptors, cell signalling proteins and adhesion molecules that are necessary for their normal function (Campisi, 1997). All tissues contain stem cells. These are undifferentiated cells that have the capacity to divide and replenish cells that have been destroyed or entered a state of senescence. With ageing, the capacity of the stem cells to regenerate tissues and restore tissue function becomes outstripped by the number of cells entering the senescent stage, and hence, functional capacity declines.

All mammalian cell types, like those of lower organisms, have the capacity to divide through the process of mitosis. Indeed, all cells will be at one of the stages in the cell cycle shown in Figure 9.2, and if they have sufficient energy and nutrients, they will continue to divide at varying rates until they reach the Hayflick limit. This limit is a set number of divisions, at which point the cell enters the senescent stage and is permanently arrested

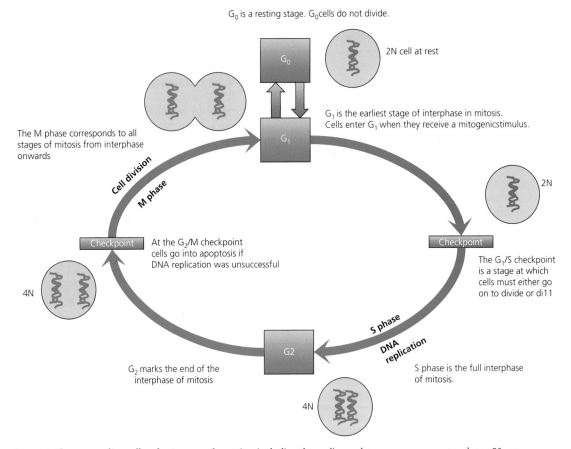

G_0 is a resting stage. G_0 cells do not divide.

2N cell at rest

G_1 is the earliest stage of interphase in mitosis. Cells enter G_1 when they receive a mitogenic stimulus.

2N

The M phase corresponds to all stages of mitosis from interphase onwards

Cell division

M phase

At the G_2/M checkpoint cells go into apoptosis if DNA replication was unsuccessful

Checkpoint

Checkpoint

The G_1/S checkpoint is a stage at which cells must either go on to divide or di11

4N

S phase

DNA replication

G_2 marks the end of the interphase of mitosis

S phase is the full interphase of mitosis.

4N

Figure 9.2 The mammalian cell cycle. A range of proteins, including the cyclins and tumour suppressors such as p53, are responsible for the regulation of cell division, ensuring that cells with damaged or incompletely replicated DNA are unable to pass through mitosis. 2N, diploid cell; 4N, tetraploid cell.

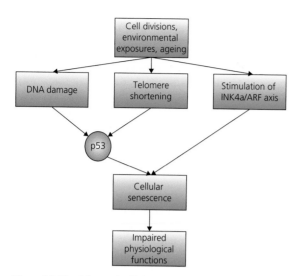

Figure 9.3 The drivers of cellular ageing. Accumulated DNA damage, including telomere shortening, activates senescence via the p53 tumour suppressor gene. The INK4a/ARF axis also has the capacity to trigger senescence.

in the G1 phase of the cycle. With the exception of stem cells, tumour cells and the germ line cells that give rise to gametes, all mammalian cells will undergo senescence once they have completed their maximal number of cell divisions (Campisi, 1997). All eukaryotic cells, with the exception of some single-celled organisms, appear to have this trait. It is now widely recognized that this control over cell division is essentially a tumour suppressor function and in fact the processes that lead to senescence and age-related degeneration are processes that prevent cancer formation (Collado *et al.*, 2007). The precise mechanisms through which senescence is induced are not fully understood, but it appears that three basic processes are involved, as summarized in Figure 9.3.

9.3.2.1 Oxidative senescence

As described in Chapter 8, DNA is highly vulnerable to damage through the actions of free radicals, reactive oxygen species (ROS), ionizing radiation and other environmental factors. While mutation and cancer is one possible outcome of this damage, ageing may also be driven by the same oxidative processes. The production of ROS is continuous throughout the lifespan since the formation of superoxide radicals and subsequently hydrogen peroxide is a normal feature of aerobic respiration. However, the rates of ROS formation appear to increase with ageing, and this results in greater levels of damage to all macromolecules within the cell, including DNA (Sohal *et al.*, 2002). Increasing ROS formation may be a consequence of damage to the mitochondria, which

are the main sources of the ROS. Some researchers argue that mutations of mitochondrial DNA may be mechanistically important in ageing, but it is unlikely that this plays more than a minor role in the process (Sohal *et al.*, 2006).

A role for oxidative processes in driving ageing has been demonstrated using transgenic mammalian and insect models. For example, *Drosophila* carrying extra copies of genes encoding antioxidant enzymes have a longer lifespan (Sohal *et al.*, 2002). Mice lacking superoxide dismutase 1 have reduced lifespan, and mice that over-express catalase specifically within mitochondria have extended longevity (Muller *et al.*, 2007). However, these animal studies do not correlate well with the normal *in vivo* situation, particularly in humans. Measurements of the levels of antioxidant protection in tissues of different species do not appear to relate to their lifespan or other markers of ageing. Importantly, interventions that extend longevity, such as caloric restriction (CR) (see Section 9.3.3), have no impact upon tissue antioxidant status.

Although antioxidant capacity is not a strong predictor of patterns of ageing, the oxidative damage theory is still considered to be of importance. Any ROS-mediated damage to DNA is likely to be repaired under normal conditions, and it is only in the older organism, where the capacity for repair is declining, that oxidative damage will begin to accumulate. It is clear that genomic instability (a loss or corruption of information carried in DNA) is a feature of ageing. There are a number of premature ageing syndromes, caused by rare mutations, that are associated with genomic instability, including xeroderma pigmentosa and ataxia telangiectasia. An imbalance between the level of oxidative damage to DNA and the capacity to repair that DNA might contribute to this instability (Muller *et al.*, 2007). The importance of these processes in individuals that do not have these rare mutations is unclear.

9.3.2.2 The role of p53 activation

p53 is a transcription factor that regulates the cell cycle. During normal cellular function, it is in an inactive state, being bound to the protein product of the human double minute 2 (Hdm2) oncogene. Cell cycle abnormalities, as seen in tumour cells, or DNA damage will result in the activation of p53, and this activation will result in one of two possible outcomes, senescence or cell death. In younger organisms, levels of p53 activation tend to be lower than in older organisms, and p53 essentially functions as a mechanism that allows damaged cells to be eliminated from healthy tissues and replaced by stem cells. In older animals, high levels of p53 activation mean that the capacity to replace and regenerate damaged tissue is insufficient to avoid loss of physiological function (Collado *et al.*, 2007).

Programmed cell death, or apoptosis, is driven by p53 through influences on the Bcl2 and Bax proteins. Bcl2 is anti-apoptotic and is down-regulated by p53, while the pro-apoptotic Bcl2-associated X protein (Bax) is up-regulated by p53. One of the actions of Bax is to increase the permeability of mitochondrial membranes. Leakage of material from the mitochondrial matrix results in the activation of the caspase system, which brings about cell death.

Senescence is driven by the activation of p53, as this protein is a key factor determining progress of the cell from the G1 to the S phase of the cell cycle (Figure 9.2). If cells become arrested at this G1/S checkpoint, then division will not occur until the DNA damage that initially activated p53 is repaired. It appears reasonable to suggest that in the ageing organism, the capacity to repair DNA damage may be outstripped by the level of oxidative processes and hence the arrest of the cell cycle is permanent. However, a more important mechanism may ensure that p53-mediated cell cycle arrest cannot be overcome once the Hayflick limit has been reached. Cells have an inbuilt 'counter' or 'clock' that measures divisions in the form of telomeres.

9.3.2.3 Telomere shortening

Telomeres are the regions of DNA that lie at the ends of the linear chromosomes in mammalian cells. They consist of long repeats of the base sequence TTAGGG and have important cellular functions, in that they prevent fusions between chromosomes, translocation of DNA from one chromosome to another and other harmful genetic defects. Telomere lengths vary widely within tissues and may be between 1.5 and 160 kilobases. Many studies have shown that the length of telomeres

shortens with ageing, and there is a clear inverse association between age and telomere length in human and animal tissues.

Telomeres provide the principal ageing clock within cells as they shorten each time the cell divides (Figure 9.4). This is because the DNA polymerases that replicate DNA during the S phase of the cell cycle are unable to faithfully copy the ends of linear DNA. The enzyme telomerase can replace some of the lost length, but as most mammalian cells have only low telomerase activity, the 3' end of the telomeres is shortened with each replication (Collado et al., 2007). Shortening of the telomeres to a critical length triggers p53 activation. This initiation of processes that result in cell cycle arrest or apoptosis most likely occurs as telomere shortening to critical levels is recognized as a form of DNA damage (Campisi, 1997). In addition to providing the equivalent of a countdown of the number of possible cell divisions remaining, telomere shortening may be a component of oxidative senescence. Experiments with cultured cells show that incubating them at low oxygen concentrations (3% O_2 instead of the usual atmospheric 21% O_2) increases the Hayflick limit and suppresses senescence. This suggests that under normal conditions, oxidative processes might cause damage to the telomeres and drive a more rapid shortening. There is some evidence that telomeric DNA is more vulnerable to oxidative damage than other regions of the chromosomes (Muller et al., 2007).

Leukocyte telomere length (LTL) is commonly reported as a biomarker of cellular ageing in human studies and has been shown to associate with age-related disease patterns. LTL is typically lower in subjects with diabetes or cardiovascular disease (Mather et al., 2011). Zhao and

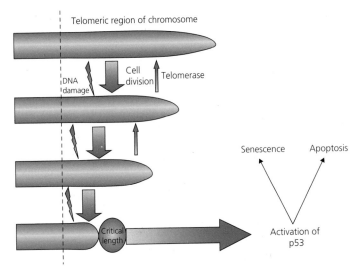

Figure 9.4 Telomere shortening is a key controller of cell division. Each mitotic division leads to loss of telomeric DNA. At critical shortening, this is recognized as DNA damage and leads to apoptosis or senescence through activation of p53. Telomeres consist of the repeated sequence TTAGGG and are between 300 and tens of thousands of bases long.

colleagues (2014) reported that in a population of over 2300 Native Americans, individuals in the lowest quartile for LTL were 83% more likely to develop type 2 diabetes in the subsequent 5.5 years than those in the highest quartile. A meta-analysis (Zhao *et al.*, 2013) confirms this association showing that shorter telomere length is significantly associated with type 2 diabetes (OR 1.29 [95% CI 1.11–1.49]). The relationship between LTL and disease may not be taken at face value, however, as disease – particularly where oxidative stress is a feature – may be a cause of telomere shortening.

Absolute telomere length is not a factor determining ageing. Mice have significantly longer telomeres than humans but live for 2–3 years rather than the 80 of our species (Gomes *et al.*, 2011). The rate at which telomeres erode is the key factor in triggering cellular senescence, and factors which limit oxidative damage or which increase telomere regeneration by telomerase are likely to have a positive impact upon cellular and physiological ageing. In an aged Italian population, high adherence to a Mediterranean dietary pattern was associated with better health longer, LTL and higher circulating telomerase activity (Boccardi and Poalisso, 2014). If telomerase is responsive to diet, then this may present a means by which prudent dietary patterns are beneficial for health and longevity.

9.3.2.4 The INK4a/ARF axis

INK4a and ARF are tumour suppressor proteins that are encoded by a single gene locus (p16INK4). Like other tumour suppressors, these proteins are known to have a pro-ageing influence by virtue of their ability to prevent cell division. Studies of cells in culture show that increased expression of the p16INK4 locus will promote senescence, even if the cells have raised activities of telomerase and long telomeres (Collado *et al.*, 2007). This indicates that the INK4a/ARF axis can override the telomere clock, and it is suggested that these proteins provide a second form of counter that monitors the number of exposures a cell has to mitogenic agents.

INK4a appears to contribute to the physiological signs of ageing by promoting the accumulation of senescent cells within tissues and by opposing regeneration of tissues by stem cells. Mice that lack p16INK4 have been shown to possess an increased capacity for regeneration (Janzen *et al.*, 2006). In tissues from aged rodents and humans, the expression of p16INK4 can be shown to be related to age, which is in keeping with the suggestion that INK4a/ARF somehow drives the ageing process. It is not clear why expression of p16INK4 increases with age, but it may be that oxidative damage, or age-dependent expression of transcriptional regulators, is responsible (Collado *et al.*, 2007).

9.3.3 Nutritional modulation of the ageing process

The long-lived nature of humans and the major difficulties of performing intervention studies that can go on for decades in order to assess the impact of nutritional factors upon the ageing process mean that most studies of nutrition and ageing have been performed using animal models. A wide variety of model systems are used including rats and mice and simpler organisms including the fruit fly *Drosophila melanogaster* and the nematode *Caenorhabditis elegans*.

9.3.3.1 CR and lifespan

It was first reported in 1935 that feeding rats a diet of reduced caloric content throughout their lives significantly extended their lifespan. Generally speaking, in mammalian models, protocols that reduce caloric intake by 60% will increase lifespan by approximately 30–40%, although, in extreme cases, the extension of longevity is closer to 50%. The same effects on lifespan are reported in yeast cells, *Drosophila* and *C. elegans*. In rodents, in addition to the extension of lifespan, the CR protocol reduces the occurrence and extent of age-related diseases, including cancer, cardiovascular disease, diabetes, autoimmune disorders and neurodegenerative problems (Young and Kirkland, 2007). Some studies of non-human primates suggest similar benefits are seen with CR in those species, and this raises the exciting possibility that human ageing might be countered by CR (Research Highlight 9.1).

The mechanism through which CR extends lifespan is not fully understood as animals that undergo CR protocols exhibit a wide range of metabolic, endocrine and physiological changes. In the early stages of CR, animals are in a state of negative energy balance and, in response, reduce their metabolic rate. Basal metabolic rates are rapidly reset, and energy balance is maintained largely through lower thermogenic capacity, resulting in a lower body temperature. Body mass is lost, and the animal maintained on CR has lower lean and fat mass. Although potentially of importance, the prevention of obesity is not, however, the sole mechanism through which health benefits and increased longevity accrue (Speakman and Hambly, 2007). CR induces major changes in endocrine axes, up-regulating the hypothalamic–pituitary–adrenal axis and suppressing the production of insulin, the thyroid hormones, the sex hormones and the somatotropic hormones (Dirks and Leeuwenburgh, 2006). At the cellular level, CR suppresses inflammatory processes and oxidative stressors while at the same time up-regulating systems involved in repair and protein synthesis.

Research Highlight 9.1 Caloric restriction, ageing and longevity in non-human primates.

The historic observations that caloric restriction (CR) could extend lifespan in invertebrates and rodents have naturally prompted speculation that similar protocols may be beneficial in human ageing. Two major studies spanning more than 20 years have examined the effects of CR in rhesus monkeys. Rhesus monkeys have a lifespan of approximately 27 years in captivity but in the wild are believed to live for up to 40 years. The Wisconsin National Primate Research Center (WNPRC) study ran from 1989 to 2009, and the National Institute on Aging (NIA) study ran over a similar period, both using cohorts of rhesus monkeys.

The WNPRC study considered the effects of 30% CR on 24 male and female monkeys compared to 18 control animals and reported a number of benefits. The CR protocol delayed the development of age-related changes in muscle including mitochondrial changes that are normally associated with ageing and sarcopenia. Additionally, the skeletal muscles of the CR monkeys maintained fibre density, and after 17 years of CR, the monkeys appeared resistant to sarcopenia (McKiernan et al., 2012). These animals also had a lower basal metabolic rate and were more metabolically efficient in their movement (Yamada et al., 2013). Most importantly, the WNPRC monkeys were less prone to age-related death than their control counterparts, with just 13% dying over the duration of the study, compared to 27% of controls.

The NIA study also used a 30% CR protocol with 23 male and female rhesus monkeys compared to 48 controls. Among monkeys introduced to CR, metabolic markers were significantly improved with lower blood glucose and cholesterol concentrations and evidence of less oxidative stress (Mattison et al., 2012). However, in the NIA study, markers of ageing, such as telomere shortening (Smith et al., 2011), were not altered by CR. There was no significant difference in age-related death or disease between the CR and control monkeys, and there was evidence of worse immune function in the CR group (Mattison et al., 2012).

Clearly, the two studies disagreed on the key finding of CR and survival, and this in itself may give a clue to the relative importance of caloric restriction in determining lifespan in primates and, therefore, humans. The NIA study authors argue that genetics and the overall composition of the diet may be more important that CR (Mattison et al., 2012). It is interesting to note that in the WNPRC study, control monkeys were fed a relatively unhealthy diet containing less minerals and vitamins, more sucrose (28.5% of diet) and a single protein source compared to NIA controls (low sucrose, varied protein sources). This may indicate that CR is only an extension of current approaches to limit weight gain and maintain healthy dietary patterns as a means of preventing disease. Both studies are ongoing and over the next 5–10 years will yield more data about the impact of CR upon ageing in non-human primates, which will inform our view of the potential risks and benefits to humans.

The extension of lifespan by CR in rodents is highly dependent upon the level of restriction and upon the timing of the introduction of the protocol. Maximal extension of lifespan is noted when rodents are fed only 35% of normal ad libitum intakes, and CR is most effective when introduced immediately after weaning. Rodent studies show that introducing CR later in life has a greatly attenuated effect or may not alter longevity at all. Speakman and Hambly (2007) used available data on rats and mice to model the anticipated benefits of CR in humans, making the assumption that humans and rodents would respond in a similar manner. On this basis, introducing a 30% CR at 16 years of age would add 11 years to life, while introducing CR at age 47 would extend life by less than 3 years (Figure 9.5). Studies of the effects of CR upon ageing in non-human primates (Research Highlight 9.1) support the view that following a lifelong CR in humans may be of minimal benefit in the absence of other forms of dietary change.

Estimates of lifespan gained based upon extrapolation from rodent experiments provide almost all that is known about the potential impact of CR in humans as there are no robust studies of populations that practise this behaviour. There are some groups that attempt CR in the hope that it will extend life, and the indications

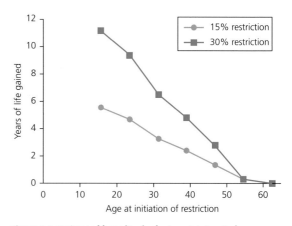

Figure 9.5 Estimated benefit of caloric restriction in humans. Adopting a more stringent reduction of energy intake at an earlier age is projected to give the optimal extension of longevity. Adapted from Banks (2010).

are that following a restricted diet for 3–15 years does improve markers of cardiovascular disease risk (Fontana et al., 2004). The population of Okinawa in Japan is renowned for its longevity, having remarkably low death rates among middle-aged men and women and the highest density of centenarians in the world. The Okinawan diet is believed to underlie this and is suggested to be similar to the CR diet protocol used with rodents, being nutrient dense and lower in energy than the diet consumed elsewhere in Japan (Dirks and Leeuwenburgh, 2006).

Despite these observations that appear to lend support to the idea that human CR might be beneficial in ageing and avoidance of age-related disease, considerable caution is needed in translating the data from CR studies in animals into humans. CR in humans would certainly have a number of adverse health effects that would offset many of the benefits. It is clear that CR would promote weight loss and excessive weight loss, and BMI of less than 20 is associated with menstrual irregularities and infertility, osteoporosis, poor wound healing and reduced capacity to metabolize drugs and toxins. Underweight is also associated with impaired immunity and hence excess levels of illness and reduced capacity for work. Mortality associated with all causes and in particular cardiovascular disease has been shown to increase when comparing BMI of less than 20 with BMI in the optimal range (Romero-Corral *et al.*, 2006). CR is also likely to result in depression and other psychological disorders (Dirks and Leeuwenburgh, 2006).

9.3.3.2 Fetal programming of lifespan

In contrast to CR in postnatal life, manipulations of the diet during early development appear to programme shorter lifespan. The feeding of maternal low-protein diets, without CR, during rat pregnancy significantly reduced the lifespan of the offspring (Aihie-Sayer *et al.*, 2001; Figure 9.6), and similar observations in mice indicate that this programming of lifespan is exacerbated by feeding an obesity-inducing diet in postnatal life (Ozanne and Hales, 2004). The mechanism through which this programming occurs has not been fully elucidated but

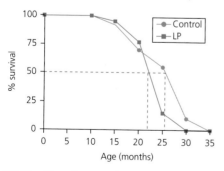

Figure 9.6 The effect of maternal protein restriction during pregnancy upon longevity in rats. Low-protein (LP) rats were exposed to an LP diet *in utero*. Fetal undernutrition reduced average lifespan by 3.5 months (10% of lifespan). Adapted from Aihie-Sayer *et al.* (2001). With permission from Karger Publishers.

appears to involve both oxidative processes and more rapid telomere shortening in key tissues such as the liver (Langley-Evans and Sculley, 2006) and kidney (Jennings *et al.*, 1999).

9.3.3.3 Supplementary antioxidants

Although it is well established that in cardiovascular disease and cancer (see Chapter 8), supplemental intakes of antioxidants are ineffective or even harmful to health, there is sufficient interest in the concept of oxidative senescence to merit experiments that consider the impact of increasing intakes of antioxidants on ageing processes. Analysis of human dietary patterns that are associated with longer life and healthier ageing shows that these diets are often rich in phytonutrients and antioxidants, in addition to unrefined carbohydrates, varied but not excessive sources of protein and low in saturated fat and this is true of the Okinawan diet (Willcox *et al.*, 2014). Given the association between oxidative stress and telomere shortening, there has been considerable attention paid to the effects of antioxidants upon longevity in mammals.

Studies in which animals are supplemented with antioxidants yield variable results. Resveratrol, derived from grapes, for example, clearly increases lifespan in yeast and *C. elegans* but in mice has no significant effect (Hector *et al.*, 2012). This agent does, however, result in attenuated age-related declines in renal and cardiovascular function and improves bone and eye health in mice (Pearson *et al.*, 2008). Massie and colleagues (1984) reported that lifelong supplementation with ascorbic acid increased lifespan in mice, but Selman *et al.* (2006) found no benefits associated with a similar protocol. Banks and colleagues (2010) reported that lifelong vitamin E supplementation increased the lifespan of mice by up to 15%. The effect of vitamin E was shown to be unrelated to the antioxidant properties of vitamin E and was instead driven by the anti-cancer action of the supplement. This and the resveratrol example (Pearson *et al.*, 2008) give a good illustration of the fact that 'antioxidant' nutrients often have physiological effects that do not depend upon their antioxidant properties.

These animal studies are largely inconclusive and have failed to establish a clear benefit of supplementary antioxidants. It is over-simplistic to assume that supplementing with a single nutrient could have any real benefit in extending lifespan, since cellular senescence and the associated tissue degeneration occur through multiple mechanisms and are the products of the balance between pro-ageing and anti-ageing processes and between cellular damage and repair. Selman *et al.* (2006) noted that supplementing mice with ascorbate apparently had no impact upon levels of oxidative injury within cells, but down-regulated genes associated with ROS scavenging and repair processes. It seems likely that any benefit attained by providing greater antioxidant protection from the diet was offset by down-regulation of endogenous systems. On this basis, antioxidant therapy to increase longevity appears unlikely to succeed in isolation.

9.4 Nutrient requirements of the elderly

9.4.1 Macronutrients and energy

As shown in Table 9.2, the requirement for energy declines with ageing, reflecting typically lower levels of energy expenditure through physical activity and a fall in basal metabolic rate. The latter is largely attributable to a loss of lean body tissue that is seen in most elderly people. Generally, there are no other major changes in the macro- or micronutrient requirements of this population, and although protein requirements, for men at least, fall slightly with age, the percentage of energy derived from protein remains relatively unchanged with ageing. With a lower energy requirement and unchanged, or in some cases increased, requirements for other nutrients, the optimal diet for the elderly needs to be nutrient dense.

9.4.2 Micronutrients

There are few micronutrients recognized within the dietary reference values of Westernized countries as being required by the elderly at greater levels of intake

Table 9.2 Dietary reference values (United Kingdom) for energy and protein.

		EAR	RNI
	Years	Energy (MJ/day)	Protein (g/day)
Males	19–29	11.0*	
	30–59	10.5*	
	60–64	9.93	
	65–75	9.71	
	75+	8.77	
	19–50		55.5
	50+		53.3
Females	19–29	9.1†	
	30–59	8.6†	
	60–64	7.99	
	65–75	7.96	
	75+	7.61	
	19–50		45.0
	50+		46.5

EAR, estimated average requirement; RNI, reference nutrient intake.
*Assumes physical activity level 1.5 and weight 70 kg.
†Assumes physical activity level 1.5 and weight 65 kg.

(Department of Health, 1999). This is surprising given the high levels of malnutrition and nutrient deficiency observed in this population and the high prevalence of chronic disease states that lead to micronutrient malabsorption. The assignment of dietary reference values that are similar to those for younger adults reflects the fact that dietary reference values are derived for healthy populations and that they were determined from relatively sparse data on the elderly. There are a number of nutrients where, despite there being no special requirement set for the elderly, special care to maintain intake at an optimal level may be worthwhile. Vitamin B6, for example, has been set a RNI value of 15 µg/g protein/day for both men and women aged 19–50 and over 50 years. This reference value reflects requirements extrapolated from studies of younger people. However, in the elderly, vitamin B6 may be of additional importance in maintaining immune function, so demands may be greater than the dietary reference values suggest. Vitamin C (RNI 40 mg/day) intakes should be comfortably maintained by most elderly individuals and therefore positively contribute to absorption of iron. However, in institutionalized settings where bulk food preparation and delivery systems necessitate maintaining food at high temperatures for long periods of time, actual intakes of ascorbate may be suboptimal. Consideration of potential raw sources of this nutrient is therefore relevant.

9.4.3 Specific guidelines for the elderly

There are few specific guidelines for the nutrition of elderly people, since in general this population is advised to follow a healthy balanced diet, as at earlier stages of adulthood. Mild–moderate physical activity is considered to be an important element of a healthy lifestyle for the elderly, since activities such as walking, climbing stairs and gardening are sufficient to increase appetite and contribute to maintenance of bone health.

In the United Kingdom and the United States, the few specific recommendations that have been made regarding intakes of elderly people relate to a narrow range of nutrients. In both countries, it is recommended that the elderly increase intakes of vitamin D either through supplementation (10 µg/day) or by increasing intakes of fortified margarines and other sources. In the United States, it is recommended that the over-50s increase their intakes of vitamin B12 through supplementation with 2.4 µg/day to offset declining absorption of this micronutrient. The US, UK and Australian guidelines for the elderly stress the need to reduce salt intake, maintain intakes of micronutrients that promote bone health and consume water to maintain hydration. Dehydration is considered to be an important issue for the elderly as fluid intakes are often poor. This may not only be partly due to declining physiological control of the thirst centre and fluid homeostasis but can also come from concerns about urinary incontinence. Dehydration can contribute to mental confusion, headaches and irritability. The elderly are recommended to consume 1.5l of fluid per day (excluding alcoholic beverages).

Maintaining the desired nutrient density for this age group might best be achieved by encouraging a diet that is rich in whole grain and nutrient-enriched breads, pasta and cereals. Using these foods to replace refined grains helps to maintain intakes of B vitamins. The elderly should favour deeply pigmented fruits and vegetables to maximize intakes of folate and antioxidant nutrients. In keeping with guidelines to prevent cardiovascular disease, choosing low-fat dairy options also maximizes intakes of calcium. Fibre is an important element of the diet in order to optimize bowel function. However, wheat bran should be avoided due to the presence of phytates that impede the absorption of iron, calcium and zinc.

Older adults tend to consume less food overall than the younger population. However, the burden of chronic diseases such as cardiovascular disease, osteoporosis and gastrointestinal disorders means that for some in this population, energy and protein requirements are actually increased. As individuals with these chronic diseases make up a high proportion of the population within long-term institutional care (e.g. nursing homes), there are major challenges in providing high-quality nutrition in these settings. As a diet rich in complex carbohydrate is bulky, attaining both the extra energy requirement and nutrient intake in frail elderly patients might best be achieved by increasing intakes of fat-rich foods.

9.5 Barriers to healthy nutrition in the elderly

9.5.1 Malnutrition and the elderly

In 2001, the Malnutrition Action Group carried out a survey of nutritional status among the elderly population of the United Kingdom. They identified high levels of malnutrition, affecting 14% of the over-65s (potentially 1.26 million people), with marked regional differences. Up to 20% of the elderly population of the northwest were malnourished, and people living in the north of England were 71% more likely to be malnourished than those in the south. It was estimated that this level of malnutrition would be associated with major ill health, costing the National Health Service up to £4 billion every year. Despite the subsequent call for action to prevent, identify and treat malnutrition in the elderly, the more recent BAPEN Nutrition Screening Survey (BAPEN, 2010) revealed that the situation had deteriorated over

the first decade of the century. This survey reported that 39% of elderly people admitted to hospital, 45% admitted to nursing homes and 30% admitted to residential care in the United Kingdom were malnourished. These are problems seen in all developed countries. Kaiser *et al.* (2010) considered malnutrition in hospitals, nursing homes and the community among elderly people from the United States, Japan, South Africa and nine European nations. In the community, 9.5% of men and 5.3% of women were malnourished with 52.6 and 29% at risk of malnutrition, and prevalence was much greater in institutionalized settings. Considering all settings, the prevalence of malnutrition in men was 28% and 20.8% in women, with close to 50% at risk. Brownie (2006) estimated that while the prevalence of malnutrition among the free-living elderly is between 5 and 10%, malnutrition is rife among the institutionalized elderly, affecting 30–65% of those in old peoples' homes or in hospital and at least 85% of those in nursing homes. Suominen and colleagues (2005) reported that among elderly people living in Finnish nursing homes, 29% were malnourished, but two-thirds were at risk of malnutrition.

It is clear that being dependent or institutionalized increases risk of malnutrition, and several lines of evidence show the decline in nutritional status as elderly people lose their independence. Eastwood and colleagues (2002) reported that institutionalized elderly had lower energy intakes than their free-living counterparts, and Hirani and Primatesta (2005) reported that elderly people living in institutions had significantly lower plasma vitamin D concentrations than those living in their own homes. A study of 14 elderly care facilities in Melbourne (Australia) found that 65% of residents had two or more indicators of undernutrition and that intake of protein and energy was below dietary reference values for 34% and 62% of residents, respectively. Low intakes of calcium, magnesium, folate and zinc and fibre were noted (Woods *et al.*, 2009).

The reasons why the elderly are so vulnerable to malnutrition are discussed in more detail in the following and include poverty, social isolation and ill health (Figure 9.5). The very high prevalence of malnutrition in institutionalized settings is both caused by, and is a contributor to, ongoing health problems. Margetts *et al.* (2003) found that while hospitalization increased risk of malnutrition (OR 1.83, 95% CI 1.03–3.16), the poor health of elderly people was in itself a major cause of their malnutrition (OR for malnutrition associated with ill health 2.34 men, 95% CI 1.20–4.58, 2.98 women, 95% CI 1.58–5.62). What is most concerning is the common failure of health professionals and nursing home staff to adequately assess the nutritional status of elderly people in their care and to set in place appropriate interventions. McWhirter and

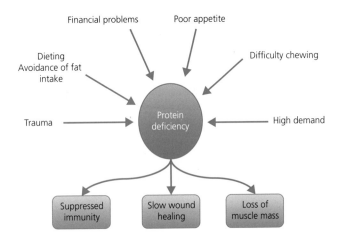

Figure 9.7 Factors leading to protein–energy malnutrition and its consequences in the elderly population.

Pennington (1994) reported that in UK hospitals, 40% of patients (mostly elderly) were malnourished on admission and that the majority went on to lose further weight during their hospital stay due to a failure to identify nutrition as an issue requiring support. Although 72% of UK hospitals now report that nutritional screening is routinely carried out on hospital admission (BAPEN, 2010), the prevalence of malnutrition remains high and clearly worsens with long-term medical and nursing care.

The consequences of malnutrition are severe as malnutrition is a cause as well as an outcome of major illness and trauma. As shown in Figure 9.7, poor nutritional status resulting from a failure to balance supply and demand establishes a vicious cycle in the elderly. Malnutrition promotes infection, which itself drives and maintains malnutrition. Undernutrition is a predictor of morbidity and mortality among the elderly. It leads to longer stays in hospital and impaired ability to recover from infections, fractures and surgery and is ultimately a major contributor to death. Sund-Levander *et al.* (2007) reported that among women living in nursing homes, survival over a 3-year period was very strongly related to nutritional status. Similarly, Gariballa and Forster (2007) found that lower serum albumin (a crude biochemical indicator of nutritional status) and lower mid-arm muscle circumference were predictors of increased risk of death over a year following admission to hospital for acute illness (e.g. stroke, falls and fractures, septicaemia and chest or urinary tract infections).

9.5.2 Poverty

The elderly are a group in the population for whom poverty is a major risk. The vast majority of elderly people are retired from full- or part-time employment and are therefore dependent upon any pension provision built up during the working years or upon state benefits.

A survey of the 28 member countries of the EU (European Commission, 2012) showed that one in six elderly people was at risk of poverty, with the highest rates of poverty in Bulgaria (59% of elderly population), Romania (35%) and Croatia (33%). The lowest rates of poverty among the elderly were noted in the Benelux countries (6%). Women may be particularly at risk of poverty as they live for longer and must therefore spread resources over a greater period of time. Levels of poverty in countries such as the United States, where the lack of a welfare state means a high proportion of pension income has to be allocated to housing costs and medical expenses, may be considerably greater. In the United States, poverty in the elderly is less prevalent than in Europe, but when the cost of private healthcare is factored in, prevalence is estimated at 16%. Low income in the United States has been shown to associate significantly with low food security (Ziliak and Gunderson, 2011).

Poverty impacts upon nutritional status in a number of ways. Primarily, a lack of money will reduce the quantity of food consumed, but importantly, it also reduces the scope for choice and variety within the diet. A study of deprivation among the elderly population of Northern Ireland showed that low consumption of fruit and vegetables was a feature of poverty in this population (Appleton *et al.*, 2009). Modern shopping practices can also make it difficult to access food without transport, and so poverty may disadvantage those unable to run a car or access public transport for shopping.

9.5.3 Social isolation

As many as one in seven elderly people will live alone, and a high proportion of these will be widowed. The sense of grief, loneliness and isolation that accompanies widowhood can be particularly great in relation to food, as the purchase of food, the preparation of food and the sharing of food at mealtimes are especially important elements of a close relationship. Pantell *et al.* (2013) reported that social isolation is more strongly associated with mortality among the elderly than high blood pressure or elevated cholesterol concentrations. Isolation is commonly associated with poverty and loss of appetite (Ramic *et al.*, 2011). Many people living alone are reluctant to invest time in cooking and eating and as a result are vulnerable to malnutrition.

Social isolation and infirmity may also make shopping difficult. The SOLINUT study of Ferry *et al.* (2005) found that in a population of 150 elderly men and women living alone, 44% could not lift a 5 kg shopping bag and therefore could not purchase adequate food supplies. 32% never shared a meal with family or friends, and 43% consumed inadequate energy to meet their requirements. Martin *et al.* (2005) identified social isolation as a major factor leading to weight loss in the elderly. Women are less vulnerable in this respect following widowhood as, for the elderly generation, they tend to have better domestic skills. Men of this generation cook less and are more dependent upon others for the acquisition and preparation of food. Hughes *et al.* (2004) studied 39 men, aged 62–94, living alone and noted that very few achieved recommended intakes for energy, trace elements and vitamins A and D. Energy intakes were highly correlated with the cooking skills of the men.

For institutionalized elderly, the opportunities for social interaction around mealtimes can be an advantage over living alone in the home setting. However, there are still factors at work that are likely to reduce intakes. In an institutional setting, individuals are no longer preparing their own food or playing a role in the purchase of food items. Regimented mealtimes that may not correspond to peaks in appetite can detract from overall intakes.

9.5.4 Education

For many elderly people, the knowledge of food and health and the cooking skills that they accrued in their younger years may be not be helpful in providing the balance of nutrients required to meet requirements. Favoured cooking and food preparation techniques may use excessive amounts of saturated fat, sugar and salt and also reduce the bioavailability of nutrients (e.g. boiling rather than steaming vegetables will reduce vitamin content). Contemporary foods (particularly foods from imported cuisines) may also be unfamiliar to some elderly people, and this reduces the number of acceptable choices when shopping and can make the diet narrow in scope. Individuals who are advised to make adjustments

to their diet to manage chronic health conditions may also struggle to meet nutrient demands due to lack of education and understanding.

9.5.5 Physical changes

Even in healthy individuals, physical changes associated with ageing will have a deleterious effect upon nutritional status. The reduced efficiency of the gastrointestinal tract leads to malabsorption and reduced bioavailability of micronutrients. The elderly may also develop a variety of conditions within the bowel that lead to discomfort and the avoidance of certain types of food. For example, the degeneration of the brush-border cells of the small intestine can limit the production of lactase, promoting lactose intolerance. Given the discomfort that will ensue with consumption of dairy products, these nutrient-rich sources will tend to be cut from the diet and not replaced with suitable alternatives. Within the mouth, periodontal disease and poorly fitted dentures can also result in avoidance of foods such as meat, which require longer mastication.

The senses of taste and smell decline with age, and this can reduce enjoyment of food and impair appetite. The sense of taste can change quite abruptly, and often, it is the sensing of sweetness and saltiness that is initially lost, effectively making food seem more bitter (Omran and Morley, 2000). Around half of the 65–80-year-old age group report reductions in the sense of smell (Griep *et al.*, 1995). These changes may be partly age related but are also brought on by medications used to manage chronic disease (e.g. phenothiazines used in treatment of mental disorders).

Physical infirmity, stemming from disability or disease, will also contribute to the development of malnutrition. Major disease states such as cancer, cardiovascular disease, renal disease and diabetes are important co-morbidities of malnutrition in the elderly. Chronic disease increases requirements for energy and protein and micronutrients such as zinc and can promote nutrient losses via the bowel and urine. In addition, these diseases and physical disability associated with musculoskeletal disorders will contribute to immobility and increase dependence upon carers. The ensuing impairment of the ability to shop, cook and self-feed and social isolation are obvious contributors to malnutrition.

9.5.6 Combating malnutrition in the elderly

The prevention and treatment of malnutrition among the elderly have to be a major public health priority in all nations. Malnutrition is clearly more prevalent among individuals who are hospitalized or otherwise institutionalized for long periods of time but is not confined to that subgroup in the population. Malnutrition is also a problem for the free-living elderly, and this group perhaps provides the greater challenge in terms of intervention.

Most malnutrition goes unnoticed, particularly among the elderly living in nursing homes (Abbassi and Rudman, 1994). The basic first step in preventing and treating malnutrition has to be the introduction of suitable tools for screening and monitoring nutritional status. The MUST, developed in the United Kingdom, is an example of such a tool (Stratton *et al.*, 2004). It uses measures of BMI, acute illness events and unplanned weight loss to assign a score that then triggers appropriate specialist referrals and interventions for the at-risk or malnourished patient.

In nursing home or hospital settings, tools such as MUST can be used for screening of the elderly on admission and for monitoring in the longer term. Having standardized measures in operation between different institutions allows for tracking of nutritional status over time and can trigger intervention at a range of different levels, up to and including oral nutritional support with fortifiers or supplements. Ideally, all staff working with institutionalized elderly patients should be trained in nutritional screening, in taking responsibility for initiating nutritional support and in carrying out basic feeding and food-related support tasks. In addition to this, there are a number of steps that can be taken to promote food intake and boost nutritional status without the need for supplemental products or specialist intervention. It is important to target the quality of the food itself,

Research Highlight 9.2 Providing nutritional support in the community.

Estimates of the prevalence of malnutrition among the elderly living in their own homes vary between countries but suggest that up to 15% are suffering from protein–energy malnutrition, micronutrient deficiency or both. Although imperfect, the detection of malnutrition through regular screening can be accomplished in nursing homes and among hospital admissions but is challenging in the community setting. Robust clinical nutritional assessment tools, such as the Malnutrition Universal Screening Tool (Todorovic *et al.*, 2003; Stratton *et al.*, 2004) or Mini Nutritional Assessment (Calvo *et al.*, 2012), are only usable when elderly people come into contact with medical professionals and have little preventive benefit. European studies suggest that among primary care professionals (mostly general practitioners), the use of routine, regular nutritional screening is uncommon as the professionals lack knowledge, motivation and time to implement it (Kennelly *et al.*, 2010; Gaboreau *et al.*, 2013) As a result, action to provide nutritional support has to have a broader nature than simply providing oral supplements to treat or reverse deficits.

Preventing malnutrition in the community requires engagement with the principal non-medical drivers of poor food intake, which are poverty and social isolation. A range of solutions is available in developed countries, including meals on wheels (MOW), cook-and-eat classes and lunch clubs. The latter two are believed to promote eating and cooking skills by creating a social environment for eating, but there is no current evidence base to support the anecdotal view that they reduce risk of malnutrition or reach those most at need.

MOW schemes are designed to provide meals to elderly people in their own homes, ensuring food intake can be maintained among individuals who struggle to shop and cook. Most MOW schemes provide one hot meal per day for 5 days per week. Extension of this to include all meals and snacks for the full week can significantly improve nutritional intakes and promote weight gain among the malnourished (Kretser *et al.*, 2003), and the inclusion of breakfast in a two-meal MOW scheme was shown to increase intakes of energy, protein, carbohydrate fibre and micronutrients; reduce depression scores; and increase enjoyment of food (Gollub and Weddle, 2004). Well-designed MOW menus can have an enhanced impact upon nutritional status. Silver *et al.* (2006) showed that by doubling the energy density of a single meal, the 24-h energy intakes of recipients could be increased by 453 kcal. There are some concerns about this form of support. The evidence that MOW does not reduce the prevalence of malnutrition among the frail elderly is weak (Roy and Payette, 2006), and there are also concerns that MOW may increase the risk of food-borne disease (Roseman, 2007). Many recipients of delivered meals do not eat them immediately and then store the whole meal, or leftovers, in unsafe conditions (Almanza *et al.*, 2007).

Other approaches to the prevention and management of malnutrition that have been attempted include the use of dietitian-led interventions and pairing newly discharged elderly hospital patients with nutrition 'buddies' who promote energy and protein intake, exercise and fluid intake for a period post-discharge (Dorner *et al.*, 2013). These approaches, which are resource intensive, have had mixed success. While Endevelt *et al.* (2011) reported increased intakes of protein, carbohydrate and B vitamins over a 6-month period in malnourished community-dwelling elderly following dietetic intervention, Locher *et al.* (2013) found limited benefits in terms of energy intake or weight gain.

The evidence suggests that frail elderly benefit most from schemes that provide nutritious meals provided in their own homes. The investment by local authorities and the availability of commercial enterprises to provide such services play an important role in maintaining elderly people in their own homes for longer periods, without risking nutritional deficits. Simply providing food, however, does not address all of the other determinants of poor appetite and nutrient availability in this vulnerable population.

ensuring that it is nutritious, varied and attractive. Carrier and colleagues (2007) found that among Canadian nursing home residents, bulk-delivery food systems, repetitious menus and provision of meals in difficult-to-open packages and dishes all decreased food intake. Large portion sizes also suppress the appetite, so provision of smaller but more frequent meals helps to increase overall intake.

The environment provided for mealtimes is also of importance. All individuals involved with the feeding of dependent elderly need to be aware of the fact that malnutrition has a multifaceted aetiology and stems not only from reduced food intake but also from all of the social, pharmacological and medical factors that contribute to reducing appetite. Eating is a social activity, so providing meals in a social, friendly and pleasant environment encourages greater intake. Mamhidir and colleagues (2007) showed that with a group of demented, hospitalized patients, providing an intervention that made the ward seem more home-like and encouraging staff and caregivers to be more attentive and responsive at mealtimes prevented weight loss over a 3-month period and in many cases promoted gains in weight. Assistance with feeding is also an essential element in the elderly care setting. This can range from physically feeding frail and dependent individuals to providing modified utensils that enable self-feeding. In all circumstances, encouragement, warmth and preservation of dignity are essential elements of maintaining a healthy intake.

In the community, the challenges are different as the level of support that can be provided is often limited. There are schemes in place in many countries that are designed to prolong the period of time that frail elderly can maintain independent living and reduce the risk of malnutrition. Meals on wheels, or community meals, is a widely used strategy. Meals are delivered directly to the homes of recipients, in a ready-to-eat form that requires no further preparation, and this has many benefits for recipients (Research Highlight 9.2).

9.6 Common nutrition-related health problems

9.6.1 Bone disorders

The degeneration of physiological function and physical well-being that is associated with ageing means that many chronic diseases first manifest in the later years of adulthood. While cardiovascular diseases and cancer are often first noted in the elderly, they are clearly also a major problem in younger adults. In contrast, there are a number of diseases of bone that are almost exclusively seen in elderly people.

9.6.1.1 Bone mineralization and remodelling

Bone has a complex structure and is a highly vascularized and innervated tissue. It essentially comprises a framework of collagen subtypes into which are deposited minerals to provide the hard, rigid structure. Most of the mineral in bone comprises calcium and phosphate, but there are many other minerals and trace elements present, including fluoride and sodium. Seventy to eighty per cent of the skeleton comprises cortical bone, which in section appears as concentric rings of bone in a bundled arrangement. The remaining bone is termed trabecular bone, which has a lattice structure, similar in nature to that of a sponge. The trabecular bone is found at the ends of the long bones, within the vertebrae and at the hips and wrist (Figure 9.8).

Bone mineralization is a process that essentially occurs during childhood and the pubertal growth spurt (Figure 9.8). As the body grows, the mass of mineral in the skeleton increases accordingly. At the end of the growth phase, coinciding with sexual maturity, there is no further net gain of mineral within the skeleton, and the individual is said to have achieved peak bone mass. Although there is now no further net gain of mineral, the skeleton is far from inert at this stage. There is a constant cycle of mineral loss and replacement taking place. This is essential not only to allow the skeleton to be repaired in the event of injury but also to allow the skeleton to be remodelled and maintained and for the release of minerals from bone to make up for any shortfall in supply for other critical processes.

The skeleton completely remodels itself every 7–10 years, and this process is driven by two cell types within the bone. Osteoclasts are cells that remove mineral from bone (Figure 9.9). They respond to hormonal signals including parathyroid hormone and vitamin D3 to release calcium from bone into the circulation. When bone is injured or fractured, they move into the damaged area to remove debris and begin the process of repair. In contrast, the osteoblasts bring about the remineralization of bone. During childhood and adolescence, osteoblast activity is in the ascendance as high concentrations of growth hormone stimulate osteoblast activity, and during puberty, rising sex steroid concentrations also promote bone mineralization. At the end of growth, the activities of osteoblasts and osteoclasts are in equilibrium, and the skeleton is maintained in a stable state through the ongoing remodelling process. With ageing, however, osteoclast activity tends to exceed the rates of

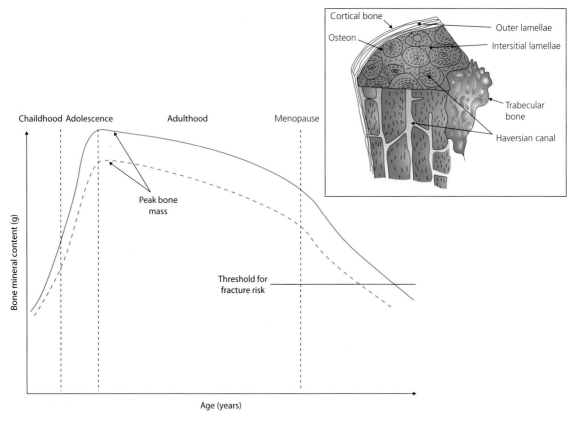

Figure 9.8 Bone mass across the lifespan. Bone mineral accrues in the first three decades of life but thereafter declines progressively. The rate of bone loss accelerates after the menopause. Inset: the structure of long bones. Spongy trabecular bone makes up the ends of the long bones, while compact cortical bone provides the main mass of the skeleton. Haversian canals contain blood vessels and nerves.

remineralization, and hence, the bone mineral content and density begin to decline (Figure 9.8). In women, the rate of decline accelerates at the menopause as the loss of oestrogen production removes the stimulatory effect upon osteoblasts. Rates of bone remodelling are not even across the whole skeleton, and trabecular bone remodels around eight times faster than cortical bone. This means that with ageing, loss of bone density from the trabecular regions is much faster, declining by up to 2.5% every year.

9.6.1.2 Osteoporosis pathology and prevalence

Osteoporosis is one of the most common causes of hospitalization among the elderly and is characterized by an increased susceptibility to bone fracture due to demineralization. In the EU, there are over a million osteoporotic fractures every year, and this number is steadily increasing. While, at the present time, most osteoporosis is noted in the developed countries, the increasing lifespan of populations in

developing countries means that the global prevalence of the condition will increase dramatically, possibly doubling over 50 years.

Osteoporosis is a serious condition, and among the elderly, a quarter of all individuals sustaining a fracture can be expected to die within 1 year. Often, the first indication of the condition comes when an elderly person has a fall and fractures a bone at one of the main trabecular bone sites, such as the hip or wrist. Fractures to the vertebrae can often go unnoticed and manifest as a loss of height or the development of a humpbacked posture. Osteoporosis is generally diagnosed through x-ray, which shows the loss of mineral from affected regions, and confirmed using the dual x-ray absorptiometry technique. This allows the determination of the total mineral present within the skeleton or specific bone regions (bone mineral content), and from this, the bone mineral density (BMD, g mineral/cm^2 bone) can be derived. BMD is the primary tool for diagnosis and monitoring of osteoporosis, with clearly characterized

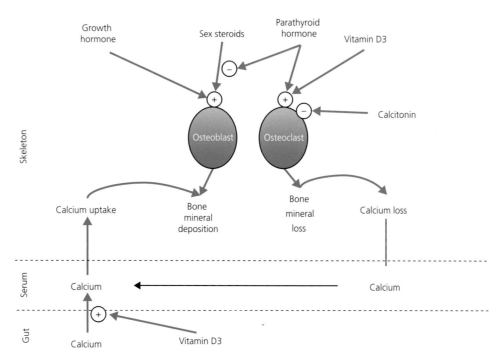

Figure 9.9 The endocrine control of bone mineralization.

thresholds for defining the progression of the disease. Markers of bone degradation (e.g. *N*-telopeptide) or formation (e.g. alkaline phosphatase activity or procollagen 1 C-terminal peptide) can also be used to monitor the disease. Although osteoporosis is seen in both men and women, it is far more common in women due to the impact of the menopause on rates of bone loss. Kanis *et al.* (2002) reported that significant risk of osteoporosis begins at around the age of 50–55 years, when up to 10% of women meet the criteria for diagnosis. By the age of 80 years, osteoporosis was seen in 47% of women and 16% of men.

9.6.1.3 Risk factors for osteoporosis

The major non-modifiable risk factors for osteoporosis include female gender, early menopause and increasing age. There is believed to be a strong genetic component underlying the risk of osteoporosis, and some twin studies suggest that this may account for as much as 50% of risk. There are a number of polymorphisms of the vitamin D receptor gene and the collagen 1α1 gene (Col1α1) that contribute to individual risk. For example, BMD tends to be lower in individuals with the ss variant of the Sp1 polymorphism of Col1α1, compared to the SS variant (Garnero *et al.*, 1998). A number of disease states will impact upon risk of osteoporosis, generally by virtue of the effects they have upon the endocrine regulation of

bone turnover or the metabolism and transport of vitamin D and calcium. These include hyperthyroidism, hyperparathyroidism, cancer, rheumatoid arthritis, coeliac disease, inflammatory bowel disorders, renal failure and anorexia nervosa. Therapies that require administration of corticosteroids or that disrupt the normal production of sex steroids will promote osteoporosis.

The level of peak bone mass attained at the end of the growth phase is considered to be an important determinant of the risk of osteoporosis later in life. Rates of bone loss are relatively constant among the population, so risk of BMD falling below the thresholds at which fractures become likely is increased in individuals for whom peak bone mass was lower (Figure 9.8). For this reason, the optimal periods for targeting interventions to prevent osteoporosis may lie during childhood and adolescence, rather than in the adult years.

The main avoidable lifestyle risk factors for osteoporosis include smoking, physical inactivity and excessive consumption of alcohol and poor dietary intakes of calcium and vitamin D. The latter two form the main targets for nutritional interventions, as will be discussed in the next section. Physical activity is important as bone mineralization occurs at faster rates around lines of stress within bone. Low-to-moderate intakes of alcohol appear to be protective against osteoporosis, but with heavy use, any benefits are lost. Alcoholics typically develop an osteopenic skeleton and suffer high rates of falls and fractures. This is because alcohol specifically blocks bone formation, while having no effect on rates of resorption (Chakkalakal, 2005).

9.6.1.4 Dietary interventions for osteoporosis prevention

Once diagnosed, osteoporosis is generally treated using pharmacological agents. Rates of bone loss can be reduced by treating with bisphosphonates, which inhibit osteoclast activity. Calcitonin has a similar effect and can be administered as a nasal spray. Bone deposition can be increased through administration of drugs that boost hormone concentrations or mimic their actions. Raloxifene, for example, is a selective oestrogen receptor modulator, which mimics oestrogen activity and helps maintain bone mass in women after the menopause (Keen, 2007). Strontium ranelate is a drug that promotes bone deposition. In addition to these pharmacological approaches, older people with osteoporosis are advised to increase intakes of calcium and vitamin D in order to limit bone loss. However, this nutritional strategy is considered to be more important in the context of osteoporosis prevention and is the cornerstone of population-wide intervention strategies.

9.6.1.4.1 Calcium and vitamin D

Calcium has been shown to be effective in increasing bone mass in individuals at any stage of life, and most observational studies are generally supportive of a role for calcium supplementation as a means of preventing osteoporosis. Stear and colleagues (2003) showed that in 17-year-old girls with good baseline calcium intakes, a 1000 mg/day calcium supplement increased whole-body BMD over a 2-year period, with particularly strong effects at the trochanter (5% increase in BMD). Among Chinese 12–15-year-olds, supplementation at a range of doses of calcium (230–966 mg/day) over 24 months increased lumbar spine and total body BMD but only in boys (Yin *et al.*, 2010). The systematic review of Huncharek *et al.* (2008) found that supplemental calcium or increasing intake of dairy foods will increase total body and lumbar spine BMD among children with low baseline calcium intakes. Studies of children generally show that initiating calcium supplementation during the pubertal growth spurt is particularly effective. Although this stage of life is well ahead of the appearance of any disease, boosting BMD at this time might enable the achievement of a greater peak bone mass.

When considering the impact of calcium supplementation in older people, the effects are less obvious. Some studies find no clear effect of calcium upon bone mineralization, although Slevin and colleagues (2014) found that bone turnover markers were increased by 800 mg

calcium per day over 2 years, in the absence of any change in BMD. Shea *et al.* (2004) performed a systematic review of the literature considering randomized clinical trials of calcium supplements (excluding calcium combined with vitamin D or other nutrients). While calcium supplementation was shown to be capable of boosting whole-body BMD by approximately 2%, with significant gains in the hip and spine, there was no benefit in terms of fracture risk. This finding was confirmed by a further meta-analysis from Rabenda *et al.* (2011) which also showed calcium increased BMD at the hip and spine but with no effect on fracture risk. While increasing BMD is desirable, fractures are the true disease outcome in osteoporosis, and any preventive or therapeutic intervention should aim to reduce their occurrence.

Epidemiological studies are similarly equivocal regarding preventive strategies that use vitamin D alone. Most vitamin D is synthesized endogenously through the action of sunlight upon the skin, and as a result, concentrations in circulation tend to vary with season, particularly among elderly people in the northern hemisphere. As vitamin D3 concentrations fall in the winter months, the risk of fracture increases. In contrast to calcium, where supplementing the elderly increases BMD, vitamin D supplements appear to have no effect on bone mineralization, except in individuals whose calcium status is poor. This is because the main function of vitamin D within bone remodelling is to reverse calcium insufficiency. A review of all randomized controlled trials using vitamin D3 in isolation showed that supplementation had no effect on BMD at any site (Reid *et al.*, 2014). However, despite this lack of effect on BMD, vitamin D supplementation of elderly women has an impact upon fracture risk, with doses of between 700 and 800 IU/day reducing risk of fractures of the hip and vertebrae by 25% (Bischoff-Ferrari *et al.*, 2004).

Most randomized controlled trials do not consider the effects of calcium and vitamin D in isolation and instead administer these two nutrients together. Di Daniele and colleagues (2004) studied 1200 women over the age of 45 years for a 30-month period and showed that combined supplements prevented the decline in BMD following the menopause and, indeed, actually increased bone mineralization. Meta-analysis (Tang *et al.*, 2007) confirms that combined supplementation with calcium (doses over 1200 mg) and vitamin D (doses over 800 IU/day) reduces bone loss at the hip and spine and reduces fracture risk by 12% (HR 0.88, 95% CI 0.83–0.95). Although relatively low-dose supplements of calcium (500 mg/day) combined with vitamin D (700 IU/day) have also been found to be effective in preventing declines in BMD and fractures among the elderly, supplementation must be maintained in the long term to preserve the benefits (Dawson-Hughes *et al.*, 2000).

Boonen *et al.* (2007) performed a meta-analysis that showed that the observed benefits of vitamin D upon fracture risk were largely dependent upon the co-administration of calcium supplements. Comparing the relative risk (RR) of hip fracture associated with combined supplements with that associated with vitamin D alone, they reported a 25% decrease (RR 0.75, 95% CI 0.58–0.90). Falls are the main cause of fractures among elderly people with osteoporosis. There is a growing body of evidence to suggest that calcium and vitamin D supplementation may contribute to reduced risk of fracture by preventing falls, in addition to increasing BMD (Research Highlight 9.3). It is suggested that vitamin D3 supplements should be targeted at the elderly population, either as a daily dose of 700–800 IU or as a large depot dose (100 000 IU) every 4 months, in order to prevent falls and fractures. Optimal strategies for delivering this on a population-wide scale have yet to be determined (Bischoff-Ferrari and Dawson-Hughes, 2007).

With increasing emphasis upon increasing calcium intake to prevent age-related bone loss and fracture, concern has been raised about potentially negative consequences. Bolland and colleagues analysed data from the US Women's Health Initiative, a study of over 144 000 women (aged 50–79 at baseline) followed longitudinally from the 1990s to 2011 (Bolland *et al.*, 2011). Women consuming supplements of calcium or calcium plus vitamin D were found to be at increased risk of myocardial infarction (HR 1.24. 95% CI 1.07–1.45). However, this observation is not widely accepted as a strong indicator of risk associated with calcium supplementation (Heaney *et al.*, 2012), as other large cohorts do not find the same risk and the Women's Health Initiative analysis did not take into account other cardiovascular risk factors.

9.6.1.4.2 Minerals and protein

Other nutrients and dietary components may be influential in determining the risk of developing osteoporosis and fractures. Iron and magnesium have both been shown to contribute to bone mineralization. Serum

Research Highlight 9.3 Vitamin D and falls in the elderly.

Vitamin D supplements appear to counter vitamin D insufficiency and reduce risk of fracture. As there appears to be no effect of vitamin D supplementation upon bone mineral density, there is considerable interest in whether it has any influence upon risk of falling. Falls are commonplace in some groups of elderly people and among populations living in nursing homes may occur at least once per year per individual. Falls are more likely with cognitive impairment, cataracts, certain medication and cardiovascular disease (Karlsson *et al.*, 2013). These falls are not trivial and are the major cause of non-vertebral fractures among individuals with osteoporosis. Vitamin D status is often poor in the elderly population, particularly during the winter months and among those living in institutions. Factors such as impaired renal function contribute further to vitamin D insufficiency (Rothenbacher *et al.*, 2014). There is evidence to suggest that individuals with higher circulating vitamin D3 concentrations suffer fewer falls (Stein *et al.*, 1999). Age at first fall tends to be earlier in those with lower vitamin D3 status (Rothenbacher *et al.*, 2014).

Many studies suggest that supplementing with vitamin D or synthetic analogues is beneficial in the elderly. This is suggested to be due to effects of supplements upon muscle function. Vitamin D increases the strength of the upper and lower limbs in the elderly (Boyé *et al.*, 2013; Sanders *et al.*, 2014). Bischoff-Ferrari *et al.* (2003) reported that administering 800 IU/day cholecalciferol (vitamin D3) with 1200 mg/day calcium to a population of 63–99-year-olds reduced risk of falling by 49%, while calcium alone increased risk. In contrast, Law *et al.* (2006) found no benefit of administering 2.5 mg of ergocalciferol (vitamin D2) every 2 months, in terms of either fracture or falls risk. The meta-analysis of Bischoff-Ferrari and colleagues (2004) concluded that providing a supplement of vitamin D could significantly reduce the risk of falling (OR 0.78, 95% CI 0.64–0.92). This benefit might be dose dependent as Broe *et al.* (2007) found that benefits were only noted when 800 IU/day was administered to elderly women at risk of falls. Lower doses appeared insufficient to significantly improve vitamin D status. The meta-analysis of Guo *et al.* (2014) confirmed the 22% reduction in falls among elderly people with or without cognitive impairment, both independently living or in institutions. However, vitamin D was no more effective than interventions based on exercise. Ringe (2012) argues that vitamin D therapy is not effective in all elderly and that the benefits depend upon basal vitamin D status before supplementation, age, mobility, renal function and the presence of co-morbidities.

The mechanism of action through which vitamin D supplements prevent falls has not been fully defined. However, there are many reports that suggest the benefits stem from improvements to musculoskeletal function. Circulating concentrations of 25-hydroxy-vitamin D are good predictors of quadriceps strength and balance in elderly people. Dhesi *et al.* (2004) recruited a population of people aged over 65 years who had previously suffered a fall. Injections of 600 000 IU ergocalciferol did not impact upon the subsequent rate of falls in the ensuing 6 months, but did significantly improve balance and reaction times. This suggests that vitamin D improves neuromuscular performance and that this mechanism could be protective in those at risk of osteoporotic fracture. Vitamin D may also promote hypertrophy of type II muscle fibres, increasing their size and maintaining strength. These effects may be mediated by the vitamin D receptor which declines in expression in bone and muscle with ageing or could be indirect benefits of improved calcium and phosphate concentrations in muscle and circulation (Sanders *et al.*, 2014).

magnesium concentrations are reported to be higher among elderly individuals with greater BMD. Iron, on the other hand, promotes bone loss but only when present in major excess, as is seen with the condition haemochromatosis. Neither of these minerals is likely to have a major influence on bone health within the normal range of dietary intakes.

Protein nutrition may also be a determinant of bone health. Availability of protein clearly plays a role in the formation of bone, and supplements are beneficial in the elderly following a fracture. Moreover, protein intake may be a determinant of muscle strength and may play a role in determining the risk of falling. Habitual protein intake may be a determinant of BMD. Rapuri and colleagues (2003) studied almost 500 elderly people (aged 65–79) with protein intakes varying between 53 and 74 g/day. Over a 3-year period, protein intake had no influence over rates of bone loss. A higher protein intake was associated with greater BMD at the spine and wrist, but only in the subjects whose calcium intake was adequate. In the Women's Health Initiative study, protein intake was not related to fracture risk at the hip, but risk of wrist fracture declined by 7% for every 20% increase in protein intake (Beasley *et al.*, 2014). Higher protein intake was also associated with total skeletal BMD and BMD at the hip.

9.6.1.4.3 Phytoestrogens

Phytoestrogens have been suggested as a safe alternative to hormone replacement therapy by virtue of their capacity to reduce bone loss after the menopause. However, their efficacy has not been firmly established, and they may only be useful as an adjunct to other therapies, such as the use of selective oestrogen receptor modulators. While some studies demonstrate benefits of isoflavones in terms of bone turnover markers (Atkinson *et al.*, 2004) or BMD at the spine (Ma *et al.*, 2008) or whole-body level (Wong *et al.*, 2009), others find no effect (Kenny *et al.*, 2009; Ricci *et al.*, 2010), and the general consensus is that the effects of isoflavones are insignificant at the important fracture-prone sites (Wong *et al.*, 2009; Taku *et al.*, 2010). To some extent, the response to phytoestrogens may depend upon the composition of the gut microflora. Intestinal bacteria metabolize the soy isoflavone daidzein to *O*-desmethylangolensin (*O*-DMA, 80–90% of population) or equol (20–30% of population). A trial of 75 mg/day isoflavones in postmenopausal women showed that bone loss was slowed significantly in equol producers, but less so among non-equol producers (Ishimi, 2010). In the placebo group, there was no difference in bone loss between equol producers and non-producers. Administration of equol can inhibit bone loss in non-equol producers (Tousen *et al.*, 2011).

9.6.1.4.4 Caffeine

Avoidance of caffeine might be advocated as a strategy to prevent bone loss in certain individuals, as there are numerous reports that high consumption interferes with calcium uptake from the gut and reduces bone mineralization (Barbour *et al.*, 2010). In a study of over 61 000 postmenopausal women in the Swedish Mammography Cohort, consumption of 4 or more cups of coffee per day was associated with a 2–4% lower BMD compared to women who consumed less than 1 cup per day (Hallström *et al.*, 2013). Coffee consumption was not related to fracture risk. The effects of caffeine upon bone health may also depend upon specific genotypes. Men with the rapid metabolizing variant of CYP1A2, the enzyme which metabolizes caffeine, showed a greater detriment of BMD when consuming more than 4 cups of coffee per day than those with the slow metabolizing variant (Hallström *et al.*, 2010). Rapuri *et al.* (2001) reported that bone loss over a 3-year period was markedly greater among postmenopausal women consuming over 300 mg caffeine (10 cups of tea, 3–5 cups of coffee) per day compared to those consuming less than 300 mg/day. However, these effects were confined to the women who expressed the tt variant of the vitamin D receptor Taq1 polymorphism. This suggests that caffeine may interfere with vitamin D metabolism via its receptor.

9.6.1.5 Paget's disease of bone

Paget's disease of bone (osteitis deformans) is a disorder that is more common among the elderly population than in younger adults. It is characterized by the development of enlarged and deformed bone, particularly in the spine and any areas adjacent to joints. This is caused by excessive remodelling of bone, with high rates of breakdown and remineralization, and leads to malformations, including curvature of the spine, and weakness of bone that increases the likelihood of fracture. In contrast to osteoporosis, Paget's disease is more common in men than in women. It is treated using bisphosphonates to inhibit osteoclast activity, and patients taking these drugs are recommended to consume calcium supplements (1000–1500 mg/day) with vitamin D (400 IU/day).

9.6.2 Immunity and infection

Nutrition, infection and immunity are closely related (Figure 9.10). Nutrient deficits, particularly protein–energy malnutrition and deficits of the B vitamins, vitamin A and trace elements, impair both passive immunity and cellular immunity and therefore reduce the capacity to resist infection. Infection promotes malnutrition by activating the acute phase response to trauma. This response is characterized by an increase in demand for energy and protein, coupled with a decrease in appetite.

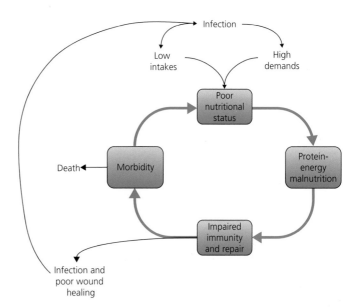

Figure 9.10 The vicious cycle of malnutrition and disease.

Chronic or recurrent infections can therefore exacerbate the effects of ongoing malnutrition. In the elderly, the relationship between nutritional status and immune function is of greater significance as the risk of malnutrition is heightened by other factors, and infection becomes more likely due to other medical conditions that either impair immune function or increased exposure to sources of infection, for example, following surgery. In developed countries, the elderly population are at two- to tenfold greater risk of death due to infectious diseases than younger adults (High, 2001). This population is also the major at-risk group for hospital-acquired infections such as multiple resistant *Staphylococcus aureus* or antibiotic-resistant strains of *Clostridium difficile* (Castle *et al.*, 2007).

While much of the increased infection risk seen among the elderly might be attributed to nutritional status or co-morbidities, it is important to appreciate that the immune system undergoes age-related changes in function that are probably greater than seen in any other tissue. Immune senescence is accompanied by complex changes to both innate and adaptive responses (Figure 9.11). Generally speaking, ageing is accompanied by a change in the profile of cytokines produced by immune cells, and increases in baseline levels of secretion of interleukin-6 and interleukin-10 create an environment that is undergoing a chronic, low-grade inflammatory response (Castle *et al.*, 2007). The lymphocyte types that are present in circulation also undergo change with senescence, and the elderly possess more memory T cells. These cells are responsible for the recognition of pathogens that the body has previously encountered and orchestrate a stronger immune response than that at the first infection. This would appear to be a feature of a more robust immune response, but it appears that the predominance of memory T cells results in reduced numbers of other T cell types, including CD4+ helper cells (which activate cytotoxic T cells) and naïve T cells. This means that there are less effective responses to new pathogens. The senescent immune system is generally less responsive to stimuli, for example, producing less interleukin-1 with an antigen challenge. Vaccinations produce lower antibody responses and are therefore less helpful. Declining functions of phagocytic cells and the complement system make the response to bacterial and viral infections less effective.

A number of studies have suggested that while nutritional status may not contribute appreciably to immune senescence, availability of nutrient supplements might lessen some of the impact. Providing nutritional support to patients in the postsurgical period can improve recovery rates, and without such support, the elderly surgical patient might be expected to lose weight for around 2 months during their convalescence (High, 2001). Multivitamin supplements are generally considered to be of greater value than supplements of single nutrients, and some trials have shown that over long periods of administration (12 months) to free-living elderly subjects, they can boost natural killer cell activity, increase expression of interleukin-2 and reduce the frequency of infectious illness (High, 2001). Among the institutionalized elderly, supplementation with zinc (20 mg/day) and selenium (100 µg/day) has been highlighted as having the potential to reduce respiratory tract and urinary tract infection rates (Girodon *et al.*, 1997). Prasad and colleagues (2007)

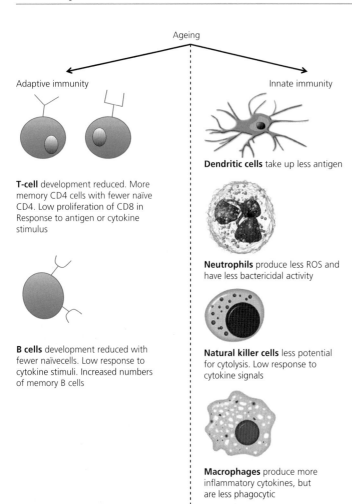

Ageing

Adaptive immunity

Innate immunity

Dendritic cells take up less antigen

T-cell development reduced. More memory CD4 cells with fewer naïve CD4. Low proliferation of CD8 in Response to antigen or cytokine stimulus

Neutrophils produce less ROS and have less bactericidal activity

B cells development reduced with fewer naïvecells. Low response to cytokine stimuli. Increased numbers of memory B cells

Natural killer cells less potential for cytolysis. Low response to cytokine signals

Macrophages produce more inflammatory cytokines, but are less phagocytic

Figure 9.11 The impact of ageing on the cellular immune system.

reported that 12-month supplementation of older adults with 45 mg zinc per day reduced the incidence of infections and pro-inflammatory tumour necrosis factor production relative to a placebo group. Production of interleukin-2 by mononuclear cells was increased. Caution is required when interpreting such findings as many trials have been poorly designed and because some nutrients may have harmful effects at higher doses. Zinc and vitamin E supplements, for example, may be effective in boosting immune responses at low-to-moderate doses, but both impair immune cell function when in excess.

Any individual who is immobilized for a long period is susceptible to the development of pressure sores, or pressure ulcers. These are areas of deep damage to skin tissue that is caused by pressure and/or friction. Such lesions are seen in up to two-thirds of all hospital

inpatients and are most likely to occur in bed-bound elderly individuals, often following other age-related injuries such as hip fracture or as a consequence of prolonged sitting and lack of physical activity (Stratton et al., 2005). Pressure ulcers carry considerable risk of further complications, extend periods of hospitalization associated with other medical problems, severely impair patients' quality of life and increase risk of death by five-fold. Malnutrition is a major risk factor for the development of pressure ulcers. This could be because there is reduced skin resistance and cushioning by body fat at areas of likely pressure in individuals of low BMI. In addition, malnutrition is associated with reduced availability of key nutrients for maintenance, repair and healing of the skin. The most effective nutritional support for those with pressure ulcers appears to be provision of oral supplements of protein and energy, which when given to at-risk patients without ulcers significantly reduce their occurrence (RR 0.75, 95% CI 0.62–0.89, Stratton *et al.*, 2005). Among elderly patients, such supplements appear to reduce the stay in hospital associated with hip fractures, presumably by lessening occurrence of complications such as pressure ulcers (Delmi *et al.*, 1990). In addition to preventing pressure ulcers, nutritional status and nutritional support are important factors in determining rates of healing (Donini *et al.*, 2005).

9.6.3 Digestive tract disorders

As described earlier in this chapter, gastrointestinal tract problems are an important contributor to undernutrition in the elderly population. There are a wide variety of different disorders that impact upon gastrointestinal function, and these affect the whole length of the tract (D'Souza, 2007).

9.6.3.1 Mouth and oesophagus

Soreness of the mouth is a common problem among the elderly. This often stems from the reduced flow of saliva or poor fitting of dentures. Clearly, this will detract from the desire to eat and can impact upon nutritional status. However, factors impacting upon oesophageal function are of much greater significance and lead to dysphagia and malnutrition. Problems with swallowing fall into two categories. Inhibition of the swallowing reflex is usually an issue in individuals who are recovering from a stroke and therefore has a clear cause and generally an acute onset. Neuromuscular disorders affecting the oesophagus and chronic conditions such as Parkinson's disease can impact upon swallowing over a much longer period and have a greater impact on general health. These conditions, and age-related declines in the peristaltic functions of the oesophagus, can induce the feeling that food is becoming stuck in transit to the stomach, and this discourages swallowing. Swallowing can also become painful due to reduced production of mucous in the oesophagus (D'Souza, 2007). Age-related loss of function in the lower oesophageal sphincter can lead to gastric reflux, and over time, the exposure to gastric secretions can promote oesophagitis.

9.6.3.2 Stomach

The inflammation of the gastric mucosa and the formation of peptic ulcers are more common among the elderly than in the younger population. There are believed to be a number of physiological reasons for this, but it should also be borne in mind that infection with *Helicobacter pylori* is also more common in the elderly. *H. pylori* infests the mucous layer of the stomach wall and generates ammonia from urea that would normally buffer stomach acids. This ammonia causes damage to the gastric epithelium. Approximately 80% of the over-65s will have *H. pylori* within the stomach, compared to 20–50% of younger adults (Marshall, 1994). Another cause of peptic ulcers is irritation of the gastric mucosa by anti-inflammatory medications. In the elderly, gastrointestinal transit times are slower, and gastric emptying is less frequent. Coupled to this, there is reduced production of mucous and gastric juices. As a result, irritants stay in the stomach for longer and undergo less dilution with stomach acid (D'Souza, 2007). With atrophy of the gastric mucosa, the capacity to repair any inflamed or damaged areas is reduced.

9.6.3.3 Small intestine

The functions of the small intestine are well preserved within the ageing gastrointestinal tract, and most of the small intestinal disorders reported in the elderly are secondary to other disease states (Hoffmann and Zeitz, 2002). Malabsorption of nutrients is a major problem in elderly patients, and it is driven by conditions such as pancreatitis, parasitic infections, inflammatory bowel disease (Crohn's disease) and coeliac disease. Bacterial overgrowth of the small intestine is another factor promoting malabsorption, which is not usually seen in younger individuals. McEvoy and colleagues (1983) reported that among a group of patients in an elderly care setting, 31% of those with malabsorption problems leading to malnutrition were showing evidence of bacterial overgrowth syndrome.

Bacterial overgrowth is most likely to occur in the elderly as a result of the other gastrointestinal and health problems that they develop. Immunosuppressive drugs, for example, will allow bacteria to resist the local immune system. The presence of blind loops formed during surgery to the small intestine, or diverticula (see following text), provides a foothold for bacterial colonization. As with all of the other causes of malabsorption, the condition is likely to manifest as abdominal pain, diarrhoea, bloating and flatulence but should be readily treatable with antibiotics.

9.6.3.4 Large intestine

Constipation is a commonly reported condition among the elderly population, with a prevalence of between 25% and 35% among the free-living population. In nursing homes, around 50–65% of nursing home residents are reported to take laxatives on a daily basis (Morley, 2007). Constipation is a serious issue and the associated pain and occasional incontinence are associated with a decline in quality of life measures. Constipation can impact upon psychological health and is noted to cause aggression and delirium in elderly people. There are many factors that promote constipation in this group. Some are related to drug treatments or nutrient supplementation for other conditions. Iron and calcium supplements, for example, lead to constipation, as do diuretics, opiate-based painkillers, many antidepressant drugs and antihypertensive agents. Lifestyle is also a major issue, and gastrointestinal transit times are lengthened by physical inactivity, poor hydration and a lack of dietary fibre. It is often suggested that the latter is a major explanation of why the elderly are more prone to constipation. It is argued that the poor dentition of the elderly can discourage intakes of fibre-rich foods. However, while the average intakes of non-starch polysaccharides among UK elderly (National Diet and Nutrition Survey, 1998) were well below the dietary reference value (intakes were on average 10–11 g/day and the EAR is 18 g/day), there is little evidence to suggest that the elderly are any different to younger adults in this respect. Indeed, the UK National Food Survey 2000 (DEFRA, 2000) showed that intakes of cereals, bread, vegetables and fruits were higher in the over-65s than in any other group of adults.

Declining peristaltic function within the large intestine contributes to constipation in the elderly. With this loss of function, the pressures generated within the colon required to keep stools moving have to increase, and this is a cause of diverticular disease (Figure 9.12). Diverticula are sacs and pouches that form within the lining of the intestine. They are present in between 50% and 80% of elderly people and in most cases are asymptomatic (in which case the condition is termed diverticulosis). In around 15–20% of cases, the condition progresses to diverticulitis in which the pouches become blocked with faecal matter. Subsequent infection leads to abdominal pain, lower gastrointestinal bleeding and

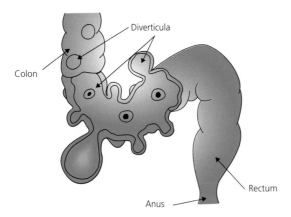

Figure 9.12 Low colonic mobility in the elderly leads to the development of diverticula. These are pockets in the colonic wall that act as a focus for the build-up of faecal material and infection.

alternating diarrhoea and constipation. Infected diverticula can ulcerate or perforate, and this can become life threatening. Diverticular disease is best avoided by following a lifestyle that prevents constipation, including increased intake of non-starch polysaccharides, physical activity and maintaining adequate hydration (D'Souza, 2007).

9.6.4 Anaemia

Anaemia is a haematological condition characterized by abnormalities of the red blood cells. It is most simply defined on the basis of haemoglobin concentrations, and the World Health Organization sets cut-off values for adults at 13 g/dl haemoglobin for men and 12 g/dl for women. As will be explained in the following, there are different forms of anaemia, and these require further examination of the red blood cells for diagnosis (Figure 9.13).

Anaemia, and in particular iron deficiency anaemia, is very common throughout the world, particularly among the female population. The elderly are especially at risk of anaemia, and many of the anaemias that are unrelated to iron deficiency are almost solely observed in older individuals. Steensma and Tefferi (2007) reported that the prevalence of anaemia in the US population was approximately 8% in the 65–74 age group (which is not significantly different to the prevalence in younger populations), 12% in the 75–84 age group and over 20% in the over-85s (26% in men, 20% in women). These figures are similar to those reported in other Westernized countries, with 20.1% of elderly British men and 13.7% of elderly British women shown to be anaemic (Mukhopadhyay and Mohanaruban, 2002). A systematic review of elderly populations across the globe suggested an overall anaemia prevalence of 17%, with greater prevalence in men relative to women and black relative to white Caucasians (Gaskell *et al.*, 2008). Prevalence of anaemia increases with age and is more prevalent in nursing homes (47%) and hospital admissions (40%) than in the community (12%).

Anaemia in general is related to a number of poor health outcomes and reduced quality of life among the elderly. It is associated with reduced mobility, greater risk of falls and osteoporotic fractures, greater frailty and reduced cognitive function (Eisenstaedt *et al.*, 2006). Moreover, mortality rates are significantly greater among the anaemic population, either due to specific causes such as cardiovascular disease or cancer or from all causes. The US Cardiovascular Health Study showed greater mortality over a 12-year period among elderly men and women in the lowest quintile of haemoglobin at baseline (Zakai *et al.*, 2005). Similarly, Izaks and colleagues (1999) reported that risk of death over a 10-year period, in a population of people aged over 85 years, was increased by 2.3-fold in men and 1.6-fold relative to those with normal haemoglobin in women with haemoglobin concentrations below 6.3 g/dl. Risk of death over a 6-year period following myocardial infarction was increased 2.3-fold (95% CI 1.2–4.36) among patients with anaemia (Tomaszuk-Kazberuk *et al.*, 2014).

There are a wide range of different anaemias, with a range of different causes (Table 9.3), but those that are most commonly observed are iron deficiency anaemia, anaemia of chronic disease and the megaloblastic anaemias (Figure 9.13). These can be diagnosed using flow

Table 9.3 Causes of anaemia in the elderly population.

Cause	Estimated % of cases
Iron deficiency	5–10
Anaemia of chronic disease	50–65
Acute haemorrhage	5–10
Vitamin B12 or folate deficiency	5–10
Myelodysplastic syndrome*	5
Leukaemia or lymphoma	5
Unknown causes	5–10

*A condition in which the bone marrow produces reduced numbers of red blood cells.

cytometry to determine the size of the red blood cells. Microcytic anaemia is diagnosed when the mean cell volume is low. This occurs when the haemoglobin concentration is low due to a failure to synthesize the protein, either due to iron deficiency or as a consequence of disordered erythropoiesis. Microcytic signs may also be noted with the anaemia of chronic disease, but this more usually manifests as a normocytic anaemia, in which the mean cell volume is in the normal range. Normocytic anaemia may also result from haemolytic anaemia in which the red cells are broken down at an abnormally high rate.

The anaemia of chronic disease is a product of inflammation and is seen commonly in patients with congestive heart failure and rheumatoid arthritis or after surgery. Approximately 65% of anaemia observed in the elderly is likely to be chronic disease related. In these situations, there are high circulating concentrations of pro-inflammatory cytokines, such as tumour necrosis factor-α, interleukin-1, and interleukin-6, and these inhibit erythropoiesis. Moreover, the production of the iron transport inhibitor hepcidin increases during chronic inflammation, and this reduces the uptake of iron across the gut (Eisenstaedt *et al.*, 2006). In chronic renal disease, the ability to produce erythropoietin is impaired, and this can produce a microcytic anaemia of chronic disease.

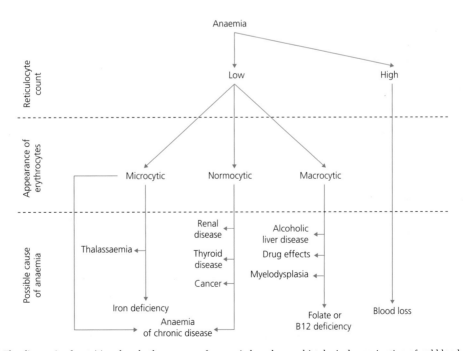

Figure 9.13 The diagnosis of nutritional and other causes of anaemia based upon histological examination of red blood cells. Reticulocytes are immature red cells.

The megaloblastic anaemias are characterized by the enlargement of red cells, which is related to the production of only immature and dysfunctional erythrocytes. The megaloblastic anaemias are the products of deficiencies of either vitamin B12 or folic acid. Megaloblastic anaemia due to vitamin B12 deficiency is often erroneously referred to as pernicious anaemia. Pernicious anaemia is a term that only applies to anaemia arising from B12 deficiency caused by atrophic gastritis or due to loss of the cells of the stomach lining, which secrete the intrinsic factor required for absorption of cobalamin. Pernicious anaemia is associated with severe neurological abnormalities that can result in sensory impairments, loss of appetite and cardiovascular and gastrointestinal problems.

9.6.4.1 Iron deficiency anaemia

Iron deficiency anaemia is relatively uncommon among the elderly populations of Westernized countries, with prevalence estimated at 3–5%. Prevalence is higher in some groups with specific conditions such as heart disease. In developing countries, iron deficiency is at a higher prevalence due to infection with malaria, hookworm, schistosomiasis and tuberculosis. In elderly patients, iron deficiency is most likely to be attributable to blood loss, and deficiency due to poor dietary intakes is rare. Villous atrophy within the intestine may be a cause of iron malabsorption, but over 60% of iron deficiency is a consequence of occult blood loss within the gastrointestinal tract (Rockey and Cello, 1993). Occult bleeding can be the result of treatment with non-steroidal anti-inflammatory drugs, but it is more often the result of underlying gastrointestinal pathologies, including gastric cancers, peptic ulcers, colonic cancers and colonic polyps. Iron deficiency in the elderly, as with younger groups, is most effectively treated through the administration of iron supplements, but given that it may indicate more sinister pathologies (Figure 9.13), this treatment should be accompanied by gastrointestinal investigations (Mukhopadhyay and Mohanaruban, 2002).

9.6.4.2 Vitamin B12 deficiency

Deficiency of vitamin B12 (cobalamin) is relatively common among the elderly population. Most estimates (Andrès *et al.*, 2004) suggest that at least 20% of the over-65s are cobalamin deficient, with greater prevalence among institutionalized elderly (30–40%) than in the community (12%). Measurements of serum homocysteine and methylmalonate provide good biomarkers of deficiency of cobalamin and folic acid. Clarke and colleagues (2003) showed that among an elderly UK population, these biomarkers indicated that 10–20% of people were at risk of cobalamin deficiency and a similar number of people were folate deficient or borderline folate deficient. Ten per cent of the cobalamin-deficient population were also folate deficient. Among elderly populations in Westernized countries, prevalence estimates for pernicious anaemia range between 50 and 300 cases per 100 000 population (Stadler and Allen, 2004), and elevated methylmalonate is seen in approximately 15% of elderly people. In some countries, the prevalence of deficiency may well be greater. Olivares *et al.* (2000) studied a group of over-60s in Chile. Chile fortifies wheat flour with iron at 30 mg/100 g flour, and so iron status was good in these elderly people. In the absence of anaemia, low serum vitamin B12 and low serum folate were noted in 50% of men and 33% of women. Iron fortification, therefore, appeared to mask the potential deleterious effects of B vitamin deficiencies.

It is rare for vitamin B12 deficiency to arise through inadequate dietary intakes, which would only be a concern in individuals consuming a strict vegetarian diet or in very severely malnourished individuals. Kwok and colleagues (2002) reported that the prevalence of deficiency was up to 75% in a population of elderly vegetarians in Hong Kong. The major causes of deficiency relate to the function of the digestive tract, which is why the elderly are a high-risk group (Stadler and Allen 2004). Cobalamin is absorbed through a complex process involving actions of the stomach and the small intestine (Andrès *et al.* 2004). Cobalamin in the diet generally enters the stomach bound to animal proteins (Figure 9.14). Pepsin and the stomach acid release the free cobalamin, which is then bound by haptocorrin, a protein released in saliva. The haptocorrin–cobalamin complex passes into the duodenum where it is degraded, again releasing free cobalamin. This is then bound by intrinsic factor, which is produced within the stomach by the gastric parietal cells. The intrinsic factor–cobalamin complex binds to cubilin receptors in the ileum, and the cobalamin is then taken up and transported around the body by the three transcobalamin transporter proteins.

In the elderly, pernicious anaemia associated with loss of gastric parietal cells accounts for 15–20% of cases of cobalamin deficiency, while most other cases are the product of malabsorption due to atrophy of cells within the gastric mucosa, atrophy of the ileum or bacterial overgrowth of the small intestine. Infection with *H. pylori* can also contribute to cobalamin malabsorption. Cobalamin deficiency can be treated, with rapid improvements in associated symptoms. Treatment protocols seek to build up and maintain cobalamin reserves through repeated high-dose depot injections, as the underlying gastrointestinal causes of deficiency are unlikely to be resolved (Reynolds, 2006).

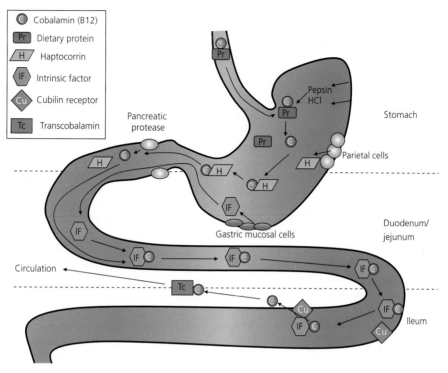

Figure 9.14 The absorption of vitamin B12 (cobalamin).

9.6.4.3 Folic acid deficiency

Folic acid deficiency is generally considered to be uncommon in Westernized countries, although in some parts of the world, prevalence may be high and related to poverty (Olivares *et al.*, 2000; Antony, 2001). Flood and Mitchell (2007) found low serum folate in 2.3% of older Australians, which is in line with estimates from elsewhere (Clarke, 2006). Unlike vitamin B12 deficiency in the elderly, folate deficiency will arise purely through inadequate intakes. It is simply treated through the administration of supplements (1 mg folic acid per day).

Any intervention to increase folic acid intakes, whether through supplementation or fortification of staple foods, in the elderly must be handled with caution. Folic acid repletion can have important consequences for the individuals in the population who are vitamin B12 deficient. B12 deficiency is often unrecognized as the clinical symptoms are often regarded as normal features of ageing. Most diagnosis is through the identification of megaloblastic anaemia in routine blood sampling, with follow-up measurements of methylmalonate, or cobalamin. Increased folic acid intakes can mask the haematological signs of vitamin B12 deficiency by resolving the megaloblastic anaemia, but do not remove the other consequences of B12 deficiency. Folic acid may also be toxic to individuals with B12 deficiency and accelerate neurological damage. For this reason, many people have expressed concerns about the general fortification of foods with folic acid, aimed at preventing spina bifida and improving population's cardiovascular health (Cuskelly *et al.*, 2007). However, evidence from the US post-introduction of folate fortification in 1998 suggests limited impact upon B12 status. Comparison of the US National Health and Nutrition Examination Surveys in 1994/1995 and 2001/2006 showed no change in the prevalence of low serum vitamin B12 among the population over 50 years of age and a decline in the prevalence of marginal deficiency post-fortification (Qi *et al.*, 2014).

9.6.4.4 Cognitive impairment and anaemia

A number of progressive disorders of the brain, including Alzheimer's disease (AZD), lead to cognitive impairments and dementia (loss of memory, reasoning and capacity to carry out mental tasks) in the elderly. Approximately 6–8% of the elderly population in Westernized countries will suffer from AZD which is characterized by the formation of neuronal tangles and plaques of amyloid protein in the brain and in particular loss of neurons in the cerebral cortex and the temporal and parietal lobes. The second most common form of dementia (vascular dementia) is associated with impaired blood flow to the brain, generally due to small strokes in regions such as the thalamus and parietal lobes. While vascular dementia is more common in people with a history of hypertension, the causes of AZD are not well understood. As the population is living longer, the numbers of affected individuals are increasing rapidly in all parts of the world. Five per cent of people aged 65–85 and 25% of the over-85s can be expected to develop cognitive impairments.

Although a range of nutritional factors have been associated with dementia (antioxidants, *n*-3 fatty acids), most interest has been directed at the possible involvement of homocysteine and the B vitamins. Homocysteine has been shown to cause neuronal death and promote formation of amyloid plaques in the brain and is seen as a risk factor for both AZD and vascular dementia (Perez *et al.*, 2012; Gillette-Guyonnet *et al.*, 2013). High circulating concentrations of homocysteine have been noted in patients with AZD and appear to precede the onset of any cognitive impairments (McCaddon *et al.*, 1998). The metabolism of homocysteine is closely associated with the dietary availability of folic acid, vitamin B12 and vitamin B6 (see Section 'Folic acid and plasma homocysteine' in Chapter 8), and as such, these nutrients are of interest in this field.

Vitamin B12 deficiency has long been associated with cognitive problems. The deficiency manifests as both haematological and neuronal abnormalities, and a high prevalence of neuropsychiatric disorders and memory impairment is seen in patients with B12 deficiency (Malouf and Areosa Sastre, 2003). Importantly, low circulating B12 is noted in individuals with AZD. Folate is also of major importance within the brain, and individuals with low folate status are at significantly greater risk of developing AZD and vascular dementia (Perez *et al.*, 2012). Other psychological disorders including depression are linked to low circulating folate, and this may reflect the role of this vitamin as a cofactor for the synthesis of certain neurotransmitters, including serotonin (Malouf *et al.*, 2003). Moreover, folate is important in the repair of DNA damage, so a limiting supply may allow the accumulation of oxidative damage associated with the amyloid beta peptide in AZD. Luchsinger *et al.* (2007) found that among 965 elderly people, those in the highest quartile of folate status had the lowest risk of AZD, while there was no significant association with B12 or B6. Although low circulating folate, B12 and B6 are often reported in elderly populations with cognitive impairment, there is a lack of convincing evidence to suggest that supplementation might be protective. McMahon *et al.* (2006) performed a double-blind randomized controlled trial over 2 years, providing subjects aged over 65 with 1 mg folate, 500 μg vitamin B12 and 10 mg vitamin B6 daily. There was no effect of the intervention upon cognitive performance. In contrast, the VITACOG study found that providing a 5 mg/day folate and 1 mg/d B12 supplement to patients with early-stage AZD over 2 years slowed cognitive decline and brain atrophy (De Jager *et al.*, 2012).

The associations between the B vitamins, AZD and dementia may not be causal, despite the plausible mechanisms that have been advanced. Individuals with dementia are highly likely to become malnourished and hence develop anaemia as a result of their psychological difficulties. Dementia impacts upon all areas of self-care, and the ability to shop, cook and feed declines. It is therefore difficult to determine whether poor intakes and absorption of B vitamins associated with anaemia promote dementia, or vice versa.

SUMMARY

- On a global scale, the numbers of elderly people in the population are increasing rapidly. Greater lifespan means that nutrition-related health problems associated with ageing are set to become more prevalent.
- Ageing-related declines in physiological functions are a product of the accumulation of cells with a senescent phenotype within tissues. Cellular senescence may be driven by oxidative processes, but telomere shortening and activation of the INK4a pathway also provide important mechanisms for limiting the normal lifespan of cellular functions.
- Caloric restriction may provide a means for extension of lifespan. However, this modulation of rates of ageing may be effective only when introduced early in life. The adverse impact of caloric restriction on human health and well-being may offset any benefit of a longer lifespan.
- The elderly have similar nutrient requirements to younger adults, but declining energy expenditure means that the optimal diet should be more nutrient dense.
- The elderly population are the main at-risk group for malnutrition in developed countries. Risk is associated with physical decline and chronic disease, with poverty, social isolation, institutionalization and a lack of knowledge of food and nutrition.
- Osteoporosis is a condition which primarily affects the elderly. Optimal intakes of vitamin D and calcium may reduce the risk of falls and fractures.
- The elderly are at high risk of gastrointestinal diseases, some of which will impact upon other aspects of health through impairment of the absorption of key micronutrients.
- There is a high prevalence of anaemia among the elderly population, with macrocytic anaemias associated with vitamin B12 and folate deficiencies predominating. Anaemia in the elderly is most commonly a product of chronic disease, but risk is also driven by malabsorption and other factors associated with malnutrition.

References

Abbassi, A.A. and Rudman, D. (1994) Undernutrition in the nursing home: prevalence, consequences, causes and prevention. *Nutrition Reviews*, **52**, 113–122.

Aihie-Sayer, A., Dunn, R., Langley-Evans, S. *et al.* (2001) Prenatal exposure to a maternal low protein diet shortens life span in rats. *Gerontology*, **47**, 9–14.

Almanza, B.A., Namkung, Y., Ismail, J.A. *et al.* (2007) Clients' safe food-handling knowledge and risk behavior in a home-delivered meal program. *Journal of the American Dietetic Association*, **107**, 816–821.

Andrès, E., Loukili, N.H., Noel, E. *et al.* (2004) Vitamin B12 (cobalamin) deficiency in elderly patients. *Canadian Medical Association Journal*, **171**, 251–259.

Antony, A.C. (2001) Prevalence of cobalamin (vitamin B-12) and folate deficiency in India–audi alteram partem. *American Journal of Clinical Nutrition*, **74**, 157–159.

Appleton, K.M., McGill, R. and Woodside, J.V. (2009) Fruit and vegetable consumption in older individuals in Northern Ireland: levels and patterns. *British Journal of Nutrition*, **102**, 949–953.

Atkinson, C., Compston, J.E., Day, N.E. *et al.* (2004) The effects of phytoestrogen isoflavones on bone density in women: a double-blind, randomized, placebo-controlled trial. *American Journal of Clinical Nutrition*, **79**, 326–333.

Banks, R., Speakman, J.R. and Selman, C. (2010) Vitamin E supplementation and mammalian lifespan. *Molecular Nutrition and Food Research*, **54**, 719–725.

BAPEN (2010) *Nutrition Screening Survey in the UK and Republic of Ireland 2010*, http://www.bapen.org.uk/pdfs/nsw/nsw10/nsw10-report.pdf (accessed 30 December 2014).

Barbour, K.E., Zmuda, J.M., Strotmeyer, E.S. *et al.* (2010) Correlates of trabecular and cortical volumetric bone mineral density of the radius and tibia in older men: the Osteoporotic Fractures in Men Study. *Journal of Bone and Mineral Research*, **25**, 1017–1028.

Beasley, J.M., Lacroix, A.Z., Larson, J.C. *et al.* (2014) Biomarker-calibrated protein intake and bone health in the Women's Health Initiative clinical trials and observational study. *American Journal of Clinical Nutrition*, **99**, 934–940.

Bischoff-Ferrari, H.A. and Dawson-Hughes, B. (2007) Where do we stand on vitamin D? *Bone*, **41** (1, Suppl. 1), S13–S19.

Bischoff-Ferrari, H.A., Stähelin, H.B., Dick, W. *et al.* (2003) Effects of vitamin D and calcium supplementation on falls: a randomized controlled trial. *Journal of Bone and Mineral Research*, **18**, 343–351.

Bischoff-Ferrari, H.A., Dawson-Hughes, B., Willett, W.C. *et al.* (2004) Effect of vitamin D on falls: a meta-analysis. *Journal of the American Medical Association*, **291**, 1999–2006.

Boccardi, V. and Poalisso, G. (2014) Telomerase activation: a potential key modulator for human healthspan and longevity. *Ageing Research Review*, **15**, 1–5.

Bolland, M.J., Grey, A., Avenell, A. *et al.* (2011) Calcium supplements with or without vitamin D and risk of cardiovascular events: reanalysis of the Women's Health Initiative limited access dataset and meta-analysis. *British Medical Journal*, **342**, d2040.

Boonen, S., Lips, P., Bouillon, R. *et al.* (2007) Need for additional calcium to reduce the risk of hip fracture with vitamin D supplementation: evidence from a comparative metaanalysis of randomized controlled trials. *Journal of Clinical Endocrinology and Metabolism*, **92**, 1415–1423.

Boyé, N.D., Oudshoorn, C., van der Velde, N. *et al.* (2013) Vitamin D and physical performance in older men and women visiting the emergency department because of a fall: data from the improving medication prescribing to reduce risk of falls (IMPROveFALL) study. *Journal of the American Geriatric Society*, **61**, 1948–1952.

Broe, K.E., Chen, T.C., Weinberg, F. *et al.* (2007) A higher dose of vitamin D reduces the risk of falls in nursing home residents: a randomized, multiple-dose study. *Journal of the American Geriatric Society*, **55**, 234–239.

Brownie, S. (2006) Why are elderly individuals at risk of nutritional deficiency? *International Journal of Nursing Practice*, **12**, 110–118.

Calvo, I., Olivar, J., Martínez, E. *et al.* (2012) MNA® Mini Nutritional Assessment as a nutritional screening tool for hospitalized older adults; rationales and feasibility. *Nutrition in Hospitals*, **27**, 1619–1625.

Campisi, J. (1997) The biology of replicative senescence. *European Journal of Cancer*, **33**, 703–709.

Carrier, N., Ouellet, D. and West, G.E. (2007) Nursing home food services linked with risk of malnutrition. *Canadian Journal of Dietetic Practice and Research*, **68**, 14–20.

Castle, S.C., Uyemura, K., Fulop, T. *et al.* (2007) Host resistance and immune responses in advanced age. *Clinics in Geriatric Medicine*, **23**, 463–479.

Chakkalakal, D.A. (2005) Alcohol-induced bone loss and deficient bone repair. *Alcoholism, Clinical and Experimental Research*, **29**, 2077–2090.

Clarke, R. (2006) Vitamin B12, folic acid, and the prevention of dementia. *New England Journal of Medicine*, **354**, 2817–2819.

Clarke, R., Refsum, H., Birks, J. *et al.* (2003) Screening for vitamin B-12 and folate deficiency in older persons. *American Journal of Clinical Nutrition*, **77**, 1241–1247.

Collado, M., Blasco, M.A. and Serrano, M. (2007) Cellular senescence in cancer and aging. *Cell*, **130**, 223–233.

Cuskelly, G.J., Mooney, K.M. and Young, I.S. (2007) Folate and vitamin B12: friendly or enemy nutrients for the elderly. *Proceedings of the Nutrition Society*, **66**, 548–558.

D'Souza, A.L. (2007) Ageing and the gut. *Postgraduate Medical Journal*, **83**, 44–53.

Dawson-Hughes, B., Harris, S.S., Krall, E.A. *et al.* (2000) Effect of withdrawal of calcium and vitamin D supplements on bone mass in elderly men and women. *American Journal of Clinical Nutrition*, **72**, 745–750.

de Jager, C.A., Oulhaj, A., Jacoby, R. *et al.* (2012) Cognitive and clinical outcomes of homocysteine-lowering B-vitamin treatment in mild cognitive impairment: a randomized controlled trial. *International Journal of Geriatric Psychiatry*, **27**, 592–600.

DEFRA (2000) *National Food Survey: 2000: Annual Report on Food Expenditure, Consumption and Nutrient Intakes*, Department of the Environment, Food and Rural Affairs, London.

Delmi, M., Rapin, C.H., Bengoa, J.M. *et al.* (1990) Dietary supplementation in elderly patients with fractured neck of the femur. *Lancet*, **335**, 1013–1016.

Department of Health (1999) *Dietary Reference Values for Food Energy and Nutrients for the United Kingdom*, The Stationery Office, London.

Dhesi, J.K., Jackson, S.H., Bearne, L.M. *et al.* (2004) Vitamin D supplementation improves neuromuscular function in older people who fall. *Age and Ageing*, **33**, 589–595.

Di Daniele, N., Carbonelli, M.G., Candeloro, N. *et al.* (2004) Effect of supplementation of calcium and vitamin D on bone mineral density and bone mineral content in peri- and postmenopause women: a double-blind, randomized, controlled trial. *Pharmacological Research*, **50**, 637–641.

Dirks, A.J. and Leeuwenburgh, C. (2006) Caloric restriction in humans: potential pitfalls and health concerns. *Mechanisms of Ageing and Development*, **127**, 1–7.

Donini, L.M., De Felice, M.R., Tagliaccica, A. *et al.* (2005) Nutritional status and evolution of pressure sores in geriatric patients. *Journal of Nutrition, Health and Ageing*, **9**, 446–454.

Dorner, T.E., Lackinger, C., Haider, S. *et al.* (2013) Nutritional intervention and physical training in malnourished frail community-dwelling elderly persons carried out by trained lay "buddies": study protocol of a randomized controlled trial. *BMC Public Health*, **13**, 1232.

Eastwood, C., Davies, G.J., Gardiner, F.K. *et al.* (2002) Energy intakes of institutionalised and free-living older people. *Journal of Nutrition, Health and Ageing*, **6**, 91–92.

Eisenstaedt, R., Penninx, B.W. and Woodman, R.C. (2006) Anemia in the elderly: current understanding and emerging concepts. *Blood Reviews*, **20**, 213–226.

Endevelt, R., Lemberger, J., Bregman, J. *et al.* (2011) Intensive dietary intervention by a dietitian as a case manager among community dwelling older adults: the EDIT study. *Journal of Nutrition Health and Ageing*, **15**, 624–630.

European Commission (2012) *People at Risk of Poverty or Social Exclusion*, http://epp.eurostat.ec.europa.eu/statistics_explained/index.php/People_at_risk_of_poverty_or_social_exclusion (accessed 30 December 2014).

Ferry, M., Sidobre, B., Lambertin, A. *et al.* (2005) The SOLINUT study: analysis of the interaction between nutrition and loneliness in persons aged over 70 years. *Journal of Nutrition Health and Ageing*, **9**, 261–268.

Flood, V. and Mitchell, P. (2007) Folate and vitamin B12 in older Australians. *Medical Journal of Australia*, **186**, 321–322.

Fontana, L., Meyer, T.E., Klein, S. *et al.* (2004) Long-term calorie restriction is highly effective in reducing the risk for atherosclerosis in humans. *Proceedings of the National Academy of Sciences of the United States of America*, **101**, 6659–6663.

Gaboreau, Y., Imbert, P., Jacquet, J.P. *et al.* (2013) What are key factors influencing malnutrition screening in community-dwelling elderly populations by general practitioners? A large cross-sectional survey in two areas of France. *European Journal of Clinical Nutrition*, **67**, 1193–1199.

Gariballa, S. and Forster, S. (2007) Malnutrition is an independent predictor of 1-year mortality following acute illness. *British Journal of Nutrition*, **98**, 332–336.

Garnero, P., Borel, O., Grant, S.F. *et al.* (1998) Collagen Ialpha1 Sp1 polymorphism, bone mass, and bone turnover in healthy French premenopausal women: the OFELY study. *Journal of Bone and Mineral Research*, **13**, 813–817.

Gaskell, H., Derry, S., Andrew Moore, R. *et al.* (2008) Prevalence of anaemia in older persons: systematic review. *BMC Geriatrics*, **8**, 1.

Gillette-Guyonnet, S., Secher, M. and Vellas, B. (2013) Nutrition and neurodegeneration: epidemiological evidence and challenges for future research. *British Journal of Clinical Pharmacology*, **75**, 738–755.

Girodon, F., Lombard, M., Galan, P. *et al.* (1997) Effect of micronutrient supplementation on infection in institutionalized elderly subjects: a controlled trial. *Annals of Nutrition and Metabolism*, **41**, 98–107.

Gollub, E.A. and Weddle, D.O. (2004) Improvements in nutritional intake and quality of life among frail homebound older adults receiving home-delivered breakfast and lunch. *Journal of the American Dietetic Association*, **104**, 1227–1235.

Gomes, N.M., Ryder, O.A., Houck, M.L. *et al.* (2011) Comparative biology of mammalian telomeres: hypotheses on ancestral states and the roles of telomeres in longevity determination. *Aging Cell*, **10**, 761–768.

Griep, M.I., Mets, T.F., Vercruysse, A. *et al.* (1995) Food odor thresholds in relation to age, nutritional, and health status. *Journal of Gerontology Series A: Biological Sciences and Medical Sciences*, **50**, B407–B414.

Guo, J.L., Tsai, Y.Y., Liao, J.Y. *et al.* (2014) Interventions to reduce the number of falls among older adults with/without cognitive impairment: an exploratory meta-analysis. *International Journal of Geriatric Psychiatry*, **29**, 661–669.

Hallström, H., Melhus, H., Glynn, A. *et al.* (2010) Coffee consumption and CYP1A2 genotype in relation to bone mineral density of the proximal femur in elderly men and women: a cohort study. *Nutrition and Metabolism*, **7**, 12.

Hallström, H., Byberg, L., Glynn, A. *et al.* (2013) Long-term coffee consumption in relation to fracture risk and bone mineral density in women. *American Journal of Epidemiology*, **178**, 898–909.

Heaney, R.P., Kopecky, S., Maki, K.C. *et al.* (2012) A review of calcium supplements and cardiovascular disease risk. *Advances in Nutrition*, **3**, 763–771.

Hector, K.L., Lagisz, M. and Nakagawa, S. (2012) The effect of resveratrol on longevity across species: a meta-analysis. *Biology Letters*, **8**, 790–793.

High, K.P. (2001) Nutritional strategies to boost immunity and prevent infection in elderly individuals. *Clinical Infectious Diseases*, **33**, 1892–1900.

Hirani, V. and Primatesta, P. (2005) Vitamin D concentrations among people aged 65 years and over living in private households and institutions in England: population survey. *Age and Ageing*, **34**, 485–491.

Hoffmann, J.C. and Zeitz, M. (2002) Small bowel disease in the elderly: diarrhoea and malabsorption. *Best Practice and Research. Clinical Gastroenterology*, **16**, 17–36.

Hughes, G., Bennett, K.M. and Hetherington, M.M. (2004) Old and alone: barriers to healthy eating in older men living on their own. *Appetite*, **43**, 269–276.

Huncharek, M., Muscat, J. and Kupelnick, B. (2008) Impact of dairy products and dietary calcium on bone-mineral content in children: results of a meta-analysis. *Bone*, **43** (2), 312–321.

Ishimi, Y. (2010) Dietary equol and bone metabolism in postmenopausal Japanese women and osteoporotic mice. *Journal of Nutrition*, **140**, 1373S–1376S.

Izaks, G.J., Westendorp, R.G. and Knook, D.L. (1999) The definition of anemia in older persons. *Journal of the American Medical Association*, **281**, 1714–1717.

Janzen, V., Forkert, R., Fleming, H.E. *et al.* (2006) Stem-cell ageing modified by the cyclin-dependent kinase inhibitor p16INK4a. *Nature*, **443**, 421–426.

Jennings, B.J., Ozanne, S.E., Dorling, M.W. *et al.* (1999) Early growth determines longevity in male rats and may be related to telomere shortening in the kidney. *FEBS Letters*, **448**, 4–8.

Kaiser, M.J., Bauer, J.M., Rämsch, C. *et al.* (2010) Frequency of malnutrition in older adults: a multinational perspective using the mini nutritional assessment. *Journal of the American Geriatric Society*, **58**, 1734–1738.

Kanis, J.A., Johnell, O., Oden, A. *et al.* (2002) Ten-year risk of osteoporotic fracture and the effect of risk factors on screening strategies. *Bone*, **30**, 251–258.

Karlsson, M.K., Vonschewelov, T., Karlsson, C. *et al.* (2013) Prevention of falls in the elderly: a review. *Scandinavian Journal of Public Health*, **41**, 442–454.

Keen, R. (2007) Osteoporosis: strategies for prevention and management. *Best Practice and Research: Clinical Rheumatology*, **21**, 109–122.

Kennelly, S., Kennedy, N.P., Rughoobur, G.F. *et al.* (2010) An evaluation of a community dietetics intervention on the management of malnutrition for healthcare professionals. *Journal of Human Nutrition and Dietetics*, **23**, 567–574.

Kenny, A.M., Mangano, K.M., Abourizk, R.H. *et al.* (2009) Soy proteins and isoflavones affect bone mineral density in older women: a randomized controlled trial. *American Journal of Clinical Nutrition*, **90**, 234–242.

Kretser, A.J., Voss, T., Kerr, W.W. *et al.* (2003) Effects of two models of nutritional intervention on homebound older adults at nutritional risk. *Journal of the American Dietetic Association*, **103**, 329–336.

Kwok, T., Cheng, G., Woo, J. *et al.* (2002) Independent effect of vitamin B12 deficiency on hematological status in older Chinese vegetarian women. *American Journal of Hematology*, **70**, 186–190.

Langley-Evans, S.C. and Sculley, D.V. (2006) The association between birthweight and longevity in the rat is complex and modulated by maternal protein intake during fetal life. *FEBS Letters*, **580**, 4150–4153.

Law, M., Withers, H., Morris, J. *et al.* (2006) Vitamin D supplementation and the prevention of fractures and falls: results of a randomised trial in elderly people in residential accommodation. *Age and Ageing*, **35**, 482–486.

Locher, J.L., Vickers, K.S., Buys, D.R. *et al.* (2013) A randomized controlled trial of a theoretically-based behavioral nutrition intervention for community elders: lessons learned from the Behavioral Nutrition Intervention for Community Elders Study. *Journal of the Academy of Nutrition and Dietetics*, **113**, 1675–1682.

Luchsinger, J.A., Tang, M.X., Miller, J. *et al.* (2007) Relation of higher folate intake to lower risk of Alzheimer disease in the elderly. *Archives of Neurology*, **64**, 86–92.

Ma, D.F., Qin, L.Q., Wang, P.Y. *et al.* (2008) Soy isoflavone intake increases bone mineral density in the spine of menopausal women: meta-analysis of randomized controlled trials. *Clinical Nutrition*, **27**, 57–64.

Malouf, R. and Areosa Sastre, A. (2003) *Vitamin B12 for cognition*. Cochrane Database of Systematic Reviews, CD004326.

Malouf, M., Grimley, E.J. and Areosa, S.A. (2003) *Folic acid with or without vitamin B12 for cognition and dementia*. Cochrane Database of Systematic Reviews, CD004514.

Mamhidir, A.G., Karlsson, I., Norberg, A. *et al.* (2007) Weight increase in patients with dementia, and alteration in meal routines and meal environment after integrity promoting care. *Journal of Clinical Nursing*, **16**, 987–996.

Margetts, B.M., Thompson, R.L., Elia, M. *et al.* (2003) Prevalence of risk of undernutrition is associated with poor health status in older people in the UK. *European Journal of Clinical Nutrition*, **57**, 69–74.

Marshall, B.J. (1994) Helicobacter pylori. *American Journal of Gastroenterology*, **89** (8 Suppl), S116–S128.

Martin, C.T., Kayser-Jones, J., Stotts, N. *et al.* (2005) Factors contributing to low weight in community-living older adults. *Journal of the American Academy of Nurse Practitioners*, **17**, 425–431.

Massie, H.R., Aiello, V.R. and Doherty, T.J. (1984) Dietary vitamin C improves the survival of mice. *Gerontology*, **30**, 371–375.

Mather, K.A., Jorm, A.F., Parslow, R.A. *et al.* (2011) Is telomere length a biomarker of aging? A review. *Journal of Gerontology A. Biological Science and Medical Science*, **66**, 202–213.

Mattison, J.A., Roth, G.S., Beasley, T.M. *et al.* (2012) Impact of caloric restriction on health and survival in rhesus monkeys from the NIA study. *Nature*, **489**, 318–321.

McCaddon, A., Davies, G., Hudson, P. *et al.* (1998) Total serum homocysteine in senile dementia of Alzheimer type. *International Journal of Geriatric Psychiatry*, **13**, 235–239.

McEvoy, A., Dutton, J. and James, O.F. (1983) Bacterial contamination of the small intestine is an important cause of occult malabsorption in the elderly. *British Medical Journal*, **287**, 789–793.

McKiernan, S.H., Colman, R.J., Aiken, E. *et al.* (2012) Cellular adaptation contributes to calorie restriction-induced preservation of skeletal muscle in aged rhesus monkeys. *Experimental Gerontology*, **47**, 229–236.

McMahon, J.A., Green, T.J., Skeaff, C.M. *et al.* (2006) A controlled trial of homocysteine lowering and cognitive performance. *The New England Journal of Medicine*, **354** (26), 2764–2772.

McWhirter, J.P. and Pennington, C.R. (1994) Incidence and recognition of malnutrition in hospital. *British Medical Journal*, **308**, 945–948.

Morley, J.E. (2007) Constipation and irritable bowel syndrome in the elderly. *Clinics in Geriatric Medicine*, **23**, 823–832.

Mukhopadhyay, D. and Mohanaruban, K. (2002) Iron deficiency anaemia in older people: investigation, management and treatment. *Age and Ageing*, **31**, 87–91.

Muller, F.L., Lustgarten, M.S., Jang, Y. *et al.* (2007) Trends in oxidative aging theories. *Free Radical Biology and Medicine*, **43**, 477–503.

National Diet and Nutrition Survey (1998) *National Diet and Nutrition Survey: People Aged 65 Years and Over*, The Stationery Office, London.

Olivares, M., Hertrampf, E., Capurro, M.T. *et al.* (2000) Prevalence of anemia in elderly subjects living at home: role of micronutrient deficiency and inflammation. *European Journal of Clinical Nutrition*, **54**, 834–839.

Omran, M.L. and Morley, J.E. (2000) Assessment of protein energy malnutrition in older persons, part I: history, examination, body composition, and screening tools. *Nutrition*, **16**, 50–63.

Ozanne, S.E. and Hales, C.N. (2004) Lifespan: catch-up growth and obesity in male mice. *Nature*, **427**, 411–412.

Pantell, M., Rehkopf, D., Jutte, D. *et al.* (2013) Social isolation: a predictor of mortality comparable to traditional clinical risk factors. *American Journal of Public Health*, **103**, 2056–2062.

Pearson, K.J., Baur, J.A., Lewis, K.N. *et al.* (2008) Resveratrol delays age-related deterioration and mimics transcriptional aspects of dietary restriction without extending life span. *Cellular Metabolism*, **8**, 157–168.

Perez, L., Heim, L., Sherzai, A. *et al.* (2012) Nutrition and vascular dementia. *Journal of Nutrition and Healthy Ageing*, **16**, 319–324.

Prasad, A.S., Beck, F.W., Bao, B. *et al.* (2007) Zinc supplementation decreases incidence of infections in the elderly: effect of zinc on generation of cytokines and oxidative stress. *American Journal of Clinical Nutrition*, **85**, 837–844.

Qi, Y.P., Do, A.N., Hamner, H.C. *et al.* (2014) The prevalence of low serum vitamin B-12 status in the absence of anemia or macrocytosis did not increase among older U.S. adults after mandatory folic acid fortification. *Journal of Nutrition*, **144**, 170–176.

Rabenda, V., Bruyère, O. and Reginster, J.Y. (2011) Relationship between bone mineral density changes and risk of fractures among patients receiving calcium with or without vitamin D supplementation: a meta-regression. *Osteoporosis International*, **22**, 893–901.

Ramic, E., Pranjic, N., Batic-Mujanovic, O. *et al.* (2011) The effect of loneliness on malnutrition in elderly population. *Medical Archives*, **65**, 92–95.

Rapuri, P.B., Gallagher, J.C., Kinyamu, H.K. *et al.* (2001) Caffeine intake increases the rate of bone loss in elderly women and interacts with vitamin D receptor genotypes. *American Journal of Clinical Nutrition*, **74**, 694–700.

Rapuri, P.B., Gallagher, J.C. and Haynatzka, V. (2003) Protein intake: effects on bone mineral density and the rate of bone loss in elderly women. *American Journal of Clinical Nutrition*, **77**, 1517–1525.

Reid, I.R., Bolland, M.J. and Grey, A. (2014) Effects of vitamin D supplements on bone mineral density: a systematic review and meta-analysis. *Lancet*, **383**, 146–155.

Reynolds, E. (2006) Vitamin B12, folic acid, and the nervous system. *Lancet Neurology*, **5**, 949–960.

Ricci, E., Cipriani, S., Chiaffarino, F. *et al.* (2010) Soy isoflavones and bone mineral density in perimenopausal and postmenopausal Western women: a systematic review and meta-analysis of randomized controlled trials. *Journal of Women's Health*, **19**, 1609–1617.

Ringe, J.D. (2012) The effect of Vitamin D on falls and fractures. *Scandinavian Journal of Clinical Laboratory Investigation Supplement*, **243**, 73–78.

Rockey, D.C. and Cello, J.P. (1993) Evaluation of the gastrointestinal tract in patients with iron-deficiency anemia. *New England Journal of Medicine*, **329**, 1691–1695.

Romero-Corral, A., Montori, V.M., Somers, V.K. *et al.* (2006) Association of bodyweight with total mortality and with cardiovascular events in coronary artery disease: a systematic review of cohort studies. *Lancet*, **368**, 666–678.

Roseman, M.G. (2007) Food safety perceptions and behaviors of participants in congregate-meal and home-delivered-meal programs. *Journal of Environmental Health*, **70**, 13–21.

Rothenbacher, D., Klenk, J., Denkinger, M.D. *et al.* (2014) Prospective evaluation of renal function, serum vitamin D level, and risk of fall and fracture in community-dwelling elderly subjects. *Osteoporosis International*, **25**, 923–932.

Roy, M.A. and Payette, H. (2006) Meals-on-wheels improves energy and nutrient intake in a frail free-living elderly population. *Journal of Nutrition Health and Ageing*, **10**, 554–560.

Sanders, K.M., Scott, D. and Ebeling, P.R. (2014) Vitamin d deficiency and its role in muscle-bone interactions in the elderly. *Current Osteoporosis Reports*, **12**, 74–81.

Selman, C., McLaren, J.S., Meyer, C. *et al.* (2006) Life-long vitamin C supplementation in combination with cold exposure does not affect oxidative damage or lifespan in mice, but decreases expression of antioxidant protection genes. *Mechanisms of Ageing and Development*, **127**, 897–904.

Shea, B., Wells, G., Cranney, A. *et al.*, Osteoporosis Methodology Group and Osteoporosis Research Advisory Group (2004) *Calcium supplementation on bone loss in postmenopausal women*. *Cochrane Database of Systematic Reviews*, CD004526.

Silver, H.J., Dietrich, M.S. and Castellanos, V.H. (2006) Increased energy density of the home-delivered lunch meal improves 24-hour nutrient intakes in older adults. *Journal of the American Dietetic Association*, **108**, 2084–2089.

Slevin, M.M., Allsopp, P.J., Magee, P.J. *et al.* (2014) Supplementation with calcium and short-chain fructo-oligosaccharides affects markers of bone turnover but not bone mineral density in postmenopausal women. *Journal of Nutrition*, **144**, 297–304.

Smith, D.L., Jr, Mattison, J.A., Desmond, R.A. *et al.* (2011) Telomere dynamics in rhesus monkeys: no apparent effect of caloric restriction. *Journal of Gerontology A. Biological Science and Medical Science*, **66**, 1163–1168.

Sohal, R.S., Mockett, R.J. and Orr, W.C. (2002) Mechanisms of aging: an appraisal of the oxidative stress hypothesis. *Free Radical Biology and Medicine*, **33**, 575–586.

Sohal, R.S., Kamzalov, S., Sumien, N. *et al.* (2006) Effect of coenzyme Q10 intake on endogenous coenzyme Q content, mitochondrial electron transport chain, antioxidative defenses, and life span of mice. *Free Radical Biology and Medicine*, **40**, 480–487.

Speakman, J.R. and Hambly, C. (2007) Starving for life: what animal studies can and cannot tell us about the use of caloric restriction to prolong human lifespan. *Journal of Nutrition*, **137**, 1078–1086.

Stabler, S.P. and Allen, R.H. (2004) Vitamin B12 deficiency as a worldwide problem. *Annual Review of Nutrition*, **24**, 299–326.

Stear, S.J., Prentice, A., Jones, S.C. *et al.* (2003) Effect of a calcium and exercise intervention on the bone mineral status of 16-18-y-old adolescent girls. *American Journal of Clinical Nutrition*, **77**, 985–992.

Steensma, D.P. and Tefferi, A. (2007) Anemia in the elderly: how should we define it, when does it matter, and what can be done? *Mayo Clinic Proceedings*, **82**, 958–966.

Stein, M.S., Wark, J.D., Scherer, S.C. *et al.* (1999) Falls relate to vitamin D and parathyroid hormone in an Australian nursing home and hostel. *Journal of the American Geriatrics Society*, **47**, 1195–1201.

Stratton, R.J., Hackston, A., Longmore, D. *et al.* (2004) Malnutrition in hospital outpatients and inpatients: prevalence, concurrent validity and ease of use of the "malnutrition universal screening tool" ("MUST") for adults. *British Journal of Nutrition*, **92**, 799–808.

Stratton, R.J., Ek, A.C., Engfer, M. *et al.* (2005) Enteral nutritional support in prevention and treatment of pressure ulcers: a systematic review and meta-analysis. *Ageing Research Reviews*, **4**, 422–450.

Sund-Levander, M., Grodzinsky, E. and Wahren, L.K. (2007) Gender differences in predictors of survival in elderly nursing-home residents: a 3-year follow up. *Scandinavian Journal of Caring Sciences*, **21**, 18–24.

Suominen, M., Muurinen, S., Routasalo, P. *et al.* (2005) Malnutrition and associated factors among aged residents in all nursing homes in Helsinki. *European Journal of Clinical Nutrition*, **59**, 578–583.

Taku, K., Melby, M.K., Takebayashi, J. *et al.* (2010) Effect of soy isoflavone extract supplements on bone mineral density in menopausal women: meta-analysis of randomized controlled trials. *Asia Pacific Journal of Clinical Nutrition*, **19**, 33–42.

Tang, B.M., Eslick, G.D., Nowson, C. *et al.* (2007) Use of calcium or calcium in combination with vitamin D supplementation to prevent fractures and bone loss in people aged 50 years and older: a meta-analysis. *Lancet*, **370**, 657–66.

Todorovic, V., Russell, C. and Elia M. (2003) *A Guide to the Malnutrition Universal Screening Tool (MUST) for Adults*. BAPEN, http://www.bapen.org.uk/pdfs/must/must_explan.pdf (accessed 8 January 2015).

Tomaszuk-Kazberuk, A., Bolińska, S., Młodawska, E. *et al.* (2014) Does admission anaemia still predict mortality 6 years after myocardial infarction? *Kardiologia Polska*, **72**, 488–493.

Tousen, Y., Ezaki, J., Fujii, Y. *et al.* (2011) Natural S-equol decreases bone resorption in postmenopausal, non-equol-producing Japanese women: a pilot randomized, placebo-controlled trial. *Menopause*, **18**, 563–574.

Willcox, D.C., Scapagnini, G. and Willcox, B.J. (2014) Healthy aging diets other than the Mediterranean: a focus on the Okinawan diet. *Mechanisms of Ageing and Development*, **136–137**, 148–162.

Wong, W.W., Lewis, R.D., Steinberg, F.M. *et al.* (2009) Soy isoflavone supplementation and bone mineral density in menopausal women: a 2-y multicenter clinical trial. *The American Journal of Clinical Nutrition*, **90** (5), 1433–1439.

Woods, J.L., Walker, K.Z., Iuliano Burns, S. *et al.* (2009) Malnutrition on the menu: nutritional status of institutionalised elderly Australians in low-level care. *Journal of Nutrition and Healthy Ageing*, **13**, 693–698.

World Health Organisation (2011) *Data and Statistics* accessed from http://www.who.int/gho/mortality_burden_disease/life_tables/en/ Page last visited 20 March 2014.

Yamada, Y., Colman, R.J., Kemnitz, J.W. *et al.* (2013) Long-term calorie restriction decreases metabolic cost of movement and prevents decrease of physical activity during aging in rhesus monkeys. *Experimental Gerontology*, **48**, 1226–1235.

Yin, J., Zhang, Q., Liu, A. *et al.* (2010) Calcium supplementation for 2 years improves bone mineral accretion and lean body mass in Chinese adolescents. *Asia Pacific Journal of Clinical Nutrition*, **19**, 152–160.

Young, G.S. and Kirkland, J.B. (2007) Rat models of caloric intake and activity: relationships to animal physiology and human health. *Applied Physiology, Nutrition, and Metabolism*, **32**, 161–176.

Zakai, N.A., Katz, R., Hirsch, C. *et al.* (2005) A prospective study of anemia status, hemoglobin concentration, and mortality in an elderly cohort: the Cardiovascular Health Study. *Archives of Internal Medicine*, **165**, 2214–2220.

Zhao, J., Miao, K., Wang, H. *et al.* (2013) Association between telomere length and type 2 diabetes mellitus: a meta-analysis. *PLoS ONE*, **8**, e79993.

Zhao, J., Zhu, Y., Lin, J. *et al.* (2014) Short leukocyte telomere length predicts risk of diabetes in American Indians: the strong heart family study. *Diabetes*, **63**, 354–362.

Ziliak, J.P. and Gunderson, C. (2011) Senior Hunger in the United States. Differences Across Rural and Urban Areas, University of Kentucky Center for Poverty Research Special Reports, Lexington, KY, USA.

Additional reading

If you would like to find out more about the material discussed in this chapter, the following sources may be of interest:

Bernstein, M. and Luggan, A. (2009) *Nutrition for the Older Adult*, Jones and Bartlett Learning, Burlington.

Caroline Walker Trust (2004) *Eating Well for Older People: Practical and Nutritional Guidelines for Food in Residential and Community Care*, Caroline Walker Trust, London.

Finch, C.E. (2010) *The Biology of Human Longevity: Inflammation, Nutrition, and Aging in the Evolution of Lifespans*, Academic Press, Amsterdam; Boston.

Stanner, S., Thompson, R. and Buttriss, J.L. (eds) (2013) *Healthy Ageing: The Role of Nutrition and Lifestyle*, Wiley-Blackwell, Chichester, UK.

APPENDIX
An introduction to the nutrients

The main body of this book is focused upon the relationship between diet and health and how that relationship changes across the lifespan. As such, the text does not deal with some of the basic principles of nutrition, or provide an overview of the biochemistry of the nutrients, the physiology of digestion or the main sources of nutrients. This Appendix is therefore intended as a very simple reference guide to the macro- and micronutrients.

A.1 Classification of nutrients

Nutrients are broadly classified into macro- and micronutrients, non-essential or essential categories. The concept of essentiality refers to the ability of the body to synthesise nutrients de novo. A nutrient that is essential has to be derived from the diet, either because there is no de novo synthesis within the human body, or because the rate of synthesis is insufficient to meet requirements. Essential nutrients may also be referred to as indispensible. By contrast, non-essential nutrients are synthesised at a level in excess of what is needed to meet requirements. Some nutrients may be considered conditionally essential, as they cannot be synthesised in sufficient amounts under certain circumstances such as pregnancy or lactation.

Macronutrient is the term used to refer to the nutrients that are consumed in large (tens of grammes per day) quantities. Generally speaking the macronutrients (carbohydrates, lipids, proteins) are required in order to meet energy requirements and provide the basic building blocks of molecules that are necessary to maintain life-critical metabolic and structural functions. *Micronutrients* are required in only small (micro- or milligrammes per day) and include the vitamins and minerals. Some minerals such as calcium, sodium, chloride, magnesium and potassium are sometimes referred to as the macro-minerals as they are required in considerably higher quantities than most other inorganic constituents in the diet. Other minerals that are required by the body in barely quantifiable amounts (chromium, boron, molybdenum) are referred to as the trace elements.

A.2 Carbohydrates

A.2.1 Major roles
Within the human body carbohydrates are principally used in energy metabolism providing around 50% of dietary energy. Glucose is the main energy substrate used for synthesis of ATP via glycolysis and the citric acid cycle. Related to this function as an energy substrate, carbohydrates (specifically glycogen) are used as a mid-term (24h) energy store.

Carbohydrates are important components and precursors of more complex molecules. The pentose sugar ribose, for example, is a component of coenzymes such as NAD and FAD and is also incorporated into the structure of ATP. Ribose also makes up the backbone of RNA, and deoxyribose provides a key structural component of DNA. Other carbohydrates form glycoproteins and glycolipids which are present on cell surfaces where they participate in intercellular signalling.

A.2.2 Structure and classification of carbohydrates
The basic structure of the carbohydrates is the monosaccharide unit. These five or six carbon units can polymerise via glycosidic bonds to form disaccharides (e.g. maltose, sucrose and lactose), oligosaccharides (e.g. inulin and raffinose) or polysaccharides (e.g. starch and glycogen). Examples of mono-, di- and polysaccharide structures are shown in Figure A.1. The most important monosaccharides

Nutrition, Health and Disease: A Lifespan Approach, Second Edition. Simon Langley-Evans.
© 2015 John Wiley & Sons, Ltd. Published 2015 by John Wiley & Sons, Ltd.
Companion website: www.wiley.com/go/langleyevans/lifespan

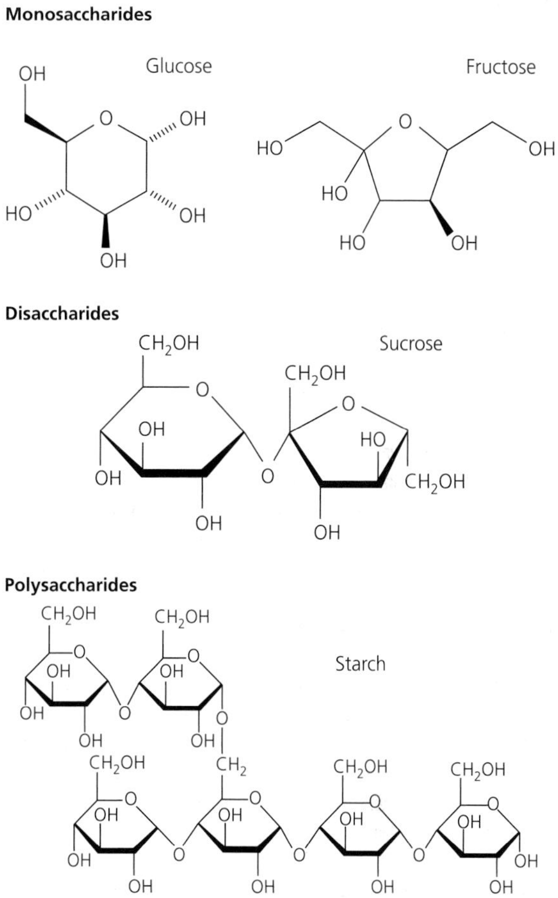

Monosaccharides

Disaccharides

Polysaccharides

Figure A.1 The structures of the carbohydrates. Carbohydrates comprise monosaccharide units which are either hexose rings (e.g. glucose) or pentose rings (e.g. fructose). These can link through glycosidic bonds to form disaccharides (e.g. sucrose), oligosaccharides (3–9 units) or polysaccharides (10+ units).

in mammalian biochemistry are glucose (the universal energy substrate), fructose, galactose and ribose.

Disaccharides are the main form in which sugars are consumed in the diet. What we describe as sugar is the disaccharide sucrose (glucose-fructose), whilst milk sugar is lactose (glucose-galactose). Increasingly fructose is consumed directly in the diet as food manufacturers use it in food processing, particularly as the basis for soft drinks and any foods that require cheap sweeteners.

Carbohydrates comprising between three and nine monosaccharide units are referred to as oligosaccharides. Within the diet these are plant-derived materials and are generally resistant to digestion. As a result, they pass through the upper digestive tract to the colon where they act as substrates for the growth of the colonic microflora. Prebiotics, which are designed to stimulate the microflora and which may improve gastrointestinal function, are generally based on oligosaccharides such as inulin.

Carbohydrates with 10 or more monosaccharide units are described as polysaccharides. These may be further

divided into digestible polysaccharides and non-starch polysaccharides (cellulose, hemicellulose, beta-glucans, pectins). The bulk of the digestible polysaccharides will be starches from plant sources. The non-starch polysaccharides, which are also referred to as dietary fibre, are resistant to digestion and pass through the gut largely unchanged. Like oligosaccharides they may be fermented by the colonic microflora, but they also make up a significant mass of faecal matter and contribute to healthy gastrointestinal function. Resistant starches, which are generally starches enclosed in indigestible structures (grain husk, unpolished rice), also contribute to the faecal bulk. Approximately 30% of ingested carbohydrate is likely to reach the colon unchanged and is available for bacterial fermentation.

A.2.3 Digestion and absorption of carbohydrates

Ingested carbohydrates undergo digestion beginning in the mouth where salivary amylase acts upon starch molecules to release maltose and oligosaccharides.

Amylase is also released in the small intestine, where hydrolysis of the polysaccharides generates disaccharides and oligosaccharides such as maltotriose and dextrins. The villi present in the small intestine express specific oligosaccharidases which hydrolyse these components to monosaccharides which can be absorbed. Lactase, for example, breaks lactose down to glucose and galactose and sucrose is hydrolysed to glucose and fructose by sucrase-isomaltase. Monosaccharides are taken up by enterocytes by both active transport and facilitated diffusion. Glucose and galactose enter via the Na^+/K^+ ATPase, SGLT1 transporter, whilst fructose is carried into the enterocyte by the GLUT5 transporter.

A.3 Lipids

A.3.1 Major roles

Lipids, derived from dietary fats, play a number of roles in cellular structure and metabolism, and have structural roles at the gross organ level. Lipids are a rich energy source (37 kJ/g fat) and are utilized in metabolic pathways that include hormone synthesis (from sterols) and phospholipid synthesis. The leukotrienes, eicosanoids and thromboxanes are all derived from fatty acids and play important roles in inflammatory processes. Lipids are also to directly modulate the expression of genes through transcription factors such as the peroxisome activated proliferator receptors. At the cellular level lipids make up the bulk of the material that comprises cell and organelle membranes. Lipids are also present in a protective role (e.g. fat pads protect the kidneys from external injury) and provide insulation as a layer within the skin. Lipids have important transport functions and provide the vehicle for uptake of fat-soluble vitamins from the diet.

A.3.2 Structure and classification of lipids

From a nutritional perspective the important lipids are the phospholipids, triacylglycerides, fatty acids and sterols. Structurally, the sterols (main representative is cholesterol) are distinct from the rest of the lipids as they comprise complex ring structures, which are the precursors for the synthesis of bile acids, vitamin D and steroid hormones. The sterols are not constructed from fatty acids.

A.3.2.1 Fatty acids

Fatty acids are the basic building blocks of triglycerides (triacylglycerides) and phospholipids. They comprise chains of between 4 and 28 carbons and are classified on the basis of the number, location and type of double bonds present within their structure (Figure A.2). Saturated fatty acids have no double bonds and are solid at room temperature. Generally they are derived from meat and milk within the human diet, but rich plant sources include palm and coconut oils. Monounsaturated fatty acids have a single double bond within their structure and tend to be oils rather than solid fats. Within the human diet most monounsaturated fatty acids are derived from rapeseed and olive oil. The polyunsaturated fatty acids have multiple double bonds and are all oils. The major dietary polyunsaturated fatty acids are in the series C18–C22 and are grouped into the n-3 and n-6 families (also referred to as omega-3 and omega-6).

The nomenclature for fatty acids indicates their structure, following the format shown below:

$$Cx : y\ n{-}z$$

where x refers to the number of carbon atoms in the chain, y is the number of double bonds and z is the first carbon in the chain to be double bonded. Hence C18:0 is the saturated fatty acid oleic acid, C18:1 n-9 is a monounsaturated fatty acid, with a double bond at carbon 9 (oleic acid) and C18:2 n-6 (linoleic acid) is a polyunsaturated fatty acid with the first double bond at carbon 6. Table A.1 gives the common name and nomenclature for some of the nutritionally important fatty acids.

There is a requirement for fatty acids within the diet and both n-6 (linoleic acid) and n-3 (alpha-linolenic acid) precursors of longer chain fatty acids are referred to as the essential fatty acids. The n-6 fatty acids are consumed in greater amounts than n-3 within the human diet (ratio of 20:1 within the Western diet), and many studies have suggested that excessive n-6 consumption may have adverse health effects. Higher consumption of n-3, particularly derived from fish, has been associated with lower risk of coronary heart disease and cancer.

The unsaturated fatty acids are also classified according to their isomeric forms as double bonds may be in a *cis-* or *trans-*orientation. This changes the overall structure of the fatty acid and trans-fatty acids have a chemical structure more akin to saturated fatty acids (Figure A.2). Trans-fatty acids are present in the diet as naturally occurring components of dietary fat in milk and meat, and are also generated during processing of food oils. To make unsaturated fats solid, or into spreadable materials such as margarines, they undergo partial hydrogenation which converts *cis-*bonds to *trans*. High intakes of trans-fatty acids produced by partial hydrogenation in industrial processing are associated with increased risk of cardiovascular disease.

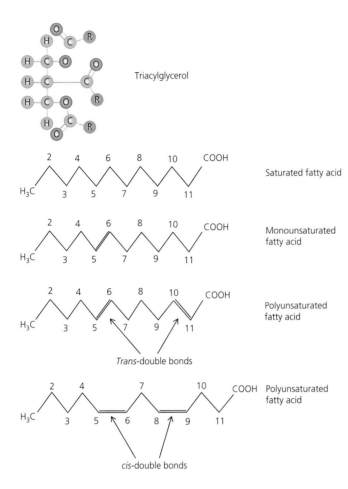

Triacylglycerol

Saturated fatty acid

Monounsaturated fatty acid

Polyunsaturated fatty acid

Trans-double bonds

Polyunsaturated fatty acid

cis-double bonds

Figure A.2 The structure and classification of triacylglycerides (triglycerides) and fatty acids. A triacylglyceride comprises a glycerol backbone conjugated to three fatty acids, which are shown here as R groups. These fatty acids may be saturated (no double bonds), monounsaturated (one double bond) or polyunsaturated (multiple double bonds). When double bonds are in the *trans*-orientation, then the overall structure of unsaturated fatty acids and the biological behaviour of those fatty acids differ significantly to when the double bonds are in the *cis*-orientation.

Table A.1 Common dietary fatty acids.

Saturated fatty acids	Monounsaturated fatty acids	Polyunsaturated fatty acids
C12:0 Lauric	C16:1 n-5 Palmitoleic	C18:2 n-6 Linoleic
C14:0 Myristic	C18:1 n-9 Oleic	C18:3 n-6 Υ-Linolenic
C16:0 Palmitic	C18:1 n-7 Vaccenic	C18:3 n-3 α-Linolenic
C17:0 Margeric	*trans* C18:1 n-9 Elaidic	C20:4 n-6 Arachadonic
C18:0 Stearic		C20:5 n-3 Eicosapentanoic
C20: Arachidic		C22:6 n-3 Docosahexanoic

A.3.2.2 Phospholipids and triglycerides

Within the body, most lipid that is present in structures such as membranes, is in the form of phospholipids. Most phospholipids comprise a glycerol backbone, which is bonded to two fatty acids (a diacylglyceride) and to a phosphate group and amino acids (e.g. phosphatidyl-*serine*), alcohols (phosphatidyl*inositol*) or vitamins (phosphatidyl*choline*). The exception to this is sphingomyelin, where glycerol is replaced by sphingosine. Phospholipids all share the property of being amphipathic, meaning that have a hydrophilic polar head and hydrophobic tail. As such they can form bilayers in cell membranes, which associate with sterols and proteins.

Fat stores within the body, lipids for transport and the vast majority of dietary fat are in the form of triglycerides. Triglycerides comprise a glycerol backbone bonded to three fatty acids (Figure A.2).

A.3.3 Digestion and absorption of lipids

Dietary fat is digested in the stomach, duodenum and ileum. Gastric processing involves the churning of food which separates the fat from the aqueous portion of the food within chyme. Emulsified fats are released from the stomach into the duodenum where they undergo lipolysis through the action of lipases (on triglycerides),

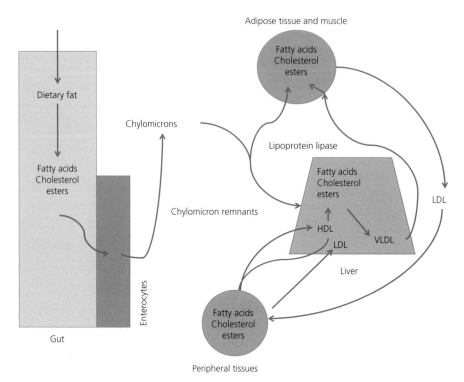

Adipose tissue and muscle

Figure A.3 The uptake and transport of fatty acids and cholesterol. Fatty acids and cholesterol esters are packaged into chylomicrons after uptake by enterocytes. Chylomicrons deliver fatty acids and cholesterol to adipose tissue and muscle with chylomicron remnants transported to the liver. Here packaging into very-low-density lipoprotein (VLDL) allows further transport of cholesterol and triglycerides to adipose tissue and muscle, where LDL picks up lipid for transport to the rest of the periphery. High-density lipoprotein (HDL) carries triglycerides and cholesterol back from the periphery to the liver.

phospholipase A$_2$ (on phospholipids) and cholesterol ester hydrolase upon cholesterol esters. Lipase action yields glycerol, monoacylglycerides and free fatty acids. Shorter chain fatty acids (<12 carbon) are absorbed directly into the portal circulation, whilst longer chain fatty acids and cholesterol are bound to bile salts and taken up by enterocytes in the ileum. Following uptake of lipids into the hepatic portal circulation or enterocytes, they are packaged into lipoproteins for transport (Figure A.3).

A.4 Proteins

A.4.1 Major roles

Protein is a basic component of all cells and is incorporated into cellular structures (cell membranes, cytoskeleton, organelles). All metabolic, physiological and endocrine functions within the body are critically dependent on the synthesis of proteins from amino acids that are derived either from the diet or produced de novo. Enzymes, neurotransmitters, peptide hormones, cell surface markers, hormone receptors and membrane transporters are all proteins that undergo constant turnover (synthesis–degradation–synthesis) to maintain cellular functions.

Dietary protein plays a different role as it is broken down into constituent parts prior to absorption. As such protein is required within the diet to meet the demands of the body for the amino acids that are required for protein synthesis, energy metabolism and other biochemical pathways. Not all dietary protein is the same, as proteins derived from some food sources contain an incomplete range of the amino acids required by humans. Whilst animal derived protein is considered 'high-quality', plant proteins may be low quality as one or more amino acids are missing or present in low quantities. For example many beans and peas lack the sulphur-amino acids cysteine and methionine, whilst maize lacks tryptophan and lysine.

A.4.2 Amino acids

The properties of proteins depend on the properties and interactions between the constituent amino acids which comprise the protein structure. There are 20 amino acids that are classically used in protein synthesis, with additional amino acids that are involved in intermediary metabolism but which do not appear in proteins (citrulline, ornithine, taurine). Amino acids have the structure shown in Figure A.4. Each comprises an amine group conjugated to a carbon that also bonds to an acid group and a side chain, or 'R group'. These R groups may be simple carbon chains (e.g. glycine), branching carbon chains (leucine, valine, isoleucine) or ring structures (e.g. tyrosine, histidine, phenylalanine). The R groups present give each amino acid its specific biochemical properties, determine how they will contribute to protein structure and what other biochemical functions may be served (e.g. glycine is a donor in methylation reactions, leucine, aspartate and alanine are nitrogen donors). As shown in Table A.2, the amino acids are classified as essential, non-essential and conditionally essential.

A.4.3 Structure of proteins

Proteins have a complex structure that is primarily based on the formation of chains of amino acids (Figure A.4). Amino acids link together by virtue of peptide bonds that form between the amine group on one moiety and the acid moiety on another. The resulting peptide or polypeptide chains have more complex structures and functions by virtue of the properties of the R-group side chains on each amino acid. Some short peptides may have important biological activity (e.g. the tripeptide antioxidant glutathione, or the octapeptide hormone angiotensin II), but most proteins would comprise 50–1000 amino acid residues.

The sequence of amino acids in a polypeptide chain provides the primary structure of a protein. The formation of cross-links between R groups, either through

Table A.2 The essential and non-essential amino acids.

Essential amino acids	Conditionally essential amino acids	Non-essential amino acids
Isoleucine	Arginine	Alanine
Leucine	Cysteine	Aspartate
Lysine	Glycine	Asparagine
Methionine	Glutamine	Glutamate
Phenylalanine	Histidine	Serine
Threonine	Proline	
Tryptophan	Serine	
Valine	Tyrosine	

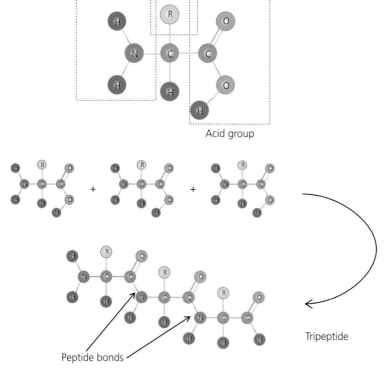

Figure A.4 The structure of amino acids and peptides. Amino acids comprise an amine group and an acid group bound to a single carbon which also bears a side chain (R). R groups may be carbon chains or ring structures. Amino acids form peptide bonds allowing them to form short chains (e.g. the tripeptide chain shown) or complex proteins with up to 1000 amino acid residues.

covalent bonds, or weak hydrogen bonds enables the chains to coil and fold into the conformation that enables biological activity. This folding and cross-linking is referred to as the secondary and tertiary structure of the protein.

A.4.4 Digestion and absorption of proteins

Dietary protein is generally broken down to dipeptides or single amino acids during digestion in the alimentary canal. Proteins are relatively resistant to digestive enzymes when in their normal conformation, as the tertiary and secondary structure limits access to the peptide bonds. Acid action in the stomach denatures these structures allowing enzymes (endopeptidases, carboxypeptidases, trypsin, chymotrypsin) to break peptide chains liberating amino acids for absorption by either passive diffusion or active transport. Small amounts of

whole proteins may pass unchanged across the gut to the circulation through the process of paracellular uptake. This movement between the tight junctions of the epithelial layer of the gut plays an important role in priming the immune system.

A.5 Micronutrients

A.5.1 Minerals

Minerals and trace elements are inorganic components of food and water intake which are required to maintain normal cellular and whole body physiological function. All of the minerals can be accumulated in storage forms, either as components of structures (e.g. bone is a reservoir for calcium, phosphorus and magnesium), or bound to proteins in a storage form (e.g. ferritin binding

Table A.3 The minerals: sources, functions and deficiency symptoms.

Mineral	Main dietary sources	Principal functions	Deficiency symptoms
Sodium	Ubiquitous, but high in cheese, processed and preserved foods	Acid–base balance Fluid balance Nerve transmission Muscle function	Low appetite, nausea and fatigue
Potassium	Fruit and vegetables	Acid–base balance Fluid balance Nerve transmission Muscle function	Confusion, muscle weakness, cardiac arrest
Calcium	Dairy produce	Bones and teeth Muscle contraction Blood clotting Nerve transmission	Convulsions, stunted growth, rickets osteoporosis
Phosphorus	Meat and fish Wholegrains Dairy produce	Bones and teeth Acid–base balance	Bone demineralization
Iron	Meat Fortified cereals Dried fruits Green vegetables	Haemoglobin synthesis	Pallor, fatigue, breathlessness
Iodine	Seafoods Iodized salt Milk (some countries)	Synthesis of thyroid hormones	Enlarged thyroid (goitre), retarded growth, foetal abnormality
Magnesium	Wholegrains Nuts Green vegetables	Bone structure DNA and protein synthesis	Neuromuscular disorders
Zinc	Meat Eggs Pulses Wholegrains	Immune function DNA synthesis Enzyme cofactor	Growth failure, reduced immunity
Copper	Meat Vegetables	Ion absorption Enzyme cofactor	Reduced immunity
Fluorine	Seafood Tea Fortified water	Maintenance of tooth enamel	Tooth decay

of iron). Approximately 3% of the mass of the human body comprises these elements.

Uptake of the minerals from the diet tends to be low and their bioavailability will be dependent on person-specific features such as age, life stage or disease, and upon the nature of the food matrix from which absorption occurs. The presence of inhibitors and enhancers of absorption from food and competition between minerals for gut transporters determines bioavailability. For example approximately 14–18% of ingested iron will be absorbed from a mixed diet, and this falls to 5–12% from a vegetarian diet.

The functions of the minerals in the body are varied and specific, but in general terms they are critical for the

Table A.4 The fat soluble vitamins: sources, functions and deficiency symptoms.

Vitamin	Main dietary sources	Principal functions	Deficiency symptoms
A: Retinol/beta carotene	Liver and fish oils (retinol) Fruits and vegetables (carotene)	Cell differentiation Antioxidant (beta carotene) Visual function	Night blindness, keratinization of the skin
D: Calciferol	Fish and fish oils Fortified cereals Fortified milk Margarine	Maintenance of calcium balance	Rickets, osteomalacia
E: Tocopherols	Vegetable oils Nuts and nut oils	Antioxidant	Rare but serious neurological symptoms
K: Phylloquinone	Green vegetables Cereals	Blood clotting	Impaired clotting

Table A.5 The water soluble vitamins: sources, functions and deficiency symptoms.

Vitamin	Main dietary sources	Principal functions	Deficiency symptoms
B1 Thiamin	Meat and fish Nuts and seeds Peas Fortified cereals and bread	Coenzyme	Peripheral nerve damage (beriberi) Central nervous system disorders (Wernicke–Korsakoff Syndrome)
B2 Riboflavin	Meat and fish Eggs Fortified cereals	Component of flavoproteins Coenzyme	Lesions of mouth, tongue and lips
Niacin	Meat and fish Nuts and seeds Fortified cereals	Component of NAD and NADP Coenzyme	Depression, photosensitive dermatitis (pellagra)
B5 Pantothenic acid	Mushrooms Oily fish Eggs	Component of coenzyme A	Peripheral nerve damage
B6 Pyridoxine	Nuts and seeds Meat and fish Fruit Fortified cereals	Coenzyme	Convulsions
B9 Folic acid	Liver Pulses and beans Green vegetables Fortified breads and cereals	Coenzyme in one carbon transfer reactions	Megalobastic anaemia
B12 Cobalamin	Liver Seafood Fortified cereals	Coenzyme in one carbon transfer reactions	Pernicious anaemia
C Ascorbic acid	Fruit and vegetables	Antioxidant Enhancer of iron uptake Collagen synthesis	Impaired wound healing, breakdown of gums and skin (scurvy)
H Biotin	Eggs Dairy products	Coenzyme	Dermatitis

formation of rigid structures such as teeth or bone; as catalytic centres for enzymes; as components of hormones; in regulation of fluid balance; in regulation of acid–base balance; and enabling muscle contraction and generating action potentials in the transmission of nervous impulses. Each mineral and trace element is associated with characteristic symptoms of deficiency as these associated functions become limited. Table A.3 lists the main minerals required within the diet, along with their main functions, dietary sources and the symptoms of deficiency.

A.5.2 Vitamins

The vitamins are organic molecules that are critical for biochemical functions by virtue of their specific characteristics as coenzymes. A number of the vitamins also have important regulatory functions, controlling gene expression (e.g. vitamin A), or regulating the uptake and excretion of minerals (e.g. vitamin D). Where vitamins are required as coenzymes, they are involved in a limited number of biochemical pathways. Thiamin, for example, is a coenzyme for just three enzymes (pyruvate dehydrogenase, alpha-ketoglutarate dehydrogenase and branched chain amino acid dehydrogenase), but this is sufficient to make it essential for normal energy and amino acid metabolism. Where the supply of vitamin is limiting the associated biochemical pathways will be affected and the resulting failure to synthesize products, or the accumulation of precursors will be drivers of deficiency symptoms and diseases.

Most of the vitamins are essential nutrients, but some can be synthesized de novo, provided that there is sufficient precursor available. Niacin, for example, is synthesized from the amino acid tryptophan. In the case of vitamin D, this de novo synthesis is far in excess of dietary intake. Several of the B vitamins and vitamin K are also synthesized by the colonic microflora, but it is believed that this bacterial synthesis is of little significance in human nutrition as there is limited uptake of these bacterial products from the gut.

The vitamins are classified according to solubility in fat or water. Several exist in multiple forms, so vitamin D, for example, comprises vitamin D2 and D3, each of which has 5–6 metabolites. Vitamin K has three vitamers (phylloquinone, menadione, menaquinone). Table A.4 summarises the functions of the fat soluble vitamins and Table A.5 describes the water-soluble vitamins.

Index

Nutrition, Health and Disease: A Lifespan Approach, Second Edition. Simon Langley-Evans.
© 2015 John Wiley & Sons, Ltd. Published 2015 by John Wiley & Sons, Ltd.
Companion website: www.wiley.com/go/langleyevans/lifespan